T0399546

Biomaterials and Materials for Medicine

Emerging Materials and Technologies

Series Editor:
Boris I. Kharissov

Biomaterials and Materials for Medicine
Innovations in Research, Devices, and Applications

Edited by
Jingan Li

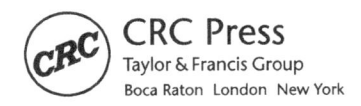

CRC Press
Taylor & Francis Group
Boca Raton London New York

CRC Press is an imprint of the
Taylor & Francis Group, an **informa** business

First edition published 2022
by CRC Press
6000 Broken Sound Parkway NW, Suite 300, Boca Raton, FL 33487-2742

and by CRC Press
2 Park Square, Milton Park, Abingdon, Oxon, OX14 4RN

ISBN: 978-0-367-75321-4 (hbk)
ISBN: 978-0-367-75323-8 (pbk)
ISBN: 978-1-003-16198-1 (ebk)

DOI: 10.1201/9781003161981

Typeset in Times
by codeMantra

Contents

Biomaterials and Materials for Medicine: Innovations in Research, Devices, and Applications

Preface

Many monographs on biomaterials have been published in recent years, which introduce the development of biomaterials from various aspects. However, biomaterials is a cutting-edge dynamic discipline. Therefore, in this book, new knowledge, technology, and concept of biomaterials worldwide, especially in developing countries, are summarized. Invited by CRC Press/Taylor & Francis's Series Editor, Prof. Boris I. Kharissov, we, together with young scientists from 13 research groups, wrote this book entitled "Biomaterials and Materials for Medicine: Innovations in Research, Devices, and Applications" to join the Emerging Materials and Technologies Book Series.

This book is application-oriented, covering nine research directions of biomaterials and medical materials, and is divided into 13 chapters. The first three chapters mainly introduce the research of vascular biomaterials, including the latest research on cardiovascular therapeutic devices, vascular patches, and biomaterials for vascular tissue engineering. Chapters 4 and 5 describe the research regarding orthopedic biomaterials in detail, including joint materials and dental materials. Chapter 6 focusses on recent research hotspots about skin tissue engineering biomaterials. Chapter 7 introduces the related research of nerve tissue engineering materials, including central nerve repair materials and peripheral nerve repair materials. Chapter 8 introduces non-mainstream biomaterials, which are special stent materials for palliative treatment of esophageal cancer and related technologies of surface modification. These design concepts and emerging technologies can also provide reference for other lumen interventions such as biliary tract and airway. Many biomaterials and related designs display high performance in drug targeting and controlled release, which will be elaborated in Chapter 9. Wearable biomedical devices is a new research field, thus its research progress is interpreted by an authoritative expert, Associate Professor Yifeng Lei from Wuhan University in Chapter 10. Micronscale and nanoscale biomaterials have been demonstrated to have a series of functions related to scale, which is discussed Chapter 11. Dr. Shuo Wang from the University of Tsukuba in Japan highlights the related research. Inspired by nature and learning from nature, the latest research progress of biomimetic materials in biomedical engineering is introduced in Chapter 12. Finally, the theoretical calculation and computer simulation of biomaterials, as a complementary discipline with physical experimental science, is elaborated in Chapter 13.

Of course, the contents we introduce in this book cannot entirely cover the current knowledge of biomaterials and materials for medicine. To be practical, it is just a drop in the ocean for this discipline. However, it represents the knowledge of first-line scientists, especially the authors of this book, in their respective fields of understanding and academic achievement. In the future, we will invite more experts and scholars from around the world to introduce new knowledge and expound their views in this series of books.

Foreword

At the invitation of Dr. Jingan Li, I am very pleased to write a foreword for the book "Biomaterials and Materials for Medicine: Innovations in Research, Devices, and Applications". Biomaterials is one of the most important frontiers and interdisciplinary fields in the world today. Almost all implant devices, medical testing equipment, and drug carriers need the development of biomaterials. The field of biomaterials covers a wide range of disciplines in science and technology, including materials, biology, iatrology, pharmacy, physics, chemistry, and mathematics. In recent years, the development of biomaterial science and technology has been progressing rapidly. At the same time, many new and detailed branches in the field of biomaterials have emerged, and these latest research achievements and technologies have not been summarized yet. Hence, it is important to provide this information to a majority of readers in a simple and easy to understand fashion. The publication of the book "Biomaterials and Materials for Medicine: Innovations in Research, Devices, and Applications" is timely, almost concluding all directions of application-oriented biomaterials, such as cardiovascular materials, bone materials, nerve scaffold materials, scaffold materials for vascular tissue engineering, controlled drug release carrier materials, wearable medical device-related materials, and research on theoretical calculation of materials.

The book is divided into 13 chapters, four of which are contributed by young scientists and teachers of Zhengzhou University. Zhengzhou University is a world-class university under the Ministry of Education of the People's Republic of China and the Henan provincial government. The disciplines of materials, chemistry, and medicine offered at the university have entered the world-class discipline construction sequence, while nine disciplines, including materials science and engineering, clinical medicine, chemistry, biology, history and culture of Central Plains, cancer prevention and treatment, resource processing and efficient utilization, engineering safety and disaster prevention, and morphology of consciousness and social governance, were selected as the first phase of the construction project of advantageous characteristic disciplines in Henan Province. Zhengzhou University also has the largest number of students in China, about 72,600 (according to statistics published in 2019). Therefore, our aptitude for science and technology is not only reflected in senior experts, scholars, and professors but also our students' desire for the latest knowledge and the most advanced technology. For Zhengzhou University, the publication of this book meets the needs of some disciplines to a certain extent, but it only meets the short-term needs of some disciplines. We welcome more books like this.

Finally, we are willing to work together with global peers to promote the rapid development of biomaterials and materials for medicine, and also wish outstanding young scientists continue on the road of science.

Shao-kang Guan
Zhengzhou University, China

Shaokang Guan
2020-9-19

Editor

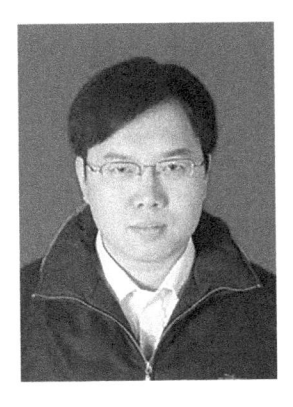

Dr. Jingan Li is a professor at Zhengzhou University, China, and his research fields include biomaterials and advanced functional materials. So far, he has published more than 70 academic papers in international academic journals as the first author or corresponding author, including *ACS Applied Materials & Interface*, *Bioactive Materials*, *Acta Biomateralia*, *Carbohydrate Polymers*, and *Journal of Materials Science & Technology*. He has served as the editorial board member of 12 journals, including *Stem Cells International* (Lead Guest Editor) and *Smart Materials in Medicine*, and is also the invited reviewer of more than 40 academic journals. Till now, he has been invited to attend more than 30 international academic conferences as plenary speaker, keynote speaker, invited speaker, organizing committee member, technical program committee, and session chair, and he was honored with "China-Korea Young Scientist Award" (2015) and "IAAM Fellow" (2020). For detailed information please see: https://www.researchgate.net/profile/Jingan_Li2.

Contributors

Hualong Bai
Department of
  Vascular and Endovascular Surgery
First Affiliated Hospital of Zhengzhou
  University
Zhengzhou, China
and
Key Vascular Physiology
  and Applied Research
  Laboratory of
  Zhengzhou City
Zhengzhou, China

Jialong Chen
Key Laboratory of Oral Diseases
  Research of Anhui Province,
  Stomatologic Hospital
  and College
Anhui Medical University
Hefei, China

Longlong Cui
School of Life Science
Zhengzhou University
Zhengzhou, China

Alan Dardik
The Vascular Biology
  and Therapeutics Program
Yale School of Medicine
New Haven, Connecticut
and
Departments of Surgery
  and of Cellular and Molecular
  Physiology
Yale School of Medicine
New Haven, Connecticut
and
Department of Surgery
Yale School of Medicine
New Haven, Connecticut

Yonghong Fan
Department of Anatomy
Third Military Medical University
Chongqing, China

Zhe Fang
School of Materials and Chemical
  Engineering
Zhongyuan University of Technology
Zhengzhou, China

Shuaimeng Guan
School of Life Science
Zhengzhou University
Zhengzhou, China

Hao He
Department of Vascular Surgery, the
  Second Xiangya Hospital
Central South University
Changsha, China

Yachen Hou
School of Material Science and
  Engineering & Henan Key
  Laboratory of Advanced Magnesium
  Alloy & Key Laboratory of Materials
  Processing and Mold Technology
  (Ministry of Education)
Zhengzhou University
Zhengzhou, China

Mujiahid Iqbal
School of Material Science and
  Engineering & Henan Key
  Laboratory of Advanced Magnesium
  Alloy & Key Laboratory of Materials
  Processing and Mold Technology
  (Ministry of Education)
Zhengzhou University
Zhengzhou, China

Quancheng Kan
Department of Pharmacy
The First Affiliated Hospital of
    Zhengzhou University
Zhengzhou, China
and
Henan Key Laboratory of Precision
    Clinical Pharmacy
Zhengzhou University
Zhengzhou, China

Yifeng Lei
School of Power and Mechanical
    Engineering & the Institute of
    Technological Science
Wuhan University
Wuhan, China

Guicai Li
University of Nantong
    University
Nantong, China

Jiankang Li
School of Life
    Science
Zhengzhou University
Zhengzhou, China

Jingan Li
School of Material Science and
    Engineering & Henan Key
    Laboratory of Advanced
    Magnesium Alloy & Key
    Laboratory of Materials
    Processing and Mold Rechnology
    (Ministry of Education)
Zhengzhou University
Zhengzhou, China

Jingwen Li
School of Power and Mechanical
    Engineering & the Institute of
    Technological Science
Wuhan University
Wuhan, China

Li Li
Key Laboratory for Advanced
    Technologies of Materials (Ministry
    of Education), School of Material
    Science and Engineering
Southwest Jiaotong University
Chengdu, China

Xiangyang Li
Key Laboratory of Oral Diseases
    Research of Anhui Province,
    Stomatologic Hospital and College
Anhui Medical University
Hefei, China

Xin Li
Department of Vascular Surgery, the
    Second Xiangya Hospital
Central South University
Changsha, China

Xinxin Li
Institute of Primate Traslational
    Medical
Kunming University of Science and
    Technology
Kunming, China

Jiaheng Liang
School of Life Science
Zhengzhou University
Zhengzhou, China

Haiyang Liu
School of Power and Mechanical
    Engineering & the Institute of
    Technological Science
Wuhan University
Wuhan, China

Xiaoxuan Lu
Key Laboratory of Oral Diseases
    Research of Anhui Province,
    Stomatologic Hospital and College
Anhui Medical University
Hefei, China

Xiao Luo
Key Laboratory for Advanced
Technologies of Materials, Ministry
of Education, School of Material
Science and Engineering
Southwest Jiaotong University
Chengdu, China

Yinhua Qin
Department of Anatomy
Third Military Medical University
Chongqing, China

Y. Ren
Department of Materials Science
and Engineering
Henan University of Technology
Zhengzhou, China

Chang Shu
Department of Vascular Surgery, the
Second Xiangya Hospital
Central South University
Changsha, China
and
Department of Vascular Surgery,
Fuwai Hospital
Chinese Academy of Medical Sciences
and Peking Union Medical College
Beijing, China

Jingjing Su
School of Life Science
Zhengzhou University
Zhengzhou, China

Hongyan Wang
School of Materials Science and
Engineering
Zhengzhou University
Zhengzhou, China

Shuo Wang
Graduate School of Science and
Technology
University of Tsukuba
Tsukuba, Japan

Xiaowei Wang
Key Laboratory of Oral Diseases
Research of Anhui Province,
Stomatologic Hospital and College
Anhui Medical University
Hefei, China

Yuhao Wang
Department of Anatomy
Third Military Medical University
Chongqing, China

Zichen Wu
Key Laboratory of Oral Diseases
Research of Anhui Province,
Stomatologic Hospital and College
Anhui Medical University
Hefei, China

Feng Wu
College of Physics and New Energy
Xuzhou University of Technology
Xuzhou, China

Yanhua Xu
Department of Internal Medicine
The First Affiliated Hospital of
Zhengzhou University
Zhengzhou, China

Youqian Xu
Department of Anatomy
Third Military Medical University
Chongqing, China

Aqeela Yasin
School of Material Science and
    Engineering & Henan Key
    Laboratory of Advanced Magnesium
    Alloy & Key Laboratory of Materials
    Processing and Mold Technology
    (Ministry of Education)
Zhengzhou University
Zhengzhou, China

Jinjie Zhang
School of Pharmacy
Zhengzhou University
Zhengzhou, China

Kun Zhang
School of Life Science
Zhengzhou University
Zhengzhou, China

Liling Zhang
University of Nantong University
Nantong, China

Yu Zhao
School of Materials Science
    and Engineering
Zhengzhou University
Zhengzhou, China

Chuhong Zhu
Department of Anatomy
Third Military Medical University
Chongqing, China

Dan Zou
Key Laboratory for Advanced
    Technologies of Materials (Ministry
    of Education), School of Material
    Science and Engineering
Southwest Jiaotong University
Chengdu, China

1 Cardiovascular Therapeutic Devices: Material and Fabrication Progress

Xiao Luo, Dan Zou, and Li Li
Southwest Jiaotong University

CONTENTS

DOI: 10.1201/9781003161981-1

1.1   INTRODUCTION

Peace and development are the main themes of the current era. In recent decades, the global social economy has developed rapidly, and the lifestyles of residents have been greatly improved. However, due to long-term unhealthy lifestyles or other congenital factors, the prevalence of cardiovascular diseases has increased significantly. According to a World Health Organization (WHO) survey, cardiovascular disease has become the leading cause of death in the global population, accounting for approximately 30% of the total deaths. Through blood circulation, the cardiovascular system provides the body with oxygen, transports nutrients, and transports metabolic waste. The stable operation of the cardiovascular system is an important guarantee for maintaining the health of the body. For patients suffering from severe heart diseases such as embolism, congenital heart defects, vascular stenosis, and heart failure (HF), effective treatments increasingly rely on therapeutic devices. During the last decades, biomaterial and medical communities have optimized and introduced various materials, as well as structure design and fabrication, approaches. These exploitations enhanced the therapeutic value of the devices, and the clinical success demonstrated great progress in reestablishing healthy blood circulation, implementing revascularization, and restoring cardiac hemodynamics.

There are various methods of cardiovascular treatment devices to deal with different cardiovascular diseases. When dealing with problems such as thrombus blood, filters are selected to remove the blood clots. When faced with tissue lesions caused by abnormal blood vessels, embolization devices are used to create thrombus to block the diseased blood vessels to maintain normal and healthy blood circulation. In dealing with vascular diseases, such as atherosclerosis, vascular stents or drug balloons are used for interventional treatment. Artificial blood vessels are selected to replace diseased blood vessels. For heart hemodynamic disorders caused by abnormal heart function and other reasons, artificial heart valves or ventricular assist devices are used for improvement, and artificial hearts are used for replacement.

In this chapter, the currently adopted/potential materials and methods that modulated the device properties of anti/pro-coagulation, anti-hyperplasia, and mechanical support are summarized and compared (Figure 1.1). The challenges cardiovascular therapeutic devices face and the opportunities that are emerging have also been identified.

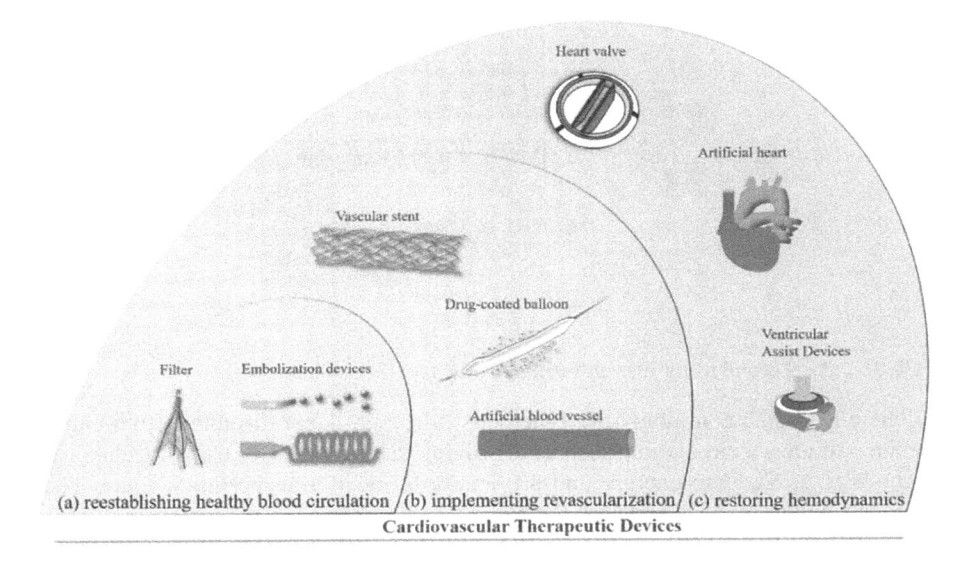

Heart valve

Artificial heart

Vascular stent

Drug-coated balloon

Ventricular
Assist Devices

Filter   Embolization devices

Artificial blood vessel

(a) reestablishing healthy blood circulation / (b) implementing revascularization / (c) restoring hemodynamics

Cardiovascular Therapeutic Devices

FIGURE 1.1   Scheme of medical devices applied to cardiovascular therapy. (a) reestablishing healthy body circulation, (b) implementing revascularization, and (c) restoring hemodynamics.

1.2   DEVICES FOR REESTABLISHING HEALTHY BLOOD CIRCULATION

Maintaining and reestablishing healthy blood circulation is the primary goal of cardiovascular therapeutic devices. There are different vascular lesions due to different causes, and therapeutic devices encounter different and complex situations. Thrombus is the most common problem that needs to be dealt with. However, thrombus plays a role as a double-edged sword that cannot be arbitrarily defined as good or bad (as shown in Figure 1.2). Under certain conditions, a filter can be applied to blood clots; and under other conditions, an embolization device can be deployed to produce the thrombus to block the diseased blood vessels.

Here, we introduce two typical cardiovascular therapeutic devices: vena cava filter (VCF) and embolization device, which were specifically used for thrombus to maintain and reestablish a healthy blood circulation.

1.2.1   VENA CAVA FILTER

Pulmonary thromboembolism (PTE) is mainly caused by deep vein thrombosis (DVT). The main pathogenic mechanism is that abnormal blood coagulation in the deep vein cavity blocks the lumen and obstructs venous reflux by forming a thrombus. Thrombus passes through the vena cava and enters the pulmonary circulation through the heart. Then, large blood clots cause blockages and insufficient blood supply to the lung.

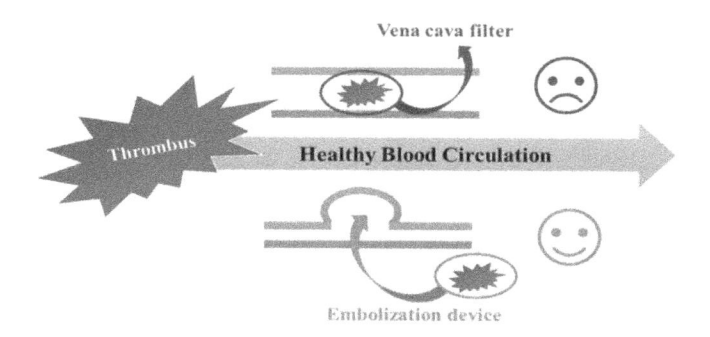

FIGURE 1.2 Thrombus for reestablishing healthy blood circulation.

There are some commonly used methods to prevent large thrombus from entering the pulmonary circulation, such as dissolving the thrombus, or using mechanical methods (e.g., VCF) to capture and artificially block its transportation route. The main principle is to place a filter in the blood vessel to catch thrombus, especially the relatively large thrombus, so that it cannot enter the heart and pulmonary circulation, thereby avoiding pulmonary embolism.

The filter has the following characteristics: (1) the filter is usually designed as an umbrella- or a cone-shaped structure which can keep the blood pressure and flow changes without any risk even it has been filled. Meanwhile, blood flow parallel to the axis can inhibit the growth of the thrombus and break the thrombus, ensuring healthy blood circulation. (2) The conveying device has a small impact. (3) The filter can stably capture thrombus. Sometimes the source of thrombosis is the thrombus that has been captured. For life-threatening thrombus, the filter should have high and stable capture efficiency. Some filters allow a small amount of other small thrombi to pass, thereby avoiding the excessive accumulation of trapped thrombus and forming the filter embolism.

According to clinical use, three types of VCF products are available in the market: permanent, temporary, and optional recyclable VCF. Their material and structural design directly affect the clinical effect.

1.2.1.1 Permanent Vena Cava Filter

Metal VCF was first used clinically in the 1980s. Once this type of filter is placed, it cannot be removed without an operation. Representative products include Greenfield [1], Bird's Nest [2], VenaTech LGM [3], Simon [4], and TrapEase [5].

1. Greenfield filter (GF)

    In 1973, Greenfield used an umbrella filter for clinical use. To date, GF is the most widely used filter available in the market and has become the reference structure for later filter designs.

    The first-generation GF filter adopts an overall tapered design, with a hook at the tail end of the strut, which is anchored on the vessel wall by the hook. It is placed by surgically incising the internal jugular vein or femoral vein. According to the geometric principle, more than 50% of the open section can still be maintained even if the thrombus fills 70% of the total length of the upper end of the cone. Therefore, the design of the GF ensures smooth blood circulation in the vena cava and captures clinically significant thrombi.

2. Bird's Nest filter (BNF)

In 1989, Cook Medical launched a new type of filter in the United States under the trade name Bird's Nest filter (BNF). The stainless steel wire of this filter is randomly bent into a net-like structure, similar to a bird's nest.

3. VenaTech LGM filter

The first-generation LGM filter was designed and developed by LG Medical and was launched in France. The filter is made of a bio-/magnetic resonance imaging-compatible alloy Phynox (cobalt, chromium, iron, nickel, molybdenum) by stamping and spot welding. Six slightly curved alloy sheet bases are connected to a flat side, and the side rails are attached to the wall of the vena cava to provide stable support.

4. Simon nitinol filter (SNF)

SNF is the first nickel-titanium alloy filter on the market. The alloy is composed of 53% nickel, 45% titanium, and 2% cobalt. This material is relatively soft at room temperature, but has thermal memory and can be restored to the original shape at body temperature. This alloy is corrosion-resistant, non-ferromagnetic, and stronger than steel, making it a suitable material for preparing VCFs.

5. TrapEase filter (TEF)

This filter is integrated by laser cutting nickel-titanium alloy tubes. It has a symmetrical design. The two sides of the head and tail are mesh baskets which are connected by six side pillars. The six side pillars are arranged into six diamonds, so the TEF becomes the center. The double basket design provides two levels of thrombus capture. The proximal and distal ends of the six side struts have straight thorns to provide the anchoring function of the filter and prevents the filter from migrating to the head or caudal side.

Compared with simple anticoagulation therapy, permanent VCF reduces the occurrence of fatal PTE; however, it increases the risk of recurrent DVT, embolism, and a series of complications over time, including filter perforation, shedding, migration, and filter breakage. These complications pose a permanent threat to the patient.

1.2.1.2 Temporary Vena Cava Filter

To solve a series of clinical deficiencies of permanent VCFs, temporary VCFs were developed. After temporary VCFs are placed, the interventional device needs to be connected to the filter and placed outside the body. At the same time, urokinase is used for thrombolysis. Generally, thrombolysis is completed after 6 hours, and then the filter is retracted through the interventional device. A representative product is Tempofilter II [6] which consists of eight Phynox and needs to be connected to a restrictive catheter. Therefore, the filter itself does not need a fixed hook to ensure correct positioning. During the placement, the degree of endothelialization is minimized, which improves the safety of recovery. However, the biggest drawback of this method is that it is easy to cause infection at the puncture site, thrombus spread along the interventional device, and filter displacement. At the same time, before the DVT is cured, the longest safe indwelling time of temporary VCFs in the body is often exceeded. Therefore, many temporary VCFs are replaced by permanent VCFs.

1.2.1.3 Retrievable Vena Cava Filter

To solve the issues with permanent VCFs, while avoiding the shortcomings of temporary VCF with many side effects, a recovery hook for recovery was added to the VCF. After being placed in the body, it no longer needs to be connected to the interventional device. It can be permanently indwelled in the body according to the patient's requirement. When the patient no longer needs the filter, it can be safely recycled. Representative products include Günther Tulip [7], Denali [8], Celect [9], and Crux Vena Cava [10].

1. Günther Tulip filter (GTF)

   GTF is made of Conichrome® (cobalt-chromium-nickel-molybdenum-iron alloy). The configuration is similar to tulip petals, hence, the name tulip. Twelve alloy wires form a cone-shaped thrombus capture net with a recovery hook on the head.

2. Denali filter

   Denali adopts the integrated manufacturing process of laser cutting nitinol tube and polishes it. Structurally, the titanium anchor on the filter wire arm is removed and the end of the leg is redesigned. There is a diverging hook at the end of each leg.

3. Celect filter

   Celect evolved from Günther Tulip. In addition to the four pillars, there are eight independent arc support rods, which cannot only capture thrombus but also support the vena cava to improve the stability and self-control of the filter.

4. Crux Vena Cava filter

   This is a novel product. It has a symmetrical double helix structure. The relatively helical self-expanding nickel-titanium alloy is connected to form a filter frame. There are five tissue anchors on the frame to optimize fixation and limit penetration.

   In recent years, biodegradable polymer materials have become a research hotspot, especially in the field of interventional devices [11]. Biodegradable materials have the characteristic of disappearing by themselves after they perform their functions, which cannot be achieved by traditional materials. This feature can meet the requirements of clinical use of VCF: VCF plays a role in filtering thrombus in the early stage of implantation; in the late stage it gradually degrades as thrombosis continues to decrease; and finally, it is completely absorbed and discharged from the body. The clinical use of degradable VCF is expected to eliminate a series of complications caused by the late stage of permanent VCF implantation; on the other hand, it is expected to eliminate the secondary trauma to patients caused by retrievable VCF. Compared with metal VCF, the structural design and mechanical properties of degradable VCF are challenging. With the development of medical materials, processing technology, and new structural design, biodegradable VCFs will be the next generation of VCF in the future.

1.2.2 EMBOLIZATION DEVICES

In the clinical treatment of intracranial aneurysms, intravascular embolization is usually required. In this situation, we need an embolization device to produce the thrombus quickly to block the blood vessels. Usually, embolic agents are injected into the supply vessels of the diseased organs or the diseased blood vessels to block them and interrupt the blood supply to control bleeding, treat vascular diseases and tumors, and eliminate the function of diseased organs.

Broadly, an embolization device includes different devices and materials which achieve embolization. The ideal embolization device needs to travel smoothly in the blood vessel and should have the following characteristics: (1) Good biocompatibility, non-toxic, and non-antigenic. (2) Easy to transmit through the catheter without sticking and blocking the tube. (3) Occlude blood vessels quickly and applicable to different calibers and different flows as needed.

An embolization device can be classified as follows: (1) According to the nature of the material, it can be divided into three categories: inactive materials, self-materials, and radioactive particles. (2) According to physical properties, it can be divided into solid and liquid embolic materials. (3) According to the duration for vascular occlusion, it can be divided into short-term, medium-term, and long-term. (4) According to whether the material can be absorbed by the body, it can be divided into absorbable and non-absorbable embolic materials.

1.2.2.1 Non-absorbable Solid Particle Embolic Material

1. Polyvinyl alcohol (PVA) particles

   PVA particles are made of PVA and formaldehyde through cross-linking, drying, crushing, and sieving. They are non-water soluble, swellable, and when exposed to aqueous liquids, their volume increases by 20%. They have good biocompatibility and are not absorbed in the body.

2. Elastic microsphere

   Poly-hydroxyethyl methacrylate (PHEMA) microsphere: the advantage of elastic microspheres is that they can be compressed in diameter and are easy to transport.

3. Shape memory polymer materials

   When processed into thin strips at low temperature, the shape of memory polymer material becomes thicker and shorter at body temperature and can be used for embolization [12,13].

1.2.2.2 Absorbable Embolic Material

1. Autologous blood clot

   An autologous blood clot is a short-term embolism, which is easy to obtain and easy to inject through a sterile and non-antigenic catheter. The disadvantage is that the time to occlude the blood vessel cannot be predicted.

2. Gelatin sponge

   Gelatin sponge is a hemostatic agent for surgical operation. It is a protein matrix sponge and can be absorbed by tissues. After the gelatin sponge blocks blood vessels, it acts as a net frame and can quickly form

a thrombus. It offers a non-permanent occlusion, which lasts from a few weeks to several months.
3. Microcollagen fiber hemostatic agent

   Microcollagen fibers, a derivative of cowhide collagen, are usually used to stop bleeding during surgery and are more effective than gelatin sponge. The advantage is that they can enter small arteries; however, they may cause extensive interruption of the collateral blood supply due to tissue ischemia infarction.
4. Alginate microspheres

   Sodium alginate microspheres have good biocompatibility, are non-toxic, non-antigenic, non-chemical, or offer immune effects after embolization. Moreover, non-toxic degradation of microspheres occurs within 3–6 months.

1.2.2.3   Mechanical Embolic Material

1. Microcoil

   According to material classification, microcoils can be divided into copper coil [14], tungsten coil [15], and platinum coil [16].
   I.   Copper coil: Copper can be easily oxidized in the body, and it has been used in neonatal Galen vein aneurysms.
   II. Tungsten coil: Tungsten is less flexible than platinum, and the friction force in the micropipette are greater; however, it remains stable after placement.
   III. Platinum coil: Platinum has good impermeability to X-ray, which can be observed on the fluorescent screen. Because platinum is very soft, when the pressure in the lumen increases slightly, the coil can adapt to the shape and size of the aneurysm very well.

   According to the control method of the coil, it can be divided into a free coil, electrolytic detachable coil [17–19], mechanical detachable spiral coil [20–22], and hydrolysis detachable coil [23–26].
   I.   Free coil: There is no connection device between the free coil and the thruster. The thruster can only push the coil and cannot withdraw. Therefore, it is dangerous and limits its application.
   II. Electrolytic detachable coil: Guglielmi's detachable coil is a representative electrolytic detachable coil. The connection between the thruster and the microcoil adopts microwelding technology. After the coil reaches the proper position, the pusher is connected to the positive electrode of the power supply and weak direct current is passed. The stainless steel surface which is not covered with the insulating layer between the platinum coil and the pusher is electrolyzed so that the coil can be released without pulling in the aneurysm. This feature can reduce the mistaken embolism caused by the coil entering the tumor-bearing artery.
   III. Mechanically detachable spiral coil: Its performance and effect are similar to the electrolytic detachable coil. The main difference is that the tungsten wire coil is released mechanically, and the coil can be pulled back or repositioned freely until the position is satisfied. At present, there are three different release devices, namely, clamp type, collar

type, and internal locking type. The internal locking type has low friction in the microcatheter and has good stability during release, which is better than the other two types.

IV. Hydrolysis detachable coil: The catheter is expanded by increasing the water pressure so that the release coil does not require an additional power supply, which is stable and reliable, and only requires two syringes. A new type of coil hydro coil is coated with a hydrogel layer. After being placed in the aneurysm, the hydrogel begins to expand and fills the aneurysm space. As the hydrogel expands, the blood promotes healing components (such as proteins) which are inhaled into the hydrogel to improve the healing rate. Matrix coil is coated with degradable polymer materials, which can block blood flow in the aneurysm, induce thrombosis, and improve the embolization effect.

Coating on the surface of the microcoil to enhance the embolization function is an efficient way to improve the clinical application value, including constructing a ciliary surface, hydrogel surface, and procoagulant protein coatings [27–30], which can effectively improve the embolization effect, promote wound repair and healing, and reduce complications.

2. Detachable balloon

There are two types of detachable balloons: latex balloon and silicone balloon. The balloon should be filled with a permanent filler during application and should be used in conjunction with the microcatheter. After the balloon enters the tumor and inflates, the catheter is gently pulled to release the balloon. At present, it is only clinically suitable for the embolization treatment of aneurysms of the basilar artery bifurcation of the skull base, ophthalmic aneurysms, occlusion tests, and internal carotid artery cavernous fistula.

3. Silk thread

Silk thread is also a type of embolic material, which plays a role in the endovascular treatment of cerebral arteriovenous malformation. It can be emblazed alone or combined with α-n-butyl cyanoacrylate.

With further understanding of the mechanism of different cardiovascular diseases, the design of the cardiovascular therapeutic device and the development of material science for maintaining and reestablishing healthy blood circulation is becoming more and more targeted, personalized, and multi-functional. Especially dealing with the complex situation caused by thrombus, a new generation of cardiovascular therapeutic device can not only solve the problem of blood circulation but also provide a bioactive surface to promote therapeutic recovery of the diseased area and achieve a better therapeutic effect.

1.3 DEVICES FOR IMPLEMENTING REVASCULARIZATION

The blood supply chain is crucial for normal body function, and a supply failure leads to tissue or organ death. Possible causes include thrombosis, vascular occlusion, vessel damage, and gangrene. Medicine, intervention, and bypass therapies are available for different lesion severity. The lesion sites are either reopened or repaired based on the existing blood vessel or are replaced by a new one. This section focuses on intervention and bypass therapies. Three major therapeutic devices for revascularization are discussed: vascular stent, drug-coated balloon, and artificial blood vessel.

1.3.1 VASCULAR STENT

In 1977, a distensible balloon was inflated to reopen the narrowed vessel, which reduced 50% vascular stenosis, and the percutaneous transluminal coronary angioplasty (PTCA) strategy emerged [31]. However, vascular elastic retraction reduced the efficacy. To prevent the retraction and provide long-term mechanical support, a vascular stent was accordingly developed, which brought a revolutionary change to vascular disease treatment. They are widely used for occlusive vessels (e.g., coronary artery, brain artery, renal artery, main aorta). Vascular stents have passed through three stages: bare-metal stent (BMS), drug-eluting stent (DES), and bioresorbable stent (BRS), and the performance of a stent platform depends on three important elements as shown in Figure 1.3. BMS (medical stainless steel, nitinol, cobalt, etc.) successfully overcame the vascular elastic retraction and dramatically reduced the second intervention rate; however, the thrombosis and in-stent restenosis issues gave way to DES [32].

1.3.1.1 Major Drugs for DES Platforms

DES consists of a BMS-based metallic backbone, extra surface coating, and drug. Clinically used DES platforms include Xience-V (Abbott Vascular), Endeavor (Medtronic), Biomatrix (Biosensors), Promus element (Boston Scientific), and Cypher (Cordis) [33]. By coating stents with drugs that prevent smooth muscle cell (SMC) proliferation, in-stent restenosis can be considerably attenuated. The major drugs

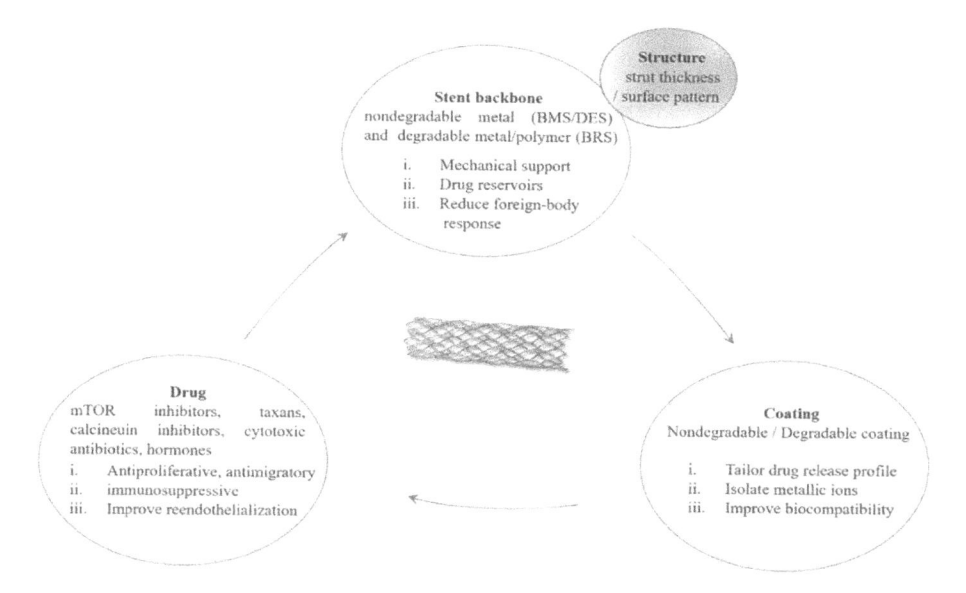

FIGURE 1.3   Vascular stents platform.

loaded to DES are mTOR inhibitors (rapamycin (sirolimus), everolimus, zotarolimus, biolimus), calcineurin inhibitors (tacrolimus, pimecrolimus), taxans (paclitaxel), hormones (estradiol), cytotoxic antibiotics (actinomycin D), and combination with tested drugs (cerivastatin, batimastat, flavopiridol, probucol, carvedilol) [34]. mTOR inhibitors showed a superior clinical effect compared to others, and the outcome of sirolimus was independent of the presence of polymer coating. Taxans also produced beneficial effect, notwithstanding that their cytotoxicity and narrow therapeutic wind brought severe side effects for peripheral artery disease such as thrombosis and inflammation [35]. However, these beneficial drugs halt the growth of endothelial cells as well as neointimal tissue, and stent struts along with the remaining coating continually stimulate the vessel wall, hence, it prolongs the chronic inflammation and delays the reendothelialization process that is vital for preventing late/very late thrombosis and in-stent restenosis.

1.3.1.2 Optimization of DES Surface Coating and Structure

To cope with these issues, varied surface coatings have been fabricated. Isolating coatings (titanium, carbon, silicon carbide, etc.) have been used to reduce the interaction between stent metal ions and blood proteins as thrombosis was originally thought to be induced by charge transfer from plasma protein to metal. Bioactive coatings (e.g., heparin, phosphorylcholine (PC), nitric oxide) were deployed to inhibit the coagulation process [32]. Degradable coatings have also been introduced: poly(L-lactic acid-co-Glycolic acid) (PLGA), PLA, and poly(L-lactic acid) (PLLA) [33]. However, all coatings must be tailored to the interfacial bonding property, fracture risk, and biocompatibility. Degradable coatings have to further balance the rate among drug-release profile, coating degradation, and stent reendothelialization.

Stent structure has also been shown to be involved in these complications. Boston refined structure from 132 μm of Taxus express to 81 μm of Promus element, and the late lumen loss was reduced more than 50% [33]. This is consistent with the finding that stent thickness is positively related to in-stent restenosis rate [36]. Firehawk (Microport Medical) was lasered with one side grooves to carry drug coating, which reduced the stimulus to blood composition and provided a comparable late thrombosis rate with Xience [37]. Nano plus (Lepu Medical) adopted nano/micropore to load drug, which thoroughly eliminated coating impacts [38].

1.3.1.3 Trials of BRS

To pursue a "leaving nothing behind" concept, the stent platform should disappear after providing transient mechanical support. To this end, polymer and metallic BRS have been developed. Most polymer BRS adopted PLLA, Poly(D, L-lactic acid) (PDLLA), proprietary tyrocore desaminotyrosine poly-carbonate (PTD-PC) as stent backbone, either fabricated with the drug directly or coated with a degradable drug film. Approximately 34 prospective polymer BRS are currently under development (e.g., Igaki-Tamai (Kyoto Medical), Absorb 1.0/2.0 (Abbott Vascular), DESolve, MeRes100 (Meril), Xinsorb (Huaan), Fortitude (Amaranth Medical), Art18AZ(ART), Ideal BioStent (Xenogenics)), wherein Abbott and Igaki-Tamai stent platforms have gained CE marks, respectively, for coronary intervention and peripheral arterial diseases [33,39]. However, in 2017, Abbott withdrew the stent from the market due to a disappointing mid-term outcome such as elevated thrombosis rate, which raised concerns about the use of polymer BRS. Despite the uncertainty, the enthusiasm for metallic biodegradable stent continued. Metallic BRS deployed magnesium, iron, and zinc as stent backbone with a polymer drug coating (e.g., Dreams (Biotronik), Unity (QualiMed), IBS(LifeTech)) [33,40]. Zinc-based alloy provides a promising platform and has just started its journey for BRS application [41]. Magmaris (DREAMS 2G) (PLLA and sirolimus) was upgraded from AMS-1, which is the only metallic BRS that has gained a CE mark so far. Through fining alloy composition, strut thickness, crown design, and adding/refreshing drug-polymer coating, Magmaris possesses similar mechanical properties to DES, a smaller strut-to-artery ratio to the Absorb, and a tailored degradation process. Ultimately, it attained a target lesion failure and target lesion revascularization within the DES ranges, which demonstrated a safe device in simple lesions [42–44].

Clinically, first-generation DES has been replaced by second and third-generation ones due to a high risk of late stent thromboses [45]. However, BMS still benefits patients under some specific conditions such as big diameter vessel disease and patients with bleeding antithrombosis conflict. Though BRS is still in its infancy, it has a promising future [46]. Among these three types of stent platforms, the average strut thickness of metallic non-biodegradable stents is smaller than that of polymeric ones; however, there is almost no difference in coating materials and drug choices among the three types of stents [33]. Therefore, it can be concluded that on the premise of the same drug choice and target function, subsequent beneficial stent relies on newly introduced stent backbone material, structure design, and tailored coating to allow rapid reendothelialization and minimize the risk of late/very late thrombosis, in-stent restenosis, and in-stent neo-atherosclerosis.

1.3.2 Drug-Coated Balloon

PTCA strategy has gone through a spiral development. Balloon's role evolved from purely reopening the vessel wall, to assisting stent implantation, to reopening and treating the diseased vessel. Due to the side effects of in-stent restenosis, late thrombosis, and long-term anti-platelet therapy, a drug-coated balloon (DCB) was developed as a non-stent therapeutic approach to the concept of "leaving nothing behind" [47]. DCB carried anti-proliferative drugs on the balloon surface and transferred them to the lesion sites by compressing the plaque, which reduced anti-platelet therapy duration as well as restenosis rate.

1.3.2.1 Approaches to Manipulate Tissue Uptake Rate of DCB Drug

To achieve therapeutic efficacy during a short contact with the vessel wall, the carried drug should be rapidly taken by the tissue. Paclitaxel was the most deployed drug for DCB as the lipophilic drug transferred easier than the hydrophilic drug. Although a dose of 2–3 $\mu g/mm^2$ was reported to successfully inhibit restenosis [48], most paclitaxel did not reach the lesion. Paclitaxel-coated drug balloon lost about 60%–80% of the drug, and only approximately 16% of the drug was transferred to the intima of target sites [35]. To overcome low transfer and high wash-off rate, one solution is avoiding unnecessary contact between drug and blood flow. DIOR had manufactured

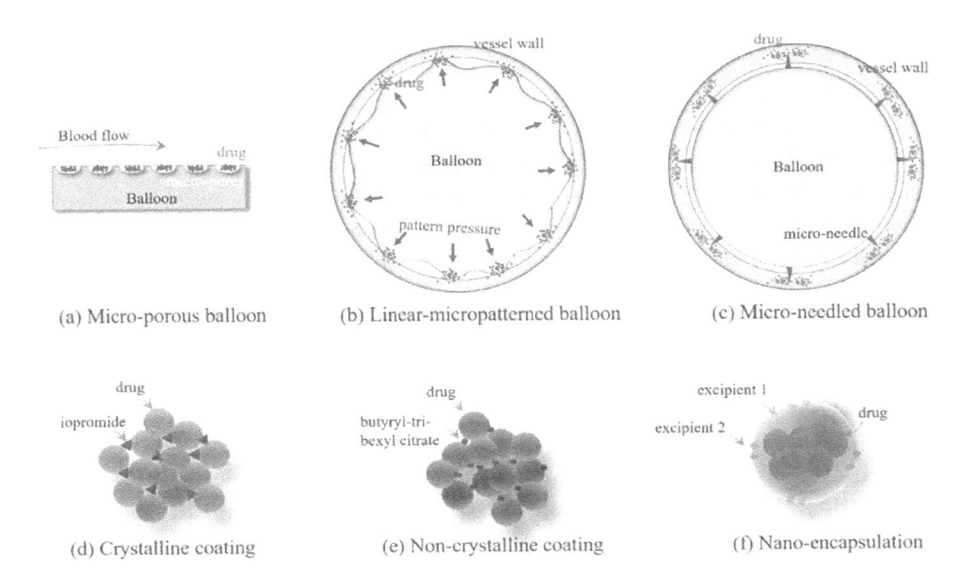

FIGURE 1.4   Methods for manipulating tissue uptake rate of DCB drug. (a) Microporous balloon, (b) linear-micropatterned balloon, (c) microneedled balloon, (d) crystalline coating, (e) non-crystalline coating, (f) nano-encapsulation.

a porous balloon with multiple micropores on the surface, with the drug embedded inside (Figure 1.4a) [49]. Another option is increasing the contact pressure. Balloon with micropatterned array has been found to have a higher contact pressure between the endothelium and balloon surface, delivering 2.3 times higher amount of drug to lesions (Figure 1.4b) [50]. Different from micropore and arrays attaching to the tissue surface, taking the drug directly into the tissue is one step further. Microneedle with a diameter of approximately 140 μm has been reported to cross the endothelium barrier into the base media and even deep into the adventitia (Figure 1.4c) [51,52]. Another unique approach is double-balloon layers. It was manufactured into an inner drug layer and an outer drug-free layer, which carried two-fold drugs (6.8 ± 0.7 μg/mm²) as normal and delivered similar amounts during each inflation [53]. Yet, both microneedle and double layers resulted in heterogeneous drug distribution.

In addition to balloon structures, tissue uptake rate can be manipulated by surface coating. Currently, based on coating structure, DCB has developed from heterogeneous crystalline coating, to homogeneous non-crystalline coating, to homogeneous encapsulated microcrystalline coating (Figure 1.4d–f) [54]. The crystalline coating usually raises the particulate issue and may cause downstream embolization [55], which was deduced as a possibility of high mortality of PCB in a meta-analysis [35]. Heterogeneous coating increased the chances of heterogeneous drug distribution in lesion sites, and a subtherapeutic dose afterward. From crystalline to non-/microcrystalline, excipients were the most common component for balloon coating, which were introduced as a hydrophilic spacer to create a high-contact surface area at lesion sites [54], and were found to enhance drug migration more than 10-fold [56]. Excipients for commercial DCB treating cardiovascular restenosis include urea (IN.

PACT, Medtronic), either polysorbate or sorbitol (Lutonix, Bard), shellac (Restore, Cardionovum), iopromide (Paccocath, Bayer AG), and butyryl trihexyl citrate (Pantera Lux, Biotronik AG) [35]. However, different coating formulations generated drug particles of different sizes. For example, IN.PACT Admiral DCB possessed larger particles than Lutonix and Ranger [54,55], whether the particle size is related to a downstream embolization is not certain so far. With or without an excipient, polymers were also deployed as a matrix to carry drugs. Poly(ethylene oxide) was designed for a two-phase drug release: small amount of drug at inflation stage and therapeutic amount at treatment stage [48]. However, a heterogeneity issue emerged on balloon surface after first-round inflation when being fabricated into double layers [53]. Recently, the possibilities of nanoparticle delivery system have been valued to improve delivery efficacy. Along with coating components, several commonly employed coating methods emerged, including dipping, spraying, surface grafting, LBL, hydrogel coating, and microsyringe. Due to poor interaction, dip coating suffered from severe wash-off rates [57,58]. Compared to dipping, precise microsyringe allowed higher coating uniformity, which significantly improved paclitaxel uptake at the proximal and distal sites, and enhanced the total tissue uptake by approximately 42% than heterogeneous coating [59]. Although paclitaxel is the default drug for most DCB that is under investigation, the different delivery efficacies between conical urea and spherical shellac, between nanoparticle carriers of UPE and PLGA, and between acrylic and LBL electrostatic coating methods illustrated the critical role that balloon coating plays in drug transfer [57,60].

1.3.2.2 Factors Relevant to Tissue Distribution and Resistance of DCB Drug

Following tissue uptake, therapeutic efficacy requires prolonged drug persistence in the vessel wall. It has been reported that only 1% drug is taken up by tissue, and the restenosis inhibition ability of paclitaxel is dose-dependent, though lower-dose PCB generates fewer peri-strut fibrin deposits [35,55]. Therefore, a subtherapeutic level of the tissue-retained drug would not work well [48]. Paclitaxel exists in three forms as amorphous solid, anhydrous crystals, and dihydrate crystals [61]. Both anhydrous and dihydrate have a higher tissue retention rate, and among mixed forms, both micro-crystalline coating and amorphous/dihydrate coating have a higher tissue retention rate. If lesions sites were premounted with stents, they can achieve a higher drug half-life of about 1.9 months [62]. High-contact pressure between tissue and balloon may also enhance drug persistence by facilitating a deeper delivery, like a balloon with microarrays [50]. Instead of drug-delivering amounts, drug penetration ability was a key factor for balloon coating, especially carriers, to achieve long drug persistence.

1.3.2.3 Alternation of DCB Drugs

Attributed to advanced coating technologies, DCB drug tends to be upgraded from paclitaxel to limus drug (sirolimus and zotarolimus) [54,63]. Paclitaxel can diffuse into the vessel wall easily because it is highly lipophilic. However, its earlier application for stent coronary interventions caused side effects of either stent thrombosis at high concentration or inflammatory response at a lower dose [35]. Furthermore, due to a higher rate of mortality caused by paclitaxel-coated balloon in femoropopliteal arteries, a hypothesis was recently concluded that paclitaxel may cause long-term focal toxicity, though the concentration of the wash-off drug in plasma was below level causing systemic toxicity. Following paclitaxel's step, focus was given to sirolimus, a default stent-carried drug wide therapeutic window. However, poorer lipophilicity limited its delivery from balloon surface to vessel wall, and normal strategies for PCB drug transfer and retention did not suit SCB [64]. A new microcrystalline and encapsulation approach was developed to improve this. Sirolimus was encapsulated in a lipophilic package with an excipient and transferred into the intima after 1 hour, media after 3 days, and adventitia after 7 days [64]. In addition sirolimus, other less toxic drugs such as metacept-3 were also under investigation [65].

In recent decades, both balloon structures and surface properties were renewed to implement a balloon-only strategy. It provided an alternative therapeutic method to stenting and presented favorable clinical results in indications of small vessel disease, de-novo coronary lesions, bifurcation lesions, patients at high bleeding risk [66], and neurovascular disease [67]. Concerns of high wash-off rate, low tissue retention, elastic recoil, coronary dissection [68], and distal embolization [69] are expected to be resolved in the future.

1.3.3 ARTIFICIAL BLOOD VESSEL

Artificial blood vessels are medical devices used to restore blood circulation in the settings of diseased or damaged arteries and veins or as hemodialysis fistula. An ideal artificial blood vessel requires good biocompatibility, especially hemocompatibility, suitable mechanical property, similar dynamics performance with host vessel, low immunogenicity, strong resistance to infection, and off-the-shelf availability [70]. Both autogenous vessels and allografts are the primary choices for artificial blood vessels, but their sources are limited and a second injury is always problematic. To overcome these, in 1952, Voorhees introduced a groundbreaking device – permeable artificial blood vessel Vinylon "N" – which was successful in both dog and human tests [71]. Since then, a variety of alternative grafts have been investigated in the past 60 years, including bioprosthetic, synthetic, and tissue-engineered grafts.

1.3.3.1 Materials for Artificial Blood Vessel Fabrication

The basic element to construct a vascular graft is bulk material. Natural polymers (e.g., collagen, cellulose, chitosan, gelatin, silk, decellularized extracellular matrix) have good biocompatibility, bioactive functions, and friendly degradation. They are an ideal scaffold for tissue-engineered/bioactive grafts, but the compositions vary with batches and the mechanical strength is weak. Synthetic materials provide a variety of alternatives and include non-resorbable materials (e.g., polytetrafluoroethylene (PTFE), polyethylene terephthalate (PET), poly(ethylene glycol) (PEG)), resorbable materials (e.g., poly(ε-caprolactone) (PCL), poly(glycerol sebacate) (PGS), polyurethane (PU), thermoplastic polyurethane (TPU), poly(d, l-lactic acid-co-glycolic acid) (PLGA), polyglycolic acid (PGA), polylactic acid (PLA), poly(l-lactic acid) (PLLA), gelatin methacrylate-GelMA). [70,72,73]. Along with both types of polymers, different fabrication methods have been developed, as is shown in Figure 1.5, including braiding and knitting, paste extrusion and expansion, electrospinning, gas foaming/particle leaching, 3D printing, cell-sheet engineering, and decellularization [74,75].

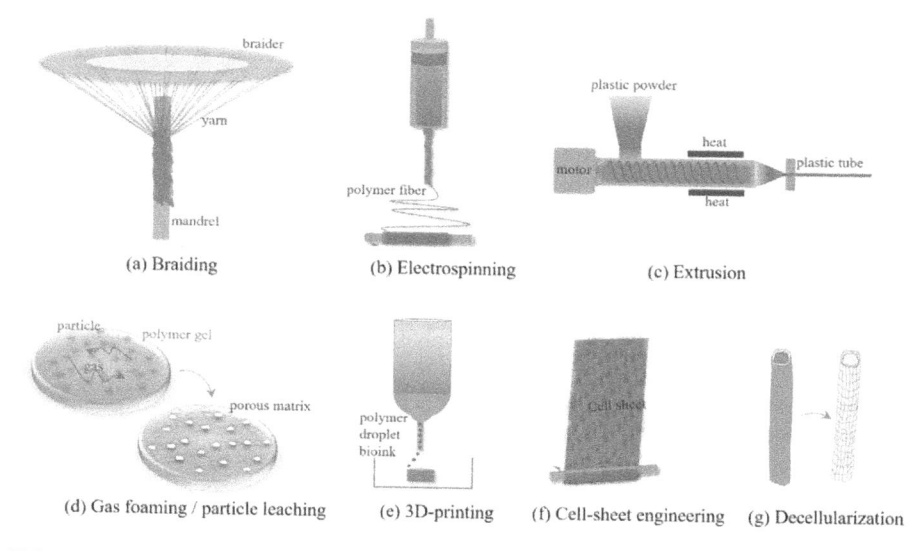

(a) Braiding   (b) Electrospinning   (c) Extrusion

(d) Gas foaming / particle leaching   (e) 3D-printing   (f) Cell-sheet engineering   (g) Decellularization

FIGURE 1.5   Commonly used methods for artificial blood vessel fabrication. (a) Braiding, (b) electrospinning, (c) extrusion, (d) gas foaming/particle leaching, (e) 3D printing, (f) Cell-sheet engineering, and (g) decellularization.

Normally, two or more mentioned approaches are adopted. However, the biocompatibility of synthetic material is limited and some exhibit mechanical issues such as incompatible compliance. Increasing fiber diameter and the porosity of the PCL sheath increase the mechanical properties and promote graft vascular remodeling [76]. United with rapid resorbable PGS core, the intima layer encourages vascular cell infiltration and matrix deposition to realize rapid cellularization [77]. For a woven graft such as PGA, looser braids lead to bleeding and early rupture due to no structural support during degradation. Moreover, changing braiding density and angle result in a different level of inflammation, elastin/collagen deposition, and neovessel distensibility [78]. Non-woven graft (ePTFE) is a node-fibril structure, and increasing the porosity from less than 30 μm to larger than 45 μm greatly facilitates cell engagement and growth without blood leakage [79]. In the setting of hemodialysis patients, an elastic layer inserted between two ePTFE layers prevents puncture-caused bleeding and allows early cannulation within 24 hours [80]. Furthermore, a sinusoidal architecture has been found to reach a mechanical strength close to the native blood vessel [81]. Therefore, both the mechanical strength and the limited biocompatibility of synthetic materials, especially anticoagulation and neo-tissue formation, can be adjusted to a certain extent through modulating the polymers' structure and composition [76]. So far, the most commonly used clinical vascular graft materials are Dacron (PET), ePTFE, polyurethane (PU), and natural silk.

1.3.3.2   Surface Modification Technologies

Surface property is another key element for a vascular graft as the substrate surface directly interacts with blood flow and native tissue to regulate the cellular events. The surface biocompatibility can be adjusted by physicochemical and bioactive modifications: (1) hydrophilic and hydrophobic surfaces [73], both of which can prevent the interaction between graft surface and blood components to reduce coagulation risk as the hydrophilic surface has a low interfacial free energy with blood and the hydrophobic surface has low surface energy [82]; (2) negative charge surface [83]: electrostatic repulsion method is based negative cell surfaces and some negative proteins such as negative ePTFE and PET surfaces; however, the immediate uncontrolled protein absorption may disturb this anti-foul process. Additionally, both (1) and (2) methods may inhibit the protein-mediated cell adhesion and proliferation; (3) microphase separation surface [84]: this kind of structure camouflages itself into a native material by inducing a site-selective absorption to different proteins; (4) grafting bioactive materials like heparin for anticoagulation, urokinase for fibrinolysis, or grafting bioactive group containing materials like sulfonic and carboxyl group [73]; (5) endothelialization: endothelial cells are a natural blood vessel barrier with ideal biofunction, a layer of which enhances biocompatibility, especially hemocompatibility. This layer can be realized either by seeding cells in vitro [85] or by presenting homing surfaces (e.g., RGD, VEGF) to recruit cells in vivo [74,86]. The latter one tends to provide a long-term functional cell layer.

1.3.3.3 Possibilities of Small Diameter Artificial Blood Vessel

Artificial blood vessels of diameter equal to and larger than 6mm have been successfully commercialized for clinical use (e.g., Atrium Advanta and Flixene (Atrium Medical Co.), Vascuted-Terumo (Vascutek), Impra & Venaflo & Carbodlo & Vectra (Bard Peripheral Vascular INC), Propaten & Gore-Tex (W.L.Gore & Associates), HeRO (Merit Medical), Acuseal (W.L. Gore)) [87]. However, the development of small diameter artificial graft (less than 6mm such as coronary artery bypass graft) remains a worldwide challenge. The compliance of widely used materials such as ePTFE, PET, PU, and PCL is not compatible with small vessels, which is always accompanied by calcification and inflammation-induced unexpected degradation. Moreover, the mismatched mechanical property together with low blood flow raises the risk of occlusive thrombus and can lead to hyperplasia [88–90]. In addition to the above-mentioned issues, there has been almost no change in the commonly used synthetic materials in the past 60 years, and the new generation of vascular graft materials have developed slowly. Therefore, manufacturing small vascular graft demands bulk material, fabrication, and surface modification.

Currently, a hybrid or tissue-engineered small diameter graft has gained a significant advantage on patency. Through biomimicking the role of SMCs in maintaining vessel homeostasis, Wang et al. bio-fabricated an elastic vessel wall in PGA scaffold using SMCs differentiated from adipose-derived stem cells [91]. Based on the native vessel wall structure, Chenxi et al. constructed a three-layered graft of 2–4mm using silk and PU: a thin dense PU intima, a thick elastic textile-PU media, and a porous silk-PU adventitia, which showed a high patency rate and is ready for clinical trial [92]. Wang et al. designed a nanotopographic intima surface to inhibit platelet adherence and activation [93]. Moreover, to ensure a native intima-like layer, Yamanaka et al. decellularized a rat rail artery of 0.6mm and modified the surface with synthesized peptide for rapid reendothelialization [94]. Xu et al. constructed a

4 mm bilayer graft of both endothelial and SMCs via 3D printing [95]. The National Cerebral and Cardiovascular Center of Japan has worked out a special approach to in situ construction. This group deployed a 0.6 mm stainless steel wire to successfully fabricate 0.6 mm collagen tubes in vivo. After transplantation, no thrombus was observed for 6 months. Recently, Yamamoto et al. revealed that shear stress (15 dynes/cm^2) activated mitochondrial ATP production of endothelial cells, and thereby the production of vasodilator and nitric oxide via Ca^{2+} signaling [96]. In this context, other key anticoagulation mechanism(s) may exist for small diameter native vessel if low shear stress failed to decrease cell membrane cholesterol. These results show great potential for brain and heart bypasses. Now, the thinnest vascular graft is around 3 mm. Only Atrium Medical Co. and Bard produce commercialized small vascular grafts. Theoretically, tissue-engineered graft is a promising approach for small diameter graft [97]; however, the production still requires further improvement in design and manufacturing techniques.

1.4 DEVICES FOR RESTORING CARDIAC HEMODYNAMICS

Valve conditions and HF seriously impede normal blood supply. For pathological valves (e.g., regurgitation and stenosis), valve substitutes, repair, or percutaneous techniques have been applied to resolve the conditions (Figure 1.6 (left)). Regarding valve replacement, numerous developers focus on the design and optimization of artificial valves (referring to the mechanical valve, biological, as well as tissue-engineering ones) for optimal therapeutic performance, high durability, low risk of thrombotic complications, and ideal hemodynamics. For treating HF, the gold standard, cardiac transplantation, is governed by the source and preservation of donor's heart (Figure 1.6 (right)). Based on this setting, total artificial heart and ventricular assist have attracted the attention of researchers. Generally, considering device

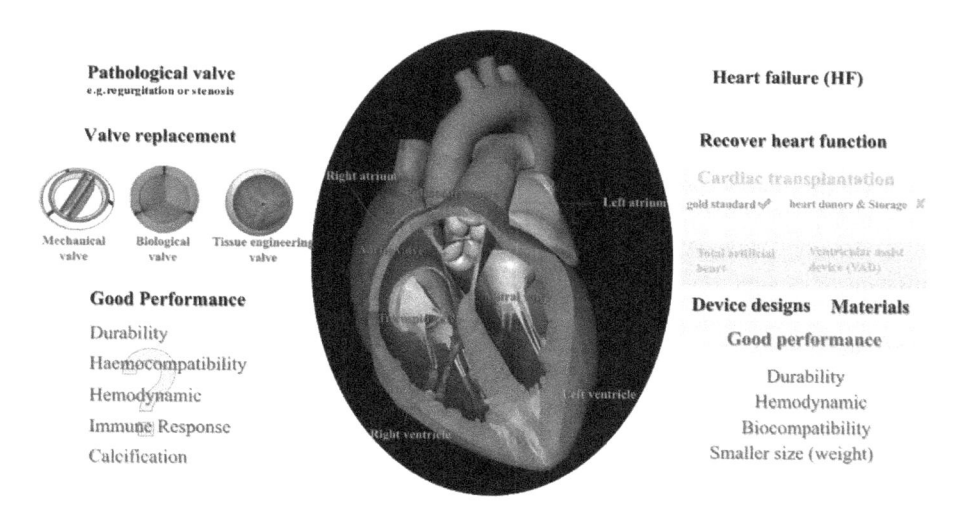

FIGURE 1.6 Typical treatments of valvular diseases (left) and heart failure (right). The heart picture in middle is from 3DBody6.0 (Free).

design and appropriate materials, excellent properties can be obtained, including good durability, smaller size or weight, and biocompatibility for human tissue.

1.4.1 ARTIFICIAL HEART VALVES REPLACEMENT

Heart valves, including pulmonary valve, tricuspid valve, aortic valve, and mitral valve, can control the flow of blood through the chamber and prevent blood reflux through the valve's "opening-closing" function. Heart valve conditions, routinely dedicated by coronary artery disease, high blood pressure, previous heart attack, or cardiomyopathy, can be resolved with valve replacement (pathological valve including regurgitation and stenosis are displaced by artificial valves), valve repair (normalizing a regurgitant valve surgically but not replacing), as well as percutaneous techniques covering percutaneous balloon valvuloplasty and transcatheter aortic valve implantation. This section discusses valves for cardiac valve replacement, primarily including mechanical valves and biological ones, the two most widely used implant valves to date. The former has the risk of thrombosis, while the latter is mainly about durability. More recent tissue-engineered valves are also discussed.

1.4.1.1 Mechanical Valves

Mechanical valves, which appeared in the 1950s, made of artificial material and comprising sewing ring, occlusion, and retaining mechanism, possessed long-term durability but high clotting risk. For common candidates, ball-cage (the earliest artificial valves), tilting disk, and bileaflet (such as the Sorin Bicarbon valve) valves were designed. Artificial materials for mechanical valves originate from metal, ceramic, and polymer (e.g., stainless steel alloys, molybdenum alloys, titanium, silicone, and pyrolytic carbon) [98]. As a typical foreign object, mechanical valves encounter thrombus, hemolysis, even resultant severe embolism and mechanical obstruction, which are induced by abnormal blood flow (including high shear stress, stagnant flow, and turbulence) related to valves' implantation and their foreign surface. Therefore, using anticoagulants (such as warfarin potassium) or lowering clotting surface or new valve design is obligatory. Patients receiving blood thinners suffer from high bleeding risk. With weakening adverse effects, coating techniques have paved the way for the ameliorative hemocompatibility of devices. As summarized by Wheatley et al., surface treatments, carbon-based coatings (e.g., depositing diamond-like carbon (DLC) coating), fluoridization, plasma and glow discharge treatment, or oxidation post-treatments, generated thrombus eradicated surface marked by fewer platelets and reduced thrombosis [99,100]. In one example, Major et al. deposited a C:H-based coating onto the thermoplastic polyurethane (TPU) substrates and subsequently confirmed that the coating could be used in blood contact circumstances with a high value of shear stress potently, increased hemocompatibility, and without causing an immune response [100]. More than surface modification, meeting mechanical design (mechanical safety) of valves and physiological requirements of the organism, new valve designs also have been attainable. Flexible valves, partly simulating native valves, guide similar hemodynamics to biological valves. Textile valves with available flexible leaflets acquire blood flow similar to natural valves with adjustable durability [101]. Different materials and manufacturing methods have been vigorously investigated, such as PET textile materials and polyester textiles [102,103]. Polynova valves provide high durability as well as low thrombogenicity, as reported by Piatti et al. [104].

1.4.1.2 Tissue Valves

Considering that the heart valves withstand repetitive "opening/closing" action about 31,536,000 times per year, high durability needs to be considered [105]. Tissue heart valves require a donor (actual valves or tissue), such as porcine (pig), bovine (cow), horse, or human, and last 10–15 years ordinarily after placing in the body [106], categorized as xenografts, allografts, and homografts. Compared with mechanical valves, bioprosthetic valves naturally instigate a more physiological blood flow with reduced clotting after replacing, while not succeeding durability and failing to meet mechanical requirements compromised by structural degradation connecting to immunoreaction and calcification [104]. Several studies have established that degeneration of tissue valves is caused by recipient and donor factors (age, disease, allograft size, body surface area of receiver), sterilization and preservation methods, and implantation techniques [107–109]. In adults, it is widely accepted that the durability of an allograft is equal to or better than that of manual bioprostheses, and slow fibrocalcific degeneration stimulates its failure [110]. Simultaneously, of note, allograft valves have ideal performance followed by normal hemodynamics and excellent freedom from infectious endocarditis and thromboembolism [111]. For allografts, the specificity of transplanted tissue can elicit an immune response, which touches on the service life of bio-valves. Compared with standard cryopreserved valved allografts, decellularized cryopreserved valve allografts with lower immunogenicity and higher durability displayed better mid-term performance in an approximately 5-year study [112]. Theoretically, thorough detachment of cellular components (cell and cellular debris) from donor tissue can lower the immunogenicity of implants, which makes implants reconfigure. Further, the remodeled patient-adapted valves can enhance durability and ameliorate degeneration and calcification [113]. Helder et al. also mentioned that acellular allografting, exhibiting fibrosis and calcification in explanted produce failure models such as standard valves, which are driven by tissue damaging through decellularization process and sterilization procedure [114]. A cryopreserved homograft is a valid option [115] because they are an imperfect but satisfactory biological material for reconstructing natural outflow [116]. Moreover, for more optimal biofunctional answering after explanting, decorating decellularized homografts have been built. In clinical practices, the problems of calcification and intimal hyperplasia impeded the outcomes of cryopreserved homografts, coating of fibronectin and stromal cell-derived factor-1a onto the cell-free ovine aortic homografts inhibited immune reaction mediated by cryopreserved heart valve, calcification, pannus formation, and accelerated re-endothelialization [117].

1.4.1.3 Tissue-Engineered Valves

Some significant advancements have been witnessed in valve explanting, from first mechanical valves and bioprosthetic valves to tissue-engineered valves. On the premise of more physiological flow patterns and affirmative blood compatibility, tissue-engineered heart valves (TEHVs) harvest durability of mechanical valves, the hemodynamic performance of biological valves, and regenerative ability of native tissues intelligently, eventually obtain the patients' valves with biocompatibility. Multitudinous TEHVs have been devised for developing "living" valves with favorable cell ingrowth and tissue remodeling, such as a scaffold integrating autologous bone marrow-derived mononuclear cells and biodegradable matrix [118]. Currently, various materials have been applied for scaffold fabrication, including natural materials (fibrin and collagen), polymeric substance (e.g., PGA and PLA or their co-polymers, and PEG-DA) and ECM from decellularized engineered tissue and decellularized donor valves [119–122]. More than materials, newer valve design emerged. In one example, Reimer and colleagues developed a tubular heart valve stemming from two cell-free extracellular matrix tubes with organized collagenous matrix. After that, exceeding recellularization and, ideally, somatic growth, these valves exhibited full leaflet opening and closing, minimal regurgitation under simulated physiological conditions, and no tissue damage after 2 million cycles of fatigue testing [120]. Cell-seeded TEHVs are another alternative. Coupling fibrin-based valves supporter and cells originating from ovine carotid artery demonstrated improved seeded cell adhesion and alignment in fibrin substrate, tuned ECM producing, and remodeled the valve matrix under given dynamic conditioning [123]. For cell-based biodegradable scaffolds, mechanical properties are dramatically determined by lost mechanical properties due to biodegradation of the scaffolds and additional counterparts involving de-novo matrix synthesis. According to Sant et al., valvular interstitial cells (VICs) entrapped into PGS–PCL (fast degrading polyglycerol sebacate (PGS) and slowly degrading polycaprolactone (PCL)) scaffolds secreted new matrix protein for rebuilding the synthetic scaffold during the old one degrading, which kept the scaffolds stable [124]. Over these, in light of structural and anisotropic mechanical characteristics of the native valve leaflets, manufacturing technologies for TEHVs are also a major research field. Existing options include bioengineering methods (decellularizing and conditioning valves successively), which reduced antigenicity and generated comparative hemodynamical with intrinsic valves [122]; multiple-step injection molding, which provided high integrity [125]; electrospinning and microfabrication techniques, which can also mimic mechanism and unique mechanical features [126]. Altogether, excimer laser microfabrication and predictive modeling are also candidates [127]. Decellularized heart valves (xenogenic or allogenic) [128] and remolded collagenous organization [120] by primitive fibrin gel holder replaced primitive cell-produced collagenous matrix served as starter matrix.

1.4.2 HEART FUNCTION RECOVERY

HF has high mortality as the 10-year lethal rates are 89% and 86% in men and women aged 65–74 years, respectively [129]. Cardiac transplantation, the gold standard for treating end-stage HF, is a highly effective solution to settle end-stage HF, but limited by the unavailability of heart donors. This drawback initiates the growing use of mechanical circulatory support. This part extensively focused on the total artificial heart and ventricular assist device (VAD) implantation, the two main options to remedy end-stage HF. Implanting a VAD also potently renews heart function, even though the device is not considered to last the entire lifecycle [130]. A large number of studies have proven that, in addition to the material itself, the hemodynamic characteristics after implantation of artificial ventricle affect the service performance of the device. Usually, hemodynamics evoke blood damage embracing different mechanisms, such as hemolysis, platelet activation, thrombosis, and emboli [131]. Given these, more than selected materials for artificial heart and VAD, extended substantial advancements have achieved optimized mechanical design.

1.4.2.1 Totally Artificial Heart

Heart transplantation is regarded as the most effective treatment for patients suffering from end-stage HF; however, unfortunately, it is obstructed by organ shortage and the source of donors. These drawbacks drive the booming of the artificial heart to minimize the need for donor hearts. Currently, total artificial heart (TAH) systems involve three blocks: pump units featuring limited durability, percutaneous tubes, as well as bulky external equipment [132]. The TAH is an extremely important curative option withstanding serious biventricular dysfunction or other aggravated structural abnormalities. From the pioneering era to date, several TAH systems have emerged. CardioWest TAH (SynCardia Systems, Inc., Tucson, AZ), the only commercially available TAH in the United States approved by the FDA, was marked completely in 2004 [133]. Copeland et al. stated that the CardioWest TAH can reduce these problems (e.g., right HF, valvular regurgitation, cardiac arrhythmias, ventricular clots) after implanting left ventricular and biventricular assist devices [134]. The AbioCor TAH, another FDA-approved TAH in 2006 [135], totally implantable, was similar to the Syncardia device with similar graft and cuff design [136], and was motor-driven without percutaneous cables, conduits, or wires [137]. The Carmat total artificial heart (C-TAH, Vélizy-Villacoublay, France), a newer heart replacement device described as an electro-hydraulically driven, pulsatile biventricular pump support containing bioprosthetic blood-contacting surfaces, was designed to weaken thromboembolism events and bleeding and save lives. The first clinical use of a bioprosthetic C-TAH has been accepted after extensive investigation. C-TAH contains ventricles, each with a blood compartment and a hydraulic fluid working on drive unit parted by hybrid membranes coming from ePTFE and bovine pericardial tissue [138,139]. Naturally, hemocompatibility and safety of hybrid membranes are vital for the performance of this device. The safety of hybrid membrane confirmed insignificant change in mechanical, physical, and chemical properties from 9 months up to 4 years of aging, eliminate membrane calcification, and no hemolysis trigger and platelet sensitization [140]. Markedly, over physiological blood dynamics, after using C-TAH, the progressive endothelialization of C-TAH has been demonstrated [141]. Pivotally, the C-TAH equipped with autoregulated mode encouraged endothelial homeostasis preservation [142]. The ReinHeart TAH, an electrically driven and fully implantable Destination Therapy TAH system, owns strong preload sensitivity and guides the integration of physiologic flow control [132,143].

1.4.2.2 Ventricular Assist Devices (VADs)

Today, over 2,000 patients receive mechanical circulatory devices annually in the United States, which relieve the pressure on the donor source [144]. VADs, a prospective lifesaving equipment, consisting of electrically powered pumps (circulating blood), controller unit (monitoring, and controlling the previous part), and power unit (supply electricity for the device), are applied to support patients until heart donation (termed as bridge-to transplantation (BTT)) or recover essential cardiac function during/after heart surgery (named as bridge-to-recovery (BTR)) [145,146]. Additionally, for destination therapy (DT), VADs also have been utilized to substitute for cardiac transplantation, permanent, or long-term application to the human body [147]. It has been seen that the usage of VADs promotes the survival rate of suffers. The study conducted by Burns and team revealed that implanting of a left ventricular assist device (LVAD) germinate beneficial reverse remodeling of myocardial structure and function [148]. VADs are divided into three categories, named LVAD, right ventricular assist device, as well as biventricular assist device [130]. The evolution of implantable blood pumps follows the rules of smaller size, lower thrombosis rate and hemolysis, high durability, fewer accessories, and low risk of postoperative infection. Progressively, first-generation VADs with pulsatile pump had limitations such as short of huge volume and blood-contacting surfaces, pro-thrombosis effects, poor durability, and infection. For thrombosis, anticoagulant therapy is necessary such as aspirin for lifelong administration after VAD implantation [149]. Further second-generation products with smaller size and high durability, engendered continuous, unidirectional blood flow, induced by their centrifugal, axial, or hybrid pumps. Seeing that hemolysis caused by contact bearings, more recent third-generation VADs use "non-contact"-bearing design, which resulted in a durable device, rapid postoperative recovery, less hemolysis, and thrombosis [130,145,150,151]. At present, implantable VAD suitable for multifarious attempts are obtainable commercially, as Heart Assist 5, Heart Mate II, and Jarvik-2000 belonging to second-generation pumps and Dura Heart belonging to third generation pump [152]. Technically, wireless transfer technology with more reliable and longer transmission distance has greatly promoted the development of mechanical circulatory supporters [153].

REFERENCES

1. G.E. Cimochowski, R.H. Evans, C.K. Zarins, C.T. Lu, T.R. DeMeester. Greenfield filter versus Mobin-Uddin umbrella: The continuing quest for the ideal method of vena cava interruption. *J. Thorac. Cardiovasc. Surg.* 79 (1980) 358–365. doi:10.1016/s0022-5223(19)37944-9.
2. Q. Chau, S.B. Cantor, E. Caramel, M. Hicks, D. Kurtin, T. Grover, L.S. Elting. Cost-effectiveness of the bird's nest filter for preventing pulmonary embolism among patients with malignant brain tumors and deep venous thrombosis of the lower extremities. *Support. Care Cancer.* 11 (2003) 795–799. doi:10.1007/s00520-003-0520-2.
3. H.J. Jaeger, S. Kolb, T. Mair, M. Geller, A. Christmann, R.K.H. Kinne, K.D. Mathias. In vitro model for the evaluation of inferior vena cava filters: Effect of experimental parameters on thrombus-capturing efficacy of the Vena Tech- LGM filter. *J. Vasc. Interv. Radiol.* 9 (1998) 295–304. doi:10.1016/S1051-0443(98)70272-6.
4. P.A. Poletti, C.D. Becker, L. Prina, P. Ruijs, H. Bounameaux, D. Didier, P.A. Schneider, F. Terrier. Long-term results of the Simon nitinol inferior vena cava filter. *Eur. Radiol.* 8 (1998) 289–294. doi:10.1007/s003300050382.
5. R.L. Leask, K.W. Johnston, M. Ojha. Hemodynamic effects of clot entrapment in the trapease inferior vena cava filter. *J. Vasc. Interv. Radiol.* 15 (2004) 485–490. doi:10.1097/01.RVI.0000124941.58200.85.

6. N.Y. Yim, N.K. Chang, J.H. Lim, J.K. Kim. Retrograde tempofilter IITM placement within the superior vena cava in a patient with acute upper extremity deep venous thrombosis: The filter stands on its head. *Korean J. Radiol.* 12 (2011) 140–143. doi:10.3348/kjr.2011.12.1.140.

7. S. Wicky, F. Doenz, J.Y. Meuwly, F. Portier, P. Schnyder, A. Denys. Clinical experience with retrievable Günther Tulip vena cava filters. *J. Endovasc. Ther.* 10 (2003) 994–1000. doi:10.1583/1545-1550(2003)010<0994:CEWRGT>2.0.CO;2.

8. S.W. Stavropoulos, J.X. Chen, R.F. Sing, F. Elmasri, M.J. Silver, A. Powell, F.C. Lynch, A.K. Abdel Aal, A. Lansky, B.E. Muhs. Analysis of the final DENALI trial data: A prospective, multicenter study of the Denali inferior vena cava filter. *J. Vasc. Interv. Radiol.* 27 (2016) 1531–1538.e1. doi:10.1016/j.jvir.2016.06.028.

9. J.C. Durack, A.C. Westphalen, S. Kekulawela, S.B. Bhanu, D.E. Avrin, R.L. Gordon, R.K. Kerlan. Perforation of the IVC: Rule rather than exception after longer indwelling times for the günther tulip and celect Retrievable Filters. *Cardiovasc. Intervent. Radiol.* 35 (2012) 299–308. doi:10.1007/s00270-011-0151-9.

10. H.B. Smouse, R. Mendes, M. Bosiers, T.G. Van Ha, T. Crabtree. The RETRIEVE trial: Safety and effectiveness of the retrievable crux vena cava filter. *J. Vasc. Interv. Radiol.* 24 (2013) 609–621. doi:10.1016/j.jvir.2013.01.489.

11. X. Zhang, B.H. Tan, Z. Li. Biodegradable polyester shape memory polymers: Recent advances in design, material properties and applications. *Mater. Sci. Eng. C.* 92 (2018) 1061–1074. doi:10.1016/j.msec.2017.11.008.

12. Q. Zhao, H.J. Qi, T. Xie. Recent progress in shape memory polymer: New behavior, enabling materials, and mechanistic understanding. *Prog. Polym. Sci.* 49–50 (2015) 79–120. doi:10.1016/j.progpolymsci.2015.04.001.

13. R.K. Avery, H. Albadawi, M. Akbari, Y.S. Zhang, M.J. Duggan, D. V. Sahani, B.D. Olsen, A. Khademhosseini, R. Oklu. An injectable shear-thinning biomaterial for endovascular embolization. *Sci. Transl. Med.* 8 (2016) 365ra156. doi:10.1126/scitranslmed.aah5533.

14. H. Jiang, J.P. Wang, Y.C. Li, Y.Y. Tong, Q. Yang, D. Yan, L.L. Ding, S.G. Yuan. Experimental study of vascular embolization with homemade second-level Copper coil. *Chinese J. Radiol.* 47 (2013) 183–187. doi:10.3760/cma.j.issn.1005-1201.2013.02.018.

15. H. Zhengsong, D. Qinshun, J. Tao, L. Junshi. Endovascular embolization of intracranial aneurysms with self-made tungsten coils in a dog model. *Chin. Med. J. (Engl).* 109 (1996) 626–630. doi:10.3171/jns.2004.101.6.0996.

16. A. Kurata, S. Suzuki, H. Ozawa, I. Yuzawa, M. Yamda, K. Fujii, S. Kan, T. Kitahara, T. Ohmomo, Y. Miyasaka. Application of the liquid coil as an embolic material for arteriovenous malformations. *Interv. Neuroradiol.* 11 (2005) 287–295. doi:10.1177/159101990501100315.

17. C.B. Luo, M.M.H. Teng, F.C. Chang, C.Y. Chang. Endovascular treatment of intracranial high-flow arteriovenous fistulas by Guglielmi detachable coils. *J. Chinese Med. Assoc.* 69 (2006) 80–85. doi:10.1016/S1726-4901(09)70118-2.

18. S. Albayram, D. Selcuk, A. Soeda, N. Sakai, K. Iihara, I. Nagata. Thromboembolic events associated with Guglielmi detachable coil embolization of asymptomatic cerebral aneurysms: Evaluation of 66 consecutive cases with use of diffusion-weighted MR imaging [3] (multiple letters). *Am. J. Neuroradiol.* 25 (2004) 159–160. PMID: 12533341.

19. W. Möller-Hartmann, T. Krings, K. Stein, H. Dreeskamp, A. Meetz, F.J. Hans, R. Thiex, J. Gilsbach, A. Thron. Treatment of experimental aneurysms in rabbits using Guglielmi detachable coils: A feasibility study. *Riv. Di Neuroradiol.* 16 (2003) 1154–1156. doi:10.1177/197140090301600631.

20. A. Tournade, P. Courtheoux, C. Sengel, S. Ozgulle, T. Tajahmady. Saccular intracranial aneurysms: Endovascular treatment with mechanical detachable spiral coils. *Radiology.* 202 (1997) 481–486. doi:10.1148/radiology.202.2.9015078.

21. H. Kiyosue, H. Mori, S. Matsumoto, Y. Hori, M. Okahara, S. Tanoue, Y. Sagara. Clinical use of a new mechanical detachable coil system for percutaneous intravenous embolization of cavernous sinus dural arteriovenous fistulas. *Radiat. Med. - Med. Imaging Radiat. Oncol.* 22 (2004) 143–147. PMID: 15287528.

22. A. Kinoshita, M. Ito, T. Skakaguchi, K. Yamada, S. Akizuki, M. Taneda, T. Hayakawa. Mechanical detachable coil as a therapeutic alternative for cerebral aneurysm. *Neurol. Res.* 16 (1994) 475–476. doi:10.1080/01616412.1994.11740277.

23. H.J. Cloft, D.F. Kallmes. Aneurysm packing with hydrocoil embolic system versus platinum coils: Initial clinical experience. *Am. J. Neuroradiol.* 25 (2004) 60–62. PMID: 14729529.

24. B.R. Bendok, K.R. Abi-Aad, J.D. Ward, J.F. Kniss, M.J. Kwasny, R.J. Rahme, S.G. Aoun, T.Y. El Ahmadieh, N.E. El Tecle, S.G. Zammar, R.J.N. Aoun, D.P. Patra, S.A. Ansari, J. Raymond, H.H. Woo, D. Fiorella, G. Dabus, G. Milot, J.E. Delgado Almandoz, J.A. Scott, A.J. Denardo, S.R. Dashti, S. Ansari, E. Deshaies, S. Lavine, H. Bozorgchami, J. Delgado, E. Veznedaroglu, F. Albuquerque, D. Fiorella, A. Boulos, M. Cortes, H. Kanaan, G. Jindal, R. Klucznik, G. Dabus, D. Kalmes, R. Tawk, J. Raymond, C. Romero, A. Xavier, M. Hussain, M. Kelly, C. Moran, I. Chaudry, A. Pandey, D. Wang, B. Van Adel, G. Milot, J. Hirsch, J. Carpenter, C. Powers, P. Jabbour, G. Luh, J. Shankar, R. Tummala, A. Patsalides, A. Evans, A. Garg, S. Dashti, S. Lee, R. James, M. Jayaraman, S. Satti, E. Sauvageau, J. Fields, T. Grobelny, J. Hartman. The Hydrogel Endovascular Aneurysm Treatment Trial (HEAT): A randomized controlled trial of the second-generation hydrogel coil. *Neurosurgery.* 86 (2020) 615–624. doi:10.1093/neuros/nyaa006.

25. W. Zhi-Gang, D. Xuan, Z. Ji-Qing, Q. Chun-Cheng, W. Cheng-Wei, H. De-Zhang, H. Xiao-Guang. HydroCoil occlusion for treatment of traumatic carotid-cavernous fistula: Preliminary experience. *Eur. J. Radiol.* 71 (2009) 456–460. doi:10.1016/j.ejrad.2008.06.009.

26. Y. Murayama, F. Viñuela, A. Ishii, Y.L. Nien, I. Yuki, G. Duckwiler, R. Jahan, Initial clinical experience with Matrix detachable coils for the treatment of intracranial aneurysms, *J. Neurosurg.* 105 (2006) 192–199.

27. L. Zhou, B. Zhong, H. Du, W. Wang, J. Shen, S. Zhang, W. Li, H. Tang, P. Zhang, W. Yang, X. Zhu. Comparison of embolic agents for varices during transjugular intrahepatic portosystemic shunt for variceal bleeding: Tissue gel or coil? *J. Interv. Med.* 3 (2020) 195–200. doi:10.1016/j.jimed.2020.08.008.

28. W. Brinjikji, A.P. Amar, J.E. Delgado Almandoz, O. Diaz, P. Jabbour, R. Hanel, F. Hui, M. Kelly, K.D. Layton, J.W. Miller, E. Levy, C. Moran, D.C. Suh, H. Woo, R. Sellar, B. Hoh, A. Evans, D.F. Kallmes. GEL THE NEC: A prospective registry evaluating the safety, ease of use, and efficacy of the HydroSoft coil as a finishing device. *J. Neurointerv. Surg.* 10 (2018) 83–87. doi:10.1136/neurintsurg-2016-012915.

29. N. Wang, X. Jiang, J. Wang, X. Hao, Study on the application of embolization materials of collagen, in: *IOP Conf. Ser. Mater. Sci. Eng.*, 2019: pp. 012005. doi:10.1088/1757-899X/587/1/012005.

30. J.J. Rong, D. Liu, M. Liang, Q.H. Wang, J.Y. Sun, Q.Y. Zhang, C.F. Peng, F.Q. Xuan, L.J. Zhao, X.X. Tian, Y.L. Han. The impacts of different embolization techniques on splenic artery embolization for blunt splenic injury: A systematic review and meta-analysis. *Mil. Med. Res.* 4 (2017). doi:10.1186/s40779-017-0125-6.

31. A.R. Grüntzig, Å. Senning, W.E. Siegenthaler. Nonoperative dilatation of coronary-artery stenosis - percutaneous transluminal coronary angioplasty. *N. Engl. J. Med.* 301 (1979) 61–68. doi:10.1056/nejm197907123010201.

32. R. Lowe, I.B.A. Menown, G. Nogareda, I.M. Penn. Coronary stents: In these days of climate change should all stents wear coats?. *Heart.* 91 (2005) 20–23. doi:10.1136/hrt.2005.060269.

33. I. Cockerill, C.W. See, M.L. Young, Y. Wang, D. Zhu. Designing better cardiovascular stent materials: A learning curve. *Adv. Funct. Mater.* 2005361 (2020) 1–23. doi:10.1002/adfm.202005361.

34. R. Wessely. New drug-eluting stent concepts. *Nat. Rev. Cardiol.* 7 (2010) 194–203. doi:10.1038/nrcardio.2010.14.

35. K. Dan, E. Shlofmitz, N. Khalid, A. Hideo-Kajita, J.P. Wermers, R. Torguson, P. Kolm, H.M. Garcia-Garcia, R. Waksman. Paclitaxel-related balloons and stents for the treatment of peripheral artery disease: Insights from the Food and Drug Administration 2019 Circulatory System Devices Panel Meeting on late mortality: Paclitaxel devices in PAD treatment. *Am. Heart J.* 222 (2020) 112–120. doi:10.1016/j.ahj.2019.12.012.

36. J. Pache, A. Kastrati, J. Mehilli, H. Schühlen, F. Dotzer, J. Hausleiter, M. Fleckenstein, F.J. Neuman, U. Sattelberger, C. Schmitt, M. Müller, J. Dirschinger, A. Schömig. Intracoronary stenting and angiographic results: Strut thickness effect on restenosis outcome (ISAR-STEREO-2) trial. *J. Am. Coll. Cardiol.* 41 (2003) 1283–1288. doi:10.1016/S0735-1097(03)00119-0.

37. A. Lansky, W. Wijns, B. Xu, H. Kelbæk, N. van Royen, M. Zheng, M. Morel, P. Knaapen, T. Slagboom, T.W. Johnson, G. Vlachojannis, K.E. Arkenbout, L. Holmvang, L. Janssens, A. Ochala, S. Brugaletta, C.K. Naber, R. Anderson, H. Rittger, S. Berti, E. Barbato, G.G. Toth, L. Maillard, C. Valina, P. Buszman, H. Thiele, V. Schächinger, A. Baumbach. Targeted therapy with a localised abluminal groove, low-dose sirolimus-eluting, biodegradable polymer coronary stent (TARGET All Comers): A multicentre, open-label, randomised non-inferiority trial. *Lancet.* 392 (2018) 1117–1126. doi:10.1016/S0140-6736(18)31649-0.

38. Y.J. Zhang, F. Chen, T. Muramatsu, B. Xu, Z.Q. Li, J.B. Ge, Q. He, Z.J. Yang, S.M. Li, L.F. Wang, H.C. Wang, B. He, K. Li, G.X. Qi, T.C. Li, H.S. Zeng, J.J. Peng, T.M. Jiang, Q.T. Zeng, J.H. Zhu, G.S. Fu, C. V. Bourantas, P.W. Serruys, Y. Huo. Nine-month angiographic and two-year clinical follow-up of polymer-free sirolimus-eluting stent versus durable-polymer sirolimus-eluting stent for coronary artery disease: The nano randomized trial. *Chin. Med. J. (Engl).* 127 (2014) 2153–2158. doi:10.3760/cma.j.issn.0366-6999.20133148.

39. Y. Katagiri, P.W. Serruys, T. Asano, Y. Miyazaki, P. Chichareon, R. Modolo, K. Takahashi, N. Kogame, J.J. Wykrzykowska, J.J. Piek, Y. Onuma, A. Kastrati. How does the failure of absorb apply to the other bioresorbable scaffolds? An expert review of first-in-man and pivotal trials. *EuroIntervention.* 15 (2019) 116–123. doi:10.4244/EIJ-D-18-00607.

40. C. Beyan, E. Beyan. Bioresorbable scaffolds: Current technology and future perspectives. *Rambam Maimonides Med. J.* 11 (2020) e0039. doi:10.5041/RMMJ.10402.

41. E. Mostaed, M. Sikora-Jasinska, J.W. Drelich, M. Vedani. Zinc-based alloys for degradable vascular stent applications. *Acta Biomater.* 71 (2018) 1–23. doi:10.1016/j.actbio.2018.03.005.

42. R.M. Waksman, PROGRESS was made toward DREAM: Magnesium Stent, report in Washington hospital center, 2012. https://bioflow.hu/dynamic/PROGRESS-to-DREAMS-Waksman-20120517-1455-RoomMaillot.pdf.

43. M. Haude, H. Ince, A. Abizaid, R. Toelg, P.A. Lemos, C. Von Birgelen, E.H. Christiansen, W. Wijns, F.J. Neumann, C. Kaiser, E. Eeckhout, S.T. Lim, J. Escaned, H.M. Garcia-Garcia, R. Waksman. Safety and performance of the second-generation drug-eluting absorbable metal scaffold in patients with de-novo coronary artery lesions (BIOSOLVE-II): 6 month results of a prospective, multicenter, non-randomised, first-in-man trial. *Lancet.* 387 (2016) 31–39. doi:10.1016/S0140-6736(15)00447-X.

44. M. Haude, H. Ince, S. Kische, R. Toelg, N.M. Van Mieghem, S. Verheye, C. von Birgelen, E.H. Christiansen, E. Barbato, H.M. Garcia-Garcia, R. Waksman. Sustained safety and performance of the second-generation sirolimus-eluting absorbable metal scaffold: Pooled outcomes of the BIOSOLVE-II and -III trials at 3 years. *Cardiovasc. Revascularization Med.* 21 (2020) 1150–1154. doi:10.1016/j.carrev.2020.04.006.

45. A.M. Galløe, H. Kelbæk, L. Thuesen, H.S. Hansen, J. Ravkilde, P.R. Hansen, E.H. Christiansen, U. Abildgaard, G. Stephansen, J.F. Lassen, T. Engstrøm, J.S. Jensen, J.L. Jeppesen, N. Bligaard, P. Thayssen, J. Aarøe, K. Saunamäki, A. Junker, H.H. Tilsted, H.E. Bøtker, S. Galatius, C.T. Larsen, S.D. Kristensen, L.R. Krusell, S.Z. Abildstrøm, M. Meng, L. Okkels. 10-Year clinical outcome after randomization to treatment by sirolimus- or paclitaxel-eluting coronary stents. *J. Am. Coll. Cardiol.* 69 (2017) 616–624. doi:10.1016/j.jacc.2016.11.055.
46. N. Rajendra, B. Wrigley, A. Gershlick. Bioabsorbable stents: Nothing from something. *Clin. Investig. (Lond).* 2 (2012) 1185–1189. doi:10.4155/cli.12.126.
47. B. Scheller, U. Speck, C. Abramjuk, U. Bernhardt, M. Böhm, G. Nickenig. Paclitaxel balloon coating, a novel method for prevention and therapy of restenosis. *Circulation.* 110 (2004) 810–814. doi:10.1161/01.CIR.0000138929.71660.E0.
48. J.A. Anderson, S. Lamichhane, T. Remund, P. Kelly, G. Mani. Preparation, characterization, in vitro drug release, and cellular interactions of tailored paclitaxel releasing polyethylene oxide films for drug-coated balloons. *Acta Biomater.* 29 (2016) 333–351. doi:10.1016/j.actbio.2015.09.036.
49. A. De Labriolle, R. Pakala, L. Bonello, G. Lemesle. Interventional rounds paclitaxel-eluting balloon : From bench to bed. *Catheter. Cardiovasc. Interv.* 652 (2009) 643–652. doi:10.1002/ccd.21895.
50. K.J. Lee, S.G. Lee, I. Jang, S.H. Park, D. Yang, I.H. Seo, S.K. Bong, D.H. An, M.K. Lee, I.K. Jung, Y.H. Jang, J.S. Kim, W.H. Ryu. Linear Micro-patterned Drug Eluting Balloon (LMDEB) for enhanced endovascular drug delivery. *Sci. Rep.* 8 (2018) 1–13. doi:10.1038/s41598-018-21649-7.
51. C.D. Owens, W.J. Gasper, J.P. Walker, H.F. Alley, M.S. Conte, S.M. Grenon. Safety and feasibility of adjunctive dexamethasone infusion into the adventitia of the femoropopliteal artery following endovascular revascularization. *J. Vasc. Surg.* 59 (2014) 1016–1024. doi:10.1016/j.jvs.2013.10.051.
52. K.J. Lee, J.Y. Lee, S.G. Lee, S.H. Park, D.S. Yang, J.J. Lee, A. Khademhosseini, J.S. Kim, W.H. Ryu. Microneedle drug eluting balloon for enhanced drug delivery to vascular tissue. *J. Control. Release.* 321 (2020) 174–183. doi:10.1016/j.jconrel.2020.02.012.
53. J.A. Anderson, S. Lamichhane, K. Fuglsby, T. Remund, K. Pohlson, R. Evans, D. Engebretson, P. Kelly, S. Falls. Development of drug-coated balloon for the treatment of multiple peripheral artery segments. *J. Vasc. Surg.* 71 (2019) 1750–1757.e7. doi:10.1016/j.jvs.2019.04.494.
54. H. Ang, T.R. Koppara, S. Cassese, J. Ng, M. Joner, N. Foin. Drug-coated balloons: Technical and clinical progress. *Vasc. Med. (United Kingdom).* 25 (2020) 577–587. doi:10.1177/1358863X20927791.
55. C.A. Gongora, M. Shibuya, J.D. Wessler, J. McGregor, A. Tellez, Y. Cheng, G.B. Conditt, G.L. Kaluza, J.F. Granada. Impact of paclitaxel dose on tissue pharmacokinetics and vascular healing a comparative drug-coated balloon study in the familial hypercholesterolemic swine model of superficial femoral in-stent restenosis. *JACC Cardiovasc. Interv.* 8 (2015) 1115–1123. doi:10.1016/j.jcin.2015.03.020.
56. T. Heilmann, C. Richter, H. Noack, S. Post, D. Mahnkopf, A. Mittag, H. Thiele, F. Hans-Reiner. Drug release profiles of different drug-coated balloon platforms. *Eur. Cardiol. Rev.* 6 (2010) 40. doi:10.15420/ecr.2010.8.2.40.
57. R. Iyer, A.E. Kuriakose, S. Yaman, L.C. Su, D. Shan, J. Yang, J. Liao, L. Tang, S. Banerjee, H. Xu, K.T. Nguyen. Nanoparticle eluting-angioplasty balloons to treat cardiovascular diseases. *Elsevier B.V.* 554 (2019) 212–223. doi:10.1016/j.ijpharm.2018.11.011.
58. T.R. Dugas, G. Brewer, M. Longwell, T. Fradella, J. Braun, C.E. Astete, M.H. Jennings, C.M. Sabliov. Nanoentrapped polyphenol coating for sustained drug release from a balloon catheter. *J. Biomed. Mater. Res. - Part B Appl. Biomater.* 107 (2019) 646–651. doi:10.1002/jbm.b.34157.

59. P.P. Buszman, A. Tellez, M.E. Afari, A. Peppas, G.B. Conditt, S.D. Rousselle, J.C. McGregor, M. Stenoien, G.L. Kaluza, J.F. Granada. Tissue uptake, distribution, and healing response after delivery of paclitaxel via second-generation iopromide-based balloon coating: A comparison with the first-generation technology in the iliofemoral porcine model. *JACC Cardiovasc. Interv.* 6 (2013) 883–890. doi:10.1016/j.jcin.2013.04.013.

60. G.H. Chang, D.A. Azar, C. Lyle, V.C. Chitalia, T. Shazly, V.B. Kolachalama. Intrinsic coating morphology modulates acute drug transfer in drug-coated balloon therapy. *Sci. Rep.* 9 (2019) 1–10. doi:10.1038/s41598-019-43095-9.

61. A.R. Tzafriri, S.A. Parikh, E.R. Edelman. Taking paclitaxel coated balloons to a higher level: Predicting coating dissolution kinetics, tissue retention and dosing dynamics. *J. Control. Release.* 310 (2019) 94–102. doi:10.1016/j.jconrel.2019.08.019.

62. U. Speck, B. Cremers, B. Kelsch, M. Biedermann, Y.P. Clever, S. Schaffner, D. Mahnkopf, U. Hanisch, M. Böhm, B. Scheller. Do pharmacokinetics explain persistent restenosis inhibition by a single dose of paclitaxel? *Circ. Cardiovasc. Interv.* 5 (2012) 392–400. doi:10.1161/CIRCINTERVENTIONS.111.967794.

63. P.M. Kitrou, K. Katsanos. Sirolimus-coated balloons for the treatment of femoro-popliteal lesions: New player in the game? *J. Endovasc. Ther.* (2020). doi:10.1177/1526602820946377.

64. S. Basavarajaiah, S. Athukorala, K. Kalogeras, V. Panoulas, B.H. Loku Waduge, G. Bhatia, R. Watkin, G. Pulikal, K. Lee, J. Ment, B. Freestone, M. Pitt. Mid-term clinical outcomes from use of sirolimus coated balloon in coronary intervention; data from real world population. *Catheter. Cardiovasc. Interv.* (2020) ccd.28998. doi:10.1002/ccd.28998.

65. H. Bin Liu, M. Byrne, P. Perlmutter, A. Walker, G.R. Sama, J. Subbiah, B. Ozcelik, R.E. Widdop, T.A. Gaspari, K. Byron, Y.C. Chen, D.M. Kaye, A.E. Dear. A novel epigenetic drug-eluting balloon angioplasty device: Evaluation in a large animal model of neointimal hyperplasia. *Cardiovasc. Drugs Ther.* 33 (2019) 687–692. doi:10.1007/s10557-019-06921-w.

66. R. V. Jeger, S. Eccleshall, W.A. Wan Ahmad, J. Ge, T.C. Poerner, E.S. Shin, F. Alfonso, A. Latib, P.J. Ong, T.T. Rissanen, J. Saucedo, B. Scheller, F.X. Kleber. Drug-coated balloons for coronary artery disease: Third report of the international DCB consensus group. *JACC Cardiovasc. Interv.* 13 (2020) 1391–1402. doi:10.1016/j.jcin.2020.02.043.

67. P. Gruber, L. Remonda. Device profile of different paclitaxel-coated balloons: Neuro Elutax SV, Elutax '3' Neuro and SeQuent Please NEO for the treatment of symptomatic intracranial high-grade stenosis: overview of their feasibility and safety. *Expert Rev. Med. Devices.* 17 (2020) 87–92. doi:10.1080/17434440.2020.1719829.

68. B. Cortese, P. Silva Orrego, P. Agostoni, D. Buccheri, D. Piraino, G. Andolina, R.G. Seregni. Effect of drug-coated balloons in native coronary artery disease left with a dissection. *JACC Cardiovasc. Interv.* 8 (2015) 2003–2009. doi:10.1016/j.jcin.2015.08.029.

69. M. Kimura, J. Shiraishi, N. Ikemura, Y. Matsubara, M. Hyogo, T. Sawada. Proximal balloon occlusion to prevent downstream embolization and thus reduce systemic adverse effects of drug-coated balloons. *Cardiovasc. Interv. Ther.* 35 (2020) 306–307. doi:10.1007/s12928-019-00595-9.

70. J. Chlupác, E. Filová, L. Bačáková. Blood vessel replacement: 50 years of development and tissue engineering paradigms in vascular surgery. *Physiol. Res.* 58 (2009) 119–140.

71. A.B. Voorhees, A. Jaretzki, A.H. Blakemore. The use of tubes constructed from vinyon "N" cloth in bridging arterial defects. *Ann. Surg.* 135 (1952) 332–336. doi:10.1097/00000658-195203000-00006.

72. J.D. Kakisis, C.D. Liapis, C. Breuer, B.E. Sumpio. Artificial blood vessel: The Holy Grail of peripheral vascular surgery. *J. Vasc. Surg.* 41 (2005) 349–354. doi:10.1016/j.jvs.2004.12.026.

73. D. Wang, Y. Xu, Q. Li, L.S. Turng. Artificial small-diameter blood vessels: Materials. fabrication, surface modification, mechanical properties, and bioactive functionalities. *J. Mater. Chem. B.* 8 (2020) 1801–1822. doi:10.1039/c9tb01849b.

74. H.J. Chung, T.G. Park. Surface engineered and drug releasing pre-fabricated scaffolds for tissue engineering. *Adv. Drug Deliv. Rev.* 59 (2007) 249–262. doi:10.1016/j.addr.2007.03.015.

75. Z. Wang, S.M. Mithieux, A.S. Weiss. Fabrication techniques for vascular and vascularized tissue engineering. *Adv. Healthc. Mater.* 8 (2019) 1–26. doi:10.1002/adhm.201900742.

76. J. Fu, M. Wang, I. De Vlaminck, Y. Wang. Thick PCL fibers improving host remodeling of PGS-PCL composite grafts implanted in rat common carotid arteries. *Small.* 16 (2020) 2004133. doi:10.1002/smll.202004133.

77. C.E.T. Stowell, X. Li, M.H. Matsunaga, C.B. Cockreham, K.M. Kelly, J. Cheetham, E. Tzeng, Y. Wang. Resorbable vascular grafts show rapid cellularization and degradation in the ovine carotid. *J. Tissue Eng. Regen. Med.* 14 (2020) 1673–1684. doi:10.1002/term.3128.

78. J.C. Zbinden, K.M. Blum, A.G. Berman, A.B. Ramachandra, J.M. Szafron, K.E. Kerr, J.L. Anderson, G.S. Sangha, C.C. Earl, N.R. Nigh, G.J.M. Mirhaidari, J.W. Reinhardt, Y.C. Chang, T. Yi, R. Smalley, P.D. Gabriele, J.J. Harris, J.D. Humphrey, C.J. Goergen, C.K. Breuer. Effects of braiding parameters on tissue engineered vascular graft development. *Adv. Healthc. Mater.* 2001093 (2020) 1–12. doi:10.1002/adhm.202001093.

79. A. Ranjbarzadeh-Dibazar, J. Barzin, P. Shokrollahi. Microstructure crystalline domains disorder critically controls formation of nano-porous/long fibrillar morphology of ePTFE membranes. *Polymer (Guildf)* 121 (2017) 75–87. doi:10.1016/j.polymer.2017.06.003.

80. M. Tozzi, M. Franchin, G. Ietto, G. Soldini, G. Carcano, P. Castelli, G. Piffaretti. Initial experience with the Gore® Acuseal graft for prosthetic vascular access. *J. Vasc. Access.* 15 (2014) 385–390. doi:10.5301/jva.5000276.

81. J. Li, Y. Long, F. Yang, H. Wei, Z. Zhang, Y. Wang, J. Wang, C. Li, C. Carlos, Y. Dong, Y. Wu, W. Cai, X. Wang. Multifunctional artificial artery from direct 3D printing with built-in ferroelectricity and tissue-matching modulus for real-time sensing and occlusion monitoring. *Adv. Funct. Mater.* 30 (2020). doi:10.1002/adfm.202002868.

82. D.J. Lyman, W.M. Muir, I.J. Lee. The effect of chemical structure and surface properties of polymers on the coagulation of blood. I. Surface free energy effects. *Trans. Am. Soc. Artif. Intern. Organs.* 11 (1965) 301–306. doi:10.1097/00002480-196504000-00056.

83. S. Srinivasan, P.N. Sawyer. Role of surface charge of the blood vessel wall, blood cells, and prosthetic materials in intravascular thrombosis. *J. Colloid Interface Sci.* 32 (1970) 456–463. doi:10.1016/0021-9797(70)90131-1.

84. A. Takahara., J. Ichi Tashita, T. Kajiyama, M. Takayanagi, W.J. MacKnight. Microphase separated structure, surface composition and blood compatibility of segmented poly(urethaneureas) with various soft segment components. *Polymer (Guildf).* 26 (1985) 987–996. doi:10.1016/0032-3861(85)90218-6.

85. S.P. Hoerstrup, I. Cummings, M. Lachat, F.J. Schoen, R. Jenni, S. Leschka, S. Neuenschwander, D. Schmidt, A. Mol, C. Günter, M. Gössi, M. Genoni, G. Zund. Functional growth in tissue-engineered living, vascular grafts: Follow-up at 100 weeks in a large animal model. *Circulation.* 114 (2006) 159–166. doi:10.1161/CIRCULATIONAHA.105.001172.

86. B. Nasiri, S. Row, R.J. Smith, D.D. Swartz, S.T. Andreadis. Cell-free vascular grafts that grow with the host. *Adv. Funct. Mater.* 30 (2020) 1–11. doi:10.1002/adfm.202005769.

87. J. DelBianco, S. Steerman, D. Dexter, S. Ahanchi, G. Stokes, S. Ongstad, O. Powell, N. Parikh, J. Panneton. Early-access upper extremity grafts offer no benefit over standard grafts in hemodialysis access. *J. Vasc. Surg.* 65 (2017) e6. doi:10.1016/j.jvs.2016.12.037.

88. S.P. Schmidt, T.J. Hunter, M. Hirko, T.A. Belden, M. Michelle Evancho, W. V. Sharp, D.L. Donovan. Small-diameter vascular prostheses: Two designs of PTFE and endothelial cell-seeded and nonseeded Dacron. *J. Vasc. Surg.* 2 (1985) 292–297. doi:10.1016/0741-5214(85)90068-0.

89. R.I. Mehta, A.K. Mukherjee, T.D. Patterson, M.C. Fishbein. Pathology of explanted polytetrafluoroethylene vascular grafts. *Cardiovasc. Pathol.* 20 (2011) 213–221. doi:10.1016/j.carpath.2010.06.005.

90. S. de Valence, J.C. Tille, D. Mugnai, W. Mrowczynski, R. Gurny, M. Möller, B.H. Walpoth. Long term performance of polycaprolactone vascular grafts in a rat abdominal aorta replacement model. *Biomaterials.* 33 (2012) 38–47. doi:10.1016/j.biomaterials.2011.09.024.

91. C. Wang, L. Cen, S. Yin, Q. Liu, W. Liu, Y. Cao, L. Cui. A small diameter elastic blood vessel wall prepared under pulsatile conditions from polyglycolic acid mesh and smooth muscle cells differentiated from adipose-derived stem cells. *Biomaterials.* 31 (2010) 621–630. doi:10.1016/j.biomaterials.2009.09.086.

92. Yang Hongjun, H. Xu. W. Xu, W. Wang, O.Y. Chenxi. Preparation of small-diameter artificial blood vessel with a biomimic structure. In: *3rd Natl. Conf. Vasc. Surg. Tissue Engineering*, Wuhan, China, 2008, issued online 2010:23–27.

93. Z. Wang, C. Liu, Y. Xiao, X. Gu, Y. Xu, N. Dong, S. Zhang, Q. Qin, J. Wang. Remodeling of a cell-free vascular graft with nanolamellar intima into a neovessel. *ACS Nano.* 13 (2019) 10576–10586. doi:10.1021/acsnano.9b04704.

94. H. Yamanaka, T. Yamaoka, A. Mahara, N. Morimoto, S. Suzuki. Tissue-engineered submillimeter-diameter vascular grafts for free flap survival in rat model. *Biomaterials.* 179 (2018) 156–163. doi:10.1016/j.biomaterials.2018.06.022.

95. L. Xu, M. Varkey, A. Jorgensen, J. Ju, Q. Jin, J.H. Park, Y. Fu, G. Zhang, D. Ke, W. Zhao, R. Hou, A. Atala. Bioprinting small diameter blood vessel constructs with an endothelial and smooth muscle cell bilayer in a single step. *Biofabrication.* 12 (2020). doi:10.1088/1758-5090/aba2b6.

96. K. Yamamoto, Y. Nogimori, H. Imamura, J. Ando. Shear stress activates mitochondrial oxidative phosphorylation by reducing plasma membrane cholesterol in vascular endothelial cells. *Proc. Natl. Acad. Sci.* 117 (2020) 33660–33667. doi:10.1073/pnas.2014029117.

97. L.E. Niklason, J.H. Lawson. Bioengineered human blood vessels. *Science.* 370 (2020) eaaw8682. doi:10.1126/science.aaw8682.

98. B. Wiatrak, Z. Rybak. History, present and future of biomaterials used for artificial heart valves. *Polim. Med.* 43(3) (2014) 183–189. PMID:24377185.

99. B.O. D.J. Wheatley, G.M. Bernacca. Cardiac surgery: Biomaterials. in: *Encyclopedia of Materials: Science and Technology*, K.H. Jürgen Buschow, R.W. Cahn, M.C. Flemings, B. Ilschner, E.J. Kramer, S. Mahajan, P. Veyssière, Elsevier, Oxford, UK, 2001: 999–1003.

100. R. Major, M. Gonsior, M. Sanak, M. Kot, R. Kustosz, J.M. Lackner. Surface modification of metallic materials designed for a new generation of artificial heart valves. *Int. J. Artif. Organs.* 41 (2018) 854–866. doi:10.1177/0391398818794064.

101. D.L. Bark, A. Yousefi, M. Forleo, A. Vaesken, F. Heim, L.P. Dasi. Reynolds shear stress for textile prosthetic heart valves in relation to fabric design. *J. Mech. Behav. Biomed. Mater.* 60 (2016) 280–287. doi:10.1016/j.jmbbm.2016.01.016.

102. A. Vaesken, F. Heim, N. Chakfe. Fiber heart valve prosthesis: Influence of the fabric construction parameters on the valve fatigue performances. *J. Mech. Behav. Biomed. Mater.* 40 (2014) 69–74. doi:10.1016/j.jmbbm.2014.08.015.

103. F. Heim, B. Durand, N. Chakfe. Textile heartvalve prosthesis: Manufacturing process and prototype performances. *Text. Res. J.* 12 (2008) 1124–1131. doi:10.1177/0040517508092007.

104. F. Piatti, F. Sturla, G. Marom, J. Sheriff, T.E. Claiborne, M.J. Slepian, A. Redaelli, D. Bluestein. Hemodynamic and thrombogenic analysis of a trileaflet polymeric valve using a fluid-structure interaction approach. *J. Biomech.* 48 (2015) 3650–3658. doi:10.1016/j.jbiomech.2015.08.009.

105. H. Tashiro, M.B. Popović, I. Dobrev, Y. Terasawa. Artificial organs, tissues, and support systems, in: *Biomechatronics*, mARKO B. POPOVIC (Ed.), Elsevier, 2019: pp. 175–199. doi:10.1016/B978-0-12-812939-5.00007-0.

106. M.F. O'Brien, D.C. McGiffin, E.G. Stafford, M.A.H. Gardner, P.F. Pohlner, G.J. McLachlan, K. Gall, S. Smith, E. Murphy. Allograft aortic valve replacement: Long-term comparative clinical analysis of the viable cryopreserved and antibiotic 4°C stored valves. *J. Card. Surg.* 6 (1991) 534–543. doi:10.1111/jocs.1991.6.4s.534.

107. P. Palka, S. Harrocks, A. Lange, D.J. Burstow, M.F. O'Brien. Primary aortic valve replacement with cryopreserved aortic allograft: An echocardiographic follow-up study of 570 patients. *Circulation.* 105 (2002) 61–66. doi:10.1161/hc0102.101357.

108. J.C. Witten, E. Durbak, P.L. Houghtaling, S. Unai, E.E. Roselli, F.G. Bakaeen, D.R. Johnston, L.G. Svensson, W. Jaber, E.H. Blackstone, G.B. Pettersson. Performance and durability of cryopreserved allograft aortic valve replacements. *Ann. Thorac. Surg.* (2020). doi:10.1016/j.athoracsur.2020.07.033. In Press Journal Pre-Proof.

109. F. Nappi, A. Nenna, T. Petitti, C. Spadaccio, I. Gambardella, M. Lusini, M. Chello, C. Acar. Long-term outcome of cryopreserved allograft for aortic valve replacement. *J. Thorac. Cardiovasc. Surg.* 156 (2018) 1357–1365. doi:10.1016/j.jtcvs.2018.04.040.

110. M.B. Forman, J.B. Atkinson, J.A. Wolfe, R.A. Hopkins. Non-bacterial thrombotic endocarditis in an adult 14 months after cryopreserved aortic allograft valve implantation. *J. Heart Valve Dis.* 16 (2007) 410–416. PMID: 17702367.

111. J.R. Doty, J.D. Salazar, J.R. Liddicoat, J.H. Flores, D.B. Doty, R.S. Mitchell, V.A. Starnes, F. Khouqeer. Aortic valve replacement with cryopreserved aortic allograft: Ten-year experience. *J. Thorac. Cardiovasc. Surg.* 115 (1998) 371–380. doi:10.1016/S0022-5223(98)70281-8.

112. M. Ruzmetov, J.J. Shah, D.M. Geiss, R.S. Fortuna. Decellularized versus standard cryopreserved valve allografts for right ventricular outflow tract reconstruction: A single-institution comparison. *J. Thorac. Cardiovasc. Surg.* 143 (2012) 543–549. doi:10.1016/j.jtcvs.2011.12.032.

113. K. Bando. A proposal for prospective late outcome analysis of decellularized aortic valves. *J. Thorac. Cardiovasc. Surg.* 152 (2016) 1202–1203. doi:10.1016/j.jtcvs.2016.04.087.

114. M.R.K. Helder, N.T. Kouchoukos, K. Zehr, J.A. Dearani, J.J. Maleszewski, C. Leduc, C.N. Heins, H. V. Schaff. Late durability of decellularized allografts for aortic valve replacement: A word of caution. *J. Thorac. Cardiovasc. Surg.* 152 (2016) 1197–1199. doi:10.1016/j.jtcvs.2016.03.050.

115. M. Vrandecic, B. Gontijo, F. Fantini, C. Acar. Homograft replacement of the mitral valve. *J. Thorac. Cardiovasc. Surg.* 112 (1996) 1678–1679. doi:10.1016/S0022-5223(96)70032-6.

116. R.A. Hopkins, A. Reyes, D.A. Imperato, G.A. Carpenter, J.L. Myers, K.A. Murphy. Ventricular outflow tract reconstructions with cryopreserved cardiac valve homografts: A single surgeon's 10-year experience. *Ann. Surg.* 223 (1996) 544–553. doi:10.1097/00000658-199605000-00010.

117. W. Flameng, G. De Visscher, L. Mesure, H. Hermans, R. Jashari, B. Meuris. Coating with fibronectin and stromal cell-derived factor-1α of decellularized homografts used for right ventricular outflow tract reconstruction eliminates immune response-related degeneration. *J. Thorac. Cardiovasc. Surg.* 147 (2014) 1398–1404. doi:10.1016/j.jtcvs.2013.06.022.

118. M.Y. Emmert, B. Weber, L. Behr, T. Frauenfelder, C.E. Brokopp, J. Grnenfelder, V. Falk, S.P. Hoerstrup. Transapical aortic implantation of autologous marrow stromal cell-based tissue-engineered heart valves: First experiences in the systemic circulation. *JACC Cardiovasc. Interv.* 4 (2011) 822–823. doi:10.1016/j.jcin.2011.02.020.

119. C. Lueders, B. Jastram, R. Hetzer, H. Schwandt. Rapid manufacturing techniques for the tissue engineering of human heart valves. *Eur. J. Cardio-Thoracic Surg.* 46 (2014) 593–601. doi:10.1093/ejcts/ezt510.

120. J.M. Reimer, Z.H. Syedain, B.H.T. Haynie, R.T. Tranquillo. Pediatric tubular pulmonary heart valve from decellularized engineered tissue tubes. *Biomaterials.* 62 (2015) 88–94. doi:10.1016/j.biomaterials.2015.05.009.

121. L.A. Hockaday, K.H. Kang, N.W. Colangelo, P.Y.C. Cheung, B. Duan, E. Malone, J. Wu, L.N. Girardi, L.J. Bonassar, H. Lipson, C.C. Chu, J.T. Butcher. Rapid 3D printing of anatomically accurate and mechanically heterogeneous aortic valve hydrogel scaffolds. *Biofabrication.* 4 (2012) 035005. doi:10.1088/1758-5082/4/3/035005.

122. R.A. Hopkins, A.A. Bert, S.L. Hilbert, R.W. Quinn, K.M. Brasky, W.B. Drake, G.K. Lofland. Bioengineered human and allogeneic pulmonary valve conduits chronically implanted orthotopically in baboons: Hemodynamic performance and immunologic consequences. *J. Thorac. Cardiovasc. Surg.* 145 (2013) 1098–1107. doi:10.1016/j.jtcvs.2012.06.024.

123. T.C. Flanagan, C. Cornelissen, S. Koch, B. Tschoeke, J.S. Sachweh, T. Schmitz-Rode, S. Jockenhoevel. The in vitro development of autologous fibrin-based tissue-engineered heart valves through optimised dynamic conditioning. *Biomaterials.* 28 (2007) 3388–3397. doi:10.1016/j.biomaterials.2007.04.012.

124. S. Sant, D. Iyer, A.K. Gaharwar, A. Patel, A. Khademhosseini. Effect of biodegradation and de novo matrix synthesis on the mechanical properties of valvular interstitial cell-seeded polyglycerol sebacate-polycaprolactone scaffolds. *Acta Biomater.* 9 (2013) 5963–5973. doi:10.1016/j.actbio.2012.11.014.

125. M. Weber, I. Gonzalez De Torre, R. Moreira, J. Frese, C. Oedekoven, M. Alonso, C.J. Rodriguez Cabello, S. Jockenhoevel, P. Mela. Multiple-step injection molding for fibrin-based tissue-engineered heart valves. *Tissue Eng. - Part C Methods.* 21 (2015) 832–840. doi:10.1089/ten.tec.2014.0396.

126. N. Masoumi, N. Annabi, A. Assmann, B.L. Larson, J. Hjortnaes, N. Alemdar, M. Kharaziha, K.B. Manning, J.E. Mayer, A. Khademhosseini. Tri-layered elastomeric scaffolds for engineering heart valve leaflets. *Biomaterials.* 35 (2014) 7774–7785. doi:10.1016/j.biomaterials.2014.04.039.

127. N. Masoumi, A. Jean, J.T. Zugates, K.L. Johnson, G.C. Engelmayr. Laser microfabricated poly(glycerol sebacate) scaffolds for heart valve tissue engineering. *J. Biomed. Mater. Res. - Part A* 101 (2013) 104–114. doi:10.1002/jbm.a.34305.

128. P.E. Dijkman, A. Driessen-Mol, L. Frese, S.P. Hoerstrup, F.P.T. Baaijens. Decellularized homologous tissue-engineered heart valves as off-the-shelf alternatives to xeno- and homografts. *Biomaterials.* 33 (2012) 4545–4554. doi:10.1016/j.biomaterials.2012.03.015.

129. K. MacIntyre, S. Capewell, S. Stewart, J.W.T. Chalmers, J. Boyd, A. Finlayson, A. Redpath, J.P. Pell, J.J.V. McMurray. Evidence of improving prognosis in heart failure: Trends in case fatality in 66 547 patients hospitalized between 1986 and 1995. *Circulation* 102 (2000) 1126–1131. doi:10.1161/01.CIR.102.10.1126.

130. S.N. Doost, L. Zhong, Y.S. Morsi. Ventricular assist devices: Current state and challenges. *J. Med. Devices, Trans. ASME.* 11 (2017) 040801. doi:10.1115/1.4037258.

131. G. Luraghi, W. Wu, H. De Castilla, J.F. Rodriguez Matas, G. Dubini, P. Dubuis, M. Grimmé, F. Migliavacca. Numerical approach to study the behavior of an artificial ventricle: Fluid–structure interaction followed by fluid dynamics with moving boundaries. *Artif. Organs.* 42 (2018) E315–E324. doi:10.1111/aor.13316.

132. B. Pelletier, S. Spiliopoulos, T. Finocchiaro, F. Graef, K. Kuipers, M. Laumen, D. Guersoy, U. Steinseifer, R. Koerfer, G. Tenderich. System overview of the fully implantable destination therapy--ReinHeart-total artificial heart. *Eur. J. Cardiothorac. Surg.* 40 (2015) 80–86. doi:10.1093/ejcts/ezu321.

133. J.A. Cook, K.B. Shah, M.A. Quader, R.H. Cooke, V. Kasirajan, K.K. Rao, M.C. Smallfield, I. Tchoukina, D.G. Tang. The total artificial heart. *J. Thorac. Dis.* 7 (2015) 2172–2180. doi:10.3978/j.issn.2072-1439.2015.10.70.

134. J.G. Copeland, R.G. Smith, F.A. Arabia, P.E. Nolan, G.K. Sethi, P.H. Tsau, D. McClellan, M.J. Slepian. Cardiac Replacement with a total artificial heart as a bridge to transplantation. *N. Engl. J. Med.* 351 (2004), 859–867. doi:10.1056/nejmoa040186.

135. G. Gerosa, S. Scuri, L. Iop, G. Torregrossa. Present and future perspectives on total artificial hearts. *Ann. Cardiothorac. Surg.* 3 (2014) 595–602. doi:10.3978/j.issn.2225-319X.2014.09.05.

136. S.D. Gregory, J. Zwischenberger, D.F. Wang, S. Liao, M. Slaughter. Chapter 18-Cannula design, in: *Mechanical Circulatory and Respiratory Support*, S.D. Gregory, M.C. Stevens, J.F. Fraser (Eds.), Academic Press, 2017: pp. 567–596. doi:10.1016/c2016-0-00501-6.

137. M.E. Stone, J. Hinchey. Mechanical assist devices for heart failure, in: *Kaplan's Essentials Cardiac Anesthesia*, 2nd ed., J.A. Kaplan (Ed.), Elsevier, 2018: pp. 51–583. doi:10.1016/B978-0-323-49798-5.00022-X.

138. A. Carpentier, C. Latrémouille, B. Cholley, D.M. Smadja, J.C. Roussel, E. Boissier, J.N. Trochu, J.P. Gueffet, M. Treillot, P. Bizouarn, D. Méléard, M.F. Boughenou, O. Ponzio, M. Grimmé, A. Capel, P. Jansen, A. Hagège, M. Desnos, J.N. Fabiani, D. Duveau. First clinical use of a bioprosthetic total artificial heart: Report of two cases. *Lancet.* 386 (2015) 1556–1563. doi:10.1016/S0140-6736(15)60511-6.

139. P. Jansen, W. van Oeveren, A. Capel, A. Carpentier. In vitro haemocompatibility of a novel bioprosthetic total artificial heart. *Eur. J. Cardio-Thoracic Surg.* 41 (2012) e166–e172. doi:10.1093/ejcts/ezs187.

140. U. Richez, H. De Castilla, C.L. Guerin, N. Gendron, G. Luraghi, M. Grimme, W. Wu, M. Taverna, P. Jansen, C. Latremouille, F. Migliavacca, G. Dubini, A. Capel, A. Carpentier, D.M. Smadja. Hemocompatibility and safety of the carmat total artifical heart hybrid membrane. *Heliyon.* 5 (2019) e02914. doi:10.1016/j.heliyon.2019.e02914.

141. D.M. Smadja, B. Saubaméa, S. Susen, M. Kindo, P. Bruneval, E. Van Belle, P. Jansen, J.C. Roussel, C. Latrémouille, A. Carpentier. Bioprosthetic total artificial heart induces a profile of acquired hemocompatibility with membranes recellularization. *J. Am. Coll. Cardiol.* 70 (2017) 404–406. doi:10.1016/j.jacc.2017.05.021.

142. D.M. Smadja, R. Chocron, E. Rossi, B. Poitier, Y. Pya, M. Bekbossynova, C. Peronino, J. Rancic, J.C. Roussel, M. Kindo, N. Gendron, L. Migliozzi, A. Capel, J.C. Perles, P. Gaussem, P. Ivak, P. Jansen, C. Girard, A. Carpentier, C. Latremouille, C. Guerin, I. Netuka. Autoregulation of pulsatile bioprosthetic total artificial heart is involved in endothelial homeostasis preservation. *Thromb. Haemost.* (2020) s-0040–1713751. doi:10.1055/s-0040-1713751.

143. M. Diedrich, S. Hildebrand, M.K. Lommel, T. Finocchiaro, E. Cuenca, H. De Ben, T. Schmitz-Rode, U. Steinseifer, S. Jansen. Experimental investigation of right-left flow balance concepts for a total artificial heart. *Artif. Organs.* (2020) 13830. doi:10.1111/aor.13830.

144. J.K. Kirklin, F.D. Pagani, R.L. Kormos, L.W. Stevenson, E.D. Blume, S.L. Myers, M.A. Miller, J.T. Baldwin, J.B. Young, D.C. Naftel. Eighth annual INTERMACS report: Special focus on framing the impact of adverse events. *J. Hear. Lung Transplant.* (2017) S105324981731896X. doi:10.1016/j.healun.2017.07.005.

145. L.E. Rodriguez, E.E. Suarez, M. Loebe, B.A. Bruckner. Ventricular assist devices (VAD) therapy: New technology, new hope? *Methodist Debakey Cardiovasc. J.* 9 (2013) 32–37. doi:10.14797/mdcj-9-1-32.

146. J. Wohlschlaeger, K.J. Schmitz, C. Schmid, K.W. Schmid, P. Keul, A. Takeda, S. Weis, B. Levkau, H.A. Baba. Reverse remodeling following insertion of left ventricular assist devices (LVAD): A review of the morphological and molecular changes. *Cardiovasc. Res.* 68 (2005) 376–386. doi:10.1016/j.cardiores.2005.06.030.

147. S.R. Wilson, M.M. Givertz, G.C. Stewart, G.H. Mudge. Ventricular assist devices. The challenges of outpatient management. *J. Am. Coll. Cardiol.* 54 (2009) 1647–1659. doi:10.1016/j.jacc.2009.06.035.

148. B.C. Blaxall, B.M. Tschannen-Moran, C.A. Milano, W.J. Koch. Differential gene expression and genomic patient stratification following Left Ventricular Assist Device support. *J. Am. Coll. Cardiol.* 41 (2003) 1096–1106. doi:10.1016/S0735-1097(03)00043-3.

149. N. Morici, M. Varrenti, D. Brunelli, E. Perna, M. Cipriani, E. Ammirati, M. Frigerio, M. Cattaneo, F. Oliva. Antithrombotic therapy in ventricular assist device (VAD) management: From ancient beliefs to updated evidence. A narrative review. *IJC Hear. Vasc.* 20 (2018) 20–26. doi:10.1016/j.ijcha.2018.06.005.

150. C. Murphy, H. Zafar, F. Sharif. An updated review of cardiac devices in heart failure. *Ir. J. Med. Sci.* 186 (2017) 909–919. doi:10.1007/s11845-017-1597-9.

151. J. Garbade, H.B. Bittner, M.J. Barten, F.W. Mohr. Current trends in implantable left ventricular assist devices. *Cardiol. Res. Pract.* 17 (2011) 290561. doi:10.4061/2011/290561.

152. S. Agarwal, K.M. High. Newer-generation ventricular assist devices. *Best Pract. Res. Clin. Anaesthesiol.* 26 (2012) 117–130. doi:10.1016/j.bpa.2012.01.003.

153. T. Wu, A.W. Khir, M. Kütting, X. Du, H. Lin, Y. Zhu, P.L. Hsu, A review of implantable pulsatile blood pumps: Engineering perspectives. *Int. J. Artif. Organs.* (2020) 039139882090247. doi:10.1177/0391398820902470.

2 Vascular Patches: Past and Future, Problems, and Solutions

Hualong Bai
First Affiliated Hospital of Zhengzhou University
Key Vascular Physiology and Applied Research
Laboratory of Zhengzhou City

Yanhua Xu
The First Affiliated Hospital of Zhengzhou University

Hao He and Xin Li
Central South University

Chang Shu
Central South University
Chinese Academy of Medical Sciences
and Peking Union Medical College

Jingan Li
Zhengzhou University

Quancheng Kan
The First Affiliated Hospital of Zhengzhou University
Zhengzhou University

Alan Dardik
Yale School of Medicine

CONTENTS

DOI: 10.1201/9781003161981-2

2.1 ANIMAL MODEL

To study neointimal hyperplasia after patch implantation in both arteries and veins, Bai et al. developed a rat model of patch angioplasty that can be used in either a vein (inferior vena cava, (IVC) venoplasty) or an artery (abdominal aorta, arterioplasty); the diameter of the vessels can range widely from less than 1 mm to larger than 2 mm [1]. The technical details are described briefly. Microsurgical procedures are performed aseptically using a dissecting microscope. The infrarenal aorta or IVC is exposed below the level of the renal arteries, and then clamped proximally and distally. A longitudinal 3-mm arteriotomy or venotomy is made on the anterior wall of the aorta or IVC. The arteriotomy or venotomy is closed with a patch using continuous 10-0 nylon sutures, and the vessel clamps are removed. The abdomen is closed, and the rat is allowed to recover; no immunosuppressive agents or heparin are administered at any time.

Because patch angioplasty is widely used in human patients after arteriotomies in medium-diameter (4–8 mm) vessels, such as after carotid artery endarterectomy (Figure 2.1a and b), our group also applied the patch angioplasty model to the rat carotid artery (Figure 2.1c). Although this model variation uses an arteriotomy on the common carotid artery that does not include the internal carotid artery, the hemodynamics in this vessel may still be a reasonable model of the hemodynamics within the carotid artery of human patients. Elastin staining shows the patch incorporated to the native carotid artery and a neointima formed on day 14 (Figure 2.2).

Compared to other models, the rat aortic and IVC patch angioplasty models have some merits: first, this model does not need to replace a segment of aorta or IVC, and thus is technically easier to perform compared to interposition grafts

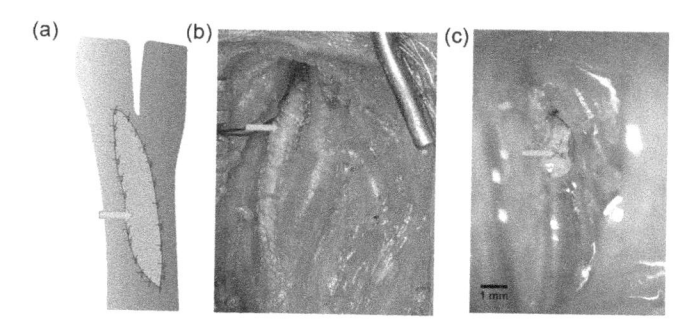

FIGURE 2.1 Photographs showing vascular patches in human and rat carotid arteries. (a) Illustration showing placement of a patch in the human carotid bifurcation (Adobe illustrator CS). (b) Intraoperative photograph showing patch angioplasty in a human carotid artery after carotid artery endarterectomy. (c) Rat carotid artery patch arterioplasty; scale bar, 1 mm. Arrows show the patches.

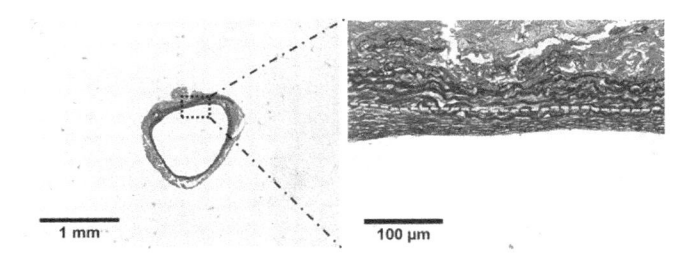

FIGURE 2.2 Verhoeff's Van Gieson staining of a rat carotid artery patch angioplasty; the patch is decellularized rat carotid artery. Scale bar, 1 mm or 100 μm; note the ratio of the width of patch to the diameter of the vessel is approximately 3. Dashed line demarcating the carotid artery patch and neointima.

models. Additionally, reduced surgical time can decrease the rate of lower limb ischemic complications. Second, compared to some other models, this model has a rapid thick neointimal formation [1,2]. Neointimal cells are found on the patch as early as day 3, and neointima is formed on day 7. Because different patch materials can influence the thickness of the neointima, different thickness of neointima is found after day 7 [3–6].

2.2 PATCH MATERIALS

Dacron and expanded polytetrafluoroethylene (ePTFE) have been used therapeutically in human patients for more than half a century, and these materials are still widely used in vascular procedures today. Whinfield and Dickinson developed the polyester fabric Dacron in 1941, and it was first used in humans as an aortic graft by Dr DeBakey in 1953 [7]. Dacron grafts can be knitted or woven; knitted grafts have better compliance but they also have larger pores that require preclotting to prevent bleeding after implantation. At present, knitted Dacron grafts are coated with albumin to prevent leakage. Dacron is estimated to last more than 30 years after implantation, but these grafts have a high risk of dilation [8]. Dacron is commonly used as a large-diameter graft in aortic and lower-extremity bypass surgery [9], and can be used in the rat patch model (Figure 2.3a).

Matsumoto and colleagues introduced ePTFE in 1973, and Gore expanded the use of this material[10]; ePTFE was found to be suitable for vascular replacement [11]. ePTFE grafts are compliant, easy to suture, and do not need to be preclotted compared to knitted Dacron grafts. ePTFE does show some suture line bleeding, and it can also induce a foreign body reaction, have a tendency toward thrombosis, and can have an increased risk of infection [9]. ePTFE can be used in the rat patch model and show increased time to hemostasis after aortic arterioplasty (Figure 2.3b).

Compared to synthetic vascular materials, decellularized tissues have a similar extracellular matrix and similar structural architecture as native vessels, but with reduced immunogenicity [5,12,13]. The pericardium is commonly used as a patch after arteriotomy during cardiovascular surgery. Compared to Dacron and ePTFE, pericardial patches have several advantages, including superior biocompatibility, easy handling, and less suture line bleeding. Li et al. showed a similar healing process of

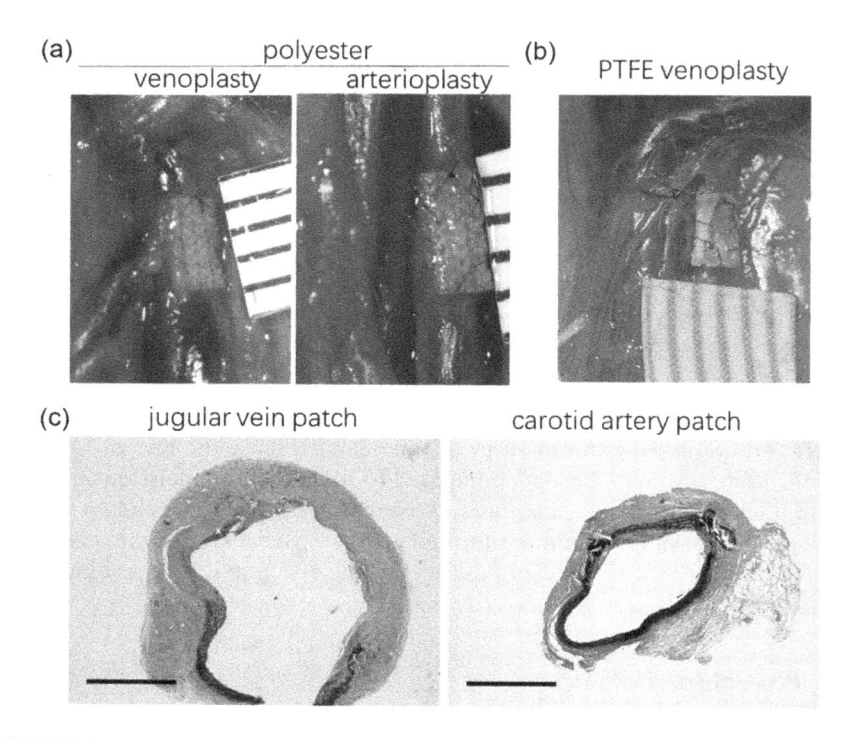

(a) polyester
venoplasty   arterioplasty

(b) PTFE venoplasty

(c) jugular vein patch   carotid artery patch

FIGURE 2.3 Patch angioplasty with different materials. (a) Polyester patch venoplasty and arterioplasty ruler marks 1 mm. (b) Rat IVC ePTFE patch venoplasty, ruler marks 1 mm. (c) Verhoeff's Van Gieson staining showing the rat autologous jugular vein and carotid artery patch angioplasty at day 14; scale bar, 1 mm.

bovine and porcine pericardial patch using the rat aortic arterioplasty model [14]. Bai et al. showed some similarities and differences in healing after arterioplasty and venoplasty in rats using pericardial patches [2].

Dacron, ePTFE, and pericardial patches show some compliance mismatch with native vessels [15–17]. To determine if decellularized vessels can minimize the compliance mismatch when used as patches, we examined decellularized human saphenous vein patches (2 mm × 3 mm) implanted to the rat aorta and IVC [5]. The healing process is similar to that of pericardial patches, despite the human saphenous vein patch being much thicker compared to the rat aorta. We similarly tested decellularized rat thoracic aorta as a patch [6]; the rat thoracic aorta and abdominal aorta have a similar thickness (150 ± 3 vs. $156 \pm 4\,\mu m$; $p = 0.2914$; t-test) and can be successfully used as a patch material [6].

In addition to the commonly used prosthetic and biological vascular materials, autologous materials are also widely used in vascular surgeries. Because autologous vascular grafts have the lowest immunoreaction and the best patency rate of all vascular grafts, we examined autologous carotid artery and jugular vein patches in the rat arterioplasty and venoplasty models; both grafts showed a similar healing process, although the jugular vein dilated as early as day 14 after implantation into the rat aorta, consistent with its high compliance (Figure 2.3c) [3].

Other materials have been tested in the patch angioplasty model. One group showed that sugarcane biopolymer membrane can be used as a patch in femoral vein angioplasty in dogs; they showed there were no cases of infection, rupture, pseudoaneurysm formation, or thrombosis. There was a chronic inflammatory reaction with lymphocytes, neutrophils, and fibrosis in the outer surface of the patches. The authors concluded that sugarcane biopolymer membrane is easily synthesized with a low cost of production and can be successfully used in femoral vein patch angioplasty [18]. However, whether this material is permanent or is resorbable in vivo is not clear and thus longer-term studies are needed.

Another group examined the peritoneum-fascia patch and found similar clot-resistant properties as polyester with superior mechanical strength compared with the pericardial patch [19]. Although this group used a peritoneum patch to repair an infected aortic stump successfully and reported this case [20], no further research was reported. However, this shows the promising application of autologous modified tissue to be used as a vascular substitute.

Glutaraldehyde fixation cross-links proteins in xenogeneic tissues, such as bovine pericardium, minimizing immune rejection and sterilizing the tissue; however, fixation may also compromise the regenerative potential of the resultant biomaterial [21,22]. One group compared SDS decellularization and glutaraldehyde fixation and showed the importance of residual antigenicity and extracellular matrix architecture preservation in modulating recipient immune and regenerative responses toward xenogeneic biomaterials [23].

Small intestinal submucosa (SIS) is a cell-free collagen matrix derived from porcine small intestine that has been used in wound healing [24], as well as a vascular patch. SIS (CorMatrix) showed no short-term adverse events when used as an aortic interposition tube graft, but there was a high rate of neointimal hyperplasia with significant stenosis in low-pressure, small-diameter conduits [25]. Clinical results using SIS have not been consistent. One group found complete incorporation and no false aneurysm formation when compared with PTFE [26]. Jacobsen et al. reported porcine SIS patches may be an appropriate tissue choice for Norwood procedures [27]. However, McCready et al. reported 7 of 76 patients developed pseudoaneurysms in less than 10 weeks [28]. Madden et al. reported using a small intestine submucosa patch after carotid artery endarterectomy and suggested further studies [29]. These different reports show the complex development of new vascular materials and suggest that well-performed, adequately powered, multi-centered clinical trials are needed.

2.3 PATCH HEALING AFTER IMPLANTATION

After implantation of prosthetics, rapid reendothelialization is critical to prevent thrombus formation. Sauvage et al. compared reendothelialization in humans, dogs, pigs, calves, and baboons, and reported that humans and dogs are limited in their ability to develop pannus ingrowth from the anastomoses, whereas pigs, calves, and baboons heal very rapidly. Healing of porous prostheses is assisted by a filamentous external surface, particularly in humans and dogs [30]. This seminal research showed the importance of neointimal reendothelialization after prosthetic implantation in vascular surgeries.

Both patch arterioplasty and venoplasty share a similar healing process; patches in the rat model show rapid reendothelialization as early as day 7, with CD34 and VEGFR2 dual-positive cells, that is, endothelial progenitor cells (EPC), located on the luminal side of the neointima [4]. EPC also display markers such as vWF and CD31 [2,31]. Below the EPC are other cell types, including SMCs, macrophages, leukocytes, mesenchymal cells, lymphocytes, CD90-positive cells, nestin-positive cells, and other cells that all potentially contribute to the neointimal formation, similar to the human process [32]. Among these cells, SMCs and macrophages play an important role in neointimal hyperplasia; we found that one-third of the SMCs [31] and half of the macrophages were PCNA- or Ki67-positive (Figure 2.4). In addition, there were more PCNA- and CD68-positive cells in the venous patches compared to arterial patches. These data suggest that both SMC and macrophages were proliferating and could be targets of anti-proliferation treatment.

Although statin drugs are commonly used for vascular disease, whether statins influence neointimal formation or arterial endothelial cell infiltration after patch angioplasty needs to be determined. In a very provocative study, Li et al. showed that atorvastatin regulates neointimal growth after pericardial patch angioplasty. This process was associated with infiltration of Ephrin-B2-positive cells, diminished ADAM10 expression, and increased Ephrin-B2 and miR-140 expression. These data show that atorvastatin can play a role in potentially enhancing endothelial repair [33]. Atorvastatin showed a higher number of infiltrating cells and a thicker patch neointima compared with control animals. These data suggest a clinical correlation, that is, patients on lower doses of atorvastatin may have thinner patch neointima, whereas higher doses of atorvastatin may be associated with increased numbers of Ephrin-B2 positive cells and thus may show more arterial-like healing.

Mature vascular endothelial cells have a vascular identity of arteries, veins, or lymphatics, and similarly, neointimal endothelial cells also acquire vascular

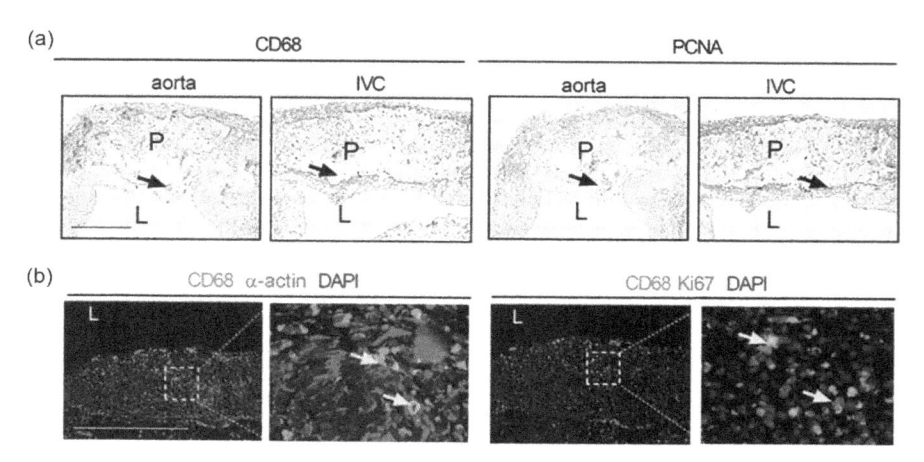

FIGURE 2.4 Proliferation and macrophage infiltration in the patch neointima on day 7. (a) Immunohistochemistry showing CD68- and PCNA-positive cells in the neointima in the arterioplasty and venoplasty on day 7. (b) Immunofluorescence showing double staining of CD68 and α-actin, CD68 and Ki67, and DAPI in the neointima. Scale bar, 100 μm.

identity depending upon their environment [34]. The Eph-ephrin family of signaling molecules was originally recognized as markers of embryonic vessel identity. Eph receptors and their membrane-associated ligands, ephrins, are now known to have a range of vital functions in vascular physiology. Interactions of Ephs with ephrins at cell-to-cell interfaces promote a variety of cellular responses such as repulsion, adhesion, attraction, and migration, and frequently occur during organ development, including vessel formation [35].

Endothelial cells express Ephrin-B2 and notch-4 but not Eph-B4 and COUP-TFII in arterial neointima, whereas endothelial cells express Eph-B4 and COUP-TFII but not Ephrin-B2 and notch-4 in venous neointima [2,14]. Previously, we showed that venous identity is lost during vein graft adaptation to the arterial environment but arterial markers were not strongly induced in the venous wall [36]. In the rat patch angioplasty model, we showed that autologous tissue patches heal by the acquisition of the vascular identity determined by the environment into which they are implanted, suggesting some plasticity of adult vascular identity [3]. In the polyester patch angioplasty model, cells in the arterial patch were Ephrin-B2- and notch-4-positive, while those in the venous patch were Eph-B4- and COUP-TFII-positive. Venous patches treated with an arteriovenous fistula (AVF) had decreased neointimal thickness. Neointimal endothelial cells expressed Ephrin-B2 and notch-4 in addition to Eph-B4 and COUP-TFII. These data suggest that synthetic patches heal by the acquisition of identity of their environment, similar to tissue patches [4]. These data suggest that endothelial cell identity plays an important role in the patch healing process. Because identity can regulate neointimal hyperplasia, patches coated with arterial or venous endothelial cells may contribute to patch healing or reendothelialization.

2.4 TISSUE-ENGINEERED VASCULAR PATCHES

Using advanced techniques of tissue engineering, vascular conduits can be modified or engineered. Tissue-engineered vascular grafts have been showing very promising results in both basic studies as well as clinical trials [12,32,37,38]. We tested several different tissue-engineered patches in the rat patch angioplasty model. We used several different patch materials [5,6] and coated the patches with drugs using hyaluronic acid (HA) solution. HA is a component of the extracellular matrix secreted from both vascular endothelial cells and vascular SMCs that plays crucial roles in cardiovascular physiology [37]. HA can inhibit SMC proliferation and synthetic phenotype change, inhibit platelet activation and aggregation, promote endothelial monolayer repair and functionalization, and prevent inflammation and atherosclerosis [39]. HA can also enhance endothelial cell adhesion, proliferation, migration, and functional factor release [39]. It is clinically used in humans to treat knee osteoarthritis [40].

Another common tool to deliver drugs locally is using nanotechnology. Nanoparticles (NP) can be made from many materials and can be used to encapsulate many types of therapeutic agents. Poly(lactic-co-glycolic acid) (PLGA) is approved for use in patients and is one of the most effective biodegradable polymeric NP in current use. We previously coated pericardial patches with PLGA NPs that released rapamycin and showed decreased neointimal thickness in the rat venoplasty model [31].

Because acute platelet accumulation can induce graft failure, and heparin is widely used clinically, we coated saphenous vein patches with heparin and showed decreased neointima in both the arterioplasty (454 ± 31 μm vs. 157 ± 31 μm) and venoplasty ($1{,}110 \pm 177$ μm vs. 227 ± 55 μm) models [5]. Heparin-coated grafts and stents are widely used in patients and show good clinical outcomes [41,42], suggesting the use of heparin as a coating for patches, especially in patients prone to thrombosis.

The feasibility of composite nanomaterial-tissue patches for vascular and cardiac reconstruction was recently assessed. Porcine vascular tissue was decellularized and conjugated with gold NPs and implanted in bilateral pig carotid arteries. The patches showed regenerating endothelial cell growth and normal healing responses, with excellent integration at 9 weeks. Histology showed cellular ingrowth without immune reactions [43]. This data show the safety of NPs and support their future application in patches. Because there are a large number of neointimal SMC after venoplasty, we conjugated PLGA NP rapamycin to the pericardial patches and implanted them into the IVC. After venoplasty, there were significantly fewer proliferating SMCs and much thinner neointima compared to the control group [31]. These data confirm the utility of NP conjugated to patches.

Because macrophages and leukocytes are also found within the neointima [6,31], we determined if manipulation of macrophages and lymphocytes would be another strategy to regulate neointimal formation. As PD-1 is expressed on macrophages and lymphocytes, we conjugated PD-1 to the surface of decellularized rat thoracic artery patches and implanted them into the rat aorta and IVC. In these composite patches, there was a much thinner neointima in the PD-1 treatment groups compared to control groups, with significantly fewer PD-1 ($p = 0.0148$), CD3 ($p = 0.0072$), CD68 ($p = 0.0001$), CD45 ($p = 0.001$), and PCNA ($p < 0.0001$)-positive cells, as well as PCNA/α-actin dual-positive cells ($p = 0.0005$) in the treated groups [6]. These data show the potential for manipulation of macrophages and leukocytes to influence the neointimal thickness.

Vascular surgeons create distal AVF in human patients to increase blood flow and patency, both in arterial [44] and venous reconstruction [45]. Similar results were shown in animal models [46,47]. We examined whether neointimal thickness that forms on a patch can be decreased with the increased velocity of an AVF (Figure 2.5) [2,4]. There was decreased neointimal thickness and a larger luminal area in the patches that had a concomitant distal AVF, which was reversible with L-NAME (Figure 2.5). Immunofluorescence showed a decreased p-eNOS expression in the AVF group with L-NAME (Figure 2.5). Other studies have also confirmed the influence of eNOS on neointimal hyperplasia [48,49]. These data suggest that strategies to increase eNOS expression may be a new method to decrease neointimal hyperplasia on patches.

2.5 COMPLICATIONS OF PATCHES

In human patients, saphenous vein patches have been used extensively, but they can result in complications such as blowout and patch rupture, which has been reported to occur in 0.5%–4% of cases [50]. Carotid blowout syndrome is a rupture of the carotid patch and is mainly associated with radiation and resection of head and neck cancers

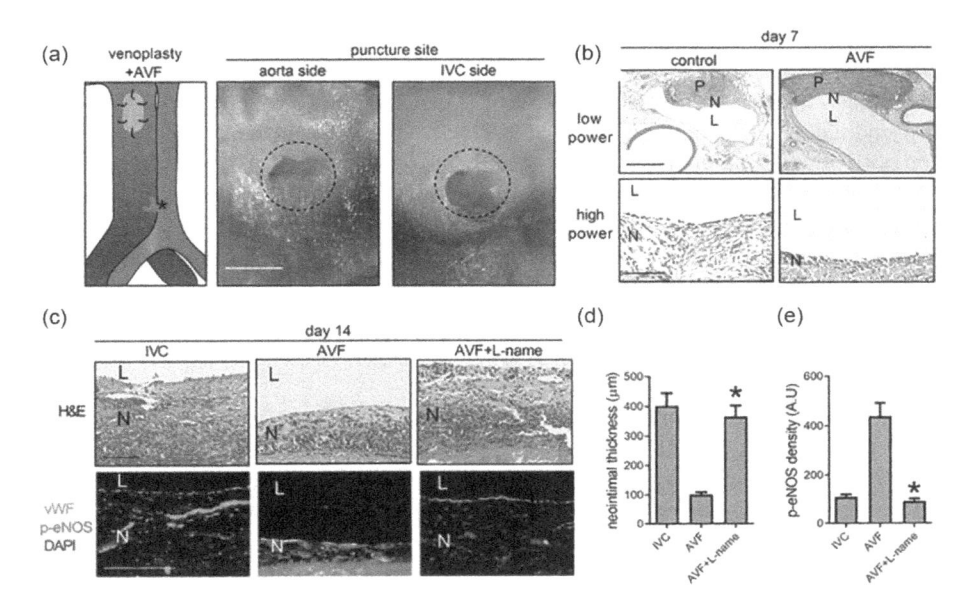

FIGURE 2.5 eNOS participates in flow-induced neointimal hyperplasia. (a) Diagram of rat venoplasty model with AVF flow; *, site of AVF creation. Side views of the IVC from the aorta and the IVC showing the fistula. Dotted circles show the fistula (day 7); scale bar, 0.5 mm. (b) H&E staining showing the venous patches with or without AVF (day 7); upper row, low power, scale bar, 1 mm; lower row, high power, scale bar, 100 μm; P, patch; N, neointima; L, lumen; n = 3–5. (c) Upper row, H&E staining showing venoplasty, AVF, and AVF with the supplement of L-NAME (day 14); low row, merge of vWF, p-eNOS and DAPI; P, patch; L, lumen; N, neointima; IVC, inferior vena cava; scale bar, 100 μm. n = 3–5. (d) Bar graph showing neointimal thickness; p = 0.0013, one-way ANOVA, *, p = 0.0031, vs. AVF; n = 3–5. (e) Bar graph showing p-eNOS density; p < 0.0001, one-way ANOVA, *, p < 0.0001, vs. AVF; n = 3–5; A.U, arbitrary units.

or direct tumor invasion of the carotid artery wall. Patch rupture is a life-threatening clinical situation [51–53]. Dr Archie suggested the use of the saphenous vein in the thigh but not the ankle to prevent blowout. He found that the use of veins with a distended diameter of ≥3.5 mm for patch reconstruction significantly reduced the probability of patch rupture [54]. In a recent systematic literature review, Dacron patches were associated with a 0.25%–0.5% rate of infection [55]; in another comprehensive review, 57 carotid pseudoaneurysms were identified, 40 of which were associated with carotid patches, of which four (10%) were infectious in etiology [56]. The etiology of pseudoaneurysm is very complex. Local factors include arterial wall degeneration, suture line disruption, prosthetic graft failure, infection or inflammation, technical errors, mechanical stress. Systemic factors include smoking, hyperlipidemia, hypertension, anticoagulation, systemic vasculitides, and generalized arterial weakness [50]. Surgical repair of pseudoaneurysms after carotid endarterectomy is frequently associated with high rates of morbidity and mortality [57].

Compared to veins, arteries are higher-pressure environments; accordingly, we noticed pseudoaneurysm formation in our patch model when patches were implanted into the aorta [57]. We noticed pseudoaneurysm formation in pericardial patches [57], polyester patches [4], decellularized human saphenous vein patches [5], and decellularized rat thoracic artery patches [6]. TGF-β1 plays a role in the progression of pseudoaneurysms and delivery of TGF-β1 via NP-stimulated smad2 phosphorylation both in vitro and in vivo and significantly decreased pseudoaneurysm formation. The decreased incidence of pseudoaneurysms in TGF-β1-treated patches may be a result of increased collagen synthesis or polarization of macrophages [57]. This data suggest that using TGF-β1-treated patches might decrease the chance of pseudoaneurysm formation in some patients at risk of poor healing.

2.6   FUTURE RESEARCH DIRECTIONS

Three-dimensional (3D) printing is a rapidly evolving technology in vascular surgery [58,59]. 3D-printed vascular patches using bio-ink (cells and biologic polymers) may be a promising technology to make patches in the future. Tissue-engineered vascular patches using advanced coating technologies are also a very promising technique. However, cost, biocompatibility, thrombogenicity, and durability remain important questions for the next generations of tissue-engineered vascular patches.

Although no vascular biomaterial currently has exactly similar characteristics to native vessels, advancement of biomaterial and engineering technologies are likely to enable new generations of vascular grafts, patches, and other implantables. These grafts may have rapid reendothelialization, less neointima hyperplasia, less foreign body reaction, similar compliance, and be easy to suture. Hopefully, these future developments will show improved long-term patency with good cost-effectiveness that will apply to all patients with vascular disease.

ACKNOWLEDGEMENTS

This study was funded by the National Natural Science Foundation of China (Grant No: 81870369; Key projects of medical science and technology in Henan Province).

DISCLOSURE

The authors have nothing to disclose.

REFERENCES

1. Bai, H., et al., Patch angioplasty in the rat aorta or inferior vena cava. *J Vis Exp*, 2017. (120).
2. Bai, H., et al., Pericardial patch venoplasty heals via attraction of venous progenitor cells. *Physiol Rep*, 2016. **4**(12).
3. Bai, H., et al., Autologous tissue patches acquire vascular identity depending on the environment. *Vasc Investig Ther*, 2018. **1**(1): pp. 14–23.
4. Bai, H., et al., Polyester vascular patches acquire arterial or venous identity depending on their environment. *J Biomed Mater Res A*, 2017. **105**(12): pp. 3422–3431.
5. Bai, H., et al., Hyaluronic acid-heparin conjugated decellularized human great saphenous vein patches decrease neointimal thickness. *J Biomed Mater Res B Appl Biomater*, 2020. **108**(6): pp. 2417–2425.

6. Bai, H., et al., Inhibition of programmed death-1 decreases neointimal hyperplasia after patch angioplasty. *J Biomed Mater Res B Appl Biomater*, 2020.

7. Eads, D. and J.S. Ikonomidis, Historical perspectives of The American Association for Thoracic Surgery: Michael E. DeBakey (1908–2008). *J Thorac Cardiovasc Surg*, 2014. **147**(4): pp. 1123–1127.

8. den Hoed, P.T. and H.F. Veen, The late complications of aorto-iliofemoral Dacron prostheses: Dilatation and anastomotic aneurysm formation. *Eur J Vasc Surg*, 1992. **6**: pp. 282–287.

9. Sidawy, A.N. and Perler, B.A, *Rutherford's Vascular Surgery and Endovascular Therapy*. 9th ed. section 9, Grafts and Devices. Elsevier, 2018.

10. 4- History of Expanded PTFE and W.L. Gore and Associates, in *Introduction to Fluoropolymers*, S. Ebnesajjad, Editor. 2013, William Andrew Publishing: Oxford. pp. 37–52.

11. Harrison, J.H., Influence of infection on homografts and synthetic (teflon) grafts; a comparative study in experimental animals. *AMA Arch Surg*, 1958. **76**(1): pp. 67–73.

12. Gutowski, P., et al., Arterial reconstruction with human bioengineered acellular blood vessels in patients with peripheral arterial disease. *J Vasc Surg*, 2020. **72**(4): pp. 1247–1258.

13. Gui, L., et al., Development of decellularized human umbilical arteries as small-diameter vascular grafts. *Tissue Eng Part A*, 2009. **15**(9): pp. 2665–2676.

14. Li, X., et al., Pericardial patch angioplasty heals via an Ephrin-B2 and CD34 positive cell mediated mechanism. *PLoS One*, 2012. **7**(6): p. e38844.

15. Gessaroli, M., et al., Prevention of neointimal hyperplasia associated with modified stretch expanded polytetrafluoroethylene hemodialysis grafts (Gore) in an experimental preclinical study in swine. *J Vasc Surg*, 2012. **55**(1): pp. 192–202.

16. Kapadia, M.R., D.A. Popowich, and M.R. Kibbe, Modified prosthetic vascular conduits. *Circulation*, 2008. **117**(14): pp. 1873–82.

17. Chang, Y., et al., Tissue regeneration patterns in a cellular bovine pericardia implanted in a canine model as a vascular patch. *J Biomed Mater Res A*, 2004. **69**(2): pp. 323–333.

18. de Barros-Marques, S.R., et al., Sugarcane biopolymer patch in femoral vein angioplasty on dogs. *J Vasc Surg*, 2012. **55**(2): pp. 517–21.

19. Sarac, T.P., et al., In vivo and mechanical properties of peritoneum/fascia as a novel arterial substitute. *J Vasc Surg*, 2005. **41**(3): pp. 490–497.

20. Sarac, T.P., et al., Use of fascia-peritoneum patch as a pledget for an infected aortic stump. *J Vasc Surg*, 2003. **38**(6): pp. 1404–1406.

21. Agathos, E.A., et al., A novel anticalcification treatment strategy for bioprosthetic valves and review of the literature. *J Card Surg*, 2019. **34**(10): pp. 895–900.

22. Lei, Y., et al., Enzyme-oxidative-polymerization method for improving glycosaminoglycans stability and reducing calcification in bioprosthetic heart valves. *Biomed Mater*, 2019. **14**(2): p. 025012.

23. Wong, M.L., et al., In vivo xenogeneic scaffold fate is determined by residual antigenicity and extracellular matrix preservation. *Biomaterials*, 2016. **92**: pp. 1–12.

24. Magden, G.K., et al., Composite sponges from sheep decellularized small intestinal submucosa for treatment of diabetic wounds. *J Biomater Appl*, 2020: p. 885328220963897.

25. Hibino, N., et al., Preliminary experience in the use of an extracellular matrix (CorMatrix) as a tube graft: Word of caution. *Semin Thorac Cardiovasc Surg*, 2015. **27**(3): pp. 288–295.

26. Jernigan, T.W., et al., Small intestinal submucosa for vascular reconstruction in the presence of gastrointestinal contamination. *Ann Surg*, 2004. **239**(5): pp. 733–738; discussion 738–740.

27. Jacobsen, R.M., et al., Porcine small intestinal submucosa may be a suitable material for Norwood arch reconstruction. *Ann Thorac Surg*, 2018. **106**(6): pp. 1847–1852.

28. McCready, R.A., et al., Pseudoaneurysm formation in a subset of patients with small intestinal submucosa biologic patches after carotid endarterectomy. *J Vasc Surg*, 2005. **41**(5): pp. 782–788.

29. Madden, N.J., D.A. Troutman, and A.J. DeMarsico, Use of a small intestine submucosa extracellular matrix patch in repeated carotid endarterectomy. *J Am Osteopath Assoc*, 2014. **114**(9): pp. 732–734.

30. Sauvage, L.R., et al., Interspecies healing of porous arterial prostheses: Observations, 1960 to 1974. *Arch Surg*, 1974. **109**(5): pp. 698–705.

31. Bai, H., et al., Covalent modification of pericardial patches for sustained rapamycin delivery inhibits venous neointimal hyperplasia. *Sci Rep*, 2017. **7**: p. 40142.

32. Kirkton, R.D., et al., Bioengineered human acellular vessels recellularize and evolve into living blood vessels after human implantation. *Sci Transl Med*, 2019. **11**(485).

33. Li, X., et al., Atorvastatin regulates pericardial patch healing via the microRNA140-ADAM10-ephrinB2 pathway. *Am J Transl Res*, 2018. **10**(12): pp. 4054–4064.

34. Wolf, K., et al., Molecular identity of arteries, veins, and lymphatics. *J Vasc Surg*, 2019. **69**(1): pp. 253–262.

35. Hashimoto, T., et al., Membrane-mediated regulation of vascular identity. *Birth Defects Res C Embryo Today*, 2016. **108**(1): pp. 65–84.

36. Kudo, F.A., et al., Venous identity is lost but arterial identity is not gained during vein graft adaptation. *Arterioscler Thromb Vasc Biol*, 2007. **27**(7): pp. 1562–1571.

37. Niklason, L.E., Understanding the extracellular matrix to enhance stem cell-based tissue regeneration. *Cell Stem Cell*, 2018. **22**(3): pp. 302–305.

38. Lawson, J.H., et al., Bioengineered human acellular vessels for dialysis access in patients with end-stage renal disease: Two phase 2 single-arm trials. *Lancet*, 2016. **387**(10032): pp. 2026–2034.

39. Li, J., et al., Controlling molecular weight of hyaluronic acid conjugated on amine-rich surface: Toward better multifunctional biomaterials for cardiovascular implants. *ACS Appl Mater Interfaces*, 2017. **9**(36): pp. 30343–30358.

40. Hohmann, E., Editorial commentary: Platelet-rich plasma and hyaluronic acid injection for knee osteoarthritis are both cost effective. *Arthroscopy*, 2020. **36**(12): pp. 3079–3080.

41. Iida, O., et al., One-year outcomes of heparin-bonded stent-graft therapy for real-world femoropopliteal lesions and the association of patency with the prothrombotic state based on the prospective, observational, multicenter viabahn stent-graft placement for femoropopliteal diseases requiring endovascular therapy (VANQUISH) study. *J Endovasc Ther*, 2020. **28**(1): pp. 123–131. doi: 10.1177/1526602820960445.

42. Bohme, T., et al., Heparin-bonded stent-graft for the treatment of TASC II C and D femoropopliteal lesions: 36-month results of the viabahn 25 cm trial. *J Endovasc Ther*, 2020. **28**(2): pp. 222–228. doi: 10.1177/1526602820965965.

43. Ostdiek, A.M., et al., Feasibility of a nanomaterial-tissue patch for vascular and cardiac reconstruction. *J Biomed Mater Res B Appl Biomater*, 2016. **104**(3): pp. 449–457.

44. Jacobs, M.J., et al., Creation of a distal arteriovenous fistula improves microcirculatory hemodynamics of prosthetic graft bypass in secondary limb salvage procedures. *J Vasc Surg*, 1993. **18**(1): pp. 1–8; discussion 8–9.

45. Menawat, S.S., et al., Effect of a femoral arteriovenous fistula on lower extremity venous hemodynamics after femorocaval reconstruction. *J Vasc Surg*, 1996. **24**(5): pp. 793–799.

46. Ellenby, M.I., et al., Role of nitric oxide in the effect of blood flow on neointima formation. *J Vasc Surg*, 1996. **23**(2): pp. 314–322.

47. Jost, C.J., et al., Surgical reconstruction of iliofemoral veins and the inferior vena cava for nonmalignant occlusive disease. *J Vasc Surg*, 2001. **33**(2): pp. 320–327; discussion 327–328.

48. Terra, M.F., et al., Physical exercises decreases thrombus and neointima formation in atherosclerotic mice. *Thromb Res*, 2019. **175**: pp. 21–31.

49. Breen, D.M., et al., Resveratrol inhibits neointimal formation after arterial injury through an endothelial nitric oxide synthase-dependent mechanism. *Atherosclerosis*, 2012. **222**(2): pp. 375–381.

50. Sidawy, A.N. and Perler, B.A, *Rutherford's Vascular Surgery and Endovascular Therapy*. 9th ed. Section 13, Cerebrovascular Diseases. 2018.

51. Kim, M., et al., Rupture of carotid artery pseudoaneurysm in the modern era of definitive chemoradiation for head and neck cancer: Two case reports. *World J Clin Cases*, 2020. **8**(20): pp. 4858–4865.

52. Alterio, D., et al., Carotid blowout syndrome after reirradiation for head and neck malignancies: A comprehensive systematic review for a pragmatic multidisciplinary approach. *Crit Rev Oncol Hematol*, 2020. **155**: p. 103088.

53. Sallustro, M., et al., Multistep and multidisciplinary management for post-irradiated carotid blowout syndrome in a young patient with oropharyngeal carcinoma: A case report. *Ann Vasc Surg*, 2020. **67**: pp. 565 e1–565 e5.

54. Archie, J.P., Carotid endarterectomy saphenous vein patch rupture revisited: Selective use on the basis of vein diameter. *J Vasc Surg*, 1996. **24**(3): pp. 346–351; discussion 351–352.

55. Knight, B.C. and W.F. Tait, Dacron patch infection following carotid endarterectomy: A systematic review of the literature. *Eur J Vasc Endovasc Surg*, 2009. **37**(2): pp. 140–148.

56. Schauber, M.D., et al., Cranial/cervical nerve dysfunction after carotid endarterectomy. *J Vasc Surg*, 1997. **25**(3): pp. 481–487.

57. Bai, H., et al., Transforming growth factor-beta1 inhibits pseudoaneurysm formation after aortic patch angioplasty. *Arterioscler Thromb Vasc Biol*, 2018. **38**(1): pp. 195–205.

58. Kocak, E., A. Yildiz, and F. Acarturk, Three dimensional bioprinting technology: Applications in pharmaceutical and biomedical area. *Colloids Surf B Biointerfaces*, 2021. **197**: p. 111396.

59. Deng, Z., T. Qian, and F. Hang, Three-dimensional printed hydrogels with high elasticity, high toughness, and ionic conductivity for multifunctional applications. *ACS Biomater Sci Eng*, 2020. **6**(12): pp. 7061–7070.

3 Biomaterials for Fabricating Vascularized Scaffolds in Tissue Engineering

Yonghong Fan and Yinhua Qin
Third Military Medical University

Xinxin Li
Kunming University of Science and Technology

Yuhao Wang, Youqian Xu, and Chuhong Zhu
Third Military Medical University

CONTENTS

DOI: 10.1201/9781003161981-3

3.1   INTRODUCTION

The clinical need for tissue repairing, regeneration, or replacing is becoming more and more exigent with the fast-growing and aging global population. Tissue engineering has been developed to restore, maintain, or improve tissue functions by combining cells, biomaterials, and biologically active molecules.[1] Tissue engineering is an interdisciplinary field that involves engineering, material science, chemistry, medicine, and life science to generate living tissue and organ replacements. Numerous people will benefit from tissue engineering-based repair and regeneration in the coming years. Although tissue engineering research is evolving rapidly, only a few engineered tissues, such as skin, cartilage, and bladder have achieved commercial success to date. Organ substitutes with complex structure are still a long way from clinical applications. There is no doubt that tissue engineering has reached some biological challenges.

One of the current limitations in engineering complex tissue is the inability to provide blood supply in the absence of perfusable vascular networks. The survival and function of cells in the living body is highly dependent on a vasculature that transports oxygen, nutrients, and metabolic waste. Due to the diffusion limit of oxygen, tissue growth beyond $100-200\,\mu m$ requires new blood vessel formation.[2] Additionally, blood circulation facilitates distal intercellular communication and enables endocrine communication by transporting soluble factors and proteins from the secretory cell to the target cell. Tissue engineering approaches rely on biomaterials to provide a three-dimensional (3D) structure to support cell survival and fulfill their biological functions. Insufficient blood supply will result in frustrated cell integration in tissue-engineered constructs. Therefore, blood supply is a major problem that must be solved to achieve successful organ replacement. To meet the demand of cell function, any reconstructed tissue or organ that exceeds $400\,\mu m$ in size must be vascularized.

It is no doubt that the injury caused by tissue transplantation induces an immune response, which results in the formation of the microvasculature. In addition, hypoxic cells in the engineered tissue can secrete angiogenic factors, such as vascular endothelial growth factor (VEGF), to help vascularization.[3] Nonetheless, the spontaneous induction of vasculature is a slow process and insufficient to supply the transplanted tissue with adequate oxygen and nutrients.[4] Clinical applications require vascularization of large tissues within a shorter time than that in development and typical physiological process. Although fabricating large vessels has achieved definite progress, many challenges exist in microvasculature construction including the complex arrangement and the fragility of the microvessels. Additional strategies should be developed to help vascular formation within the engineered tissue constructs.

In the past few years, numerous attempts have been made to vascularize engineered constructs, with varying degrees of success. Generally, the current technologies for generating vascularized tissue can be divided into two groups: in vitro prevascularization and in vivo vascularization. All approaches are related to the fabrication of scaffolds, the delivery of growth factors (GFs), the induction of cell differentiation and organization, and the elaborate design of biomaterials. In this chapter, we focus on natural and synthetic biomaterials for vascularization in tissue engineering, as well as the fabrication technologies of these biomaterials. This chapter also serves to highlight the physicochemical, mechanical and biological design of biomaterials to promote vascularization. Furthermore, the current limitations and challenges will be explored.

3.2 BIOMATERIALS FOR VASCULARIZATION

The ability to generate functional tissue-engineered constructs highly depends on integrating cells with biomaterials in 3D morphology. In the past years, scientists have made great progress in tissue engineering and regenerative medicine. This may be largely attributed to the development of biomaterials which are designed to exert mechanical and biochemical cues for guiding cell behaviors.[5] These biocompatible, biodegradable, bioadhesive, mechanically sound, low immunogenic biomaterials that support and enhance vascular network formation can be divided into natural polymers and synthetic biomaterials. In this section, we will describe some representative biomaterials for vascularization and their recent applications.

3.2.1 NATURAL POLYMERS

3.2.1.1 Natural Proteins

3.2.1.1.1 Collagen

Collagen is the primary component of the extracellular matrix (ECM) in tissues and organs. It plays critical roles in molecular and cellular interactions in the ECM, as well as defining the shape and form of tissues. Collagen has a unique conformation which is made from three left-handed polyproline-like chains twisted together into a right-handed triple-helix. There are 29 types of collagen, and all of them can be degraded by collagenase.[6] Collagen hydrogel has been used to study the key steps of vascular morphogenesis by Bayless et al.[7]. They found that the integrin and Rho GTPase-dependent pinocytic vacuole mechanism controls capillary lumen formation in collagen matrices. The secretion of collagen IV is speculated to support blood vessel formation and maturation in vivo,[8] and can stabilize aorta-derived neovessels to prevent vascular regression.[9] Due to its pronounced biocompatibility, biodegradability, and stability arising from its self-aggregation and cross-linking, collagen has been extensively used to fabricate scaffolds for vascularization through fabrication processes such as lyophilization, electrospinning, and 3D bioprinting.

In 2019, Lee et al. presented a suspended 3D-printing method to engineer components of the human heart at various scales, from capillaries to the full organ using collagen.[10] By controlling the pH-driven gelation process, this approach provides a porous microstructure that enables rapid cellular infiltration and microvascularization, as well as mechanical strength for the fabrication and perfusion of multiscale vasculature and tri-leaflet valves. The collagen scaffolds also facilitate vascularization to achieve a perfusable platform through embedding vascular cells.[11] These perfusable scaffolds can maintain the survival of the seeding cells. It is well known that pancreatic islets are fragile cell clusters and vascularization determines the survival of the transplanted isolated islets. Hence, an endothelialized collagen scaffold has been used to create a perfusable vascularized scaffold to support insulin-secreting beta-cell survival in subcutaneous engraftment.[12] To generate vascularized bone graft, Vuornos et al. have developed a 3D gellan gum and collagen type I hydrogel mixture to culture human adipose stem cells (hASCs) and human umbilical vein endothelial cells (HUVECs) for osteogenic differentiation and microvascularization. Strong production of CD31 and elongated tube-like structures were found to be apparent in the EGM-2 culture medium.[13] The collagen-based biomaterials are also harnessed to generate systems for the local delivery of angiogenic agents such as GFs. The keratinocyte GF (KGF or FGF-7) and basic fibroblast GF (bFGF or FGF-2)-released chemically modified collagen membranes have been reported to facilitate skin wound healing.[14] This dual-GFs releasing collagen scaffold showed more highly developed vascular networks and organized epidermal regeneration in the wounds after being transplanted into an excisional wound healing model.

Moreover, the mechanical properties of the collagen scaffolds can be enhanced through combination with other stiff materials for applications such as bone repair. Baheiraei et al. developed collagen/beta-tricalcium phosphate (β-TCP) scaffolds by freeze-drying.[15] The composite scaffolds can promote vascularization and achieved good integration with the surrounding tissue. Inducing β-TCP powder into the porous collagen matrix effectively improved the mechanical and biological properties of the collagen scaffolds, making these scaffolds potential bone substitutes in orthopedic and dental applications. The silicification[16] and biomimetic mineralization[17] methods have also been reported to fabricate collagen-based scaffolds for promoting vascular formation and bone generation.

3.2.1.1.2 Fibrin

Fibrin is one of the main components in the coagulation cascade and is derived from soluble fibrinogen. After the injury, the thrombin binds to the E domain of fibrinogen, resulting in the proteolytic cleavage of fibrinopeptide A (FPA) and fibrinopeptide B (FPB) from the fibrinogen, thus initiating the fibrin polymerization process to form an insoluble fibrin mesh.[18] The fibrin network is rich in binding sites for cells and GFs that promote angiogenesis and cell adhesion, proliferation, and migration. Its degradation products also encourage cell infiltration and the subsequent tissue remodeling.[19] A detailed study of two naturally occurring variants of fibrin revealed that a high-molecular-weight fibrin matrix shows increased cell and tubular structure ingrowth, whereas the ingrowth of tubular structures in a low-molecular-weight fibrin matrix is decreased when compared with unfractionated fibrin.[20]

The fibrin matrix facilitates endothelial cell (EC) migration during angiogenesis through integrin $\alpha5\beta1$ and $\alpha v\beta3$ interactions, as well as nonintegrin receptors such as VE-cadherin.[21,22] During wound healing, GFs such as FGF-2 and VEGF can bind specifically to fibrin, allowing these factors to promote cell regeneration and angiogenesis in sites of tissue damage.[23] In addition, fibrin can be harvested from the patient's blood to avoid immune or foreign body reactions. The polymerization, structural, mechanical, and biological properties of fibrin can be modified in a multitude of ways to achieve desired properties such as altering fibrin and thrombin ratios, adding bioactive factors, creating fibrin–protein composites, and introducing fibrin-binding modifying agents to the polymerizing fibrin network.[24]

Fibrin is an excellent material for making scaffolds to promote vascularization. After the culture of vascular cells in the fibrin gels, the scaffolds can be easily prevascularized with capillary networks. After being implanted, rapid inoculation and perfusion of the microvessels have achieved in the fibrin-based tissues. [25] This demonstrated that prevascularization of a fibrin-based tissue with well-formed capillaries can accelerate anastomosis with the host vasculature. Lee et al. examined the potential utility of prevascularized mucosal cell sheets in oral wound healing.[26] The cell sheets were generated using cultured keratinocytes and a mixture of fibrin, fibroblasts, and ECs. In the oral wound model, the vascularized cell sheets exhibit rapid wound closure more prominently. Furthermore, fibrin scaffolds have been applied in generating prevascularized cardiac patches,[27] adipose tissues,[28] tracheal mucous[29], and pancreatic islets.[30] The preformed vascular networks in fibrin scaffolds also enhanced the performance of engineered bone.[31] Not only that, the fibrin matrices have been used to control the release of GFs to induce salivary gland regeneration by promoting vascularization.[32] However, fibrin has limited mechanical strength and is too weak to resist dynamic physiological conditions.[33]

3.2.1.1.3 Fibronectin

Fibronectin is another ECM glycoprotein and can modulate cell adhesion and migration, proliferation, and differentiation.[34] Fibronectin promotes tissue assembly through binding cell-surface receptors and ECM proteins simultaneously. Studies have shown that the fibronectin-null mice displayed developmental abnormalities in hearts and vessels, indicating the importance of fibronectin in mediating EC interactions.[35] Due to the specific collagen-binding domains in fibronectin, these two ECM proteins can form hydrogels conveniently.[36] Schechner et al. have reported the formation of functional vasculature in collagen-fibronectin gels using genetically modified HUVECs with Bcl-2 overexpression.[37] Similar observations have been presented by Shepherd et al. who reported that the embedding of Bcl-2-transduced HUVECs and human aortic SMCs in a poly(glycolic acid)/collagen/fibronectin scaffold can accelerate vessel formation in vivo in a mouse model.[38] Furthermore, the vascularization ability of hASCs has been tested in the collagen-fibronectin gel by Zhou et al.[39]. hASCs cultured in the 3D scaffolds have shown to promote vascularization with ECs both in vitro and in vivo, and bone morphogenetic protein (BMP-4) protein further help to drive the process. Fibronectin also contains GF-binding sites which can modulate the activity of the GFs such as VEGF and hepatic growth factor (HGF) to enhance angiogenesis, which makes fibronectin an excellent carrier to deliver GF for engineering vascularized scaffolds.[40] Fibronectin on poly(ethyl acrylate) results in a spontaneous fibrillar organization, and the GF binding which makes integrin-binding sites simultaneously available on fibronectin fibrils. Then, fibronectin binds to BMP-2 or VEGF to enhance osteogenesis[41] or angiogenesis[42] at low GF concentration, respectively. The fibronectin-based 3D scaffold with controlled stiffness and degradability enabled the solid-phase presentation of GFs in a physiological manner.[43] In addition, preconditioning of the TCP scaffolds with fibronectin facilitates the adhesion of endothelial progenitor cells (EPCs)[44], and promotes vascularization and bone formation after implantation.[45]

3.2.1.1.4 Gelatin

Gelatin material is derived from denatured collagen in the presence of a dilute acid and shares similar properties with its precursor collagen, and is easily cross-linked to form hydrogels.[46] The gelatin solution has the unique property of gelation at low temperatures to form physically cross-linked hydrogels.[47] RGD (sequence of arginine, glycine, aspartic acid) motifs in gelatin that enhance cell attachment, and the matrix metalloproteinase (MMP) target sequences makes gelatin suitable for cell remodeling.[48] Gelatin has better solubility and less antigenicity than collagen, and these characteristics make gelatin a good candidate for tissue engineering applications.[49] The gelatin scaffolds can induce endothelial differentiation of mesenchymal stem cell (MSCs) and then promote perfusable blood vessel formation in vitro and in vivo via purely material-driven effects.[50] The GFs such as bFGF,[51] histatin-1,[52] and VEGF[53] have achieved controlled delivery from the gelatin scaffolds for increasing neovascularization. Gelatin has a greater degradation rate, which allows increasing the porosity of the scaffold during remolding after being integrated into degradation-resistant materials.[54,55] Moreover, the gelatin can be melted and flushed from the bulk scaffolds. By creating patterned sacrificial gelatin structures in the material, it is easy to form complex, interconnected, 3D perfusable channels after being seeded with ECs.[56] Methacrylamide groups and a minority of methacrylate groups are often introduced into gelatin to form gelatin methacryloyl (GelMA), which undergoes photoinitiated radical polymerization to generate covalently cross-linked hydrogels. GelMA retains most of the functional amino acid motifs such as the RGD motifs and MMP-degradable motifs and has been thoroughly studied as scaffolds for vascularization.[57–59] GelMA also enables the fabrication of scaffolds with specific shapes and structures through 3D printing or electrospinning to mediate vasculogenesis for bone and skin regeneration.[60,61]

3.2.1.1.5 Silk

Silk proteins are naturally occurring proteins that can be found in a wide variety of insects such as spiders and silkworm. Silk is lightweight, extremely strong and elastic, and can be spun as fibers at room temperature with ambient pressure using water as the solvent.[62] The silk scaffold has the ability to entrap cells during fabrication, as well as provide a porous matrix to facilitate nutrient/waste transportation and intercellular communication.[63] Silk is also a material with slow degradation and low immunogenicity, rendering it an attractive biomaterial for tissue engineering applications.[64] Ghanaati et al. have created a silk fibroin scaffold with preseeded osteoblasts for in vivo vascularization.[65] The scaffold was found to achieve rapid and thorough vascularization by the host blood capillaries in vivo, and the osteoblasts produced soluble factors to instruct host ECs to migrate, proliferate, and initiate the process of scaffold vascularization. Similarly, a silk fibroin scaffold with human dental pulp stem cells and gingival fibroblasts has the ability to attract vessels ingrowth to promote vascularization and integrate into the host tissues.[66] Due to the slow degradation of silk, the ingrowth of blood vessels depends significantly on the microchannels in the scaffold. Therefore, most of the silk scaffolds used for engineering vascularized tissues are fabricated to have a high porosity[67] and/or 3D channels.[68–70] Porous silk scaffolds with microchannels can significantly increase vascular volume and vascular density without affecting overall tissue infiltration.[71,72] The hierarchical microstructure of silk-based matrices has a noticeable influence on vascularization. As reported by Lu et al., the anisotropic SF scaffolds alone, without requiring GFs and cells, promoted significant cell migration, vascularization, and skin regeneration and may have the potential to effectively treat dermal wounds.[73] Silk has been combined with additional materials, GFs, or functional motifs to successfully modulate vascular cell response and improve vascularization.[74–78] Moreover, the ingrowth of host blood vessels may be induced by the mild inflammatory response to silk.[79] The injectable silk hydrogels have also been prepared to control neovascularization in specific tissues.[80,81] However, most of the silk-based scaffolds are treated to achieve water insolubility usually with a higher stiffness than that required for vascularization. Han et al. have developed a new method for preparing water-insoluble silk protein scaffolds with vascularization capacity using an all-aqueous process.[82] In the lyophilization process, acid is added temporarily to help scaffold formation directly. Their silk scaffold shows appropriate softer mechanical property to promote cell differentiation into endothelial cells and enhance neovascularization and tissue ingrowth in vivo without the addition of GFs (Table 3.1).

3.2.1.2 Polysaccharides

3.2.1.2.1 Chitosan

Chitosan (CS) is a linear polysaccharide composed of N-glucosamine and N-acetyl-glucosamine units. CS is derived from chitin molecule after N-deacetylation, and its degree of deacetylation and molecular weight depend upon the source and preparation procedure. The degradation of CS mainly depends on the enzymatic hydrolysis of lysozyme. CS has been proven to be abundant, biocompatible, biodegradable, and chemically versatile. However, unmodified CS does not contain cell-binding motifs and have been reported to contribute little to vascularization.[83] Therefore, CS materials are often blended with other biomaterials to help vascularization of the scaffolds, including collagen,[84–87] hydroxyapatite,[88] alginate,[89] or gelatin.[90] The abundant hydroxyl and amino groups in CS provide reactive sites that allow for tailoring the biological properties of the CS-based scaffolds. For example, the RoY peptide has been conjugated onto the CS chain via amide linkages to form a thermosensitive hydrogel for cardiac repair.[91] The introduction of RoY peptide not only improved angiogenesis but also improved cardiac functions. Sulfated chitosan (SCS) is a heparin-like polysaccharide and has been used in tissue engineering to

TABLE 3.1

Summary of Natural Proteins for Engineering Scaffolds with Enhanced Vascularization

Material	Modification	Fabrication	Cells	Application	Reference
Collagen	Loading of fibronectin and VEGF	Suspended 3D printing	hESC-CMs HUVECs	Rebuild components of the human heart	[10]
Collagen	--	Gelation and drawning	MSCs HUVECs	Pseudo-islets	[12]
Collagen	Mix with gellan gum	Gelation and casting	hASCs HUVECs	Bone graft	[13]
Collagen	KGF and bFGF loading	Stacking and cross-linking	--	Wound healing	[14]
Collagen	Mix with β-TCP	Freeze-drying	BMMSCs	Bone regeneration	[15]
Fibrin	--	Cross-linking	Keratinocytes Fibroblasts EPCs	Oral wound healing	[26]
Fibrin	Addition of SCF, IL-3, and SDF-1α	Gelation and molding	BOECs	Cardiac patch	[27]
Fibrin	--	Gelation	MVFs	Adipose tissue	[28]
Fibrin	Blend with agarose and type I collagen	Molding	Fibroblasts Respiratory epithelial cells ECs	Mucosal substitute	[29]
Fibrin	--	Gelation	MSCs Fibroblasts HUVECs iPSC-ECFCs	Pancreatic islet	[31]
Fibrin	YIGSR grafting, VEGF, and FGF loading	Chemical cross-linking	--	Salivary gland regeneration	[32]
Fibronectin	Mix with collagen	Gelation	HUVEC	Synthetic skin	[37]

(Continued)

TABLE 3.1 (*Continued*)

Summary of Natural Proteins for Engineering Scaffolds with Enhanced Vascularization

Material	Modification	Fabrication	Cells	Application	Reference
Fibronectin	Supported by PEA and load BMP-2	Dip-coating	HUVEC MSCs	Osteogenesis	[41]
Fibronectin	PEGylation, and VEGF and BMP-2 loading	Cross-linking and gelation	--	Osteogenesis	[43]
Fibronectin	Supported by β-TCP	Dip-coating	EPCs MSCs	Osteogenesis	[44]
Gelatin	Phenol conjugation	Enzymatic cross-linking	MSCs	Angiogenesis	[50]
Gelatin	bFGF loading	Chemical cross-linking	--	Intestinal anastomotic healing	[51]
GelMA	Histatin-1 loading	Photo-cross-linking	--	Burn wound therapy	[52]
Gelatin	Heparinized and VEGF loading	Chemical cross-linking	--	Angiogenesis	[53]
Gelatin	Mix with PCCP	Extrudation	--	Osteoconductivity	[54]
GelMA	--	Photo-cross-linking	HUVECs BMSCs	Vascularization	[57]
GelMA	Scaffold with microcavitary	Photo-cross-linking	EPOCs	Vascularization	[58,59]
GelMA/ gelatin	--	Extrusion-based bioprinting	DMECs ASCs	Bone tissue	[60]
GelMA	--	Electrospinning	--	Skin flap regeneration	[61]
Silk	--	Acid treating	Osteoblasts	Bone regeneration	[65]
Silk	--	Acid treating and casting	hDPSCs Gingival fibroblasts	Bone regeneration	[66]
Silk	--	Acid treating, casting, and lyophilization	HUVECs	Spinal cord regeneration	[67]
Silk	--	Molding and lyophilization	HUVECs	Fabrication of vascular channels	[68]

(*Continued*)

TABLE 3.1 (Continued)
Summary of Natural Proteins for Engineering Scaffolds with Enhanced Vascularization

Material	Modification	Fabrication	Cells	Application	Reference
Silk	--	Molding and lyophilization	--	Fabrication of vascular microchannels	[69,71,72]
Silk	Electrical field pretreating	Lyophilization	--	Healing of skin wounds	[73]
Silk	Mix with chitosan	Lyophilization and cross-linking	--	Angiogenesis	[74]
Silk	RGD motif	Foaming	MSCs, DMECs	Islet-like clusters	[76]
Silk	REDV grafting	Lyophilization	--	Angiogenesis	[77]
Silk	Desferrioxamine loading	Gelation	--	Healing of skin wounds	[80]
Silk	IKVAV peptide	Chemical cross-linking	BOECs, MSCs	Angiogenesis	[81]
Silk	--	Lyophilization	BMSCs	Angiogenesis	[82]

hESC-CMs: human embryonic stem cell-derived cardiomyocytes; BOECs: human blood outgrowth endothelial cells; SCF: stem cell factor; IL-3: interleukin-3; SDF-1a: stromal-derived factor 1a; MVFs: microvascular fragments; iPSC-ECFCs: induced pluripotent stem cell-derived endothelial colony-forming cells; PCCP: partially crystallized calcium phosphate; EPOC: endothelial progenitor outgrowth cell; DMECs: dermal microvascular endothelial cells; hDPSCs: human dental pulp stem cells stimulate angiogenesis.[92–95] Sulfonate groups can be grafted directly to free amino groups or hydroxyl groups to produce sulfamate products ($-NH-SO_3^-$)[96] or sulfated products($-O-SO_3^-$), respectively.[97] Han et al. have compared the proliferation of HUVECs in three types of SCS with different sulfonic group sites on the molecular chain, and found that the 2,6-SCS had a more obvious performance on vascularization.[98] Notably, SCS-coated scaffolds exhibit an ability to capture VEGF in vivo, resulting in a concentrated VEGF microenvironment in specific domains to accelerate angiogenesis and wound healing.[95] The cationic chains of CS can complex with several types of negatively charged biomolecules or with DNA, enhancing its ability of vascularization.[99] Anionic glycosaminoglycans (GAG) such as heparin can form ionic complexes with CS, thereby imparting upon the CS material the ability to bind and deliver heparin-binding angiogenic GFs.[100–102] In addition, CS elicits a minimal foreign body reaction, and the interaction of CS oligosaccharides with immune cells may stimulate helpful wound healing processes such as cell proliferation and enhanced angiogenesis.[103]

3.2.1.2.2 Hyaluronic Acid

Hyaluronic acid (HA) is part of the GAG component in ECM and is synthesized by HA synthases at the inner wall of the plasma membrane. HA is a negatively charged linear polysaccharide composed of N-acetylglucosamine and glucuronic acid. The hyaluronan receptor CD44[104] and the receptor for HA-mediated motility (RHAMM or CD168)[105] are the most widely studied cell-surface hyaladherins which bind to HA. The biological functions of HA depend on its molecular weight, especially angiogenic properties. Low-molecular-weight HA significantly enhances EC adhesion, proliferation, migration, and functional factors release, as well as stimulates capillary growth and tube formation.[106] Conversely, high-molecular-weight HA can inhibit angiogenic processes.[107] HA in combination with some adult cells has been shown to promote neovascularization.[108,109] Injection of HA along with ECs promotes the retention and growth of transplanted cells, thus improving angiogenesis and arteriogenesis in a mouse model of hind limb ischemia.[110] Moreover, some GFs or cytokines have been incorporated into HA to increase its bioactivity for vascularization.[111–113] However, the half-life of HA is very short in the presence of hyaluronidase, which leads to transient neovascularization. Marques's group have developed some gellan gum-doped HA scaffolds with controllable degradation rate by varying the HA content.[114] Their scaffolds showed no effect on microvascular endothelial cells in vitro, but neovascularization and blood perfusion were attained in ischemic mice hind limbs after implantation.[115] In addition, HA can be chemically modified for controlled degradation and stability.[116] Carboxylic acid, hydroxyl groups, or acetamido groups are principal targets for the chemical modification of HA. After grafting methacrylate groups to the HA molecule, the scaffolds can be prepared via photo-cross-linking. This approach has the advantage of allowing the encapsulation of vascular cells during gelation,[117] and then enables the direct formation of microvessel-like structures.[118] In addition, HA is often copolymerized with other biomaterials for prolonged degradation and better mechanical property. Hozumi et al. have developed an injectable gelatin/HA hydrogel with low degradability, which consists of carbohydrazide-modified gelatin (Gel-CDH) and HA monoaldehyde (HA-mCHO).[119] The prolonged degradation is suitable for inducing angiogenesis and makes these hydrogels stable during the angiogenesis process. In another work, HA has been added into fibrin to form an interpenetrating hydrogel. This hydrogel provides higher mechanical strength, and shows better vascularization and cell recruitment.[120]

3.2.1.2.3 Alginate

Alginate is found in the cell walls of brown algae, and is a linear, unbranched block copolymer. Due to its biocompatibility, abundance, low cost, and mild cross-linking mechanism, alginate has been widely used in tissue engineering applications. However, unmodified alginate materials are considered relatively inert because they do not possess bioactive sequence for cell attachment.[121] Alginate materials are amenable to form scaffolds with angiogenic GFs, peptides, or proteins.[122,123] A biocompatible composite bilayer scaffold has been fabricated for dermatology reconstruction and burn treatment using alginate as base component while collagen and fibrinogen as minor additives in variable concentrations.[124] Manipulating the material ratio enables the sponge scaffolds with highly interconnected porous structures, thus enhancing their vascularization ability. Another work shows that the alginate/CS scaffold with fucoidan addition displays better hemostatic and antibacterial performances, as well as promotes vascularization by upregulating the expression of CD31.[125] Alginate can rapidly form hydrogels upon exposure to divalent cations such as Ca^{2+}, even in the presence of cells or sensitive biomolecules. This mild gelation mechanism facilitates the entrapment of vascular cells and angiogenic GFs into the alginate scaffolds to promote vascular formation.[126–128] Delivering droplets of laminin-modified alginate solution into a calcium chloride solution has been used as a facile and rapid method to encapsulate ADSCs and Rg1 for breast reconstruction after lumpectomy by promoting vascularization.[129] Moreover, alginate cannot be degraded enzymatically in mammals, but the chelating agents (such as citrate or EDTA) can increase the susceptibility to hydrolysis by displacing the cross-linking ions in the ionic cross-linked alginate. Particularly, the ionic cross-linked alginate has been used as a sacrificial template to obtain a hollow vascularizable channel inside the gelatin hydrogel by selectively dissolving the Ca^{2+} ions.[130] Different cation sources can be used to control the mechanical and biological properties of alginate hydrogel. Zhou et al. have compared the mechanical performance, swelling ratio, antibacterial properties, and biocompatibility of alginate-polyacrylamide hydrogels which use copper, zinc, strontium, or calcium as cation source.[131] The results show that copper ion cross-linking exhibit the maximum breaking strength, while strontium and zinc ion cross-linked hydrogels exhibit excellent mechanical strength. The zinc cross-linked hydrogel has a spectrum of antibacterial activities, cell viability, mechanical strength, and the ability of wound closure by promoting fibroblasts migration, vascularization, collagen deposition, and formation of granulation tissue.

3.2.1.2.4 Dextran

Dextran is a natural glucose-containing polysaccharide derived from bacteria and is degradable in the presence of dextranase. Dextran-based hydrogels are biocompatible and biodegradable which can be generated by chemoenzymatic cross-linking methods.[132] Similar to the other polysaccharide materials mentioned before, dextran is naturally resistant to protein adsorption and cell adhesion. Therefore, physical or chemical modifications are required to improve the angiogenic effects of this biomaterial, such as peptide binding, GF delivery, cell encapsulation, cross-linking, and physical mixture.[108,133–136] In 2007, Ferreira et al. developed a dextran-based hydrogel with immobilized RGD peptide and microencapsulated $VEGF_{165}$ to enhance the vascular differentiation of human embryonic stem cells (hESCs).[137] Furthermore, a methacrylated dextran hydrogel with controllable swelling upon equilibrium hydration has been used to identify material properties that impact angiogenesis. By tuning degradability independently from the matrix stiffness of this scaffold, the results suggest that ECM degradability is a key regulator of the collective nature of the multicellular invasion.[138] When treating third-degree burn wounds, dextran hydrogels composed of dextran-allyl isocyanate-ethylamine (Dex-AE) and polyethylene glycol diacrylate (PEGDA) can serve as instructive scaffolds to promote neovascularization and skin regeneration.[139] This hydrogel scaffold facilitates early inflammatory cell infiltration, leads to rapid degradation of dextran, and enhances the infiltration of angiogenic cells into the healing wounds. The ECs can be recruited into the hydrogel scaffold to enable neovascularization, resulting in increased blood flow. Further works by the same group have proposed a synergistic delivery of angiogenic GFs from dextran scaffolds to promote vascularization.[140] Co-delivery of GFs such as VEGF, angiopoietin-1, insulin-like GF, and stromal cell-derived factor-1(SDF-1) induces more and larger blood vessels than any individual GF, while the combination of all GFs dramatically increases the size and number of newly formed functional vessels. The oxidized dextran, dextran aldehyde, is capable of generating hydrogel with succinylated CS. Subsequently, HUVECs and functional peptides have been embedded into the hydrogel as a bioink to prepare regenerative, prevascularized constructs using the 3D printing method.[141] Pullulan is another natural water-soluble polysaccharide and has been explored to form hydrogels with dextran using the cross-linker sodium trimetaphosphate.[142] Rujitanaroj et al. have prepared pullulan/dextran electrospun fibers with the addition of fucoidan through a one-step electrospinning process. The angiogenic factor VEGF can be incorporated into polysaccharide electrospun fibers by taking advantage of the interactions between VEGF and fucoidan. This work demonstrates the potential of pullulan/dextran material with fucoidan as tunable reservoirs for the effective delivery of VEGF to control vascularization of tissue-engineered constructs.[143]

3.2.1.3 Decellularized Extracellular Matrix

Tissues not only consist of cells but are also filled with networks of proteins that are generally known as ECM. Cells divide and integrate into tissues and organs with distinct functions by ceaselessly remolding the ECM into specific 3D architectures and compositions. ECM provides 3D structural support for cell encapsulation and protects cells from deforming damage by acting as a compression buffer. In addition, the biological cues in the ECM play a crucial role in supporting cell survival, organization, and differentiation.[144,145] In the ECM, the proteins, proteoglycans, and glycosaminoglycans are arranged in a fibrous network, and this specific 3D structure provides topographical signaling cues to mediate the behaviors of vascular cells, as well as interconnected channels for diffusion and convection of nutrients and oxygen.

[146] The ECM also serves as an adhesive substrate not only for cell attachment and migration but also as a local depot of GFs, cytokines, and morphogens that provide a microenvironment for cell differentiation and maintenance of tissue-specific cell phenotypes and functions.[5] Therefore, the ECM is a promising biomaterial for fabricating scaffolds to promote vascularization.

To maintain the structural, biochemical, and biomechanical properties and to remove all cells and genetic components of the native ECM, a decellularization process is often performed to produce dECM for further use. The decellularization protocols have been widely described, and these techniques are usually a combination of physical, chemical, and enzymatic strategies.[147] Physical methods are auxiliary means to accelerate the decellularization process, which include freeze-thaw processing, stirring, ultrasonication, and oscillation. The chemical reagents such as peracetic acid, sodium hydroxide, hypotonic and hypertonic solutions, ionic or nonionic detergents, and chelating agents are used to lyse cell membranes and remove cytosolic and genomic materials. In addition, enzymes such as trypsin, dispase, thermolysin, RNase, and DNase are used to digest cell debris and nucleic acids.[148] Specifically, the selection of decellularization reagents or methods highly depends on the source of tissue. Then, the dECM can be fabricated as scaffolds using electrospinning, 3D printing, molding, or gelation methods (Figure 3.1).

The dECM material for vascularization has been extensively explored. Zhao's group has fabricated a prevascularized hMSC/ECM sheet by the combination of hMSCs, ECs, and a naturally derived nanofibrous ECM scaffold.[149] The cell sheets were cultured under low oxygen to promote hMSCs to secrete angiogenic factors, and then included to form microvessels under normal oxygen. A branched and mature vascular network then formed in the scaffolds. Because oriented ECM nanofibrous scaffold guides neovascular network formation, another work from Zhao's group has created an oriented and dense microvessel network with physiological myocardial microvascular features using highly aligned decellularized human dermal fibroblast sheets.[150] They found that the ECM topography influenced ECs organization via CD166 tracks and significantly improved hMSC-EC crosstalk and vascular network formation. In addition, the aligned ECM nanofibers enhanced the length and density of the networks compared to randomly organized ECM.

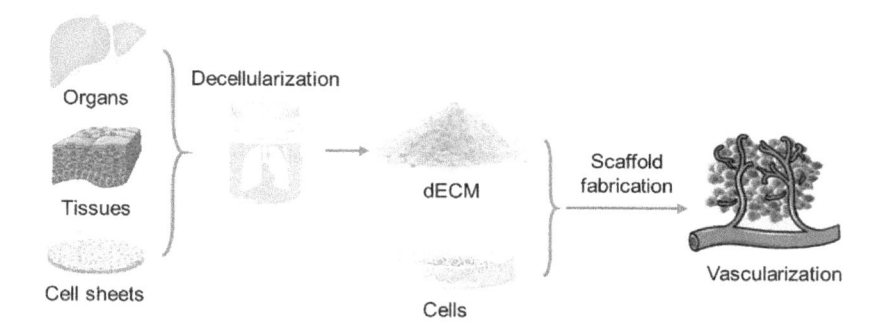

FIGURE 3.1 Decellularized ECM for fabricating vascularized scaffolds.

These vascularized cell/ECM scaffolds are capable of mimicking vasculatures in vitro and delivering cells for therapeutic applications in soft tissue injury.[151–153] Recently, Zhu et al. have engineered ECM scaffolds with parallel microchannels by subcutaneous implantation of sacrificial templates, followed by template removal and decellularization. The scaffolds provide cells with guidance cues for directional migration and spatial organization, and enhance vascularization upon in vivo implantation. Vascularized neo-muscle and neo-nerve were observed after implantation in their animal models, that confirmed the versatility and flexibility of these dECM scaffolds.[154] Furthermore, genetically engineered animals have been demonstrated to create decellularized biologic scaffolds with favorable properties. Morris et al. utilized skin from thrombospondin (TSP)-2 KO mice to derive various decellularized products. This ECM is able to promote vascularization over wild-type ECM. In a diabetic wound model, the genetically engineered ECM showed great ability to accelerate wound healing, and exhibited enhanced remodeling and vascular maturation.[155] Even better, decellularized whole tissues or organs can retain intact vascular networks from the main blood vessels to capillaries while this perfusion system is hard to be fabricated based on current technologies. Therefore, the decellularized whole matrix holds great potential as a technology for developing a theoretically limitless supply of functional vascularized organs.[156]

Although the dECM has gained extensive attention in promoting vascularization due to its dramatic bioactivity, major hurdles remain for the widespread clinical translation of these biomaterials. During the decellularization process, the structure and composition of ECM were disrupted invariably. Immoderate decellularization results in a large loss of bioactivity. Furthermore, inefficient decellularization has detrimental effects on tissue remodeling after implantation.[157] Hence, it is important to optimize the decellularization process for achieving a balance between the preservation of native ECM and the removal of antigenic substances. Specific ECM-derived molecules that modulate the immune response should be identified and removed to avoid a pro-inflammatory immune response following implantation.

3.2.2 SYNTHETIC BIOMATERIALS

3.2.2.1 Poly(Ethylene Glycol)

Poly(ethylene glycol) (PEG) is a biocompatible material that has been approved by the FDA for many certain applications. Introducing diacrylate groups to the ends of the chain allows producing PEGDA, which can be cross-linked to generate hydrogel scaffolds via a light or other chemical approaches. However, PEG is hydrophilic and essentially a bioinert polymer nonadhesive to cells and proteins. This material provides a blank platform for incorporating bioactive molecules to induce vascularization.

Some bioadhesive ligands, enzyme-sensitive motifs, or angiogenic peptides have been used to modify the PEG material.[158–160] The RGD-functionalized PEG scaffold with 3D channels enables endothelialization and can be perfused with blood under high-pressure pulsatile flow.[161] Using the perfusion-based frontal photopolymerization method, Turturro et al. have created a PEGDA hydrogel with mechanical and biofunctional gradients.[162] The gradients of elastic modulus, immobilized MMP sensitivity, and YRGDS cell adhesion ligands in the hydrogel are capable of directing 3D vascular sprout formation in tissue-engineered scaffolds. Glucagon-like peptide 2(GLP-2) has also been integrated into high-molecular-weight PEG, and this scaffold show an additive effect on EC proliferation, tissue growth, histomorphology, and vascularization.[163] Furthermore, GFs and/or angiogenic cells have been incorporated into the PEG-derived materials for vascularizing the scaffolds. Covalent immobilization of VEGF into the PEG hydrogel allows for protease degradation-dependent release of the GF while maintaining its bioactivity.[164] Co-culture of hBM-MSCs and HUVECs in biological inert PEG matrices can be directed toward vascularized bone and bone marrow-like 3D tissue constructs.[165] A semi-interpenetrating polymer network generated from the mixture of vinyl sulfone-terminated PEG (PEG-VS) and sodium polymethacrylate (PMAA-Na) has been used as an injectable carrier to deliver cells and generate blood vessels. Islets embedded in this hydrogel were viable and responsive to glucose stimulation, and the results showed that the generated vessels were perfused and connected to the host vasculature as early as seven days after transplantation.[166] Another work demonstrated that VEGF and pancreatic islets encapsulated PEG-maleimide hydrogel prolonged the in vivo release of GF and enhanced graft vascularization.[167]

To increase the stability of natural biomaterials, PEG is often combined with HA,[168] collagen,[169] CS,[170] or fibrin[171] materials to yield hybrid scaffolds that possess improved mechanical and biological performance. Jiang et al. have developed a fibrin-loaded PEG hydrogel for vascularized tissue formation.[172] The porous PEG hydrogels can serve as scaffolds for mechanical and structural support, and fibrin is loaded within the pores to induce vascularization and increase hydrogel mechanical stiffness. PEG-fibrin hydrogels are also reported to store and release VEGF-A in a sustained and controlled fashion and improve arteriogenesis and cardiac performance.[173] Using PEG to modify fibrinogen can increase scaffold longevity, and human amniotic fluid-derived stem cells (AFSC) cultured in the PEG-fibrin hydrogel have the potential to form 3D vascular-like networks in vitro. Subcutaneously injecting the AFSC-encapsulated hydrogels can induce a fibrin-driven angiogenic response and promote in situ AFSC-derived neovascularization.[174] The four-arm PEG acrylate can form cryogels with methacrylated gelatin and methacrylated HA using cryopolymerization.[168] The addition of four-arm PEG acrylate improves the scaffold robustness and mechanical properties. This cryogel facilitates the co-culture of HUVECs while loading with human adipose progenitor cells and helps the formation of capillary-like networks.

3.2.2.2 Polycaprolactone

Polycaprolactone (PCL) is another polyester that has been approved by the FDA. PCL is relatively flexible but degrades very slowly due to its hydrophobicity. PCL scaffolds that promote vascularization have been fabricated by electrospinning, 3D printing, micropatterning, and casting, whether alone or mixed with other angiogenic materials. In a dorsal skinfold chamber model, CS-modified PCL fibrous mats have shown to increase vascularization, as well as reduce the activation of immune cells. [175,176] PCL nanofiber mats embedded with placental-derived bioactive molecules can attract, stimulate, and support vascularization, and then facilitate wound closure with well-organized dermis and epidermis.[177] In addition, the angiogenic GFs such as VEGF and PDGF have been delivered from PCL scaffolds to help vascular formation. Simultaneous deposition of HA, PCL, and collagen allows the dual loading and controlled release of these two GFs with intact bioactivity.[178] While PCL scaffold coated by only collagen does not change the release kinetics of loaded VEGF.[179] Alternatively, heparinized PCL-derived scaffolds provide binding sites for VEGF and enable the sustained release of GF.[180,181] EPCs seeded on the heparinized PCL scaffold with VEGF show significantly high density of blood vessel formation. These vessels have been found to anastomose with the host circulatory system as evidenced by the presence of murine erythrocytes in the lumen of human-CD31 positive vessels.[181] More recently, an endothelial-specific fusion protein (VEGF-Fc) has been designed and used to construct a bioactive interface by steeping in a porous PCL scaffold.[182] The hydrophobic binding of the Fc domain allows to form uniform VEGF coating throughout the PCL scaffolds without affecting their surface morphology and mechanical properties. These VEGF functionalized PCL scaffolds are suggested to promote the migration of HUVECs into the pores and support vascularization. Moreover, the VEGF can be integrated into the PCL scaffolds by hydrophobin HGFI protein, thus enhancing the adhesion, migration, and proliferation of HUVECs.[183,184] Some inorganic materials such as calcium carbonate,[185] hydroxyapatite,[186,187] β-TCP,[188] europium hydroxide nanorods,[189] and copper nanoparticle decorated reduced graphene oxide[190] have also been used to enhance vascularization in PCL scaffolds.

3.2.2.3 Polyglycolide, Polylactide, and Their Copolymer Poly(Lactide-Co-Glycolide)

Polyglycolide (PGA), polylactide, and PLA their copolymer poly(lactide-co-glycolide) (PLGA) are well known for their good biocompatibility. These polymers can be degraded by hydrolysis at different rates, and PLA and PGA possess a relatively high rate of degradation. The degradation of PLGA depends on the glycolic acid content. Higher glycolic acid content allows faster degradation. Importantly, fast degradation of these materials may result in local toxicity even the degradation products are considered to be biocompatible.

These materials have been used to create porous or fibrous scaffolds individually or in combination with other bioactive materials to induce vascularization.[191–194] Human ADSCs on the PGA/PLA meshes have been found to obtain a mature endothelial phenotype while the alpha-SMA expression was markedly suppressed in the 3D-cultured hADSCs.[195] The PGA fibrous scaffold shows to facilitate the attachment of ECs to the islet surface, and then enhances the function, survival, and vascularization of isolated islets in vitro and in vivo.[196] Moreover, the cell-free biomimetic PLA scaffolds consisting of radially aligned electrospun fibers have been demonstrated to support neuronal migration and complete vascularization.[197] However, these polymers are stiff and mismatch with the ECM of soft tissues; hence, most of these scaffolds are used for bone repair. Kim et al. have fabricated a porous PLA graft for bone repair by salt leaching technique. The VEGF achieved more effective loading capacity after modifying the PLA surface with calcium phosphate mineral, and profiled sustainable release of VEGF for up to a couple of weeks. This scaffold presents significantly improved proliferation of primary ECs and vascularization.[198] Furthermore, the PLA scaffolds that combine with nanohydroxyapatite phosphate,[199] calcium phosphate,[200,201] Ti-doped calcium phosphate,[202] or bioglasses[203] can promote vascularization and bone formation. The supercritical carbon dioxide foaming technique is another method to fabricate mesoporous scaffolds. Using this approach, bioactive glasses and PLGA have been blended to form composite scaffolds with appropriate mechanical and degradation properties.[204] This foamed porous scaffold incorporated with bioactive lipids achieve desirable vascularization-coupled bone formation and could be a promising strategy for bone regenerative medicine. Seeding angiogenic cells on these polymers can help the formation of vascular-like structures.[205–210] The ECs with supporting cells on PLLA/PLGA scaffolds treated with tropoelastin elicit a more expanded, complex, and developed vascularization.[211] Furthermore, co-culture of HUVECs and MSCs on a VEGF-loaded PLGA fiber promotes angiogenesis of MSCs, indicating a good strategy for vascularization in bone tissue engineering.[212] Similar vascularization can be achieved while using aortic fragments and osteoblast-like cells in matrigel-filled PLGA scaffolds.[213]

Moreover, the PGA, PLA, and PLGA materials are suitable for 3D printing and micropatterning.[214,215] In a neovascularized implantable cell homing and encapsulation system (NICHE), the 3D-printed PLA scaffolds were prepared as vascularized cell encapsulation devices.[216] The elaborate PLA scaffolds were modified by platelet-rich plasma hydrogel coating and filling. First, scaffolds were completely vascularized by stimulating angiogenesis after subcutaneous implantation. Then, the cells were transcutaneously inserted via injection. Finally, the NICHE was harvested and enabled the transplantation of Leydig cells along with the scaffold.

3.2.2.4   Poly(Glycerol Sebacate)

Poly(glycerol sebacate) (PGS) is a novel thermoset bioelastomer, and is constructed by hydrolysable ester bonds which degrade in the physiological environment. PGS shows a linear in vivo degradation profile with preservation of geometry and retention of mechanical strength.[217] Glycerol and sebacic acid are the basic building blocks of PGS, and the potential degradation products of PGS are nontoxic. In vitro and in vivo studies show that the PGS has good biocompatibility.[218] The mechanical properties of PGS are similar to those of soft tissues, making this material suitable for preparing scaffolds for implantation in dynamic mechanical environments.[219] Photolithographic tools have been used to generate capillary networks of PGS.[220] The microchannels can be endothelialized by HUVECs under flow culture conditions, suggesting that this approach can generate tissue-engineered microvasculature. In another work, PGS has been made into 3D microfluidic networks through tailored microfabrication processes. The hepatocyte cell line (HepG(2)) was cultured in this scaffold with long-term perfusion to create vascularized liver constructs.[221] A mechanically robust, elastomeric, biodegradable microvessel scaffold made from PGS has also been reported to induce the differentiation of human skeletal muscle cells.[222] After implantation, substantial biodegradation of the PGS scaffold was found to be in association with host blood cell infiltration of the microvessels. Furthermore, the mechanical and biological properties of PGS can be readily modulated to match those of specific tissues, enabling the fabrication of vascularized scaffolds for repairing bone,[223,224] tracheal,[225] myocardium,[226] endometrium,[227] and valves.[228]

3.3 FABRICATION TECHNIQUES FOR ENGINEERING VASCULARIZED SCAFFOLDS

Vascularization of tissue-engineered constructs relies on the ability of engineers to recreate the ECM-mimetic microenvironment and microstructure in the biomaterials. The scaffolds not only provide mechanical support but also present topological and biological cues to promote vascular formation. Therefore, it is important to choose the appropriate processing method according to the type of biomaterial and the target tissue (Table 3.2).

3.3.1 ELECTROSPINNING

Electrospinning is a manufacturing technique involving an electrostatic-driven process used to produce nano and microscale polymer fibers. During the process, a stream of polymer which, generally diluted with a solvent or plasticizer, is stretched into a solution jet by a high enough charge density and then be accelerated through a voltage differential toward a collecting plate, finally be solidified to form fibrous scaffolds. The morphology of electrospun fibers is affected by multiple parameters, including polymer flow rate, tip-to-collector distance, supplied voltage, humidity, and temperature.[229] The diameter of the fibers can be adjusted by the device, ranging from several microns to several nanometers. Scaffolds prepared through electrospinning with characteristics of high surface-area-to-volume ratio, high porosity, and suitability for cell attachment and proliferation. Most biocompatible polymers have been used as the sole component or in combination to fabricate aligned or randomly deposited fibers, including synthetic polymers, such as PCL, PGA, PLA, PLGA, and natural polymers, such as silk, gelatin, collagen, chitosan, fibrin, and HA.[230] For example, natural polymers mainly of collagen and elastin fibrils can be tailored by electrospinning to resemble the ECM structure, supporting ECs and SMCs to form capillary networks. The 3D fibrin hydrogel spun meshes can increase ECM deposition and allow for the creation of self-supporting multilayered microvasculature with a distinct circular.[231] In addition, the microvascular networks can be fabricated by sacrificial electrospinning techniques. The sacrificial polymers for generating microchannel patterns are collected and then embedded onto an ECM scaffold. Finally, a perfusbale network is obtained after elution.[232] Gualandi et al. used electrospun nonwoven mats as sacrificial fibers to generate 3D vascularized scaffolds containing interconnected networks.[233] Jeffries et al. have prepared micropatterning fibrous scaffolds through electrospinning using vascular-like branching poly(vinyl alcohol) (PVA) as templates.[234] After dissolving PVA in water, microvascular patterns were transferred onto fibrous scaffolds. More recently, Han's group has fabricated a novel scaffold of dimpled/hollow electrospun fibers that enables the formation of highly mature vasculatures with adequate dimensions by rapid degradation in the tissue.[235] This unique scaffold-based vasculature can hold implanted cells and tissue constructs for a prolonged duration while minimizing cellular loss.

TABLE 3.2

Advantages and Disadvantages of Scaffold Fabrication Techniques for Vascularization

Technique	Advantages	Disadvantages
Electrospinning	• Versatile and cost-effective • Fabrication of interconnected microchannels	• Random arrangement channels • Complex manual processes
Micropatterning	• Able to fabricate highly ordered microstructures • High-precision and resolution • Simple to create microchannels	• Unable to fabricate 3D vascular networks
Micromolding	• Fabrication of interconnected microchannels with desired size and shape	• Hard to create microvasculature and hierarchical networks • Complex operational processes
Gelation	• Fast and simple process for fabrication of 3D vascular networks • Excellent biocompatibility to the incorporated cells • Fabrication of intricate vasculature	• Random arrangement of channels • Poor mechanical stability and suboptimal durability
Particle leaching	• Easy fabrication of interconnected microchannels with controlled size and porosity	• Low cell viability • Limited porogen particles
Inkjet bioprinting	• Fast fabrication speed • High resolution and scalability	• Nozzle clogging • Hard to create 3D microvasculature
Extrusion bioprinting	• Versatile and cost-effective • Great flexibility in terms of materials choice	• Nozzle clogging • Hard to create microvasculature and hierarchical networks
Laser-assisted bioprinting	• Fast process for microvasculature • High precision and resolution • Relatively low or no damage to the incorporated cells	• Increased fabrication time for hierarchical networks • Limited thickness of fabricated tissue • Limited scalability • High cost
Stereolithography bioprinting	• Generation of intricate networks of channels with varying diameters • Excellent resolution	• Cytotoxicity • High cost

3.3.2 MICROFABRICATION

Microfabrication is defined as a process that can fabricate complex microstructure with multiple materials. This approach is of interest to construct 3D multilayer perfusable tissue scaffolds as they can create complex microgeometries resembling the natural tissue environment. A series of microfabrication techniques include photolithography, rapid prototyping, soft lithography, and hierarchical assembly have emerged in engineering vascularized scaffolds. The biodegradable polymers such as PLA, PGA, PLGA, collagen, fibrin, and alginate have been applied in this field.[236]

3.3.2.1 Micropatterning

Micropatterning is a powerful tool to create highly ordered microstructures by photolithography. This method is often related to a photomask that has the desired micropattern. The UV light through the mask induces a cross-linking reaction of liquid-based, photosensitive monomers. Consequently, the micropattern is cured and can be transferred onto the materials to form perfusable channels.[237] Many studies have used collagen, fibronectin, or HA to fabricate micropatterned structures to investigate the role of EC morphology in migration, ECM deposition, alignment, proliferation, lumen formation and tube-like structure development. A laser-guided, noncontact, high-precision micropatterning method has been reported to create highly ordered 3D nanofibrous tubes in the biomaterial.[238] This technique may present a powerful approach for the generation of functional tissues with well-organized microvessels.

3.3.2.2 Micromolding

Using a mold to produce polymer-based scaffolds with customized size and shape is a highly efficient and reproducible method. Micromolding allows researchers to create microfeatures, typically ranging from 1 to 1000 µm in size.[239] Accurate and high-resolution micromolds can be fabricated by the photolithography method.[240,241] Sacrificial molding is well known for its convenience in creating microfluidic channels and biomimetic microstructures in biomaterials. This approach often entails a sequential process of sacrificial template fabricating, soft polymer casting, and mold etching. Particularly, sacrificial molding is suitable for fabricating tubular-shaped vascular grafts or complex branching vasculatures.[242] Wang et al. have described a method to rapidly cast interconnected 3D vascular networks in hydrogels using a cross-linked sodium alginate lattice as a biocompatible sacrificial template.[243] Dissolving the template with EDTA solution generates interconnected 3D microfluidic channels for EC culture and vascular simulation. Moreover, the 3D printing micromolds have been used in engineering vascularized constructs. Jordan et al. first reported the rapid casting of patterned vascular networks through sacrificial molding using a 3D printing template. By combining the micromolding and 3D printing techniques, this approach allows independent control of network geometry, endothelialization and the extravascular tissue. It is compatible with a wide variety of cell types, synthetic or natural ECM, and the cross-linking strategies.
[161] In another work, Luiz et al. have printed agarose template fibers that could simply be removed to form a cell-laden hydrogel material for generating microchannel networks which populated with human ECs.[244]

3.3.3 GELATION

Gelation is the process of forming a gel from polymer sol. This process can be initiated by physical cross-linking or chemical cross-linking. The gels often have high water-holding capacity, high permeability, and excellent biocompatibility, making this technique useful for replicating the characteristics of native ECM when building vascularized tissues.[245] Natural biomaterials that can form hydrogels include matrigel, collagen, HA, fibrin, dextran and alginate. Zimmermann et al. have created a microvascularized and functional cardiac construct by mixing cardiac myocytes with collagen I and matrigel gel in a circular mold.[246] Montaño et al. have reported the construction of a network with highly organotypic capillaries in fibrin-based hydrogels.[247] To generate a prevascularized network, Heo et al. have employed collagen/fibrin hydrogel as an encapsulation matrix for the incorporation of MSCs/HUVECs spheroids.[248] However, some natural materials have limitations such as poor mechanical stability and suboptimal durability.[249] Accordingly, cell-compatible synthetic materials have lent themselves to form hybrid gels with natural materials to remedy these limitations. Also the naturally occurring hydrogels can be modified with functional groups to improve their properties, for example, GelMA.[250,251] This photo-cross-linkable hydrogel has been widely used for generating functional vascular networks.[252] With the help of emerging techniques such as micromolding, 3D printing, or coaxial microfluidic spinning, hydrogels provide a great versatile platform for generating complex vasculature within engineered tissues in the presence of functional motifs, GFs, and seeding cells.[253,254]

3.3.4 PARTICLE LEACHING

Particle leaching is the most common technique that generates porous scaffolds. First, the polymer solution is uniformly mixed with porogen particles and shaped into desired geometry. Then the solvent is removed by vacuum drying or lyophilization, and the porogen particles are leached out with water to produce a 3D porous scaffold.[255] The porogen particles are mainly known as salt particles; besides, sugar, glucose, paraffin, gelatin, and ammonium chloride are also used.[256] Depending on the shape, dimension, and amount of the added porogen, the pore size and porosity of the materials can be controlled. The porous scaffolds are crucial in tissue engineering for cell penetration, tissue ingrowth, vascularization and nutrient delivery.[257] Due to its ease of fabrication and creation of a specific 3D interconnected structure for vascular formation, this strategy has been extensively explored to prepare vascularized scaffolds in combination with freeze-drying, compression molding, gas foaming, photopolymerization and soft lithographic techniques.[258]

3.3.5 BIOPRINTING

Bioprinting is a 3D fabrication technology that uses a computer-aided, layer-by-layer deposition approach for the fabrication of living tissue and organ analogs from cells and other biologics [259–261]. Due to its precision, 3D bioprinting is one of the most promising technologies to create vascularized constructs. This method enables the encapsulation of cells and GFs into the scaffolds during fabrication to help vascular formation. However, no single bioprinting technique has enabled the production of all scales and complexities of synthetic tissues to date.[262] Current printing strategies for generating vascularized constructs include inkjet bioprinting, extrusion bioprinting, and laser-assisted bioprinting.

3.3.5.1 Inkjet Bioprinting

Inkjet bioprinting is the first bioprinting technology and is similar to conventional 2D inkjet printing. A hydrogel solution with encapsulated cells (called a bioink) is stored in the ink cartridge. The cartridge is then connected to a printer head and generates droplets with controllable size. Intricate hierarchical architectures can be rapidly fabricated by controlling the dropwise deposition of cell-laden bioinks. Many studies have reported the creation of customized tissue-engineered vascular networks through this method. Lee et al. have fabricated a perfused vascular channel within a thick collagen scaffold by inkjet bioprinting.[263] After being covered by ECs, the perfused functional channel presented barrier functions for both plasma protein and dextran molecule and could support the viability of tissue up to 5 mm in distance. In another study, thermal inkjet bioprinting was used to fabricate successive layers of cellular aggregates such as microvasculature by depositing bioink consisting of human microvascular ECs and fibrin.[264] While using electrohydrodynamic (EHD) inkjet printing to create hydrogel-based microvascular tissues with hierarchical and branching channels, the minimum feature size achieved was 30 μm which close to the physical scale of native capillary blood vessels.[265]

3.3.5.2 Extrusion Bioprinting

Extrusion bioprinting is a modified method of inkjet bioprinting, which uses either an air-forced pump or a mechanical screw plunger to dispense bioinks. This method can print uninterrupted cylindrical lines rather than a single bioink droplet. Most biomaterials with variable viscosity can be printed by extrusion bioprinting, even hydrogels with high cell density.[266] While using sacrificial bioinks such as Pluronic F-127 (PLU), carbohydrate-glass, gelatin, and agarose, it is possible to create hollow channels directly. Kang et al. have used collagen and alginate solutions to prepare hepatocyte-laden bioink and EC-laden bioink to print highly vascularized complex tissue. The cell-free alginate bioink was used as the sacrificial material, and the well-organized ECs formed a lumen and finally interconnected from the lumen to the exterior of the construct.[267] More recently, the use of support bath materials has allowed the generation of more complex 3D vascular networks via extrusion bioprinting. Hinton et al. have proposed a freeform reversible embedding of suspended hydrogels technique, which enables 3D printing of hydrated materials with an elastic modulus of <500 kPa, including alginate, collagen, and fibrin.[268] The authors printed a perfusable structure using MRI data of part of the right coronary artery vascular tree and obtained a hollow lumen with a wall thickness of <1 mm.

3.3.5.3 Laser-Assisted Bioprinting

Laser-assisted bioprinting uses a laser pulse to detach cells from a donor slide and deposits them on a substrate following a specific pattern. This approach is highly monochromatic, focused, and coherent.[269] Laser-assisted bioprinting can avoid direct contact between the dispenser and the bioink, which allows achieving higher cell viability. In addition, laser-assisted printing has greater accuracy and more types of bioinks can be used than inkjet printing. Currently, this approach has been demonstrated to be a valuable technique to preorganize ECs into high cell density patterns to create a vascular network with defined architecture in tissue-engineered constructs. Wu et al. have fabricated a branch/stem structure of HUVEC and human umbilical vein smooth muscle cells (HUVSMC) by laser-assisted bioprinting. This simple structure mimics the vascular networks in natural tissue but also allows cells to develop new, finer structures away from the stem and branches.[270] In another work, ECs and MSCs were printed in a collagen hydrogel scaffold to create microvascular networks by laser-assisted bioprinting.[271] Then, this vascularized scaffold has been used to investigate the effect of distance between printed cell islets and the influence of coprinted mesenchymal cells on migration.[272]

3.3.5.4 Stereolithography Bioprinting

Stereolithography is maskless photolithography which induces photopolymerization in the desired regions to produce individual shape for each layer of the scaffold. Bioprinting through projection-based stereolithography has emerged as a high-throughput digital light processing technique that overcomes some momentary technical limitations. This method offers great biocompatibility for cell encapsulation and is superior to other bioprinting techniques.[273] It enables the generation of intricate channels with variable diameters. Therefore, stereolithography bioprinting has great potential to create perfusable cell-laden constructs with physiological complexity. Thomas et al. have designed a system of HA-based enzymatically degradable bioinks to produce perfusable vascular channels using a projection-based multimaterial stereolithographic bioprinting platform.[273] After embedding HUVECs, the vascular networks can remain stable for 28 days, which established a new strategy for 3D bioprinting of complex tissue models.

3.4 MODULATING THE PROPERTIES OF BIOMATERIALS

The scaffolds are fabricated to serve as provisional matrices for supporting cell survival and function. Materials themselves influence vascularization through regulating cell behaviors. Their physicochemical and mechanical properties have profound effects on protein adsorption and, consequently, cell binding, spreading, migration, differentiation and ECM secretion. Ideal biomaterials should provide an instructive microenvironment that responds to changes during vascularization. Modulating the material properties in terms of microstructure, bioactivity, biodegradation, mechanical property and gradient fabrication is in favor of promoting vascularization.

3.4.1 MODULATING THE MICROSTRUCTURES

Natural ECM defines a specific microstructure that can accommodate cells and allows cells to respond, maintain, and remodel their surroundings. Vascularization relies on the cues and signaling events that occur in the microenvironment. Therefore, successful construction of scaffolds to support vascularization requires the recapitulation of in vivo microenvironmental factors.[274] The scaffolds should have similar microstructures that match the porosity and topography of the native ECM, enhancing cell attachment and proliferation, and providing space for tubule formation.

The porosity of scaffold determines the total surface for cellular attachment. Proper pore size is required to allow cells to migrate into the structure, and establishing a sufficiently high specific surface for enough cells binding to the scaffold. According to O'Brien et al., the optimum pore size of a collagen scaffold for cell adhesion and migration is ~100 μm. The cell viability decreased with increasing mean pore size, but increasing linearly with the specific surface area.[275] The scaffold for skin regeneration has been proved to be inactive when the mean pore size was either lower than 20 μm or higher than 120 μm.[276] Meanwhile, the porosity of a scaffold should be not too large in case it weakens its mechanical strength.[277] These results suggest that porosity plays a key role in inducing vascularization of engineered constructs. Various processing techniques, such as salt leaching, gas foaming, freeze-drying, colloidal templating, and phase separation have been developed to control the porosity of the scaffolds. Ma and co-workers have created macroporous gelatin scaffolds by combining a thermally induced phase separation technique with a porogen-leaching process.[278] The resulting scaffolds represent a high surface area, porosity, and well-connected macropores. In bone tissue engineering, submicron-scale, pore-sized silk fibroin has been wildly attempted. A silk fibroin containing salt-leached PDLLA sponge has been developed by Stoppato et al. to mimic both porous and fibrous topographical features of natural ECM. The scaffold with multilevel pore sizes enhanced the mechanical properties and heightened its capacity to support ECs in vitro and to promote vascularization in vivo.[78] Another work has suggested that tunable pore size guides the fate of BMSCs toward chondrogenesis and endochondral ossification, and is a critical design parameter to mediate neotissue vascularization. The pore interconnectivity is critical to promote capillary ingrowth, and vascularization results in endochondral ossification and mineralized bone formation.[279]

Moreover, ECM proteins are usually assembled into 3D structures in vivo with typical topographies in the range of nano- to micrometer-scale sizes.[280] The topography of ECM, such as collagen-fiber alignment, provides guiding cues for tissue development. Nanogrooves have been found to enhance cell adhesion on the patterned surfaces. The ECs prefer to adhere and cover the aligned nanometer-scaled patterns rather than the larger micrometer-scale patterns and random nanostructured surfaces.[281] Moreover, nanofabricated substrates are demonstrated to promote the organization of EC lineages into well-defined tubular structures in vitro by inducing the contact guidance phenomenon.[282,283] Bettinger et al. found that EPCs responded to ridge-groove grating and enhanced capillary tube formation and organization.[284] Later, Dickinson and co-workers guided the ordered adhesion and tube formation of human EPCs using optimized, patterned fibronectin surfaces.[285] These approaches remind us to develop well-organized patterned nanostructures to help tubular formation. Electrospinning is often used to produce fibers that mimic the fibrillar structure of ECM. The topologies can be easily controlled by altering the diameter and arrangement of fibers. The long fibrillar structure is similar to the nano-grooves which induces alignment and directional growth of the cells and contributes to tubular formation and host blood vessel ingrowth. Barreto-Ortiz et al. represented an electrospun 3D fibrin microfiber scaffold as a novel in vitro model of microvasculature formation. Their scaffold can induce longitudinal adhesion and alignment of endothelial colony-forming cells (ECFCs), and promote these cells to deposit circumferentially organized ECM. This work demonstrated the important role of microfiber in regulating organized cell arrangement and ECM deposition.[286] In another work,

Gugutkov et al. have developed a new type of hybrid fibrinogen–PLA scaffold with random or aligned nanofibers. They found that the HUVECs showed an elongated cell shape and significantly increased cell mobility in aligned scaffolds. Significantly faster recoverage of HUVECs on aligned samples was observed while almost absent directional migration on random ones.[287,288]

However, the aforementioned works lack control over pore geometry and porous interconnectivity in the scaffold, the vascular structures formed on these porous materials are randomly organized. Some specific tissues such as cardiac and skeletal muscles have highly organized and aligned microvascular networks,[289] indicating that regular channels should be involved when fabricating scaffolds. Photo-cross-linking has been widely used to cross-link light-sensitive materials through a photomask to create open channels. To create highly aligned capillary-like networks, Nikkhah et al. have used cell-loaden GelMA to develop rectangular channels via photo-cross-linking. The result showed that highly aligned and stable capillary-like structures with circular lumens were obtained.[290] Similar capillary-like structures have been developed using PEGDA via photo-cross-linking.[291] Laser photolithography is a highly precise method that can create microchannels with defined geometrical parameters in the scaffold.[292] This approach has been used to micropattern cell adhesive ligand in hydrogels to guide cell migration along predefined 3D pathways.[293] The encapsulated fibroblasts were found to undergo guided 3D migration only onto the RGDS-patterned regions of the hydrogels, suggesting that this approach is also applicable in guiding EC growth to create a highly aligned microvascular network in 3D scaffolds. Moreover, recent advancements in high-resolution microscopy and imaging techniques enabled the development of biomimetic microvascular networks in vitro.

3.4.2 IMPROVE THE BIOACTIVITY OF SCAFFOLDS

The bioactivity of scaffolds reflects the capability of a material to affect cell behaviors.[294] Vascular cells sense their surrounding microenvironment through integrin receptors, which represent the first crucial step in vascular morphogenesis. Cell attachment is primarily mediated by integrins that bind to adhesive motifs present in various ECM proteins in the scaffolds, including fibronectin, vitronectin, laminin, and collagen.[295] Following ligand binding, the integrin cluster and cytoskeletal proteins form "focal adhesions" to provide anchorage forces and activate signaling pathways, followed by regulating the cell behavior.[296] Cell adhesion and migration depend on the available ligands exposed to cells. The ligand density is mainly determined by the composition of the scaffold. Many ECM proteins are well known to promote vascular cell adhesion, growth, migration, and survival while supporting tube formation and stabilizing blood vessels, thus incorporating ECM proteins into scaffolds may promote vascularization. Clark and co-workers have found that collagen and fibrin display synergistic effects in regulating sprouting angiogenesis. Moreover, the fibrin is essential for sprouting in the presence of angiogenic factors.[23] It seems that the addition of fibrin is conducive to promote vascularization when preparing collagen scaffolds.

One of the primary mechanisms of revascularization at ischemic sites is the secretion of GFs. These soluble GFs are crucial to recruit and differentiate vascular progenitor cells, as well as to start tube formation and stabilization. Controlled delivery of angiogenic GFs has been established as an effective method to improve vascularization of the scaffolds. The major GFs important in vascularization include isoforms of VEGF, angiopoietins (Ang), platelet-derived growth factor (PDGF-BB), bFGF, transforming growth factor-β1 (TGF-β1), HGF, and interleukin-8 (IL-8).[297] Among them, VEGF is well known to promote angiogenesis. Under the cross-linking action of calcium ions, a 3D fibrin gel with VEGF delivery has been constructed by Tan et al.[298] VEGF differentiates BMSC into CD31+ and vWF+ EC in fibrin gel and showed the potential to promote neovascularization at the injured site. After neovascular formation, the GFs secreted by both ECs and prevascular cells are responsible for tube stabilization. PDGF and TGF-β1, which are produced by the nascent blood vessel, are strong stimulators of mural cell recruitment and differentiation. The mural cells secrete Ang-1 to suppress EC apoptosis and promote lumen stabilization. Then, the ECM deposition is enhanced by TGF-β and Ang-2 to induce vessel stabilization and maturation. Therefore, it is of great concern to achieve a dynamic balance between tube formation and stabilization by delivering multiple GFs simultaneously or sequentially. Richardson et al. have reported a GF-doped PLGA scaffold with a VEGF and PDGF-BB controlled release which significantly increased the size and distribution of blood vessels.[299] Co-delivery of PDGF-BB and TGF-β1 from an injectable fibrin hydrogel stabilized neovascularization in the treatment of ischemic tissue, and the release of GFs could be controlled by modulating the degradation rate of the PEGylated scaffold.[300] Benefitting from the different affinities of VEGF and PDGF with alginate hydrogels, Hao et al. have constructed a matrix with sequential GF delivery property that could induce greater angiogenic effect and functional improvement than single factor after myocardial infarction.[301] However, the biological activity of GFs is easily lost, especially undergoing a complex manufacturing process. For heparin-binding GFs, it is a great method to stabilize the GF through binding them to a biocompatible substrate with heparin. Pieper et al. have used heparan sulfate to increase the bFGF binding capacity in collagen matrices, the more gradual and sustained release of bFGF achieved a highly vascularized scaffold after implantation.[302] Due to the short half-life and narrow therapeutic dosage of VEGF, designing biomaterials with the right spatiotemporal release of VEGF is crucial for angiogenesis.[303] Covalent immobilization can prolong the bioactivity of VEGF and Ang-1, and mature blood vessels can be found in the collagen scaffold after one-week implantation.[304] Additionally, the therapeutic potential of GFs is reported to be maximized by embedding GF-loaded particles in the biomaterials.[305]

Moreover, many peptides have been identified and have shown a promising effect on vascularization, and different types of peptide sequences have been incorporated into the scaffolds, including GF-mimicking and ECM protein-mimicking motifs.[306] The VEGF-mimicking pentadecapeptide QK can mediate ERK1/2 and Akt phosphorylation similar to full-length growth factor, as well as induce EC proliferation and migration effectively. The QK peptide was grafted to a PEG hydrogel scaffold by photo-cross-linking and showed increased bioactivity to promote microvasculature formation.[307] QK is more stable than full-length VEGF. Even so, the half-life of QK in serum is only ~4 hours, and elaborate selected carrier material and/or controlled release system is required to maintain therapeutic levels of bioactive peptide. Both matrigel and Pluronic gels have been used to sustain the release of QK, and the scaffolds showed increasing vessel density and wound closure rate.[308] Mulyasasmita et al. have extended the QK peptide with the proline-rich sequence to create bifunctional peptide conjugates capable of specific binding to a mixing-induced, two-component hydrogel scaffold while preserving their angiogenic bioactivity. Mixing of the modified QK peptide with the matrix results in an extended-release rate and exhibit vasculogenic facilitation by promoting cell migration and organization.[309] The peptide PAB2-1c has been designed to mimic PDGF, promoting sprouting, pericyte recruitment, and vessel maturation and remodeling. PBA2-1c also stimulated an increase in cell proliferation, cell migration, and collagen gel contraction. Additionally, PAB2-1c has a heparin-binding domain and that could be exploited for controlled release purposes.[310] The GHK peptide is a copper-binding sequence that comes from the cleavage of secreted protein acidic and rich in cysteine. GHK is well known to have numerous pro-angiogenic effects, including mediating VEGF and FGF secretion from fibroblast, increasing ECM production and remodeling, and promoting vessel formation.[311] After being covalently coupled to alginate hydrogel, the GHK can upregulate secretion of pro-angiogenic factors from human MSCs in culture, followed by increased EC proliferation, migration and tubule formation.[312] In addition, several cell-binding motifs based on ECM protein-mimicking peptides have been developed to modulate cell adhesion and spreading. IKVAV is derived from the α-chain of laminin and has been identified to induce EC adhesion and neovascularization. The IKVAV-grafted collagen type I scaffolds show great potential to stimulate EC migration, adhesion, and capillary network formation.[313] The integrin receptor-ligand YIGSR has been found in the β chain of laminin and plays a key role in EC interactions and tubule formation. Covalently immobilized PEG-YIGSR has resulted in significant microvascular network formation in tissue-engineered constructs.[314] The tripeptide RGD is a short biomimetic integrin-bounding motif. The binding of integrins onto the RGD motif triggers the activation of downstream signaling events mediated by Rho GTPase, Cdc42, and Rac1, which are required for lumen formation.[315] The RGD-dependent pinocytosis contributes to the formation of vacuoles and then coalesce into a developing lumen.[316] A PEG hydrogel scaffold functionalized with protease-cleavable peptide sequences and RGDs facilitated initial cell adhesion, while degradation of the polymer promoted the formation of vascular networks in cocultures of endothelial and MSC progenitor cells.[317] Even though the RGD sequence is conducive to lumen formation, it is well acknowledged that the amount of this motif can determine the extent of vascular morphogenesis. Appropriate RGD density induces cell binding and vacuole formation, but suppresses branching and sprouting with excessive RGD motifs.

3.4.3 TUNING THE BIODEGRADATION PROPERTY

The formation and stabilization of vascular networks depend on the migration and ECM remodeling of ECs and the supporting cells. Ideally, the scaffold degrades over time to allow cellular infiltration, vessel formation, and ECM secretion. It is generally accepted that the degradation rate of scaffolds should match the regeneration rate of the engineered tissue. The mechanical support of the scaffold is closely related to material degradation and ECM deposition. If ECM deposition is insufficient to support the physical entity of the scaffold, degradation of the matrix results in significant decrease of mechanical properties and finally causes scaffold disintegration. Meanwhile, the mesh size increases with the degradation process, then facilitates the diffusion of nutrients and migration of the cells. Therefore, the degradation rate should be fine-tuned to meet the scaffold remolding, so that the physical properties of the matrix remain unchanged during vascularization.

Forming chemical bonds between the polymer chains in the scaffold is a useful method in tissue engineering applications to control the degradation rate of biomaterials. Fibrin gels can support vascularization but the gels are degraded by enzyme within 2 weeks *in vivo*. By using PEGDA to create photo-cross-linkable hydrogels with fibrinogen domains, the angiogenesis of the fibrin scaffold has been enhanced while inhibiting fibrinolysis.[318] Seliktar's group has created PEGylated-fibrin constructs, and the elastic moduli (0.01–10 kPa), degradation rates, and cellular invasion kinetics can be adjusted by simply modulating the size of PEG and the ratio of fibrin to PEG.[318]

Alternatively, functional groups or enzymes can be incorporated into the scaffolds, rendering the resulting matrices achieve rational degradation behavior. ECM proteins in the scaffolds are known to be digested by MMPs. Therefore, some enzyme-cleavable peptide sequences have been identified and used to modify the matrices to enable cell-mediated proteolysis. By altering the inserted motif, the materials can be degraded under the action of target enzyme but remain stable in the presence of other enzymes.[319] Furthermore, the product of enzymolysis allows activating GFs to promote vascularization. Moreover, if an adhesive sequence is simultaneously involved, the scaffolds can promote cell migration through a cell-mediated matrix remodeling. As reported by Zisch et al., an MMP-degradable sequence was introduced into VEGF-bearing PEG scaffolds as a cross-linker, the resulting scaffolds are conducive to promote vascular healing and therapeutic angiogenesis.[320] The incorporation of non-natural amino acids has expanded our ability to control the degradation rate of the biomaterials. This approach has been demonstrated to disturb the enzymolysis and then delay material degradation. Self-assembled peptide scaffold has obtained great concern to promote vascularization, but these peptides are often associated with poor proteolytic stability. Malhotra et al. have developed self-assembled peptide/CS gels, Boc-D-Phe-γ^4-L-Phe-PEA (NH007)/CS and Boc-L-Phe-γ^4-L-Phe-PEA (NH009)/CS by complexing dipeptide NH007 or NH009 with CS in DMSO/acetic acid. Incorporating non-natural amino acids into the peptides and then complexation with CS led to an increase in stability against proteolytic degradation.[321] More recently, by using a different configuration of amino acids, Xu and co-workers have synthesized four types of polyamide-imides (PAIs) containing dipeptides of LL, DL, LD, and DD configurations. It was found that the PAIs based on the natural LL configuration of dipeptide structure are much more readily biodegradable than those based on non-natural LD, DL, and DD configuration of dipeptides.[322]

Unlike ECM components, most of the synthetic polymers are designed to degrade by ester hydrolysis. Some synthetic materials can be remolded to be biodegradable by introducing hydrolytically labile motifs such as ester bonds or cyclic acetal linkages. The degradation rate can be tailored by optimizing the hydrolyzable blocks.[323] However, the process of ester hydrolysis is uncommon in vivo, resulting in a slow degradation rate.

3.4.4 ENGINEERING SCAFFOLDS WITH RATIONAL MECHANICAL PROPERTIES

The formation of different tissues relies on the different cell types and their surroundings. In addition to chemical components, the mechanical properties of biomaterials are known to modulate cellular events, thus playing a profoundly influential role in controlling vascularization.

Dynamic material-integrin binding leads to cyclic cell adhesion and deadhesion to the scaffold, in concert with cytoskeletal contraction, the traction forces are generated and promote cell migration. Cells can sense the biomechanical properties of the scaffolds and adjust their phenotype accordingly. The substrate stiffness plays a crucial role in regulating the cell cycle through Rac1-mediated Cyclin D upregulation. The speed of cell migration reaches its maximum at an intermediate stiffness level and the cell apoptosis is enhanced on the compliant substrates.[324] Furthermore, the differentiation of cells is known to be more preferable on materials that have stiffness similar to natural tissues.[325] Matrix stiffness can regulate cell response to soluble GFs, as well as morphogenesis during angiogenic sprouting. A decrease in matrix stiffness changes the force transduction of integrin receptors, increases cell tension, and results in cytoskeletal arrangement to form branching networks.[326] Sieminski et al. cultured HUVEC in a collagen gel and found an increase in capillary branching, elongated tubes, and enlarged lumen structures when decreasing the matrix stiffness.[327] The same phenomenon has been observed in fibrin gels,[328] self-assembling peptides, and HA hydrogels.[329] By contrast, the ECs cultured on stiff substrates failed to form networks even in the presence of VEGF. In addition, the EC function was found to be influenced by matrix stiffness. Cell proliferation and migration increased with stiffness, while displaying higher endothelial function on the soft substrate, for example, nitric oxide (NO) release. VEGF treatment increases EC migration and NO release in a stiffness-dependent manner.[330,331] Due to the paracrine role in supporting endothelial tubulogenesis and vascular network formation, ASC is a promising cell source for vascular tissue engineering. Unlike EC, endogenous VEGFA expression in ASCs is enhanced on the stiff substrate, and the stiff substrate could promote angiogenesis of ASCs in the form of more ring-like formations in 2D and vessel-like structure formations in 3D compared to that of the soft substrate using ectogenic VEGFA.[332] These discoveries suggest the importance of engineering scaffolds with appropriate stiffness to support cell growth and transmit the external mechanical forces to the encapsulated cells to promote tubular network formation. Cross-linking of the biomaterial is easily manipulated to control matrix stiffness for directing vascularization. Sungwoo et al. have reported the combining of chemical cross-linking and photo-cross-linking methods to engineer dual-layer CS lactide hydrogel constructs with graded stiffness for inducing microvascular networks formation. The photo-cross-linked hydrogel is relatively stiff and possessed more compact networks, denser surface texture, and lower enzymatic degradation rates than the relatively soft, chemically cross-linked hydrogel. This dual-layer hydrogel construct enabled a lasting HUVEC aggregate-induced microvascular network due to the combination of stable substrate, enriched cell adhesion molecules, and ECM proteins.[333] Additionally, the incorporation of nanoparticles into soft materials results in increasing stiffness. Wenz et al. developed a co-culture system with two scaffolds that have different stiffness to improve vasculogenesis and bone matrix formation. GelMA with a high degree of methacrylation, methacryl-modified hyaluronic acid (HAM), and added hydroxyapatite (HAp) nanoparticles were used to prepare stiffer "bone hydrogels" for hASCs.[334] While GelMA with a lower degree of methacryloylation was used to prepare softer "vascularization hydrogels" for the encapsulation of human dermal microvascular ECs and supporting hASCs. Then the scaffolds were separated by a transwell to build a co-culture system. After 14 days, the hASC in the stiffer scaffold expressed matrix proteins like collagen type I and fibronectin, as well as bone-specific proteins osteopontin and alkaline phosphatase. Within the soft vascularization gels, the formed capillary-like networks were significantly longer after 14 days of co-culture than the structures in the control gels. In addition, the stability, as well as the complexity of the vascular networks, were significantly increased by co-culture.

Mechanical strength of biomaterials ensures the morphology of tissue-engineered constructs during fabrication and implantation. Natural proteins are widely used to produce vascularized tissues, but most of them lack mechanical strength. Hence, incorporating additional components may increase the mechanical and biological potential of the scaffold. The blended scaffolds can retain the properties of each composing material. Lesman et al. developed a fibrin-PLLA/PLGA scaffold to support in vitro construct vascularization and to enhance neovascularization upon implantation. The synthetic PLLA/PLGA sponges increased the mechanical strength of the scaffold and facilitated vessels-like networks maturation.[335] Physically cross-linked collagen hydrogels compact rapidly and exhibit limited strength, as major obstacles to generating vascular networks. To address this issue, an interpenetrating polymer network (IPN) hydrogel comprising collagen and norbornene-modified HA (NorHA) has been synthesized.[336] This dual-network hydrogel with higher strength is capable of supporting vasculogenesis. Upon iPSC-derived EPCs encapsulation, robust, and lumenized microvascular networks were found to form in IPN hydrogels over 2 weeks. Producing vascularized bone and cartilage implants has remained a challenge in the field of tissue engineering, while the mixture of materials serves as a solution to provide mechanical support and biological clues. To address this challenge, Correa and co-workers have developed an interconnected foam structure of Ti-6Al-4V within the extracellular matrix-based hydrogel. The scaffold has high porosity and tensile strength, and finally forms an endothelial network in the metal foam.[337]

Elasticity is another important mechanical property for biomaterials. Elasticity allows transmitting mechanical stimulation to the adhered cells and promotes tissue morphogenesis. Many cell behaviors are greatly influenced by elasticity such as cytoskeleton organization, cell attachment, migration, and differentiation. A scaffold with elastic properties matching the native vascular tissue produces a biomimetic environment to help tube formation and lumen stabilization. Early in 1989, Folkman's group investigated the mechanochemical switching between growth and differentiation during FGF-stimulated angiogenesis in vitro. They claimed that angiogenesis is controlled by both molecular signals and the viscoelastic properties of the surrounding matrix.[338] Byfield et al. have demonstrated that EC is sensitive to changes in substrate elasticity as low as 400 Pa after being seeded in a 3D scaffold.[339] Similar phenomenon has been observed for ECs grown on substrates of varied elasticity.[340,341] Subsequent studies have found that the vascular SMCs spreading increased quantitatively with substrate elasticity.[342] Moreover, MSCs can differentiate into SMC or EC-like cells and secret pro-angiogenic factors such as VEGF under the guidance of substrate elasticity. Lower elasticity suppresses MSCs proliferation but contributes to higher VEGF secretion activity and EC marker expression, conversely, higher elasticity leads to differentiation into SMA$^+$ cells.[343] Electrospinning and photopolymerization techniques have been used to fabricate 3D PEGDA nanofiber scaffolds with tunable elasticity. This could be a potential strategy to regulate human stem cells for generating vascularized tissues. Both collagen and elastin fibers provide tensile strength and elasticity of blood vessels, respectively. Therefore, scaffolds composed of collagen and elastin have been fabricated to replicate the elasticity of native ECM in vascular tissue engineering.[344]

3.4.5 GRADIENTS FABRICATION OF TISSUE-ENGINEERED SCAFFOLDS

The vascularization of engineered tissue either through an assembly process or via the ingrowth of a preexisting capillary network is motivated by the signals involved in the surrounding matrices.[345] During vasculogenesis, the related vascular cells respond to gradients of GFs, mechanical and physical properties of the scaffold, as well as blood flow. Typically, EC migration relies on the gradients of soluble chemoattractants, ligands, mechanical forces, and matrix properties. The development of biomimetic matrices with the spatiotemporal presentation of these gradient cues may control and guide the vascularization processes.[346] A variety of material approaches have been used to fabricate a microenvironment that induces vascular cells response to gradients, including modulation of the GFs density and oxygen diffusion, as well as the stiffness, microstructures, and binding ligands of the scaffold. Regardless of the approach, optimization of the spatial presentation of these gradient cues is important to promote vascular ingrowth and vascularization of the tissue-engineered constructs.

In the early stage of vasculogenesis, the EC in response to a gradients stimulus of angiogenesis-promoting signals such as VEGF,[347] and then differentiates to enable migration, proliferation, lumen formation, and vessel assembly. Subsequently, gradients of other GFs, for example, PDGF and TGF, are responsible for the maturation of newly formed vessels. Finally, the vessels undergo anastomosis to form a perfused vascular network. Therefore, the guided EC migration and stable neovascularization are highly dependent on GF gradients in the 3D local microenvironment. The creation of GF gradients within scaffolds for the promotion of vascularization has been achieved through the spatial distribution of GFs in biomaterials or the controlled release from GF-loaded particles. The use of microfluidic techniques allows to create stable gradients of soluble GFs in the tissue-engineered constructs for in vitro vascularization through variations in input and output flow rates and channel geometry, even the scaffolds themselves are not fabricated to contain the desired gradient.[348] Shin et al. have developed a unique 3D hydrogel scaffold with a precise gradient of soluble angiogenic factors (VEGF and Ang-1) in a microfluidic system to mimic the physiological microenvironment and found that VEGF gradient alone was sufficient in inducing a greater number of tip cells while the addition of Ang-1 to the VEGF gradient enhanced the connection of the stalk cells with the tip cells.[349] Microfluidic systems provide effective platforms for introducing GF gradients into scaffolds, but this technique was restricted to in vitro culture rather than to in vivo applications. The alternative approach that allows the spatiotemporal release of loaded GFs is controlling the properties of biomaterials or embedding particle carriers. Mooney's group has developed porous PLGA scaffolds for delivering spatial gradients of VEGF,[350] and their scaffolds led to more vasculature formation in ischemic mouse hind limbs compared to scaffolds without VEGF and scaffolds with uniformly distributed VEGF. Furthermore, to mimic the spatial and temporal signaling of multiple GFs which present in the angiogenic process, they have designed a bilayered PLGA scaffold that allowed for the sequential delivery of VEGF and PDGF.[351] The VEGF was loaded in the pores of the scaffold, and PDGF was encapsulated by PLGA microspheres in the scaffold to achieve sequential delivery. In vivo experiments showed that sequential delivery of VEGF and PDGF led to a slightly lower blood vessel density; however, vessel size and maturity were significantly enhanced. Many other publications have also suggested the importance of the gradient slope of multiple GFs in controlling vascularization.[352,353]

In addition to the GF gradients, the gradients of specific peptides or ECM proteins have been shown to guide neovascular formation. For example, the gradients of RGD motif promote preferential cell adhesion with increased ligand density.[354] Sundararaghavan et al. have created RGD gradients that vary with depth in fibrous methacrylated hyaluronic acid scaffolds by electrospinning and photopolymerization.[355] Increased cellular infiltration was found in low to high RGD gradient scaffolds compared to the high-to-low RGD gradients and uniform high RGD or uniform low RGD control scaffolds. Gradients of other ECM components, such as HA, have been shown to promote EC sprouting in vitro.[356]

Because matrix stiffness and elasticity significantly influence cell behaviors, gradients of these properties have been introduced into the scaffolds. Cross-linking is often used to fabricate gradients of stiffness by combining with precision manufacturing technologies. For example, the biomaterials and initiator were mixed to generate a concentration gradient through a microfluidic device firstly, and then the mixture can be photo-cross-linked to form stiffness gradients.[357] Moreover, the two-photon laser scanning lithography allows precise controlling to create microscale gradients.[358] Patterned gradients in ECM elasticity was demonstrated to guide SMC migration according to Wong and co-workers; hence, elasticity may be another key design parameter for modulation of cell migration for vascularization of tissue-engineered scaffolds.[359] Studies have found that the migration speed of SMC shows to have a nonlinear manner correlation with elasticity, and the optimal substrate stiffness was found to depend on the density of adhesive ligands.[360]

The microstructures of scaffolds provide specific gradients for vascular cells to organize into tubular structures. It is well known that the unique orientation, organization, and nanotopography of fibronectin is inductive of integrin-mediated vascular morphogenesis.[361] Therefore, the biomaterials were electrospun to produce fibers to control scaffold geometry and micropatterning.[362] In addition, microsphere-based scaffold fabrication techniques have been used to create structural gradients. By changing the size and distribution of microspheres, it is easy to produce scaffolds with heterogeneous porosity, microarchitecture, and spatial GF delivery. Scott et al. have fabricated a scaffold with the homogeneous presentation of RGD motifs and gradients of porosity by using microsphere-based approaches.[363] Varying the buoyancy results in controlled distribution of the microspheres, followed by microsphere leaching, gradients in porosity were created within the scaffold. The engineered scaffold showed enhanced EC infiltration from highly porous regions to the lower porous region. These studies suggest the importance of structural gradients in scaffolds for promoting vascularization.

Another gradient in scaffold fabrication is the distribution of oxygen along the scaffolds. The ECs have a signaling pathway to compensate for lower oxygen consumption, which is known as hypoxia-inducible factor-1a (HIF-1a). This transcription factor plays a critical role in both angiogenesis and vasculogenesis by upregulating the secretion of VEGF and other angiogenic cytokines. These GFs and cytokines promote the migration of ECs, as well as the mobilization and recruitment of other prevascular cells. Hence, to create an oxygen gradient in tissue-engineered constructs could, in turn, enhance vascularization.

Because multiple types of gradients influence vascularization, it is important to introduce multiple gradients of biological, mechanical, and physicochemical clues into the scaffolds simultaneously. Approaches focusing on the fabrication of controllable gradients in physicochemical and mechanical properties of the scaffolds include precise control of cross-link density, porosity, stiffness, degradation, and topographical features. While the biological gradients consist of GFs, binding motifs, ECM proteins, and cytokines. The combination of these gradients will provide effective force for promoting scaffold vascularization.

3.5   CURRENT LIMITATION AND FUTURE DIRECTIONS

Various studies have shown that vascularization can improve the survival, integration, and functionality of the newly implanted tissue-engineered constructs. Creating functional vasculature is a fundamental challenge that should be addressed when developing large-sized tissue-engineered constructs. In vitro prevascularization is expected to achieve immediate blood supply after implantation thanks to surgical anastomosis. Recent developments in this field have allowed researchers to create complex tubular structures by combining advanced manufacturing technologies and biomaterials. Unfortunately, the biological functions of these tubular networks are now far insufficient to meet the requirements of in vivo transplantation. To achieve adequate blood supply, the main vessels are demanded to be anastomosed with autogenous artery and vein. There are very few artificial vascular networks that have achieved successful perfusion in vivo because most of the engineered tissues do not have enough mechanical strength for suturing and perfusion. Furthermore, the long-term patency of these vascular constructs is essential to maintain the survival of seeded cells before scaffold remolding. It depends on the progress in constructing small-dimeter tissue-engineered blood vessels.[364] Also in vitro prevascularization is often associated with a complex in vitro culture period that might not be easy to perform in a standard hospital situation.[365] Moreover, the size, shape, and branching of the vascular networks need to be precisely controlled to fit the principle of hemodynamics and the specific shape of engineered tissue.

Recently, suspension 3D printing has provided an applicable method to generate spatially distributed vascular networks according to the natural organs.[366] However, delicate capillaries are hard to be produced as limited by the print resolution. While the main blood vessels are responsible for distributing blood in the large tissues and organs, more complex microvasculature is required for nutrients, gas, and waste diffusion between the blood and the cells of vascularized tissues. By comparison, in vivo vascularization is demonstrated to form such a mature and organized capillary network by promoting angiogenesis. Following the angiogenic process, blood circulation can be built without sewing. However, this spontaneous vascular ingrowth is a time-consuming process that relies on blood vessels to invade the scaffold from the host vasculature. In vivo vascularization is inapplicable to build large tissues with more than several millimeters as this strategy is often limited to the long time needed for complete vascularization of the whole implant. Insufficient vascularization will lead to nutrient deficiencies and/or hypoxia deeper in the scaffold due to the time-consuming process.[367] Therefore, in vivo vascularization could be a complementary means to in vitro vascularization.

Another challenge is to design a biomaterial that can satisfy the needs of mechanical and biological properties for vascularization both in vitro and in vivo. First, the biomaterial should provide morphological characteristics and sewing strength of the fabricated main vessels, supporting the attachment and function of vascular cells to maintain blood flow without thrombosis. Then, the scaffold is responsible to start cell differentiation and organization to form capillary-like structures and accelerate host vasculature ingrowth simultaneously. Finally, vascularization of the whole implant further facilitates scaffold remolding to achieve a functionalized tissue. Recent developments in biomaterials have attempted multiple strategies for improving vascularization. The biomaterials are deliberately tailored to induce cell differentiation, migration, organization, and sprouting with specific mechanical and degradation property. Furthermore, individualized microfabricating technologies for each biomaterial have been tested for constructing scaffolds and/or complex vascular networks. Further study of the biological clues in angiogenesis will give us some insights into biomaterial design. The morphogens, GFs, and scaffold remolding function sequentially and are critical guidance for vascularization. Precise control over these factors spatiotemporally by appropriate material design is known to permit specific management of vascularization. However, the traditional method to develop new biomaterials is incremental and involves iterative experiments to improve its performance. Nowadays, high-throughput methods with automatic high content image analysis can parallelly assay the cell behavior on thousands of materials.[368] Using this approach, Anderson et al. have identified polymers that control embryonic stem cell adhesion, spreading, and differentiation. This work proved that the high-throughput methods enable rapid screening of suitable materials by increasing complexity. In addition, by combining computer modeling, experimentation, and data, the material genome initiative (MGI) may cut in half the time it takes to get a newly designed biomaterial with greater vascularization for tissue engineering. MGI can increase the number of new biomaterials available in the library and lower the R&D costs.[369] Besides, whole-genome sequencing can detect early changes in cell adhesion, metabolism, proliferation, and differentiation. This advanced technology will undoubtedly speed up the process of biomaterial design to produce precisely tailored scaffolds for vascularization. To increase the chances of success and reduce the waste of time and resources, researchers should not focus on only one of these strategies. Instead, an integrated approach is encouraged in material design to foster strengths and circumvent weaknesses, and then provide a real solution in the near future.

ACKNOWLEDGEMENTS

This work was supported by the National Natural Science Foundation of China (82001966), China Postdoctoral Science Foundation (2020M673653), National Science Foundation of Chongqing, China (cstc2020jcyj-bshX0063), National Science Fund for Distinguished Young Scholars (31625011), National Key K&D Program of China (2016YFC1101100), and Key Project of the National Natural Science Foundation of China (81830055). Particularly, Yonghong Fan thanks the Science and Technology Innovation Enhancement Project of Third Military Medical University (2020XQN03), Youqian Xu thanks the Scientific Research Foundation of Third Military Medical University.

REFERENCES

1. Langer R, Vacanti J P. Tissue engineering. *Science*, 1993, 260(5110): 920–926.
2. Carmeliet P, Jain R K. Angiogenesis in cancer and other diseases. *Nature*, 2000, 407(6801): 249–257.
3. Laschke M W, Harder Y, Amon M, et al. Angiogenesis in tissue engineering: Breathing life into constructed tissue substitutes. *Tissue Engineering*, 2006, 12(8): 2093–2104.
4. Hanjaya-Putra D, Wanjare M, Gerecht S. Biomaterials approaches in vascular engineering: A review of past and future trends, Burdick J A, Mauck R L, editor, *Biomaterials for Tissue Engineering Applications: A Review of the Past and Future Trends*, Vienna: Springer Vienna, 2011: pp. 457–487.
5. Hussey G S, Dziki J L, Badylak S F. Extracellular matrix-based materials for regenerative medicine. *Nature Reviews Materials*, 2018, 3(7): 159–173.
6. Chattopadhyay S, Raines R T. Collagen-based biomaterials for wound healing. *Biopolymers*, 2014, 101(8): 821–833.
7. Davis G E, Bayless K J. An integrin and Rho GTPase-dependent pinocytic vacuole mechanism controls capillary lumen formation in collagen and fibrin matrices. *Microcirculation*, 2003, 10(1): 27–44.
8. Zhou Z, Pausch F, Schlötzer-Schrehardt U, et al. Induction of initial steps of angiogenic differentiation and maturation of endothelial cells by pericytes in vitro and the role of collagen IV. *Histochemistry and Cell Biology*, 2016, 145(5): 511–525.
9. Bonanno E, Iurlaro M, Madri J A, et al. Type IV collagen modulates angiogenesis and neovessel survival in the rat aorta model. *In Vitro Cellular & Developmental Biology - Animal*, 2000, 36(5): 336–340.
10. Lee A, Hudson A R, Shiwarski D J, et al. 3D bioprinting of collagen to rebuild components of the human heart. *Science*, 2019, 365(6452): 482–487.

11. Hertweck J, Ritz U, Götz H, et al. CD34+ cells seeded in collagen scaffolds promote bone formation in a mouse calvarial defect model. *Journal of Biomedical Materials Research Part B: Applied Biomaterials*, 2018, 106(4): 1505–1516.
12. Vlahos A E, Kinney S M, Kingston B R, et al. Endothelialized collagen based pseudo-islets enables tuneable subcutaneous diabetes therapy. *Biomaterials*, 2020, 232: 119710.
13. Vuornos K, Huhtala H, Kääriäinen M, et al. Bioactive glass ions for in vitro osteogenesis and microvascularization in gellan gum-collagen hydrogels. *Journal of Biomedical Materials Research Part B: Applied Biomaterials*, 2020, 108(4): 1332–1342.
14. Qu Y, Cao C, Wu Q, et al. The dual delivery of KGF and bFGF by collagen membrane to promote skin wound healing. *Journal of Tissue Engineering and Regenerative Medicine*, 2018, 12(6): 1508–1518.
15. Baheiraei N, Nourani M R, Mortazavi S M J, et al. Development of a bioactive porous collagen/β-tricalcium phosphate bone graft assisting rapid vascularization for bone tissue engineering applications. *Journal of Biomedical Materials Research Part A*, 2018, 106(1): 73–85.
16. Sun J L, Jiao K, Song Q, et al. Intrafibrillar silicified collagen scaffold promotes in-situ bone regeneration by activating the monocyte p38 signaling pathway. *Acta Biomaterialia*, 2018, 67: 354–365.
17. França C M, Thrivikraman G, Athirasala A, et al. The influence of osteopontin-guided collagen intrafibrillar mineralization on pericyte differentiation and vascularization of engineered bone scaffolds. *Journal of Biomedical Materials Research Part B: Applied Biomaterials*, 2019, 107(5): 1522–1532.
18. Litvinov R I, Gorkun O V, Galanakis D K, et al. Polymerization of fibrin: Direct observation and quantification of individual B:b knob-hole interactions. *Blood*, 2006, 109(1): 130–138.
19. Laurens N, Koolwijk P, De Maat M P M. Fibrin structure and wound healing. *Journal of Thrombosis and Haemostasis*, 2006, 4(5): 932–939.
20. Kaijzel E L, Koolwijk P, Van Erck M G M, et al. Molecular weight fibrinogen variants determine angiogenesis rate in a fibrin matrix in vitro and in vivo. *Journal of Thrombosis and Haemostasis*, 2006, 4(9): 1975–1981.
21. Sahni A, Sahni Sanjeev K, Francis Charles W. Endothelial cell activation by IL-1β in the presence of fibrinogen requires αVβ3. *Arteriosclerosis, Thrombosis, and Vascular Biology*, 2005, 25(10): 2222–2227.
22. Altieri D C, Plescia J, Thornton G B, et al. Structural recognition of a novel fibrinogen chain sequence (117133) by intercellular adhesion molecule-1 mediates leukocyte-endothelium interaction. *Journal of Biological Chemistry*, 1995, 270(2): 696–699.
23. Feng X, Tonnesen M G, Mousa S A, et al. Fibrin and collagen differentially but synergistically regulate sprout angiogenesis of human dermal microvascular endothelial cells in 3-dimensional matrix. *International Journal of Cell Biology*, 2013, 2013: 231279–231290.
24. Sproul E, Nandi S, Brown A. Fibrin biomaterials for tissue regeneration and repair, Barbosa M A, Martins M C L, editor, *Peptides and Proteins as Biomaterials for Tissue Regeneration and Repair*. Cambridge, UK: Woodhead Publishing, 2018: pp. 151–173.
25. Chen X, Aledia A S, Ghajar C M, et al. Prevascularization of a fibrin-based tissue construct accelerates the formation of functional anastomosis with host vasculature. *Tissue Engineering Part A*, 2008, 15(6): 1363–1371.
26. Lee J, Kim E H, Shin D, et al. Accelerated oral wound healing using a pre-vascularized mucosal cell sheet. *Scientific Reports*, 2017, 7(1): 10667–10667.
27. Riemenschneider S, Mattia D, Wendel J, et al. Inosculation and perfusion of pre-vascularized tissue patches containing aligned human microvessels after myocardial infarction. *Biomaterials*, 2016, 97: 51–61.

28. Acosta F M, Stojkova K, Brey E M, et al. A straightforward approach to engineer vascularized adipose tissue using microvascular fragments. *Tissue Engineering Part A*, 2020, 26(15–16): 905–914.

29. Kreimendahl F, Ossenbrink S, Köpf M, et al. Combination of vascularization and cilia formation for three-dimensional airway tissue engineering. *Journal of Biomedical Materials Research Part A*, 2019, 107(9): 2053–2062.

30. Rambøl M H, Han E, Niklason L E. Microvessel network formation and interactions with pancreatic islets in three-dimensional chip cultures. *Tissue Engineering Part A*, 2019, 26(9–10): 556–568.

31. Roux B M, Akar B, Zhou W, et al. Preformed vascular networks survive and enhance vascularization in critical sized cranial defects. *Tissue Engineering Part A*, 2018, 24(21–22): 1603–1615.

32. Nam K, Dean S M, Brown C T, et al. Synergistic effects of laminin-1 peptides, VEGF and FGF9 on salivary gland regeneration. *Acta Biomaterialia*, 2019, 91: 186–194.

33. Shaikh F M, Callanan A, Kavanagh E G, et al. Fibrin: A natural biodegradable scaffold in vascular tissue engineering. *Cells Tissues Organs*, 2008, 188(4): 333–346.

34. Vogel V, Baneyx G. The tissue engineering puzzle: A molecular perspective. *Annual Review of Biomedical Engineering*, 2003, 5(1): 441–463.

35. Astrof S, Crowley D, Hynes R O. Multiple cardiovascular defects caused by the absence of alternatively spliced segments of fibronectin. *Developmental Biology*, 2007, 311(1): 11–24.

36. An B, Abbonante V, Yigit S, et al. Definition of the native and denatured type II collagen binding site for fibronectin using a recombinant collagen system. *Journal of Biological Chemistry*, 2014, 289(8): 4941–4951.

37. Schechner J S, Nath A K, Zheng L, et al. In vivo formation of complex microvessels lined by human endothelial cells in an immunodeficient mouse. *Proceedings of the National Academy of Sciences of the United States of America*, 2000, 97(16): 9191–9196.

38. Shepherd B R, Jay S M, Saltzman W M, et al. Human aortic smooth muscle cells promote arteriole formation by coengrafted endothelial cells. *Tissue Engineering Part A*, 2008, 15(1): 165–173.

39. Zhou C, Cai X, Grottkau B E, et al. BMP4 promotes vascularization of human adipose stromal cells and endothelial cells in vitro and in vivo. *Cell Proliferation*, 2013, 46(6): 695–704.

40. Wijelath Errol S, Rahman S, Namekata M, et al. Heparin-II domain of fibronectin is a vascular endothelial growth factor-binding domain. *Circulation Research*, 2006, 99(8): 853–860.

41. Llopis Hernández V, Cantini M, Gonzalez-Garcia C, et al. Material-driven fibronectin assembly for high-efficiency presentation of growth factors. *Science Advances*, 2016, 2: e1600188–e1600188.

42. Moulisová V, Gonzalez-García C, Cantini M, et al. Engineered microenvironments for synergistic VEGF - Integrin signalling during vascularization. *Biomaterials*, 2017, 126: 61–74.

43. Trujillo S, Gonzalez-Garcia C, Rico P, et al. Engineered 3D hydrogels with full-length fibronectin that sequester and present growth factors. *Biomaterials*, 2020, 252: 120104.

44. Störmann P, Kupsch J, Kontradowitz K, et al. Cultivation of EPC and co-cultivation with MSC on β-TCP granules in vitro is feasible without fibronectin coating but influenced by scaffolds' design. *European Journal of Trauma and Emergency Surgery*, 2019, 45(3): 527–538.

45. Seebach C, Henrich D, Kähling C, et al. Endothelial progenitor cells and mesenchymal stem cells seeded onto β-TCP granules enhance early vascularization and bone healing in a critical-sized bone defect in rats. *Tissue Engineering Part A*, 2010, 16(6): 1961–1970.

46. Nair L S, Laurencin C T. Polymers as biomaterials for tissue engineering and controlled drug delivery, Lee K, Kaplan D, editor, *Tissue Engineering I*, Berlin, Heidelberg: Springer Berlin Heidelberg, 2006: 47–90.
47. Djabourov M, Papon P. Influence of thermal treatments on the structure and stability of gelatin gels. *Polymer*, 1983, 24(5): 537–542.
48. Van Den Steen P E, Dubois B, Nelissen I, et al. Biochemistry and molecular biology of Gelatinase B or Matrix Metalloproteinase-9 (MMP-9). *Critical Reviews in Biochemistry and Molecular Biology*, 2002, 37(6): 375–536.
49. Gorgieva S, Kokol V. Collagen- vs. Gelatine-based biomaterials and their biocompatibility: Review and perspectives, Pignatello R, editor, *Biomaterials Applications for Nanomedicine. London, UK*: InTechOpen, 2011:17_52.
50. Lee Y, Balikov D A, Lee J B, et al. In situ forming gelatin hydrogels-directed angiogenic differentiation and activity of patient-derived human mesenchymal stem cells. *International Journal of Molecular Sciences*, 2017, 18(8): 1705.
51. Hirai K, Tabata Y, Hasegawa S, et al. Enhanced intestinal anastomotic healing with gelatin hydrogel incorporating basic fibroblast growth factor. *Journal of Tissue Engineering and Regenerative Medicine*, 2016, 10(10): E433–E442.
52. Zheng Y, Yuan W, Liu H, et al. Injectable supramolecular gelatin hydrogel loading of resveratrol and histatin-1 for burn wound therapy. *Biomaterials Science*, 2020, 8(17): 4810–4820.
53. Claaßen C, Sewald L, Tovar G E M, et al. Controlled release of vascular endothelial growth factor from heparin-functionalized gelatin type A and albumin hydrogels. *Gels*, 2017, 3(4): 35.
54. Yu T, Dong C, Shen Z, et al. Vascularization of plastic calcium phosphate cement in vivo induced by in-situ-generated hollow channels. *Materials Science and Engineering: C*, 2016, 68: 153–162.
55. Zhong M, Wei D, Yang Y, et al. Vascularization in engineered tissue construct by assembly of cellular patterned micromodules and degradable microspheres. *ACS Applied Materials & Interfaces*, 2017, 9(4): 3524–3534.
56. Chrobak K M, Potter D R, Tien J. Formation of perfused, functional microvascular tubes in vitro. *Microvascular Research*, 2006, 71(3): 185–196.
57. Liu J, Chuah Y J, Fu J, et al. Co-culture of human umbilical vein endothelial cells and human bone marrow stromal cells into a micro-cavitary gelatin-methacrylate hydrogel system to enhance angiogenesis. *Materials Science and Engineering: C*, 2019, 102: 906–916.
58. Fu J, Wiraja C, Muhammad H, et al. Improvement of endothelial progenitor outgrowth cell (EPOC)-mediated vascularization in gelatin-based hydrogels through pore size manipulation. *Acta Biomaterialia*, 2017, 58: 255–237.
59. Leong W, Fan C, Wang D-A. A novel gelatin-based micro-cavitary hydrogel for potential application in delivery of anchorage dependent cells: A study with vasculogenesis model. *Colloids and Surfaces B: Biointerfaces*, 2016, 146: 334–342.
60. Leucht A, Volz A-C, Rogal J, et al. Advanced gelatin-based vascularization bioinks for extrusion-based bioprinting of vascularized bone equivalents. *Scientific Reports*, 2020, 10: 5330.
61. Sun X, Lang Q, Zhang H, et al. Electrospun photocrosslinkable hydrogel fibrous scaffolds for rapid in vivo vascularized skin flap regeneration. *Advanced Functional Materials*, 2017, 27(2): 1604617.
62. Hinman M B, Jones J A, Lewis R V. Synthetic spider silk: A modular fiber. *Trends in Biotechnology*, 2000, 18(9): 374–379.
63. Chen X, Zaro J L, Shen W-C. Fusion protein linkers: Property, design and functionality. *Advanced Drug Delivery Reviews*, 2013, 65(10): 1357–1369.

64. Thurber A E, Omenetto F G, Kaplan D L. In vivo bioresponses to silk proteins. *Biomaterials*, 2015, 71: 145–157.
65. Ghanaati S, Unger R, Webber M, et al. Scaffold vascularization in vivo driven by primary human osteoblasts in concert with host inflammatory cells. *Biomaterials*, 2011, 32: 8150–8160.
66. Woloszyk A, Buschmann J, Waschkies C, et al. Human dental pulp stem cells and gingival fibroblasts seeded into silk fibroin scaffolds have the same ability in attracting vessels. *Frontiers in Physiology*, 2016, 7: 140–140.
67. Zhong J, Xu J, Lu S, et al. A prevascularization strategy using novel fibrous porous silk scaffolds for tissue regeneration in mice with spinal cord injury. *Stem Cells and Development*, 2020, 29(9): 615–624.
68. Zhang W, Wray L, Rnjak-Kovacina J, et al. Vascularization of hollow channel-modified porous silk scaffolds with endothelial cells for tissue regeneration. *Biomaterials*, 2015, 56: 68–77.
69. Rnjak-Kovacina J, Wray L S, Golinski J M, et al. Arrayed hollow channels in silk-based scaffolds provide functional outcomes for engineering critically sized tissue constructs. *Advanced Functional Materials*, 2014, 24(15): 2188–2196.
70. Baptista M, Joukhdar H, Alcala-Orozco C R, et al. Silk fibroin photo-lyogels containing microchannels as a biomaterial platform for in situ tissue engineering. *Biomaterials Science*, 2020, 8(24): 7093–7105.
71. Rnjak-Kovacina J, Gerrand Y-W, Wray L S, et al. Vascular pedicle and microchannels: Simple methods toward effective in vivo vascularization of 3D scaffolds. *Advanced Healthcare Materials*, 2019, 8(24): 1901106.
72. Tang F, Manz X D, Bongers A, et al. Microchannels are an architectural cue that promotes integration and vascularization of silk biomaterials in vivo. *ACS Biomaterials Science & Engineering*, 2020, 6(3): 1476–1486.
73. Lu G, Ding Z, Wei Y, et al. Anisotropic biomimetic silk scaffolds for improved cell migration and healing of skin wounds. *ACS Applied Materials & Interfaces*, 2018, 10(51): 44314–44323.
74. Ding Z Z, Ma J, He W, et al. Simulation of ECM with silk and chitosan nanocomposite materials. *Journal of Materials Chemistry B*, 2017, 5(24): 4789–4796.
75. Yao D, Qian Z, Zhou J, et al. Facile incorporation of REDV into porous silk fibroin scaffolds for enhancing vascularization of thick tissues. *Materials Science and Engineering: C*, 2018, 93: 96–105.
76. Johansson U, Shalaly N D, Hjelm L C, et al. Integration of primary endocrine cells and supportive cells using functionalized silk promotes the formation of prevascularized islet-like clusters. *ACS Biomaterials Science & Engineering*, 2020, 6(2): 1186–1195.
77. Yao D, Peng G, Qian Z, et al. Regulating coupling efficiency of REDV by controlling silk fibroin structure for vascularization. *ACS Biomaterials Science & Engineering*, 2017, 3(12): 3515–3524.
78. Stoppato M, Stevens H, Carletti E, et al. Effects of silk fibroin fiber incorporation on mechanical properties, endothelial cell colonization and vascularization of PDLLA scaffolds. *Biomaterials*, 2013, 34(19): 4573–4581.
79. Wang Y, Yao D, Li L, et al. Effect of electrospun silk fibroin-silk sericin films on macrophage polarization and vascularization. *ACS Biomaterials Science & Engineering*, 2020, 6(6): 3502–3512.
80. Ding Z, Zhou M, Zhou Z, et al. Injectable silk nanofiber hydrogels for sustained release of small-molecule drugs and vascularization. *ACS Biomaterials Science & Engineering*, 2019, 5(8): 4077–4088.
81. Sun W, Motta A, Shi Y, et al. Co-culture of outgrowth endothelial cells with human mesenchymal stem cells in silk fibroin hydrogels promotes angiogenesis. *Biomedical Materials*, 2016, 11(3): 035009.

82. Han H, Ning H, Liu S, et al. Silk biomaterials with vascularization capacity. *Advanced Functional Materials*, 2016, 26(3): 421–432.
83. Sheehy E, Mesallati T, Vinardell T, et al. Engineering cartilage or endochondral bone: A comparison of different naturally derived hydrogels. *Acta Biomaterialia*, 2014, 13: 245–253.
84. Deng C, Vulesevic B, Ellis C, et al. Vascularization of collagen–chitosan scaffolds with circulating progenitor cells as potential site for islet transplantation. *Journal of Controlled Release*, 2011, 152: e196–e198.
85. Ellis C, Suuronen E, Yeung T, et al. Bioengineering a highly vascularized matrix for the ectopic transplantation of islets. *Islets*, 2013, 5(5): 216–225.
86. Ahtzaz S, Waris T, Shahzadi L, et al. Boron for tissue regeneration-it's loading into chitosan/collagen hydrogels and testing on chorioallantoic membrane to study the effect on angiogenesis. *International Journal of Polymeric Materials and Polymeric Biomaterials*, 2020, 69: 525–534.
87. Ahmadi A, Vulesevic B, Ruel M, et al. A collagen-chitosan injectable hydrogel improves vascularization and cardiac remodeling in a mouse model of chronic myocardial infarction. *Canadian Journal of Cardiology*, 2013, 29(10): S203–S204.
88. Liu C, Liu Y, Li S, et al. Bioprinted chitosan and hydroxyapatite micro-channels structures scaffold for vascularization of bone regeneration. *Journal of Biomaterials and Tissue Engineering*, 2017, 7: 28–34.
89. Zhang W, Choi J, He X. Engineering microvascularized 3D tissue using alginate-chitosan microcapsules. *Journal of Biomaterials and Tissue Engineering*, 2017, 7: 170–173.
90. Linh N T B, Abueva C D G, Lee B-T. Enzymatic in situ formed hydrogel from gelatin–tyramine and chitosan-4-hydroxylphenyl acetamide for the co-delivery of human adipose-derived stem cells and platelet-derived growth factor towards vascularization. *Biomedical Materials*, 2017, 12(1): 015026.
91. Shu Y, Hao T, Yao F, et al. RoY peptide modified chitosan based hydrogel to improve angiogenesis and cardiac repair under hypoxia. *ACS Applied Materials & Interfaces*, 2015, 7(12): 6505–6517.
92. Han G, Zheng Z, Pan Z, et al. Sulfated chitosan coated polylactide membrane enhanced osteogenic and vascularization differentiation in MC3T3-E1s and HUVECs co-cultures system. *Carbohydrate Polymers*, 2020, 245: 116522.
93. Yu Y, Chen J, Chen R, et al. Enhancement of VEGF-mediated angiogenesis by 2-N, 6-O-Sulfated Chitosan-coated hierarchical PLGA scaffolds. *ACS Applied Materials & Interfaces*, 2015, 7(18): 9982–9990.
94. Chen Z, Wang W, Guo L, et al. Preparation of enzymatically cross-linked sulfated chitosan hydrogel and its potential application in thick tissue engineering. *Science China Chemistry*, 2013, 56: 1701–1709.
95. Wang C, Yu Y, Chen H, et al. Construct cytokine reservoirs based on sulfated chitosan hydrogels for the capturing of VEGF in situ. *Journal of Materials Chemistry B*, 2019, 7: 1882–1892.
96. Yang J, Xie Q, Jianfeng Z, et al. Preparation and In vitro antioxidant activities of 6-amino-6-deoxychitosan and its sulfonated derivatives. *Biopolymers*, 2015, 103: 539–549.
97. Qu G, Wu X, Yin L, et al. N-octyl-O-sulfate chitosan-modified liposomes for delivery of docetaxel: Preparation, characterization, and pharmacokinetics. *Biomedicine & Pharmacotherapy = Biomédecine & Pharmacothérapie*, 2012, 66: 46–51.
98. Han G, Xia X, Pan Z, et al. Different influence of sulfated chitosan with different sulfonic acid group sites on HUVECs behaviors. *Journal of Biomaterials Science, Polymer Edition*, 2020, 31: 1–17.
99. Li W, Wu D, Tan J, et al. A gene-activating skin substitute comprising PLLA/POSS nanofibers and plasmid DNA encoding ANG and bFGF promotes in vivo revascularization and epidermalization. *Journal of Materials Chemistry B*, 2018, 6(43): 6977–6992.

100. Tan Q, Tang H, Hu J, et al. Controlled release of chitosan/heparin nanoparticle-delivered VEGF enhances regeneration of decellularized tissue-engineered scaffolds. *International Journal of Nanomedicine*, 2011, 6: 929–942.
101. Choi J, Yoo H. Chitosan/pluronic hydrogel containing bFGF/heparin for encapsulation of human dermal fibroblasts. *Journal of Biomaterials Science. Polymer Edition*, 2013, 24: 210–223.
102. Parajó Y, D'angelo I, Welle A, et al. Hyaluronic acid/Chitosan nanoparticles as delivery vehicles for VEGF and PDGF-BB. *Drug Delivery*, 2010, 17: 596–604.
103. Kim I Y, Seo S-J, Moon H-S, et al. Chitosan and its derivatives for tissue engineering applications. *Biotechnology Advances*, 2008, 26: 1–21.
104. Wu S-C, Chen C-H, Chang J-K, et al. Hyaluronan initiates chondrogenesis mainly via CD44 in human adipose-derived stem cells. *Journal of Applied Physiology*, 2013, 114(11): 1610–1618.
105. Missinato M, Tobita K, Romano N, et al. Extracellular component hyaluronic acid and its receptor Hmmr are required for epicardial EMT during heart regeneration. *Cardiovascular Research*, 2015, 107(4): 487–498.
106. Li J, Wu F, Zhang K, et al. Controlling molecular weight of hyaluronic acid conjugated on amine-rich surface: Toward better multifunctional biomaterials for cardiovascular implants. *ACS Applied Materials & Interfaces*, 2017, 9(36): 30343–30358.
107. Monzack E, Rodriguez K, Mccoy C, et al. Natural materials in tissue engineering application, Burdick J A, Mauck R L, editors, *Biomaterials for Tissue Engineering Applications: A Review of the Past and Future Trends*. Vienna: Springer, 2011: pp. 209–241.
108. Portalska K, Moreira Teixeira L, Leijten J, et al. Boosting angiogenesis and functional vascularization in injectable dextran-hyaluronic acid hydrogels by endothelial-like mesenchymal stromal cells. *Tissue engineering. Part A*, 2013, 20(3–4): 819–829.
109. Yee D, Putra D, Bose V, et al. Hyaluronic acid hydrogels support cord-like structures from endothelial colony-forming cells. *Tissue engineering. Part A*, 2011, 17: 1351–1361.
110. Tang Z, Liao W-Y, Tang A, et al. The enhancement of endothelial cell therapy for angiogenesis in hindlimb ischemia using hyaluronan. *Biomaterials*, 2010, 32: 75–86.
111. Peattie R, Rieke E, Hewett E, et al. Dual growth factor-induced angiogenesis in vivo using hyaluronan hydrogel implants. *Biomaterials*, 2006, 27: 1868–1875.
112. Peattie R, Fisher R. Effect of gelatin on heparin regulation of cytokine release from hyaluronan-based hydrogels. *Drug Delivery*, 2008, 15:363–371.
113. Elia R, Fuegy P, Vandelden A, et al. Stimulation of in vivo angiogenesis by in situ cross-linked, dual growth factor-loaded, glycosaminoglycan hydrogels. *Biomaterials*, 2010, 31: 4630–4638.
114. Cerqueira M, Silva L, Santos T, et al. Gellan gum-hyaluronic acid spongy-like hydrogels and cells from adipose tissue synergize promoting neoskin vascularization. *ACS Applied Materials & Interfaces*, 2014, 6(22): 19668–19679.
115. Silva L, Pirraco R, Santos T, et al. Neovascularization induced by the hyaluronic acid-based spongy-like hydrogels degradation products. *ACS Applied Materials & Interfaces*, 2016, 8(49): 33464–33474.
116. Prestwich G, Kuo J-W. Chemically-modified HA for therapy and regenerative medicine. *Current Pharmaceutical Biotechnology*, 2008, 9: 242–245.
117. Jiang L, Luo Y. Guided assembly of endothelial cells on hydrogel matrices patterned with microgrooves: A basic model for microvessel engineering. *Soft Matter*, 2012, 9: 1113–1121.
118. Zhang Q, Wei X, Ji Y, et al. Adjustable and ultrafast light-cured hyaluronic acid hydrogel: Promoting biocompatibility and cell growth. *Journal of Materials Chemistry B*, 2020, 8(25): 5441–5450.

119. Hozumi T, Kageyama T, Ohta S, et al. Injectable hydrogel with slow degradability composed of gelatin and hyaluronic acid cross-linked by Schiff's base formation. *Biomacromolecules*, 2017, 19(2): 288–297.

120. Lin H, Wang C-K, Tung Y-C, et al. Increased vasculogenesis of endothelial cells in hyaluronic acid augmented fibrin-based natural hydrogels - from in vitro to in vivo models. *European Cells & Materials*, 2020, 40: 133–145.

121. Augst A, Kong H, Mooney D. Alginate hydrogels as biomaterials. *Macromolecular Bioscience*, 2006, 6: 623–633.

122. Wang B, Wang W, Yu Y, et al. The study of angiogenesis stimulated by multivalent peptide ligand-modified alginate. *Colloids and Surfaces B: Biointerfaces*, 2017, 154: 383–390.

123. Hartrianti P, Nguyen L, Johanes J, et al. Fabrication and characterization of a novel cross-linked human keratin-alginate sponge. *Journal of Tissue Engineering and Regenerative Medicine*, 2016, 11(9): 2590–2602.

124. Solovieva E, Teterina A Y, Klein O, et al. Sodium alginate-based composites as a collagen substitute for skin bioengineering. *Biomedical Materials*, 2020, 9(1): 015002.

125. Hao Y, Zhao W, Zhang L, et al. Bio-multifunctional alginate/chitosan/Fucoidan sponges with enhanced angiogenesis and hair follicle regeneration for promoting full-thickness wound healing. *Materials & Design*, 2020, 193: 108863.

126. Liu Q, Huang Y, Lan Y, et al. Acceleration of skin regeneration in full-thickness burns by incorporation of bFGF-loaded alginate microspheres into a CMCS-PVA hydrogel. *Journal of Tissue Engineering and Regenerative Medicine*, 2015, 11(5): 1562–1573.

127. Quinlan E, López-Noriega A, Thompson E M, et al. Controlled release of vascular endothelial growth factor from spray-dried alginate microparticles in collagen–hydroxyapatite scaffolds for promoting vascularization and bone repair. *Journal of Tissue Engineering and Regenerative Medicine*, 2017, 11(4): 1097–1109.

128. Guerreiro S, Oliveira M, Barbosa M, et al. Neonatal human dermal fibroblasts immobilized in RGD-alginate induce angiogenesis. *Cell Transplantation*, 2013, 23(8): 945–957.

129. Yang I H, Chen Y-S, Li J-J, et al. The development of laminin-alginate microspheres encapsulated with ginsenoside Rg1 and ADSCs for breast reconstruction after lumpectomy. *Bioactive Materials*, 2021, 6: 1699–1710.

130. Contessi Negrini N, Bonnetier M, Giatsidis G, et al. Tissue-mimicking gelatin scaffolds by alginate sacrificial templates for adipose tissue engineering. *Acta Biomaterialia*, 2019, 87: 61–75.

131. Zhou Q, Kang H, Bielec M, et al. Influence of different divalent ions cross-linking Sodium Alginate-Polyacrylamide hydrogels on antibacterial properties and wound healing. *Carbohydrate Polymers*, 2018, 197: 292–304.

132. Ferreira L, Rafael A, Lamghari M, et al. Biocompatibility of chemoenzymatically derived dextran-acrylate hydrogels. *Journal of Biomedical Materials Research. Part A*, 2004, 68: 584–596.

133. Sun X, Zhang H, He J, et al. Adjustable hardness of hydrogel for promoting vascularization and maintaining stemness of stem cells in skin flap regeneration. *Applied Materials Today*, 2018, 13: 54–63.

134. Weber D, Torger B, Richter K, et al. Interaction of poly(l-lysine)/polysaccharide complex nanoparticles with human vascular endothelial cells. *Nanomaterials*, 2018, 8: 358.

135. Tang R, Xin W, Zhang H, et al. Promoting early neovascularization of SIS-repaired abdominal wall by controlled release of bioactive VEGF. *RSC Advances*, 2018, 8: 4548–4560.

136. Stahl P, Chan T, Shen Y I, et al. Capillary Network-Like Organization of Endothelial Cells in PEGDA Scaffolds Encoded with Angiogenic Signals via Triple Helical Hybridization. *Advanced Functional Materials*, 2014, 24(21): 3213–3225.

137. Ferreira L, Gerecht S, Fuller J, et al. Bioactive hydrogel scaffolds for controllable vascular differentiation of human embryonic stem cells. *Biomaterials*, 2007, 28: 2706–2717.
138. Trappmann B, Baker B, Polacheck W, et al. Matrix degradability controls multicellularity of 3D cell migration. *Nature Communications*, 2017, 8(1): 371.
139. Sun G, Zhang X, Shen Y I, et al. Dextran hydrogel scaffolds enhance angiogenic responses and promote complete skin regeneration during burn wound healing. *Proceedings of the National Academy of Sciences of the United States of America*, 2011, 108: 20976–20981.
140. Sun G, Shen Y-I, Kusuma S, et al. Functional neovascularization of biodegradable dextran hydrogels with multiple angiogenic growth factors. *Biomaterials*, 2011, 32(1): 95–106.
141. Turner P, Murray E, Mcadam J, et al. Peptide chitosan/dextran core/shell vascularized 3D constructs for wound healing. *ACS Applied Materials & Interfaces*, 2020, 12(29): 32328–32339.
142. Simon-Yarza T, Labour M-N, Aid R, et al. Channeled polysaccharide-based hydrogel reveals influence of curvature to guide endothelial cell arrangement in vessel-like structures. *Materials Science and Engineering: C*, 2020, 118: 111369.
143. Rujitanaroj P-O, Aid R, Chew S Y, et al. Polysaccharide electrospun fibers with sulfated poly(fucose) promote endothelial cell migration and VEGF-mediated angiogenesis. *Biomaterials Science*, 2014, 2: 843.
144. Cox T, Erler J. Remodeling and homeostasis of the extracellular matrix: Implications for fibrotic diseases and cancer. *Disease Models & Mechanisms*, 2011, 4: 165–178.
145. Mecham R P. Overview of extracellular matrix. *Current Protocols in Cell Biology*, 2012, 57(1): 10.11.11–10.11.16.
146. Young J, Holle A, Spatz J. Nanoscale and mechanical properties of the physiological cell-ECM microenvironment. *Experimental Cell Research*, 2015, 343(1): 3–6.
147. Keane T, Swinehart I, Badylak S. Methods of tissue decellularization used for preparation of biologic scaffolds and in-vivo relevance. *Methods (San Diego, Calif.)*, 2015, 84: 25–34.
148. Crapo P, Gilbert T, Badylak S. An overview of tissue and whole organ decellularisation processes. *Biomaterials*, 2011, 32: 3233–3243.
149. Zhang L, Qian Z, Tahtinen M, et al. Prevascularization of natural nanofibrous extracellular matrix for engineering completely biological three-dimensional prevascularized tissues for diverse applications. *Journal of Tissue Engineering and Regenerative Medicine*, 2018, 12(3): e1325–e1336.
150. Qian Z, Sharma D, Jia W, et al. Engineering stem cell cardiac patch with microvascular features representative of native myocardium. *Theranostics*, 2019, 9: 2143–2157.
151. Du P, Suhaeri M, Ha S S, et al. Human lung fibroblast-derived matrix facilitates vascular morphogenesis in 3D environment and enhances skin wound healing. *Acta Biomaterialia*, 2017, 54: 333–344.
152. Aurora A, Wrice N, Walters T, et al. A PEGylated platelet free plasma hydrogel based composite scaffold enables stable vascularization and targeted cell delivery for volumetric muscle loss. *Acta Biomaterialia*, 2017, 65: 150–162.
153. Bejleri D, Streeter B, Nachlas A, et al. A bioprinted cardiac patch composed of cardiac-specific extracellular matrix and progenitor cells for heart repair. *Advanced Healthcare Materials*, 2018, 7: 1800672.
154. Zhu M, Li W, Dong X, et al. In vivo engineered extracellular matrix scaffolds with instructive niches for oriented tissue regeneration. *Nature Communications*, 2019, 10(1): 4620.
155. Morris A, Stamer D, Kunkemoeller B, et al. Decellularized materials derived from TSP2-KO mice promote enhanced neovascularization and integration in diabetic wounds. *Biomaterials*, 2018, 169: 61–71.

156. Shaheen M, Joo D J, Ross J, et al. Sustained perfusion of revascularized bioengineered livers heterotopically transplanted into immunosuppressed pigs. *Nature Biomedical Engineering*, 2020, 4: 1–9.

157. White L, Taylor A, Faulk D, et al. The impact of detergents on the tissue decellularization process: A ToF-SIMS study. *Acta Biomaterialia*, 2016, 50: 207–219.

158. Delong S, Moon J, West J. Covalently immobilized gradients of bFGF on hydrogel scaffolds for directed cell migration. *Biomaterials*, 2005, 26: 3227–3234.

159. Vigen M, Ceccarelli J, Putnam A. Protease-sensitive PEG hydrogels regulate vascularization in vitro and in vivo. *Macromolecular Bioscience*, 2014, 14(10): 1368–1379.

160. Weaver J, Headen D, Hunckler M, et al. Design of a vascularized synthetic poly(ethylene glycol) macroencapsulation device for islet transplantation. *Biomaterials*, 2018, 172: 54–65.

161. Miller J, Stevens K, Yang M, et al. Rapid casting of patterned vascular networks for perfusable engineered 3D tissues. *Nature Materials*, 2012, 11: 768–774.

162. Turturro M, Christenson M, Larson J, et al. MMP-sensitive PEG diacrylate hydrogels with spatial variations in matrix properties stimulate directional vascular sprout formation. *PLoS One*, 2013, 8: e58897.

163. Sueyoshi R, Ralls M, Teitelbaum D. Glucagon-like peptide 2 increases efficacy of distraction enterogenesis. *The Journal of Surgical Research*, 2013, 184(1): 365–373.

164. García J R, Clark A Y, García A J. Integrin-specific hydrogels functionalized with VEGF for vascularization and bone regeneration of critical-size bone defects. *Journal of Biomedical Materials Research Part A*, 2016, 104(4): 889–900.

165. Blache U, Metzger S, Vallmajo-Martin Q, et al. Dual role of mesenchymal stem cells allows for microvascularized bone tissue-like environments in PEG hydrogels. *Advanced Healthcare Materials*, 2015, 5(4): 489–498.

166. Mahou R, Zhang D, Vlahos A, et al. Injectable and inherently vascularizing semi-interpenetrating polymer network for delivering cells to the subcutaneous space. *Biomaterials*, 2017, 131: 27–35.

167. Phelps E, Templeman K, Thule P, et al. Engineered VEGF-releasing PEG–MAL hydrogel for pancreatic islet vascularization. *Drug Delivery and Translational Research*, 2013, 5(2): 125–136.

168. Qi D, Wu S, Kuss M, et al. Mechanically robust cryogels with injectability and bioprinting supportability for adipose tissue engineering. *Acta Biomaterialia*, 2018, 74: 131–142.

169. Singh R, Seliktar D, Putnam A. Capillary morphogenesis in PEG-collagen hydrogels. *Biomaterials*, 2013, 34(37): 9331–9340.

170. Jafari A, Hassanajili S, Azarpira N, et al. Development of thermal-crosslinkable chitosan/maleic terminated polyethylene glycol hydrogels for full thickness wound healing: In vitro and in vivo evaluation. *European Polymer Journal*, 2019, 118: 113–127.

171. Zamora D, Natesan S, Becerra S, et al. Enhanced wound vascularization using a dsASCs seeded FPEG scaffold. *Angiogenesis*, 2013, 16(4): 745–757.

172. Jiang B, Waller T, Larson J, et al. Fibrin-loaded porous poly(ethylene glycol) hydrogels as scaffold materials for vascularized tissue formation. *Tissue Engineering Part A*, 2013, 19: 224–234.

173. Rufaihah A J, Vaibavi S R, Plotkin M, et al. Enhanced infarct stabilization and neovascularization mediated by VEGF-loaded PEGylated fibrinogen hydrogel in a rodent myocardial infarction model. *Biomaterials*, 2013, 34(33): 8195–8202.

174. Benavides O, Brooks A, Cho S, et al. In Situ vascularization of injectable fibrin/poly(ethylene glycol) hydrogels by human amniotic fluid-derived stem cells. *Journal of Biomedical Materials Research Part A*, 2015, 103(8): 2645–2653.

175. Gniesmer S, Brehm R, Hoffmann A, et al. Vascularization and biocompatibility of poly(ε-caprolactone) fiber mats for rotator cuff tear repair. *PLoS One*, 2020, 15: e0227563.

176. Gniesmer S, Brehm R, Hoffmann A, et al. In vivo analysis of vascularization and bio-compatibility of electrospun polycaprolactone fibre mats in the rat femur chamber. *Journal of Tissue Engineering and Regenerative Medicine*, 2019, 13(7): 1190–1202.

177. Rameshbabu A, Datta S, Bankoti K, et al. Polycaprolactone nanofibers functionalized with placental derived extracellular matrix for stimulating wound healing activity. *Journal of Materials Chemistry B*, 2018, 6(42): 6767–6780.

178. Ekaputra A, Prestwich G, Cool S, et al. The three-dimensional vascularization of growth factor-releasing hybrid scaffold of poly(3-caprolactone)/collagen fibers and hyaluronic acid hydrogel. *Biomaterials*, 2011, 32: 8108–8117.

179. Singh S, Wu B, Dunn J. Delivery of VEGF using collagen-coated polycaprolactone scaffolds stimulate angiogenesis. *Journal of Biomedical Materials Research. Part A*, 2012, 100: 720–727.

180. Wang K, Chen X, Pan Y, et al. Enhanced vascularization in hybrid PCL/gelatin fibrous scaffolds with sustained release of VEGF. *BioMed Research International*, 2015, 2015: 865076.

181. Singh S, Wu B, Dunn J. Accelerating vascularization in polycaprolactone scaffolds by endothelial progenitor cells. *Tissue Engineering. Part A*, 2011, 17: 1819–1830.

182. Xu K, Zhu C, Xie J, et al. Enhanced vascularization of PCL porous scaffolds through VEGF-Fc modification. *Journal of Materials Chemistry B*, 2018, 6(27): 4474–4485.

183. Zhao L, Ma S, Pan Y, et al. Functional modification of fibrous PCL scaffolds with fusion protein VEGF-HGFI enhanced cellularization and vascularization. *Advanced Healthcare Materials*, 2016, 5(18): 2376–2385.

184. Wang K, Zhang Q, Zhao L, et al. Functional modification of electrospun poly(ε-caprolactone) vascular grafts with the fusion protein VEGF–HGFI enhanced vascular regeneration. *ACS Applied Materials & Interfaces*, 2017, 9(13): 11415–11427.

185. Saveleva M, Ivanov A N, Kurtukova M O, et al. Hybrid PCL/CaCO$_3$ scaffolds with capabilities of carrying biologically active molecules: Synthesis, loading and in vivo applications. *Materials Science and Engineering: C*, 2018, 85: 57–67.

186. Ji X, Yuan X, Ma Limin, et al. Mesenchymal stem cell-loaded thermosensitive hydroxy-propyl chitin hydrogel combined with a three-dimensional-printed poly(ε-caprolactone)/nano-hydroxyapatite scaffold to repair bone defects via osteogenesis, angiogenesis and immunomodulation. *Theranostics*, 2020, 10(2): 725–740.

187. Milovac D, Gallego Ferrer G, Ivanković or Opalički M, et al. PCL-coated hydroxyapa-tite scaffold derived from cuttlefish bone: Morphology, mechanical properties and bio-activity. *Materials Science & Engineering. C, Materials for Biological Applications*, 2014, 34C: 437–445.

188. Shanjani Y, Kang Y, Zarnescu L, et al. Endothelial pattern formation in hybrid con-structs of additive manufactured porous rigid scaffolds and cell-laden hydrogels for orthopedic applications. *Journal of the Mechanical Behavior of Biomedical Materials*, 2016, 65: 356–372.

189. Augustine R, Nethi S, Kalarikkal N, et al. Electrospun polycaprolactone (PCL) scaf-folds embedded with europium hydroxide nanorods (EHNs) with enhanced vascular-ization and cell proliferation for tissue engineering applications. *Journal of Materials Chemistry B*, 2017, 5(4): 4660–4672.

190. Chakka L J, Kumar S, Chatterjee K. Multi-biofunctional polymer graphene composite for bone tissue regeneration that elutes copper ions to impart angiogenic, osteogenic and bactericidal properties. *Colloids and Surfaces B: Biointerfaces*, 2017, 159: 293–302.

191. Kobayashi H, Terada D, Yokoyama Y, et al. Vascular-inducing poly(glycolic acid)-collagen nanocomposite-fiber scaffold. *Journal of Biomedical Nanotechnology*, 2013, 9: 1318–1326.

192. Li W, Huang L, Zhang J, et al. PLLA/POSS nanofibers loaded with multitargeted pANG composite nanoparticles for promotion of vascularization in shear flow. *Macromolecular Bioscience*, 2019, 20: 1900204.

193. Yu M, Huang J, Zhu T, et al. Liraglutide-loaded PLGA/Gelatin electrospun nanofibrous mats promote angiogenesis to accelerate diabetic wound healing via the modulation of miR-29b-3p. *Biomaterials Science*, 2020, 8(15): 4225–4238.
194. Wang X, Li Q, Hu X, et al. Fabrication and characterization of poly(L-lactide-co-glycolide) knitted mesh-reinforced collagen-chitosan hybrid scaffolds for dermal tissue engineering. *Journal of the Mechanical Behavior of Biomedical Materials*, 2012, 8: 204–215.
195. Deng M, Gu Y, Liu Z, et al. Endothelial differentiation of human adipose-derived stem cells on polyglycolic acid/polylactic acid mesh. *Stem Cells International*, 2015, 2015: 1–11.
196. Li Y, Ping F, Ding X-M, et al. Polyglycolic acid fibrous scaffold improving endothelial cell coating and vascularization of islet. *Chinese Medical Journal*, 2017, 130: 832.
197. Álvarez Z, Castaño O, Castells A A, et al. Neurogenesis and vascularization of the damaged brain using a lactate-releasing biomimetic scaffold. *Biomaterials*, 2014, 35(17): 4769–4781.
198. Kim J-H, Kim T-H, Jin G-Z, et al. Mineralized poly(lactic acid) scaffolds loading vascular endothelial growth factor and the in vivo performance in rat subcutaneous model. *Journal of Biomedical Materials Research. Part A*, 2013, 101(5): 1447–1455.
199. Wang H, Chang X, Qiu G, et al. Vascularization of nanohydroxyapatite/collagen/poly(L-lactic acid) composites by implanting intramuscularly in vivo. *International Journal of Polymer Science*, 2014, 2014: 1–5.
200. Majchrowicz A, Roguska A, Krawczyńska A, et al. In vitro evaluation of degradable electrospun polylactic acid/bioactive calcium phosphate ormoglass scaffolds. *Archives of Civil and Mechanical Engineering*, 2020, 20: 50.
201. Vila O, R. Bago J, Navarro M, et al. Calcium phosphate glass improves angiogenesis capacity of poly(lactic acid) scaffolds and stimulates differentiation of adipose tissue-derived mesenchymal stromal cells to the endothelial lineage. *Journal of Biomedical Materials Research. Part A*, 2013, 101(4): 932–941.
202. Sachot N, Castano O, Oliveira H, et al. A novel hybrid nanofibrous strategy to target progenitor cells for cost-effective: In situ angiogenesis. *Journal of Materials Chemistry B*, 2016, 43: 6967–6978.
203. Eldesoqi K, Seebach C, Nguyen Ngoc C, et al. High calcium bioglass enhances differentiation and survival of endothelial progenitor cells. Inducing early vascularization in critical size bone defects. *PLoS One*, 2013, 8: e79058.
204. Li S, Song C, Yang S, et al. scCO2 foamed composite scaffolds incorporating bioactive lipids promote vascularized bone regeneration via Hif-1α upregulation and enhanced type H vessel formation. *Acta Biomaterialia*, 2019, 94: 253–267.
205. Hegen A, Blois A, Tiron C, et al. Efficient in vivo vascularization of tissue engineering scaffolds. *Journal of Tissue Engineering and Regenerative Medicine*, 2011, 5: e52–e62.
206. Jehn P, Winterboer J, Kampmann A, et al. Angiogenic effects of mesenchymal stem cells in combination with different scaffold materials. *Microvascular Research*, 2019, 127: 103925.
207. Zhao X, Liu L, Wang J, et al. In vitro vascularization of a combined system based on a 3D printing technique. *Journal of Tissue Engineering and Regenerative Medicine*, 2016, 10(10): 833–842.
208. Kim J-S, Jung Y, Kim S H, et al. Vascularization of PLGA-based bio-artificial beds by hypoxia-preconditioned mesenchymal stem cells for subcutaneous xenogeneic islet transplantation. *Xenotransplantation*, 2019, 26(1): e12441.
209. Schumann P, Von See C, Kampmann A, et al. Comparably accelerated vascularization by preincorporation of aortic fragments and mesenchymal stem cells in implanted tissue engineering constructs. *Journal of Biomedical Materials Research. Part A*, 2011, 97: 383–394.

210. Kampmann A, Lindhorst D, Schumann P, et al. Additive effect of mesenchymal stem cells and VEGF to vascularization of PLGA scaffolds. *Microvascular Research*, 2013, 90: 71–79.

211. Landau S, Szklanny A, Yeo G, et al. Tropoelastin coated PLLA-PLGA scaffolds promote vascular network formation. *Biomaterials*, 2017, 122: 72–82.

212. Lv L, Deegan A, Musa F, et al. The effects of biomimetically conjugated VEGF on osteogenesis and angiogenesis of MSCs (human and rat) and HUVECs co-culture models. *Colloids and Surfaces B: Biointerfaces*, 2018, 167: 550–559.

213. Schumann P, Kampmann A, Sauer G, et al. Accelerated vascularization of tissue engineering constructs in vivo by preincubated co-culture of aortic fragments and osteoblasts. *Biochemical Engineering Journal*, 2015, 105: 230–241.

214. Pizzicannella J, Diomede F, Gugliandolo A, et al. 3D printing PLA/gingival stem cells/ EVs upregulate miR-2861 and -210 during osteoangiogenesis commitment. *International Journal of Molecular Sciences*, 2019, 20: 3256.

215. Zhao D, Jiang W, Wang Y, et al. Three-dimensional-printed Poly-L-Lactic acid scaffolds with different pore sizes influence periosteal distraction osteogenesis of a rabbit skull. *BioMed Research International*, 2020, 2020: 1–14.

216. Farina M, Chua C, Ballerini A, et al. Transcutaneously refillable, 3D-printed biopolymeric encapsulation system for the transplantation of endocrine cells. *Biomaterials*, 2018, 177: 125–138.

217. Wang Y, Kim Y, Langer R. In vivo degradation characteristics of poly(glycerol sebacate). *Journal of Biomedical Materials Research. Part A*, 2003, 66: 192–197.

218. Wang Y, Ameer G, Sheppard B, et al. A tough biodegradable elastomer. *Nature Biotechnology*, 2002, 20: 602–606.

219. Lee M-C, Haut R. Strain rate effects on tensile failure properties of the common carotid artery and jugular veins of ferrets. *Journal of Biomechanics*, 1992, 25: 925–927.

220. Fidkowski C, Mofrad M, Borenstein J, et al. Endothelialized microvasculature based on a biodegradable elastomer. *Tissue Engineering*, 2005, 11: 302–309.

221. Bettinger C, Weinberg E, Kulig K, et al. Three-dimensional microfluidic tissue-engineering scaffolds using a flexible biodegradable polymer. *Advanced Materials (Deerfield Beach, Fla.)*, 2006, 18: 165–169.

222. Ye X, Lu L, Kolewe M, et al. A biodegradable microvessel scaffold as a framework to enable vascular support of engineered tissues. *Biomaterials*, 2013, 34(38): 10007–10015.

223. Faria Bellani C, Yue K, Flaig F, et al. Suturable elastomeric tubular grafts with patterned porosity for rapid vascularization of 3D constructs. *Biofabrication*, 2021, 13: 035020..

224. Liang B, Shi Q, Xu J, et al. Poly (glycerol sebacate)-based bio-artificial multiporous matrix for bone regeneration. *Frontiers in Chemistry*, 2020, 8: 603577.

225. Wu W, Jia S, Chen W, et al. Fast degrading elastomer stented fascia remodels into tough and vascularized construct for tracheal regeneration. *Materials Science and Engineering: C*, 2019, 101: 1–14.

226. Rai R, Tallawi M, Frati C, et al. Bioactive electrospun fibers of poly(glycerol sebacate) and poly(ε-caprolactone) for cardiac patch application. Advanced healthcare materials, 2015, 4(13): 2012–2025.

227. Xiao B, Yang W, Lei D, et al. PGS scaffolds promote the in vivo survival and directional differentiation of bone marrow mesenchymal stem cells restoring the morphology and function of wounded rat uterus. *Advanced Healthcare Materials*, 2019, 8(5): 1801455.

228. Gaharwar A, Nikkhah M, Sant S, et al. Anisotropic poly (glycerol sebacate)-poly (ε-caprolactone) electrospun fibers promote endothelial cell guidance. Biofabrication, 2015, 7: 015001.

229. Wang Z, Mithieux S, Weiss A. Fabrication techniques for vascular and vascularized tissue engineering. *Advanced Healthcare Materials*, 2019, 8: 1900742.

230. Awad N, Niu H, Ali U, et al. Electrospun fibrous scaffolds for small-diameter blood vessels: A review. *Membranes*, 2018, 8(1): 15.

231. Barreto-Ortiz S, Fradkin J, Eoh J, et al. Fabrication of 3-dimensional multicellular microvascular structures. *FASEB Journal: Official Publication of the Federation of American Societies for Experimental Biology*, 2015, 29(8): 3302–3314.

232. Martinez-Rivas A, Gonzalez-Quijano G, Proa-Coronado S, et al. Methods of micropatterning and manipulation of cells for biomedical applications. *Micromachines*, 2017, 8: 347.

233. Gualandi C, Zucchelli A, Fernández Osorio M, et al. Nanovascularization of polymer matrix: Generation of nanochannels and nanotubes by sacrificial electrospun fibers. *Nano Letters*, 2013, 13(11): 5385–5390.

234. Jeffries E, Nakamura S, Lee K, et al. Micropatterning electrospun scaffolds to create intrinsic vascular networks. *Macromolecular Bioscience*, 2014, 14(11): 1514–1520.

235. Said S, Yin H, Elfarnawany M, et al. Fortifying angiogenesis in ischemic muscle with FGF9-loaded electrospun poly(ester amide) fibers. *Advanced Healthcare Materials*, 2019, 8(8): e1801294.

236. Wray L, Tsioris K, Gi E, et al. Microfabricated porous silk scaffolds for vascularizing engineered tissues. *Advanced Functional Materials*, 2013, 23: 3404–3412.

237. Cha C, Piraino F, Khademhosseini A. Chapter 9 - Microfabrication technology in tissue engineering, Blitterswijk C a V, De Boer J, editor, *Tissue Engineering (Second Edition)*, Oxford: Academic Press, 2014: pp. 283–310.

238. Ma C, Qu T, Chang B, et al. 3D maskless micropatterning for regeneration of highly organized tubular tissues. *Advanced Healthcare Materials*, 2017, 7: 1700738.

239. Simmons B A. Micromolding (injection and compression molding), Li D, editor, *Encyclopedia of Microfluidics and Nanofluidics*, New York: Springer, 2014: pp. 1–10.

240. Aldana A A, Malatto L, Rehman M a U, et al. Fabrication of Gelatin Methacrylate (GelMA) scaffolds with nano- and micro-topographical and morphological features. *Nanomaterials*, 2019, 9(1): 120.

241. Hwang C, Sim W Y, Lee S H, et al. Benchtop fabrication of PDMS microstructures by an unconventional photolithographic method. *Biofabrication*, 2010, 2: 045001.

242. Papautsky I, Peterson E T K. Micromolding, Li D, editor, *Encyclopedia of Microfluidics and Nanofluidics*, Boston, MA: Springer US, 2008: 1256–1267.

243. Wang X-Y, Jin Z-H, Gan B-W, et al. Engineering interconnected 3D vascular networks in hydrogels using molded sodium alginate lattice as the sacrificial template. *Lab on a Chip*, 2014, 14(15): 2709–2716.

244. Bertassoni L, Cecconi M, Manoharan V, et al. Hydrogel bioprinted microchannel networks for vascularization of tissue engineering constructs. *Lab on a Chip*, 2014, 14(13): 2202–2211.

245. Xie R, Zheng W, Guan L, et al. Engineering of hydrogel materials with perfusable microchannels for building vascularized tissues. *Small*, 2019, 16(15): e1902838.

246. Zimmermann W, Schneiderbanger K, Schubert P, et al. Tissue engineering of a differentiated cardiac muscle construct. *Circulation Research*, 2002, 90: 223–230.

247. Montaño I, Schiestl C, Schneider J, et al. Formation of human capillaries in vitro: The engineering of prevascularized matrices. *Tissue Engineering. Part A*, 2009, 16: 269–282.

248. Heo D N, Hospodiuk M, Ozbolat I T. Synergistic interplay between human MSCs and HUVECs in 3D spheroids laden in collagen/fibrin hydrogels for bone tissue engineering. *Acta Biomaterialia*, 2019, 95: 348–356.

249. Helary C, Bataille I, Abed A, et al. Concentrated collagen hydrogels as dermal substitutes. *Biomaterials*, 2009, 31: 481–490.

250. Putra D, Bose V, Shen Y I, et al. Controlled activation of morphogenesis to generate a functional human microvasculature in a synthetic matrix. *Blood*, 2011, 118: 804–815.

251. Nichol J, Koshy S, Bae H, et al. Cell-laden microengineered gelatin methacrylate hydrogels. *Biomaterials*, 2010, 31: 5536–5544.

252. Chen Y-C, Lin R-Z, Qi H, et al. Functional human vascular network generated in photocrosslinkable gelatin methacrylate hydrogels. *Advanced Functional Materials*, 2012, 22: 2027–2039.

253. Mansoorifar A, Tahayeri A, Bertassoni L E. Bioinspired reconfiguration of 3D printed microfluidic hydrogels via automated manipulation of magnetic inks. *Lab on a Chip*, 2020, 20(10): 1713–1719.

254. Zhang Y, Pi Q, Van Genderen A M. Microfluidic bioprinting for engineering vascularized tissues and organoids. *Journal of Visualized Experiments*, 2017, 2017(126): 55957.

255. Liao C-J, Chen C F, Chen J-H, et al. Fabrication of porous biodegradable polymer scaffolds using a solvent merging/particle leaching method. *Journal of Biomedical Materials Research*, 2002, 59: 676–681.

256. Raeisdasteh V, Davaran S, Ramazani A, et al. Design and fabrication of porous biodegradable scaffolds: A strategy for tissue engineering. *Journal of Biomaterials Science, Polymer Edition*, 2017, 28: 1–47.

257. Hu C, Uchida T, Tercero C, et al. Development of biodegradable scaffolds based on magnetically guided assembly of magnetic sugar particles. *Journal of Biotechnology*, 2012, 159: 90–98.

258. Haider A, Haider S, Rao Kummara M, et al. Advances in the scaffolds fabrication techniques using biocompatible polymers and their biomedical application: A technical and statistical review. *Journal of Saudi Chemical Society*, 2020, 24(2): 186–215.

259. Xing F, Xiang Z, Rommens P, et al. 3D bioprinting for vascularized tissue-engineered bone fabrication. *Materials*, 2020, 13: 2278.

260. Tomasina C, Bodet T, Mota C, et al. Bioprinting vasculature: Materials. Cells and emergent techniques. *Materials*, 2019, 12: 2701.

261. Bova L, Billi F, Cimetta E. Mini-review: Advances in 3D bioprinting of vascularized constructs. *Biology Direct*, 2020, 15: 22.

262. Mandrycky C, Wang D Z, Kim K, et al. 3D bioprinting for engineering complex tissues. *Biotechnology Advances*, 2015, 34(4): 422–434.

263. Lee V, Kim D, Ngo H, et al. Creating perfused functional vascular channels using 3D bio-printing technology. *Biomaterials*, 2014, 35(28): 8092–8102.

264. Campbell A, Mohl J E, Gutierrez D A, et al. Thermal bioprinting causes ample alterations of expression of LUCAT1, IL6, CCL26, and NRN1L genes and massive phosphorylation of critical oncogenic drug resistance pathways in breast cancer cells. *Frontiers in Bioengineering and Biotechnology*, 2020, 8: 82.

265. Fei Z, Brian D, Jason W. Fabrication of microvascular constructs using high resolution electrohydrodynamic inkjet printing. *Biofabrication*, 2020, 13: 035006.

266. Pati F, Jang J, Lee J W, et al. Chapter 7- Extrusion bioprinting, Atala A, Yoo J J, editor, *Essentials of 3D Biofabrication and Translation*, Boston, MA: Academic Press, 2015: pp. 123–152.

267. Kang D, Hong G, An S, et al. Bioprinting of multiscaled hepatic lobules within a highly vascularized construct. *Small*, 2020, 16: 1905505.

268. Hinton T, Jallerat Q, Palchesko R, et al. Three-dimensional printing of complex biological structures by freeform reversible embedding of suspended hydrogels. *Science Advances*, 2015, 1: e1500758–e1500758.

269. Jana S, Lerman A. Bioprinting a cardiac valve. *Biotechnology Advances*, 2015, 33(8): 1503–1521.

270. Wu P, Ringeisen B. Development of human umbilical vein endothelial cell (HUVEC) and human umbilical vein smooth muscle cell (HUVSMC) branch/stem structures on hydrogel layers via biological laser printing (BioLP). *Biofabrication*, 2010, 2: 014111.

271. Kérourédan O, Bourget J-M, Rémy M, et al. Micropatterning of endothelial cells to create a capillary-like network with defined architecture by laser-assisted bioprinting. *Journal of Materials Science: Materials in Medicine*, 2019, 30(2): 28.

272. Bourget J-M, Kérourédan O, Medina M, et al. Patterning of endothelial cells and mesenchymal stem cells by laser-assisted bioprinting to study cell migration. *BioMed Research International*, 2016, 2016: 1–7.

273. Thomas A, Orellano I, Lam T, et al. Vascular bioprinting with enzymatically degradable bioinks via multi-material projection-based stereolithography. *Acta Biomaterialia*, 2020, 117: 121–132.

274. Lutolf M P, Hubbell J A. Synthetic biomaterials as instructive extracellular microenvironments for morphogenesis in tissue engineering. *Nature Biotechnology*, 2005, 23(1): 47–55.

275. O'brien F, Harley B, Yannas I V, et al. The effect of pore size on cell adhesion in collagen-GAG scaffold. *Biomaterials*, 2005, 26: 433–441.

276. Yannas I V, Lee E, Orgill D P, et al. Synthesis and characterization of a model extracellular matrix that induces partial regeneration of adult mammalian skin. *Proceedings of the National Academy of Sciences*, 1989, 86(3): 933.

277. Chan B, Leong K. Scaffolding in tissue engineering: General approaches and tissue-specific considerations. *European Spine Journal: Official Publication of the European Spine Society, the European Spinal Deformity Society, and the European Section of the Cervical Spine Research Society*, 2008, 17(Suppl 4): 467–479.

278. Liu X, Ma P. Phase separation, pore structure, and properties of nanofibrous gelatin scaffolds. *Biomaterials*, 2009, 30: 4094–4103.

279. Gupte M, Swanson W, Hu J, et al. Pore size directs bone marrow stromal cell fate and tissue regeneration in nanofibrous macroporous scaffolds by mediating vascularization. *Acta Biomaterialia*, 2018, 82: 1–11.

280. Janson I, Putnam A. Extracellular matrix elasticity and topography: Material-based cues that affect cell function via conserved mechanisms. *Journal of Biomedical Materials Research. Part A*, 2015, 103(3): 1246–1258.

281. Lu J, Rao M, Macdonald N, et al. Improved endothelial cell adhesion and proliferation on patterned titanium surfaces with rationally designed, micrometer to nanometer features. *Acta Biomaterialia*, 2008, 4: 192–201.

282. Bettinger C, Orrick B, Misra A, et al. Microfabrication of poly (glycerol-sebacate) for contact guidance applications. *Biomaterials*, 2006, 27: 2558–2565.

283. Wu S, Peng H, Li X, et al. Effect of scaffold morphology and cell co-culture on tenogenic differentiation of HADMSC on centrifugal melt electrospun poly (L-lactic acid) fibrous meshes. *Biofabrication*, 2017, 9: 044106.

284. Bettinger C, Zhang Z, Gerecht S, et al. Enhancement of in vitro capillary tube formation by substrate nanotopography. *Advanced Materials*, 2007, 20: 99–103.

285. Dickinson L, Moura M, Gerecht S. Guiding endothelial progenitor cell tube formation using patterned fibronectin surfaces. *Soft Matter*, 2010, 6: 5109–5119.

286. Barreto-Ortiz S, Zhang S, Davenport M, et al. A novel in vitro model for microvasculature reveals regulation of circumferential ECM organization by curvature. *PLoS One*, 2013, 8(11): e81061.

287. Gugutkov D, Gustavsson J, Cantini M, et al. Electrospun fibrinogen-PLA nanofibres for vascular tissue engineering. *Journal of Tissue Engineering and Regenerative Medicine*, 2016, 11(10): 2774–2784.

288. Ren X, Han Y, Wang J, et al. An aligned porous electrospun fibrous membrane with controlled drug delivery - An efficient strategy to accelerate diabetic wound healing with improved angiogenesis. *Acta Biomaterialia*, 2018, 70: 140–153.

289. Kaneko N, Matsuda R, Toda M, et al. Three-dimensional reconstruction of the human capillary network and the intramyocardial micronecrosis. *American Journal of Physiology. Heart and Circulatory Physiology*, 2010, 300: H754–H761.

290. Nikkhah M, Eshak N, Zorlutuna P, et al. Directed endothelial cell morphogenesis in micropatterned gelatin methacrylate hydrogels. *Biomaterials*, 2012, 33: 9009–9018.

291. Moon J, Hahn M, Kim I, et al. Micropatterning of poly(ethylene glycol) diacrylate hydrogels with biomolecules to regulate and guide endothelial morphogenesis. *Tissue engineering. Part A*, 2008, 15: 579–585.

292. Sharma D, Ross D, Wang G, et al. Upgrading prevascularization in tissue engineering: A review of strategies for promoting highly organized microvascular network formation. *Acta Biomaterialia*, 2019, 95: 112–130.

293. Lee S-H, Moon J, West J. Three-dimensional micropatterning of bioactive hydrogels via two-photon laser scanning photolithography for guided 3D cell migration. *Biomaterials*, 2008, 29: 2962–2968.

294. Stratton S, Shelke N, Hoshino K, et al. Bioactive polymeric scaffolds for tissue engineering. *Bioactive Materials*, 2016, 1(2): 93–108.

295. Geiger B, Bershadsky A, Pankov R, et al. Transmembrane crosstalk between the extracellular matrix–cytoskeleton crosstalk. *Nature Reviews Molecular Cell Biology*, 2001, 2: 793–805.

296. Barrias C, Martins M C, Almeida-Porada G, et al. The correlation between the adsorption of adhesive proteins and cell behaviour on hydroxyl-methyl mixed self-assembled monolayers. *Biomaterials*, 2008, 30: 307–316.

297. Li J, Zhang Y-P, Kirsner R. Li J, Zhang Y P, Kirsner R S. Angiogenesis in wound repair: Angiogenic growth factors and the extracellular matrix. *Microscopy Research and Technique*, 2003, 60: 107–114.

298. Tan J, Li L, Wang H, et al. Biofunctionalized fibrin gel co-embedded with BMSCs and VEGF for accelerating skin injury repair. *Materials Science and Engineering: C*, 2021, 121: 111749.

299. Richardson T, Peters M, Ennett A, et al. Polymeric system for dual growth factor delivery. *Nature Biotechnology*, 2001, 19: 1029–1034.

300. Drinnan C, Zhang G, Alexander M, et al. Multimodal release of transforming growth factor-beta 1 and the BB isoform of platelet derived growth factor from PEGylated fibrin gels. *Journal of Controlled Release: Official Journal of the Controlled Release Society*, 2010, 147: 180–186.

301. Hao X, Silva E A, Månsson-Broberg A, et al. Angiogenic effects of sequential release of VEGF-A165 and PDGF-BB with alginate hydrogels after myocardial infarction. *Cardiovascular Research*, 2007, 75(1): 178–185.

302. Pieper J, Hafmans T, Wachem P, et al. Loading of collagen-heparan sulfate matrices with bFGF promotes angiogenesis and tissue generation in rats. *Journal of Biomedical Materials Research*, 2002, 62: 185–194.

303. Ferrara N, Gerber H-P, Lecouter J. The biology of VEGF and its receptors. *Nature Medicine*, 2003, 9: 669–676.

304. Chiu L, Radisic M. Scaffolds with covalently immobilized VEGF and Angiopoietin-1 for vascularization of engineered tissues. *Biomaterials*, 2010, 31: 226–241.

305. Hoare T, Kohane D. Hoare TR, Kohane DS. Hydrogels in drug delivery: Progress and challenges. *Polymer*, 2008, 49: 1993–2007.

306. Van Hove A, Benoit D. Depot-based delivery systems for pro-angiogenic peptides: A review. *Frontiers in Bioengineering and Biotechnology*, 2015, 3: 102.

307. Leslie-Barbick J E, Saik J E, Gould D J, et al. The promotion of microvasculature formation in poly(ethylene glycol) diacrylate hydrogels by an immobilized VEGF-mimetic peptide. *Biomaterials*, 2011, 32(25): 5782–5789.

308. Santulli G, Ciccarelli M, Palumbo G, et al. In vivo properties of the proangiogenic peptide QK. *Journal of Translational Medicine*, 2009, 7: 41.

309. Mulyasasmita W, Cai L, Hori Y, et al. Avidity-controlled delivery of angiogenic peptides from injectable molecular-recognition hydrogels. *Tissue engineering. Part A*, 2014, 20(15–16): 2102–2114.
310. Lin X, Takahashi K, Liu Y, et al. A synthetic, bioactive PDGF mimetic with binding to both α-PDGF and β-PDGF receptors. *Growth Factors (Chur, Switzerland)*, 2007, 25: 87–93.
311. Pickart L. The human tri-peptide GHK and tissue remodeling. *Journal of Biomaterials Science. Polymer edition*, 2008, 19: 969–988.
312. Jose S, Hughbanks M, Binder B, et al. Enhanced trophic factor secretion by mesenchymal stem/stromal cells with Glycine-Histidine-Lysine (GHK)-modified alginate hydrogels. *Acta Biomaterialia*, 2014, 10(5): 1955–1964.
313. Nakamura M, Mie M, Mihara H, et al. Construction of multi-functional extracellular matrix proteins that promote tube formation of endothelial cells. *Biomaterials*, 2008, 29: 2977–2986.
314. Ali S, Saik J, Gould D, et al. Immobilization of cell-adhesive laminin peptides in degradable PEGDA hydrogels influences endothelial cell tubulogenesis. *BioResearch Open Access*, 2013, 2: 241–249.
315. Davis G, Koh W, Stratman A. Mechanisms controlling human endothelial lumen formation and tube assembly in three-dimensional extracellular matrices. *Birth Defects Research. Part C, Embryo Today: Reviews*, 2007, 81: 270–285.
316. Kopan R. Notch: A membrane-bound transcription factor. *Journal of Cell Science*, 2002, 115: 1095–1097.
317. Moon J, Saik J, Poche R, et al. Biomimetic hydrogels with pro-angiogenic properties. *Biomaterials*, 2010, 31: 3840–3847.
318. Dikovsky D, Bianco-Peled H, Seliktar D. The effect of structural alterations of PEG-fibrinogen hydrogel scaffolds on 3-D cellular morphology and cellular migration. *Biomaterials*, 2006, 27: 1496–1506.
319. West J, Hubbell J. Polymeric biomaterials with degradation sites for proteases involved in cell migration. *Macromolecules*, 1998, 32(1): 241–244.
320. Zisch A, Lutolf M, Hubbell J. Biopolymeric delivery matrices for angiogenic growth factors. *Cardiovascular Pathology: The Official Journal of the Society for Cardiovascular Pathology*, 2003, 12: 295–310.
321. Malhotra K, Shankar S, Chauhan N, et al. Design, characterization, and evaluation of antibacterial gels, Boc-D-Phe-γ4-L-Phe-PEA/chitosan and Boc-L-Phe-γ4-L-Phe-PEA/chitosan, for biomaterial-related infections. *Materials Science and Engineering: C*, 2020, 110: 110648.
322. Xu X, He F, Yang W, et al. Effect of homochirality of dipeptide to polymers' degradation. *Polymers*, 2020, 12(9): 2164.
323. Benoit D, Durney A, Anseth K. Manipulations in hydrogel degradation behavior enhance osteoblast function and mineralized tissue formation. *Tissue Engineering*, 2006, 12: 1663–1673.
324. Humphrey J D, Dufresne E R, Schwartz M A. Mechanotransduction and extracellular matrix homeostasis. *Nature Reviews Molecular Cell Biology*, 2014, 15(12): 802–812.
325. Discher D, Janmey P, Wang Y-L. Tissue cells feel and respond to the stiffness of their substrate. *Science (New York, N.Y.)*, 2005, 310: 1139–1143.
326. Ingber D. Mechanical signaling and the cellular response to extracellular matrix in angiogenesis and cardiovascular physiology. *Circulation Research*, 2002, 91: 877–887.
327. Sarang-Sieminski A, Hebbel R, Gooch K. The relative magnitudes of endothelial force generation and matrix stiffness modulate capillary morphogenesis in vitro. *Experimental Cell Research*, 2004, 297: 574–584.

328. Stephanou A, Meskaoui G, Vailhé B, et al. The rigidity in fibrin gels as a contributing factor to the dynamics of in vitro vascular cord formation. *Microvascular Research*, 2007, 73: 182–190.

329. Hanjaya-Putra D, Yee J, Ceci D, et al. Vascular endothelial growth factor and substrate mechanics regulate in vitro tubulogenesis of endothelial progenitor cells. *Journal of Cellular and Molecular Medicine*, 2010, 14(10): 2436–2447.

330. Jannatbabaei A, Tafazzoli-Shadpour M, Seyedjafari E. Effects of substrate mechanics on angiogenic capacity and nitric oxide release in human endothelial cells. *Annals of the New York Academy of Sciences*, 2020, 1470(1): 31–43.

331. Chang H, Zhang H, Hu M, et al. Stiffness of polyelectrolyte multilayer film influences endothelial function of endothelial cell monolayer. *Colloids and Surfaces B: Biointerfaces*, 2016, 149: 379–387.

332. Xie J, Zhang D, Ling Y, et al. Substrate elasticity regulates vascular endothelial growth factor A (VEGFA) expression in adipose-derived stromal cells: Implications for potential angiogenesis. *Colloids and Surfaces B: Biointerfaces*, 2019, 175: 576–585.

333. Kim S, Kawai T, Wang D, et al. Engineering a dual-layer chitosan-lactide hydrogel to create endothelial cell aggregate-induced microvascular networks in vitro and increase blood perfusion in vivo. *ACS Applied Materials & Interfaces*, 2016, 8(30): 19245–19255.

334. Wenz A, Tjoeng I, Schneider I, et al. Improved vasculogenesis and bone matrix formation through coculture of endothelial cells and stem cells in tissue-specific methacryloyl gelatin-based hydrogels. *Biotechnology and Bioengineering*, 2018, 115(10): 2643–2653.

335. Lesman A, Koffler J, Atlas R, et al. Engineering vessel-like networks within multicellular fibrin-based constructs. *Biomaterials*, 2011, 32: 7856–7869.

336. Crosby C, Hillsley A, Kumar S, et al. Phototunable interpenetrating polymer network hydrogels to stimulate the vasculogenesis of stem cell-derived endothelial progenitors. *Acta Biomaterialia*, 2020, 122: 133–144.

337. Correa V, Garza K, Murr L. Vascularization in interconnected 3D printed Ti-6Al-4V foams with hydrogel matrix for biomedical bone replacement implants. *Science China Materials*, 2017, 61: 565–578.

338. Ingber D E, Folkman J. Mechanochemical switching between growth and differentiation during fibroblast growth factor-stimulated angiogenesis in vitro: Role of extracellular matrix. *The Journal of Cell Biology*, 1989, 109: 317–330.

339. Byfield F, Reen R, Shentu T P, et al. Endothelial actin and cell stiffness is modulated by substrate stiffness in 2D and 3D. *Journal of Biomechanics*, 2009, 42: 1114–1119.

340. Pompe T, Glorius S, Bischoff T, et al. Dissecting the impact of matrix anchorage and elasticity in cell adhesion. *Biophysical Journal*, 2009, 97: 2154–2163.

341. Hong Z, Ersoy I, Sun M, et al. Influence of membrane cholesterol and substrate elasticity on endothelial cell spreading behavior. *Journal of Biomedical Materials Research. Part A*, 2013, 101A: 1994–2004.

342. Engler A J, Griffin M A, Sen S, et al. Myotubes differentiate optimally on substrates with tissue-like stiffness: Pathological implications for soft or stiff microenvironments. *Journal of Cell Biology*, 2004, 166(6): 877–887.

343. Wingate K, Bonani W, Tan Y, et al. Compressive elasticity of three-dimensional nanofiber matrix directs mesenchymal stem cell differentiation to vascular cells with endothelial or smooth muscle cell markers. *Acta Biomaterialia*, 2012, 8: 1440–1449.

344. Boland E. Electrospinning collagen and elastin: Preliminary vascular tissue engineering. *Frontiers in Bioscience*, 2004, 9: 1422–1432.

345. Geudens I, Gerhardt H. Coordinating cell behaviour during blood vessel formation. *Development (Cambridge, England)*, 2011, 138: 4569–4583.

346. Biondi M, Ungaro F, Quaglia F, et al. Controlled drug delivery in tissue engineering. *Advanced Drug Delivery Reviews*, 2008, 60: 229–242.

347. Germain S, Monnot C, Muller L, et al. Hypoxia-driven angiogenesis: Role of tip cells and extracellular matrix scaffolding. *Current Opinion in Hematology*, 2010, 17: 245–251.
348. Rich M, Kong H. Biomaterials for cell-based therapeutic angiogenesis, Reinhart-King C A, editor, *Studies in Mechanobiology, Tissue Engineering and Biomaterials*, Berlin: Springer, 2013: pp. 247–259.
349. Shin Y, Jeon J, Han S, et al. In vitro 3D collective sprouting angiogenesis under orchestrated ANG-1 and VEGF gradients. *Lab on a Chip*, 2011, 11: 2175–2181.
350. Chen R, Silva E, Yuen W, et al. Integrated approach to designing growth factor delivery systems. *FASEB Journal: Official Publication of the Federation of American Societies for Experimental Biology*, 2008, 21: 3896–3903.
351. Chen R, Silva E, Yuen W, et al. Spatio–temporal VEGF and PDGF delivery patterns blood vessel formation and maturation. *Pharmaceutical Research*, 2007, 24: 258–264.
352. Tayalia P, Mooney D. Controlled growth factor delivery for tissue engineering. *Advanced Materials (Deerfield Beach, Fla.)*, 2009, 21: 3269–3285.
353. Guo X, Elliott C, Li Z, et al. Creating 3D angiogenic growth factor gradients in fibrous constructs to guide fast angiogenesis. *Biomacromolecules*, 2012, 13: 3262–3271.
354. He J, Du Y, Villa-Uribe J L, et al. Rapid generation of biologically relevant hydrogels containing long-range chemical gradients. *Advanced Functional Materials*, 2010, 20(1): 131–137.
355. Sundararaghavan H, Burdick J. Gradients with depth in electrospun fibrous scaffolds for directed cell behavior. *Biomacromolecules*, 2011, 12: 2344–2350.
356. Borselli C, Oliviero O, Battista S, et al. Induction of directional sprouting angiogenesis by matrix gradients. *Journal of Biomedical Materials Research. Part A*, 2007, 80: 297–305.
357. Isenberg B, Dimilla P, Walker M, et al. Vascular smooth muscle cell durotaxis depends on substrate stiffness gradient strength. *Biophysical Journal*, 2009, 97: 1313–1322.
358. Hahn M, Miller J, West J. Three-dimensional biochemical and biomechanical patterning of hydrogels for guiding cell behavior. *Advanced Materials*, 2006, 18: 2679–2684.
359. Wong J, Velasco A, Rajagopalan P, et al. Directed movement of vascular smooth muscle cells on gradient-compliant hydrogels. *Langmuir*, 2003, 19(5): 1908–1913.
360. Peyton S, Putnam A. Extracellular matrix rigidity governs smooth muscle cell motility in a biphasic fasion. *Journal of Cellular Physiology*, 2005, 204: 198–209.
361. Romer L, Birukov K, Garcia J. Focal adhesions paradigm for a signaling nexus. *Circulation Research*, 2006, 98: 606–616.
362. Igarashi S, Tanaka J, Kobayashi H. Micro-patterned nanofibrous biomaterials. *Journal of Nanoscience and Nanotechnology*, 2007, 7: 814–817.
363. Scott E, Nichols M, Willits R, et al. Modular scaffolds assembled around living cells using poly(ethylene glycol) microspheres with macroporation via a non-cytotoxic porogen. *Acta Biomaterialia*, 2009, 6: 29–38.
364. Zeng W, Li Y, Wang Y, et al. Tissue engineering of blood vessels, Reis R L, editor, *Encyclopedia of Tissue Engineering and Regenerative Medicine*. Salt Lake City, UT: American Academic Press, 2019: pp. 413–424.
365. Rouwkema J, Rivron N C, Van Blitterswijk C A. Vascularization in tissue engineering. *Trends in Biotechnology*, 2008, 26(8): 434–441.
366. Grigoryan B, Paulsen S J, Corbett D C, et al. Multivascular networks and functional intravascular topologies within biocompatible hydrogels. *Science*, 2019, 364(6439): 458.
367. Malda J, Rouwkema J, Martens D, et al. Oxygen gradients in tissue-engineered PEGT/PBT cartilaginous constructs: Measurement and modeling. *Biotechnology and Bioengineering*, 2004, 86(1): 9–18.
368. Ghosh R, Lapets O, Haskins J. Characteristics and value of directed algorithms in high content screening. *Methods in Molecular Biology (Clifton, N.J.)*, 2007, 356: 63–81.
369. Widener A. Materials genome initiative. *Chemical & Engineering News Archive*, 2013, 91(31): 25–27.

4 Biomaterials and Coatings for Artificial Hip Joints

Y. Ren
Henan University of Technology

CONTENTS

DOI: 10.1201/9781003161981-4

4.1　INTRODUCTION: BACKGROUND OF HIP JOINT REPLACEMENT

Nowadays, due to increasing population, increasing average weight of people, and larger number of accidental injuries, especially among young people, more and more load-bearing joint replacements, particularly hip joint replacements, are required. Moreover, about 10% of patients require second replacements. In addition, diseases such as arthritis also require joint replacement due to worn cartilage. The normal hip displays healthy articular cartilage, and the diseased hip joint shows damaged cartilage, as seen in Figure 4.1.

Therefore, more and more implants have been placed in human bodies, and more than 250,000 total hip replacements (THRs) are performed annually in the United States. Not only replacement surgeries have increased, but also revision surgeries of hip implants. The total number of hip revision surgeries is expected to increase by 137% between 2005 and 2030.[1]

A total hip arthroplasty (THA), or THR, is a surgical procedure to replace the hip joint with an artificial prosthesis, which is considered to be one of the greatest achievements in the field of biomaterials and bioengineering in the 20th century.[2] Although THA has provided good results for over 40 years, the choice of the optimal bearing surface remains controversial.

Clinical studies have shown that the service life of traditional artificial joints (metal ultra-high-molecular-weight polyethylene (UHMWPE) and metal-metal components) is only 10–15 years. However, with an aging population and the significant increase in the average life span of human beings, people have put forward

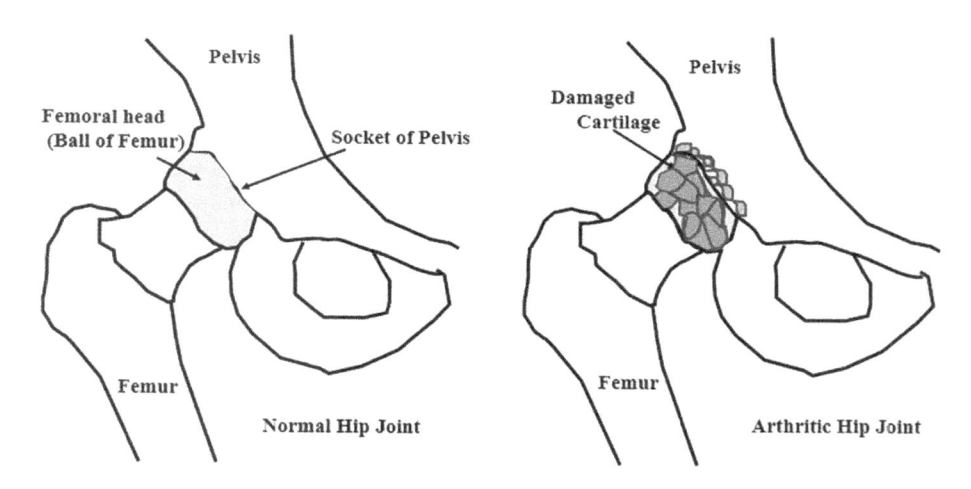

FIGURE 4.1　Normal hip joint and arthritic hip joint.

higher requirements for the life span of artificial joints. At present, researchers are working hard to develop materials for long life implantation in the human body. This is because commercial biomaterials have exhibited tendencies to fail after long-term use due to various reasons such as low fatigue strength, high modulus compared to that of bone, low wear and corrosion resistance, and lack of biocompatibility.[3,4] The development of appropriate materials with high longevity and excellent biocompatibility is crucial.

4.2 NORMAL HIP JOINT AND ARTIFICIAL HIP JOINT

4.2.1 COMPOSITION OF HIP JOINT

Figure 4.2 shows a schematic of a normal hip joint and an artificial hip joint. In the human body, the normal hip joint mainly consists of the femur, femoral head (ball), and the cup-shaped acetabulum (cup) in the pelvis (see Figure 4.2a). Figure 4.2b shows the structure of the corresponding artificial hip joint. The artificial joint friction pair is a convex–concave socket structure, and the joint rotation, rotation, and swing are realized through the relative movement of the femoral head and the socket.

Ligaments as bands of tissue connect the femur to the acetabulum and help to keep them steady. Articular cartilage, a smooth and tough substance, covers the surfaces of the femoral head (ball) and the acetabulum (cup). Additionally, the cartilage cushions the bones like a shock absorber which allows smooth movement, so that bones can move easily. The rest of the surfaces of the hip joint are covered by the synovial membrane, which is a thin and smooth tissue liner. The synovial membrane produces a small amount of the synovial fluid that acts as a lubricant to reduce friction between bones. The capsule surrounds the joint and keeps the synovial fluid from leaking.

The artificial hip joint consists of an acetabular cup made of UHMWPE, steel, ceramic, or polyethylene (PE) inner, femoral head made of steel or ceramic, as well as the femoral stem. UHMWPE acetabular cup is sometimes not covered with a metal shell. In joint prosthesis, polymers are used for one of the articulating surface components. Therefore, these polymers must have a low friction coefficient and low

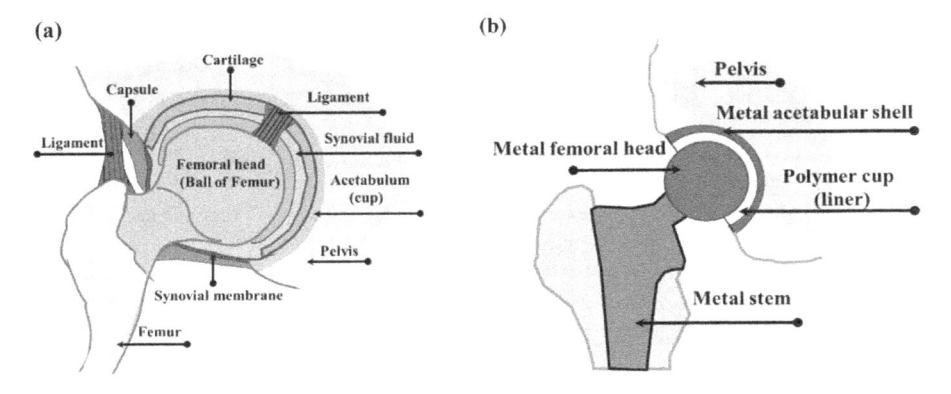

FIGURE 4.2 Schematic of the composition of hip joints:(a) normal hip joint; (b) artificial hip joint.

wear rate when they are in contact with the opposing surface, which is usually made of metal (e.g., cobalt-chromium alloys or titanium alloys) or ceramics such as alumina (Al_2O_3) and zirconia. These alloys are based on titanium, iron (surgical steel), cobalt, chromium, nickel (may cause allergies), zirconium, tantalum, noble metals, and carbon in different forms.[5]

According to the different materials of the femoral head and socket, there are three main types of artificial joints: metal (or ceramic)-on-polyethylene (MOP or COP), ceramic-on-ceramic (COC), and metal-on-metal (MOM).[6] As seen in Table 4.1, there are advantages and disadvantages of traditional artificial joints. Although ceramic joints have excellent biocompatibility and wear resistance, their wide application is limited due to their low toughness. Compared with MOP, the wear rate of MOM joints is reduced by two orders of magnitude; however, high concentration of metal ions can cause poisoning. Therefore, the vast majority of artificial joints available in the market are MOP joints.

Currently, the lifetime of such artificial joints is only about 15 years. Therefore, some (10%) patients require second replacements. It is currently an urgent need to extend the life expectancy, especially for patients aged <50 years.

4.2.2 CAUSES OF IMPLANT FAILURE

There are various causes for failure of implants that lead to revision surgery, such as particulate debris generation and accumulation in the human tissue resulting in hypersensitivity, inflammation due to rejection, low fatigue strength or low fracture toughness composed with bone, and mismatch in modulus of elasticity between the bone and implant.[3] However, it has been confirmed that wear debris is the main factor limiting the lifetime of the implants. Especially particulates that are phagocytosed by macrophages result in granulomatosis lesions, osteolysis, and bone resorption, causing pain and aseptic loosening of the prosthesis.[9,10]

TABLE 4.1
Comparison of Traditional Artificial Joints[7,8]

Hip Joints	Materials	Advantages	Disadvantages
MOP	Austenitic stainless steel; Co-Cr or Ti-Al alloy	0.1 mm/y of the line wear rate of polyethylene; better histocompatibility	Low friction coefficient
COP	Al_2O_3 ZrO_2	Excellent biocompatibility and wear resistance; 0.05 mm/y of the line wear rate	Low toughness
COC	Al_2O_3	No allergic reaction to metal ions; 0.001 mm/y of line wear rate	Ceramic fragmentation; abnormal sound; dislocation of prosthesis
MOM	Co-Cr alloy	0.005 mm/y of the line wear rate; joint dislocation rate reduced	High concentration of metal ions

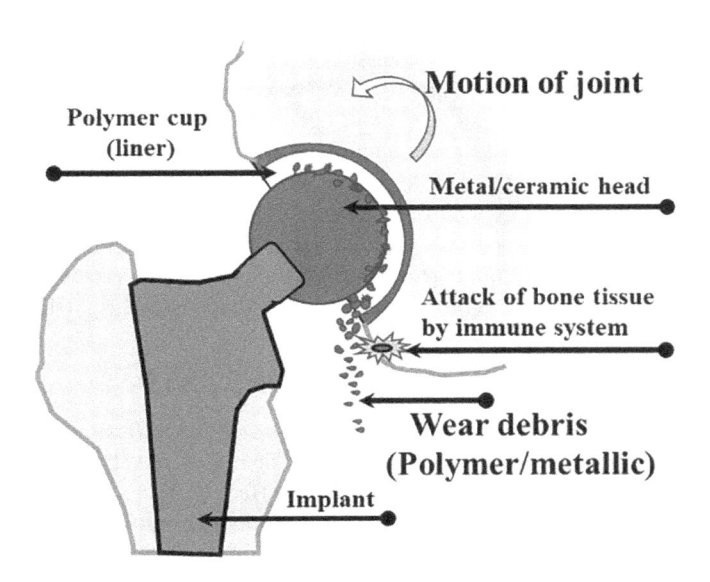

FIGURE 4.3 Wear of artificial hip joints.

Implant debris generated by wear and corrosion is a prominent cause of joint replacement failure. Figure 4.3 shows that during joint motion, wear particles are generated and shed into the surrounding synovial fluid and tissues, which initiates a macrophage-mediated inflammatory response, leading to osteoclast cell activation. Biological interaction with particles then occurs. The body's immune system attempts to digest the wear particles as it would be a bacterium or virus; meanwhile, enzymes are released that result in osteolysis. Over time, sufficient bone is resorbed around the implant to cause aseptic implant loosening.[11–13] If the particles are toxic, they cause a series of morphological changes in macrophages, including retraction of pseudopodia, blebbing and smoothing of the surface, and finally, cell destruction.[14]

Murray et al.[15] concluded that if there are enough particles, macrophages phagocytosing foreign particles become activated and release mediators (soluble factors) that stimulate bone resorption even though there is no toxic effect. Following this, the implant is loosened as its bony support is lost, which indicates the importance of the number of particles during implant loosening. Several studies have demonstrated that the composition and the volume of particles affect the macrophage response to particles.[16–20] Meanwhile, few researchers have proposed that the size of particles is also one of the critical factors associated with aseptic loosening,[19,21] and have demonstrated that submicron particles play a major role in wear particle-induced osteolysis.[17] Moreover, the large number of these particles, their size, as well as their ability to adsorb endotoxins can induce inflammatory reactions resulting in bone resorption. The onset of osteolysis is closely linked to both the volume and size of the wear debris produced.[22,23] The volume of debris generated is inversely proportional to the hardness of the materials; hence, hard-on-hard bearings have also been investigated.[24]

Hirayama et al.[25] have shown that particle size can affect the differentiation of macrophages into osteoclasts. The results show that the particles in the size range of 1~10 μm enhance the process of macrophage–osteoclast differentiation. Other studies[26–28] have shown that phagocytosis can occur with particles in the size range of 0.5~12 μm. There are two different mechanisms to internalize foreign bodies: phagocytosis and pinocytosis. In contrast to phagocytosis, particles with the size of 0.1 μm are thought to be taken in by macrophages via pinocytosis, which is less active than phagocytosis.[25] Therefore, particle size is also a very important factor for artificial hip joint loosening. In addition, research has shown that contact conditions and material parameters significantly influence the size and shape of wear particles.

4.3   BIOMATERIALS FOR ARTIFICIAL HIP JOINTS

Biomaterials refer to a class of materials with special properties and functions that are used for artificial organs, surgical repair, physical therapy rehabilitation, diagnosis, and treatment of diseases without adversely affecting human tissues. Currently, different kinds of synthetic materials and natural polymer materials, metal and alloy materials, ceramics and carbon materials, various composite materials, and their finished products are widely used in clinical and scientific research. The biomaterials used for artificial hip joints not only have good compatibility but also need to have high strength and good wear resistance.

4.3.1   METALLIC BIOMATERIALS FOR ARTIFICIAL HIP JOINT

Biomedical metallic materials are metals or alloys used as biomedical materials. Due to the high mechanical strength and anti-fatigue properties, metallic biomaterials are the most wildly used load-bearing implant material in clinical applications. Although some pure metals have excellent characteristics for use as load-bearing implants, most metallic implants are made from alloys, namely, medical-grade stainless steels (SS316L), cobalt-chromium alloys, and titanium alloy (e.g., Ti6Al4V, Ti6Al7Nb).[29] The Ni-free CrMnMo-steel X13CrMnMoN18-14-3 (1.4452, brand name: P2000) with high nitrogen (about 1%), due to high strength in combination with superior ductility[30] and better corrosion resistance,[31] has attracted more and more research interest.[32,33] Metal implants are essential tools for the treatment of bone fractures and joint replacements.

4.3.1.1   Biocompatibility of Metal Implants

All materials implanted in the human body must be non-toxic and biocompatible. The biological biocompatibility of any implant, which is defined by its toxicity, carcinogenicity, and metal sensitivity from the release of metal ions, must be quantified to reduce the patient's risk and failure of implants.[3] In other words, these materials are considered chemically stable with respect to the internal chemistry of the human body (i.e., good chemical biocompatibility).

The main elements of metal implants include cobalt, chromium, molybdenum, nickel, titanium, vanadium, and aluminum. The cytotoxicity of typical surgical implant alloys and pure metals have been studied by many researchers, as reported by Seinemann et al.[34] Ti, Zr, Nb, and Ta are low cytotoxic elements, exhibit an inert behavior, and have excellent biocompatibility; nevertheless, steel 316L and Co-Cr alloy are encapsulated by a tissue membrane and their behavior is not inert.[35]

However, it is observed that the blood levels of metal ions released from the metal joint are increased, which may negatively influence the hemocompatibility of the surface and cause a delayed-type metal hypersensitivity.[5,36] Additionally, the number of allergies is increasing at a rate of about 10% each year, and many people have allergies to implant metals or metallic particles (Cr, Co, Nic, and V).[36] Nickel is also a known allergenic carcinogen element that exhibits one of the highest sensitivities in metallic allergen tests.[37] Vanadium is classified in the sterile abscess group and aluminum in the capsule (scar tissue) group.[3] Al is involved in severe neurological disorders, for example, Alzheimer's disease, and metabolic bone diseases, for example, osteomalacia.[38]

The ideal biomaterial should possess good biological biocompatibility by being free of toxic elements. Therefore, stainless steel, Co-Cr-based and Ti-6Al-4V alloys, the most common implant alloys, are not the ideal alloys to be used for long-term implantation in the human body from a biological point of view due to their high content of high cytotoxic elements such as V, Ni, and Co.[3] Therefore, the development of Ni-free, Co-based, and Ti-based alloys is ongoing, as well as V- and Al-free Ti alloys are being developed as well. The nickel-free, high-nitrogen austenitic steel P2000 not only performed improved mechanical properties and high corrosion resistance but also displayed good biocompatibility and hemocompatibility compared to 316L, Ti6Al4V, or CoCrMo.[32] Ti-13Nb-13Zr alloy free of toxic elements shows improved bone biocompatibility and corrosion resistance compared to that of Co-Cr-based and Ti-6Al-4V alloys.[39]

4.3.1.2   Mechanical Properties of Metal Implants

Metal implants, especially as load-bearing joints, in many cases, should not only avoid short-term rejection and infection but also provide long-term biocompatibility and avoid long-term material limitations. Cyclic loading is applied to artificial implants during body motion, resulting in alternating plastic deformation of microscopically small zones of stress concentration produced by notches or microstructural inhomogeneities.[3] Therefore, in addition to the biological biocompatibility discussed above, mechanical properties are essential for long-term implantation.

The microstructure and mechanical properties of some common alloys commercially used in biomedical applications are listed in Table 4.2. Stainless steel shows moderate mechanical properties and is more resistant to a broad range of corrosive environments (e.g., human body fluid) due to the high Cr content of the steel. It allows the formation of a firmly adherent, self-healing, and corrosion-resistant coating oxide of Cr_2O_3.[42] Therefore, it is most often used in implants that are intended to help in fracture repairs, such as bone plants, bone screws, pins, and rods. Despite these properties, stainless steel implants are degraded because of pitting, crevice, corrosion fatigue, fretting corrosion, stress corrosion cracking, and galvanic corrosion in the body.[43] The elastic modulus of stainless steel is about 200 GPa higher than that of bone, as shown in Table 4.2. Moreover, when stainless steel is used as an MOM or MOP joint, a large amount of wear particles generated during body motion leads to aseptic loosening of the joint, and the wear resistance is relatively weak.

TABLE 4.2

Mechanical Properties of Metal Implants and Human Bone[30,40,41]

Material	Microstructure	Elastic Modulus (GPa)	Vickers Hardness(Hv)	Yield Strength (MPa)	Ultimate Tensile Strength (MPa)	Fatigue Limit (GPa)
Bone	Viscoelastic composite	30	26.3	-	90-140	-
SS316L[a]	Austenite	211	190	280	480	0.28
P2000	Ni-free Austenite	-	259	590	1030	0.30
CoCrMo	Austenite	541	450	1050	565	0.49
Ti-6Al-4V	α+β	121	-	970	780	0.40

[a] annealed

Compared to 316 steel, P2000 also provides better corrosion resistance, which accounts for the high nitrogen content.[31] Nanoindentation hardness tests of 316L, CoCrMo, and P2000 specimens exposed an indentation hardness of about 4, 5.6, and 7.5 GPa, respectively. Becerikli et al. [34] demonstrated the advantages of P2000 against titanium, 316L, or CoCrMo. They concluded that P2000 is available and has processing similar to that of other steels, and can therefore be used directly. Moreover, it can be a promising alternative candidate for applications in bone surgery.

Cobalt-chromium alloys have excellent mechanical properties, as shown in Table 4.2, such as higher hardness and high fatigue resistance, but relatively high strength compared to that of bone;[44] hence, they are used in various joint replacement implants, as well as some fracture repair implants that require a long service life. It is well known that the higher the fatigue strength of an alloy is, the longer is the lifetime of the implant. However, CoCrMo implants have been related to metal hypersensitivity, local adverse tissue reactions, and implant failure.[45–47] Adverse biological effects of chromium and cobalt ions from CoCrMo implants have been also reported.[48,49]

At present, titanium alloys are extensively used as bone replacement implants due to their excellent mechanical properties, corrosion resistance, and biocompatibility compared to other metallic materials, accounting for the enhanced utilization of these alloys in medical applications.[50] Moreover, they are excellent biomaterials due to their light weight (the density is half of the CoCrMo alloy) and the high yield strength, as well as their relatively low elastic modulus, making it an ideal material for long-term implantation.[51] However, titanium and titanium alloys show relatively high elastic modulus (about 120 GPa) resulting from α or α+β phase existing in the alloy compared with that of human bone (maximum 30 GPa), as shown in Table 4.2. Moreover, they display a relatively poor tribological performance, which limits their use in medical fields. To decrease the elastic modulus of implants, various β-type titanium alloys with a low elastic modulus have been developed such as Ti-29Nb-13Ta-4.5Zr (TNTZ)[52,53] and Ti-35Nb-5Ta-7Zr (TNZT).[34,54] Although the elastic modulus of these β-type titanium alloys is as low as about 60 GPa close to that of human bone, they are expensive due to the low abundance of these elements in the earth's crust.

Furthermore, titanium and its alloys can easily react with oxygen to form TiO_2, Ti_3O_2, and TiO in a physiological environment. Although this oxidation film possesses good corrosion resistance and displays a biologically inert property, it spalls during contact friction because of the complexity of human body fluid, continuous external force, and poor wear resistance. Consequently, this film fails to provide efficient protection. Spalling oxide also participates in the wear of a friction pair, resulting in abrasive wear. In addition, Ti6Al4V releases numerous metal ions when this alloy is exposed to constant wear; these ions then accumulate around joint tissues and induce abnormal reactions in the human body, thereby causing aseptic loosening and failure.[55–57]

4.3.1.3 Tribocorrosion Properties of Metal Implants

Although metals used in implants are corrosion-resistant, there are still some interchanges of metal ions into the tissues or tissue fluids, which is related to the corrosion resistance of the metal, environmental conditions, mechanical factors, electrochemical effects, and dense cell concentrations around implants.

Tribology is fundamental to the function and long-term survival of orthopedic implants. Tribocorrosion can be defined as the study of the influence of environmental factors (chemical and/or electrochemical) on the tribological behavior of surfaces, which refers to synergistic effects of wear and corrosion on metals with passive films.[58,59] Much tribocorrosion research work are *in-vitro* experiments, investigated with laboratory tribometer machines or hip simulators integrated with a three-electrode electrochemical setup, as shown in Figure 4.4.[58] The metal disk is used as the working electrode (WE). A platinum wire is a typical counter electrode (CE), and RE stands for a reference electrode.

The tribological test refers to a rotating disk and sliding pin, which has been described as "pin-on-disk" or "pin-on-plate". The disk-on-disk test with a Wazau TRM 1000 tribometer (Berlin, Germany) was also used to study the tribological properties and generate wear particles, where a rotary disk is located above and pressed against a stationary disk with a defined normal force.[60] The biotribocorrosion setup is commonly used to study the wear and corrosion of metallic implants *in-vitro* tests. Both tribological and corrosion (electrochemical) were studied using

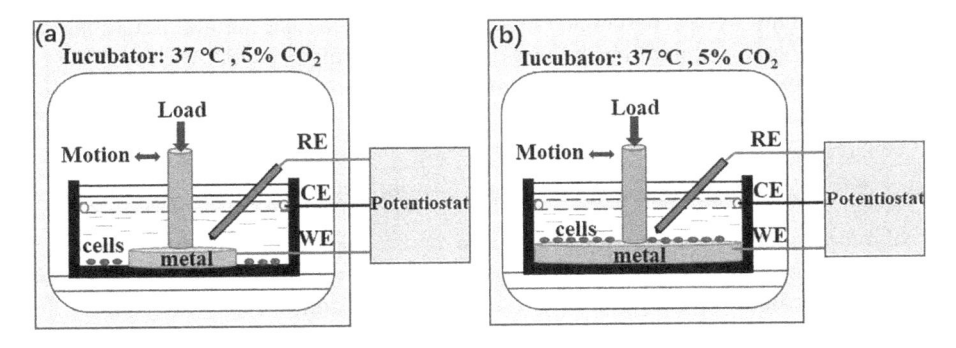

FIGURE 4.4 Schematic of the biotribocorrosion test system: (a) cells cultured near the metal surface; (b) cells cultured on the metal surface.[58]

the schematic diagrams shown in Figure 4.4. There are many parameters during the biotribocorrosion process, for example, load or amplitude and frequency in oscillation wear, as well as the duration of the wear test affecting the living cell culture, and so on.

Figure 4.4 shows two setups depending on the place where the cells are cultured. The left setup corresponds to having cell culture dishes located near the metal, where the tribocorrosion process takes place, which primarily addressed the issue of cells' response to wear and corrosion debris.[61-63] Researchers successfully implemented fretting tests within a cell culture (L929 mouse fibroblasts) and using stainless steel, Co-Cr alloy, and Ti6Al4V as orthopedics plates and screws. This setup was found to generate corrosion debris with resulting metal ion release, rather than metallic debris from wear.[61,62] Impergre et al.[63] studied cell viability test, cell cytotoxicity, PE wear rate, PE wear debris analysis, metal ion release, and inflammatory cytokine measurements by building up inside a clean room within a custom thermostatic enclosure for a controlled atmosphere replacing the incubator in the context of an orthopedic system simulating the wear in total ankle prostheses.

Another one corresponds to having cells cultured directly on the metal, thus directly involved in the electrochemical (corrosion) processes occurring at the metallic surface, which investigated issues related to the fixation interface of implants, that is, the question of biocompatibility and osseointegration of modified surfaces.[64-68] Cells cultured directly in the wear contact were seen as a lubricant component.[65] This experimental setup was used first in 2007 by Shi et al.[64] Frictional properties and wettability of Ni samples under dry and lubricated conditions were studied. It was reported that cells did not attach to the Ni-matrix, and a lower and more constant friction coefficient was noted with cells cultured on the Ni-matrix compared to BSA solution.[64] The problem of implant fixation at the bone–stem interface in THR was addressed by Runa et al. [67,68] In a study by Runa et al.,[67] the influence of an osteoblastic layer on the tribocorrosion behavior of Ti6Al4V alloy was demonstrated.

They showed that metals and metal alloys used in implants are generally well tolerated in most orthopedic clinical cases. However, the use of metal implant components has not been free from complications resulting from inflammatory and immune reactions. In addition to the increased osteolytic activity caused by wear particles, the current evidence strongly suggests that the released metal ions stimulate the immune system and bone metabolism through a series of direct and indirect pathways, thereby promoting the pathophysiological mechanism of aseptic loosening. The occurrence of such complications can be reduced by choosing a metal alloy for joint replacement.

4.3.2 POLYMER BIOMATERIALS FOR ARTIFICIAL HIP JOINTS

Polymer materials, due to their low cost and a wide range of mechanical and physical properties, are popular for various applications, including the biomedical field. According to their durability in biological environments, biodegradable and biostable polymers can be implanted into the human body.[69] Poly(e-caprolactone) (PCL), poly(glycolic acid) (PGA), poly(lactic acid) (PLA), and poly(lactic-co-glycolic acid), as biodegradable polymers, have been widely used as sutures,

TABLE 4.3
Mechanical Properties of Polymer Implants[72]

Material	Elastic Modulus (GPa)	Tensile Strength (MPa)
PE	0.88	35
UHMWPE	0.96	48
PMMA	2.55	59
PEEK	8.3	139

membranes to support wound healing, stents, and patches.[70] They are resorbable, that is, they can break down gradually in the physiological environment of the body into biocompatible products.

For longer-term applications, such as osteosynthesis plates, pins, and screws, these implants not only have biological properties but also have mechanical properties. Table 4.3 shows the mechanical properties of polymer implants. These implants can degrade predictably and yet maintain their mechanical strength over an extended period. Poly-β-hydroxybutyrate (PHB) as a degradation product shows good tissue response to the material and was considered for use in the fabrication of long-term resorbable implants or drug delivery systems.[71] The second class of biostable polymers are PE or UHMWPE, polymethyl-methacrylate (PMMA), and polyetheretherketone (PEEK), which are used in hip and dental implants. UHMWPE has been used extensively for hip and knee joints as well. In 1962, PMMA was used as bone cement fixation with a metal stem in MOP hip prostheses, where a UHMWPE was chosen as the acetabulum.

4.3.2.1 Ultra-High-Molecular-Weight Polyethylene (UHMWPE)

UHMWPE consisting of only hydrogen and carbon, as a linear homopolymer with outstanding physical and mechanical properties, has excellent biocompatibility, wear resistance, and corrosion resistance. This polymer is a high-molecular-weight PE with extremely long chains (between 2 and 6 million atomic mass units). It is an ideal material for biomedical implants, especially used in orthopedics as a bearing material in artificial joints. The commonly used prosthetic nucleus pulposus has an outer layer of UHMWPE and a hydrophilic hydrogel core. Therefore, UHMWPE is usually used to simulate the outer layer as the sample ball in tribocorrosion research for friction pairs. The ball indentation hardness of UHMWPE is about 78 MPa, and the elastic modulus is about 1.52 GPa.

As working implant and bone are unevenly loaded, polymers as low modulus material are suitable, but low modulus associated with little strength restricts the potential use of polymers.[73] For long-term applications, researchers have suggested reinforcing polymer with carbon fibers to improve its creep resistance, stiffness, and strength.[71] It has been reported that reinforcing PEEK with carbon fiber (CF/PEEK) offers superior wear resistance compared to unfilled UHMWPE when rubbed against either metal or ceramic.[74,75] Additionally, the mismatch of the stiffness of femur bone and prosthesis is another serious problem associated with THR. Metal alloys as commercial hip joint stems are 5–6 times stiffer than bone, which leads to aseptic loosening and failure of the joint.[73] Some composite polymers, such as CF/epoxy and CF/UHMWPE, can provide tailor implant with selecting material ingredients and controlling ingredient composition, which helps to manage strength and modulus according to requirement.[76,77] Therefore, the composite polymers are suitable for artificial hip joint stems. CF/PEEK composite stem possess a mechanical behavior similar to that of the femur.[77] Compared to pure UHMWPE, the addition of multi-walled carbon nanotube (MWCNT) to UHMWPE can improve the mechanical characteristics and superior wear behavior.[78] The strain energy density, ductility, and tensile strength were increased significantly. The wear volume and wear coefficient were decreased.[79] However, few animal studies have observed adverse effects of MWCNT on the lung, liver, and kidney.[42]

4.3.2.2 Highly Cross-Linked Polyethylenes (HXLPEs)

Highly cross-linked polyethylenes (HXLPEs), developed in the 1990s by cross-linking polymer chains and forming bonds between them, allows the modification of the molecular structure of the PE.[80] Cross-linking is done by free radical reactions that are achieved by irradiation using either electron beams or gamma rays.[80] Some researchers introduced vitamin E to exhibit signs of HXLPEs oxidation before the molding process.[81,82] This new structure leads to a significantly higher resistance against abrasive and adhesive wear, which has been confirmed by initial clinical studies and makes researchers interested in its studies as artificial joint friction pairs. Additionally, lower revision rate for HXLPE compared with standard PE for metal-on-HXLPE and ceramic-on-HXLPE has been reported. However, the survival advantages of HXLPE will inevitably need to be determined in large cohorts, and long observation periods will be required.

4.3.3 CERAMIC BIOMATERIALS FOR ARTIFICIAL HIP JOINTS

Ceramic materials, due to good biocompatibility, ultra-high hardness, wear resistance, and corrosion resistance, can solve the problem of osteolysis caused by the wear particles of metal and polymer prosthetic materials, and can also overcome the problem of metal ions released from prostheses in the body. Furthermore, ceramic materials have good hydrophilic ability and can ensure the lubricity of joints as artificial joints. Usually, this kind of ceramic materials is defined as "bioceramics".

Ceramics are a crystalline structure where atoms are held together by ionic and covalent bonds, which gives these compound high compressive strength, hardness, and chemical inertness. Ceramics are categorized as oxidized ceramics (Al_2O_3, ZrO_2) and non-oxidized ceramics (Si_3N_4, SiC). Alumina-zirconia composite known as zirconia-toughened alumina (ZTA) has also been used in hip replacement.[83] As seen in Table 4.4, there are mechanical properties of Al_2O_3, ZTA, and Si_3N_4.

Alumina is the most frequently used in THA owing to its low friction, low wear coefficient, and better biocompatibility than metals and PE materials. The first-generation alumina (Al_2O_3) ceramic product was first applied to artificial hip replacements by a French doctor Boutin in the 1970s, in which wear resistance was better than traditional metal and PE materials.[84] However, under microseparation conditions, one study showed that the wear rate increased to almost $2\,mm^3$/ million cycles.[85] Due to

TABLE 4.4
Mechanical Properties of Ceramics[42]

Material	Vickers Hardness (GPa)	Elastic Modulus (GPa)	Tensile Strength (MPa)	Compressive Strength (MPa)
Al_2O_3	14–16	400–450	250–300	2,000–3,000
ZTA^a	19.1	350	-	2,400
Si_3N_4	13–16	300–320	350–400	2,500–3,000

a 20 Vol% ZrO_2

the brittle nature of alumina components and the catastrophic consequences of a possible fracture with the generation of a large number of small alumina fragments, the use of alumina-on-alumina bearing was not widespread until the early 2000s when the new composite ceramic ZTA (82% alumina and 17% zirconia) was introduced.[86] Despite its improved strength and toughness, ZTA is still unstable and prone to low-temperature degradation (aging) in most environments.[87]

Compared with Al_2O_3, zirconia (ZrO_2) as the most fracture-resistant ceramic offers two to three times more flexure strength and fracture toughness. Due to its excellent mechanical properties, zirconia material has become one of the important materials in the field of oral restoration. However, pure zirconia is unstable and transforms from one form to another, leading to a change in shape and volume. Therefore, zirconia composite was developed to control its phase transformation by adding stabilizing materials such as magnesia (MgO), calcium oxide (CaO), and yttria (Y_2O_3). Additionally, zirconia is also an effective additive for strengthening and toughening ceramic materials. ZTA ceramics, dispersing the stabilized zirconia nanoparticles in an alumina matrix, can effectively inhibit the growth of the crystal grains of the alumina and are also beneficial to the existence of the metastable zirconia phase.

Silicon nitride is biocompatible but is widely used in various industrial applications and is reliable under extreme conditions in a space vehicle and aircraft due to low friction and corrosion resistance.[88] Some researchers investigated that Si_3N_4 presented low coefficient of friction and low wear during sliding against itself in water or in the presence of bovine serum and PBS, and there were no adverse effects when silicon nitride was implanted in spinal surgery in the last 4 years.[89–93] Bonshitskaya et al. found that Si_3N_4 wear particles would be biodegradable and suggested that Si_3N_4 can be used in hip joint replacement because silicon nitride was less prone to wear and silicon nitride powder can dissolve in blood serum, gastric juice, and synthetic biochemical media at pH 7.4.[90] Compared with alumina sliding against alumina bearing, silicon nitride sliding against itself or Co-Cr alloy showed the lowest wear rate.[94] Therefore, silicon nitride is a very good alternative for hip joint replacement.

Silicon carbide ceramics not only have excellent normal temperature mechanical properties, such as high bending strength, excellent oxidation resistance, good corrosion resistance, high wear resistance, and low friction coefficient but also high-temperature mechanical properties (strength, creep resistance).[95] However, the disadvantage of SiC ceramics is lower fracture toughness, that is, higher brittleness.

Therefore, SiC is widely used in high-temperature bearings, high-temperature corrosion-resistant parts, and some high-temperature electronic equipment parts, but is rarely used as artificial joint ceramics. Meanwhile, ceramic heads with titanium alloy inner sleeves may reduce the risk of recurrence of corrosion issues at the level of the taper compared to Co-Cr heads, but this remains unconfirmed.[96,97]

In conclusion, the ideal THR material still needs to be evaluated with the modifying metal surface, improving the PE and developing composite ceramic. Coating or addition of boron nitride in nonoxide ceramic-like silicon nitride implant material also presents an opportunity for the development of future materials.

4.4 CLASSIFICATION FOR ARTIFICIAL HIP JOINTS

4.4.1 Metal Femoral Heads Articulating Against Polyethylene Cups (MOP)

In the early 1960s, MOP bearings as hip implants began to be used, but cases of aseptic loosening of prostheses started to be seen toward the beginning of the 1970s. Figure 4.5 shows the components of the MOP hip implant. The convex femoral stem and femoral head are constructed using metal (usually a cobalt chrome alloy) and the concave cup liner is made of PE. After several years of investigation, it was confirmed that the observed cases of aseptic loosening could be explained by a concept they described as "particle disease".[98]

PE debris particles are generated in the absence of fluid film lubrication between the femoral head and the acetabular cup due to abrasive and adhesive wear caused by the relative movements between the two surfaces. Wear particles trigger a series

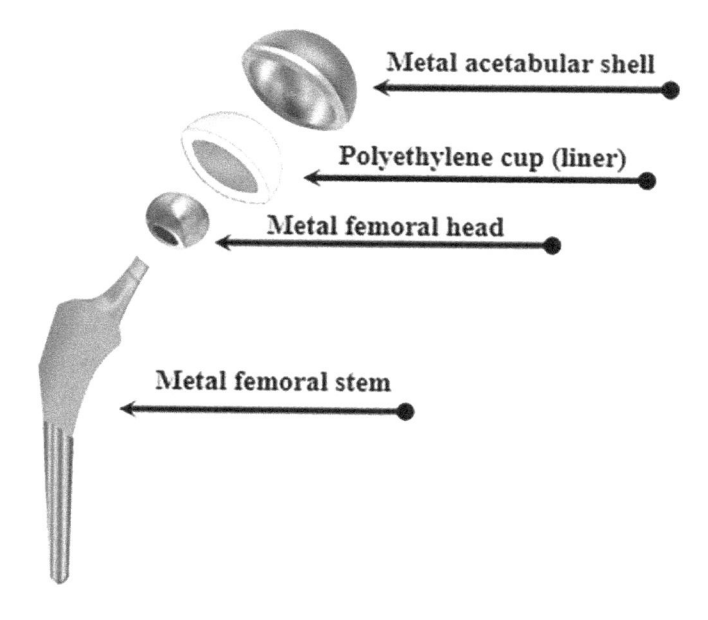

Metal acetabular shell

Polyethylene cup (liner)

Metal femoral head

Metal femoral stem

FIGURE 4.5 Components of metal-on-polyethylene hip implant.

of biochemical reactions, which change the dynamic balance between osteoblasts and osteoclasts. The enhanced osteoclast activity results in osteolysis in the areas affected by a high number of wear particles. This resorption of bone eventually leads to aseptic loosening of implants in the long term. Osteolysis is directly correlated with the amount of debris particles.

However, about 10^{10}–10^{11} PE wear debris is generated, which weakens the surrounding bone causing bone resorption and loosening of the prosthesis and ultimate failure.[99–101] In addition, the average wear rate of the polymer cup ranges 20–60 mm³/year for the MOP hip joint. To maximize implant survival, articulating components should minimize the generation of wear particles of a biologically critical size, which is, according to Green et al., between 0.3 and 10 μm.[102]

Generally, the most common materials used in orthopedic implants are metals and UHMWPE. These two material types are combined in most joint implants. Traditional metal femoral heads articulating against UHMWPE acetabular cups are widely employed in prosthetic hip replacements and most of them are successful clinically.[103] Although some pure metals have excellent characteristics for use as implants, most metallic implants are made from alloys, namely, stainless steels, cobalt-chromium alloys, and titanium alloys. According to Long et al., [104] cobalt-base alloys are the most commonly used metals for current MOP implants. The oxide surface layer on titanium alloy (Ti-6Al-4V) femoral heads result in high UHMWPE wear due to the breakdown of the titanium surface.

Metal-on-UHMWPE bearings are still commonly used today as conventional artificial hip joints. The standard head diameters range between 22 mm and 32 mm. Linear wear of metal-on-UHMWPE bearings is typically within the range of 100–300 μm/year, which corresponds to volumetric wear of around 20–150 mm³/year for 28 mm heads.[105,106] Previous research has suggested that linear wear rates for 22 mm, 28 mm, and 32 mm do not vary significantly.[107]

Comparing with the conventional PE, the highly cross-linked PE (HXLPE) showed good wear resistance. The metal-on-HXLPE first used for total hip prosthesis was introduced at the end of the 1990s and showed a significant wear reduction.[2] For metal-on-HXLPE bearings, linear wear rates ranged between 2 and 20 μm/year, and volumetric wear rates were substantially lower than 1 mm³/year for 28 mm prosthetic femoral heads.[108–111] The Australian National Joint Replacement Registry reported that the 14-year cumulative revision rate for metal-on-HXLPE compared with conventional PE decreased from 9.9% to 5.4%.[2]

Adverse soft tissue reactions and pain can occur in metal-on-highly cross-linked polyethylene (MOP) THA, and histopathological study on MOP THA was confirmed to be pseudotumor associated with corrosion products released from the head–neck junction.[97]

4.4.2 METAL FEMORAL HEADS ARTICULATING AGAINST METAL CUPS (MOM)

The hip implants of metal femoral heads articulating against metal cups have been used even longer than MOP implants. Only MOM components allow the largest heads throughout the entire range of implant sizes. Figure 4.6 shows the MOM hip joint. With MOM implants, liners may be eliminated allowing surgeons to use large femoral heads.

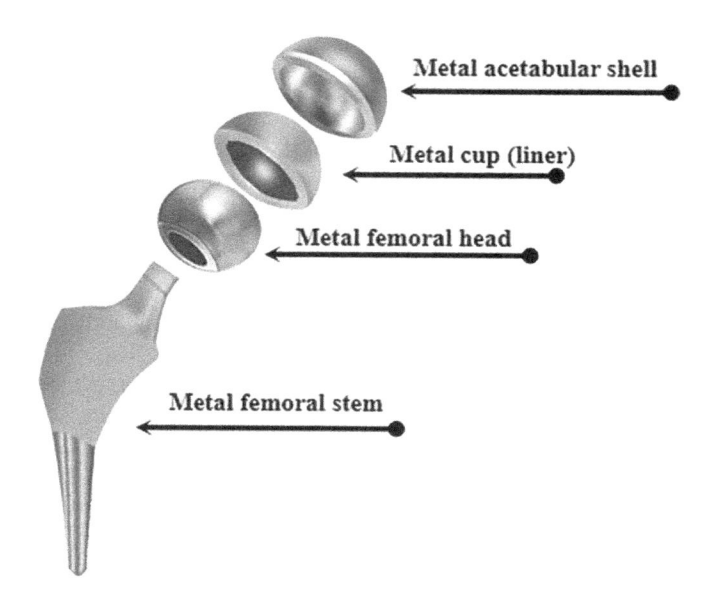

FIGURE 4.6   Metal-on-Metal hip joint.

The MOM articulation was THA's first bearing when it was first implanted by Wiles in 1938. The cast CoCrMo alloys were widely used as the main material for these bearings between the 1950s and 1970s. However, these long-established bearings had largely unsatisfactory clinical results, such as increased wear and friction.[112] Although the MOM THR was introduced in the 1960s, the early failure rate of this implant is higher than that of the prosthesis based on MOP joints due to bearing irregularities and impingement. At the 20-years follow-up, it was found that the survival rate of MOM is no longer lower than that of MOP prosthesis, which is 77% and 73%, respectively.[113]

Debris generated from THA is known to trigger adverse soft tissue reaction. Recently, academic attention has focused on MOM bearings.[114] Compared with UHMWPE, MOM hip joints have a lower rate in the range of 1–5 mm³/year, and the wear debris particles are reduced, smaller than those of UHMWPE in metal-on-UHMWPE and ceramic-on-UHMWPE implants.[101,104,115] Although wear is reduced with MOM implants, wear products about 10^9 in size (submicroscopic particulates, soluble metal ions) are distributed throughout the body. This has raised concerns about long-term biocompatibility.

For MOM bearings, the debris was generated from modular junctions or metal interfaces, which caused adverse soft tissue reactions. The mechanism may be fretting, crevice corrosion, or a mixture of both.[116,117] The concept that corrosion may occur at the mixed alloy modular head–neck taper junction in hip arthroplasty was first introduced over 30 years ago. Mechanical disruption of the passivation layer and crevice corrosion were suggested as potential causes.[118] The effect may be time-dependent and is greater in mixed alloys.[116,118] Once initiated, crevice corrosion may continue even in the absence of loading.[119]

Patients with an adverse reaction to metal debris have a variable presentation of pain, soft tissue pseudotumor, instability, or asymptomatic lesions. The presentation may be confused with periprosthetic joint infection.[120] In 2011, Bolland et al. reported the mid-term results of a large-bearing hybrid MOM THR (cobalt chrome) in 199 hips (185 patients) with a mean follow-up of 62 months. A high failure rate was observed, with evidence of high wear at the trunnion–head interface and passive corrosion of the stem surface, which resulted from the use of large heads on conventional 12/14 tapers. Additionally, there was a significant increase in Co levels, but no significant rise in Cr or Mo ion levels. This effect has been attributed to debris produced from the head–neck taper junction rather than the bearing surface.[97,121]

However, for MOM implants, although there is no conclusion on whether the worn heavy metal ions will cause harm to the human body, they may have an impact on fetal development. Because heavy metal ions are mainly excreted through the kidneys, the MOM bearings are not suitable for patients with renal insufficiency. Moreover, wear particles produced during the motion of the joint have been identified as the main factor limiting the lifetime of the implants, the number of wear particles have attracted research attention. As described above, the volume of debris is inversely proportional to the material's hardness, thus hard-on-hard bearings have also been investigated.[26]

4.4.3 CERAMIC FEMORAL HEADS ARTICULATING AGAINST POLYETHYLENE CUPS (COP)

Due to excellent biocompatibility and low friction coefficient, ceramic materials have been used instead of a metallic femoral head for artificial joints.[122] COP is a good combination of two very reliable materials and currently accounts for around one in seven hip replacements in the UK according to the report of the National Joint Registry of England and Wale. Figure 4.7 shows the COP hip joint. Ceramic heads are harder than metal and are the most scratch-resistant implant material. The hard, ultra-smooth surface can greatly reduce the wear rate on the PE bearing. The potential wear rate for this type of implant is less than MOP.

Hip simulator studies have shown variable results depending on the lubricant used between the two surfaces. Compared to the traditional metal and PE materials, the average wear rate of the UHMWPE can be decreased by 50% when a ceramic femoral head articulates against UHMWPE.[123,124] However, these results have been brought into doubt as the saline used for the lubricant allows for virtually no PE wear to occur. Clarke used different concentrations of lubricants, showing that an alumina head using bovine serum as lubricants can reduce wear by an average of 50%.[125] Retrieval studies have found that alumina heads, although worn, remained smoother than new cobalt chrome heads, which indicated a significant reduction of PE wear when using COP.[126]

There are some *in-vivo* studies evaluating wear rates of COP compared with other artificial hip joints. Compared with standard MOP implants, alumina femoral heads have been documented to induce lower rates of linear and volumetric wear (0.03–0.1 mm per year) *in vivo* resulting in significantly lower rates of osteolysis and revision surgery.[127–129] When discarding studies which include zirconia ceramic implants, the difference is more pronounced.

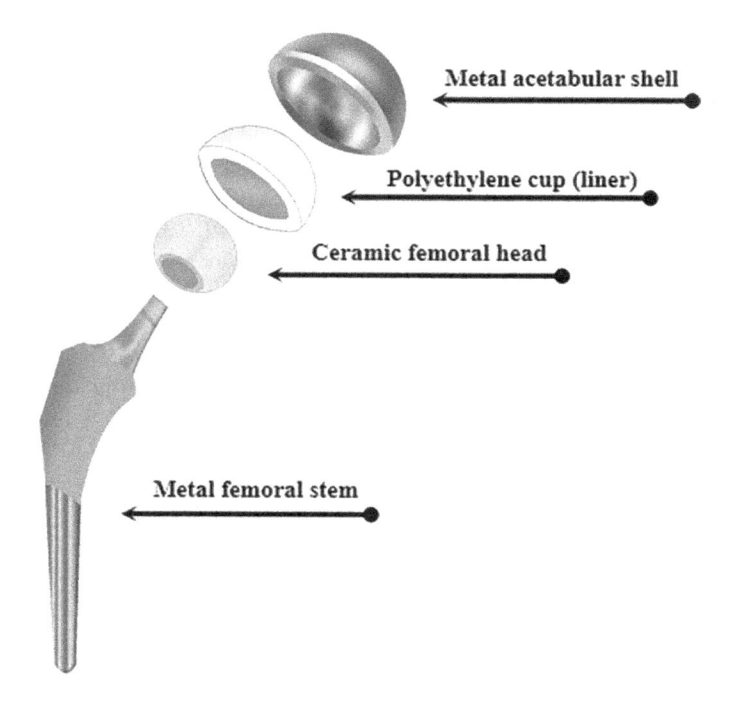

FIGURE 4.7   Ceramic-on-polyethylene hip joint.

Considering the number of wear particles, a major step has been taken using highly cross-linked PE as an inlay material in combination with a ceramic joint head. It was found that acetabular wear rates were reduced by 50% and the rate of osteolysis was zero compared with 25% for the standard polyethylene.[130] Additionally, the highly cross-linked PE shows very little wear at 5 million cycles even at thicknesses of 4 mm even when it is eccentrically loaded.[131]

Although ceramic materials generate significantly less PE debris when used in conjunction with PE acetabular components in bearing couples, there is still a large number of particles. Additionally, stress shielding due to the high elastic modulus of ceramic materials may be responsible for cancellous bone atrophy and loosening of the acetabular cup in older patients with senile osteoporosis or rheumatoid arthritis.[132] Therefore, the new PE and alumina ceramics have good mid-term outcomes and reduce the risk of catastrophic failure.[133] Of cause, COP should be seriously considered especially in younger patients, but long-term research using newer implant materials must be conducted.

4.4.4   CERAMIC FEMORAL HEADS ARTICULATING AGAINST CERAMIC CUPS (COC)

COC articulation, as shown in Figure 4.8, developed in 1970 was another "alternative" bearing to the MOP.[84,134] Al_2O_3 and ZrO_2 ceramic are usually used in THA, where alumina is the most frequently used of the two because it is chemically more stable *in vivo*.

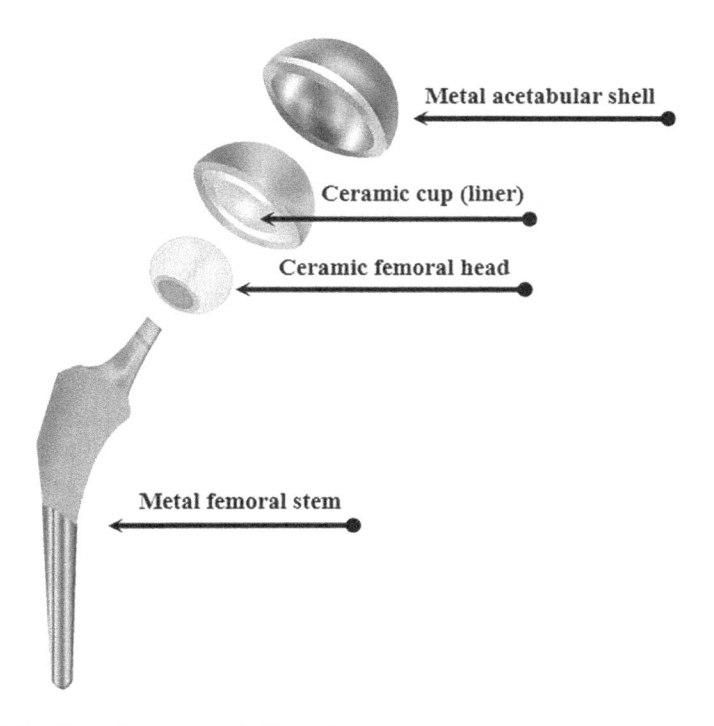

FIGURE 4.8 Ceramic-on-ceramic hip replacement.

However, the early alumina ceramic total hip joint had problems in the quality of ceramic materials, fixation of the ceramic acetabulum on the pelvic bone, and connection between ceramic head and femoral stem prosthesis; hence, it has not been promoted clinically. By the 1980s, improvements in material quality and processing technology, as well as further development of ceramic design, made second-generation alumina parts have better wear resistance. COC hip joints, where an alumina femoral head is combined with an alumina acetabular cup, show very low wear in the range of 0.05 mm³/year [123] and reduce the wear rate to just 0.032 mm³/million cycles. However, due to the brittle nature of alumina, zirconia nanoparticles were introduced to the alumina matrix to improve the toughness of COC bearings. For example, COC articulation (82% Al_2O_3 and 17% ZrO_2) has twice the tenacity of pure alumina, which reduces the risk of *in vivo* fracture.[86] Fracture rates of the femoral head have reduced from 0.021% for alumina-on-alumina to 0.003% for COC articulation (82% Al_2O_3 and 17% ZrO_2).[135]

Furthermore, the use of COC hip joint not only resolves the problems caused by wear debris but also alleviates any concerns about metal ion release into the body compared to other hip joint systems discussed above. Long-term clinical results for alumina COC have shown a cumulative survival rate of 99% at 10-year follow-up and 84.4% survival after 21 years.[136–138] There was no osteolysis, loosening, fractures, or squeaking at a minimum follow-up of 4.5 years in young patients (<30 years).[139,140] Moreover, it was reported that large-diameter COC articulation (up to 48 mm) did not have higher wear rate comparing with small bearings (up to 32 mm) after an *in vitro* study, and remains low even under edge-loading conditions.[141] Therefore, it is very popular with a patient population requiring large-diameter femoral heads, although it is still essential to avoid malposition.[142] First results from the Australian National Joint Replacement Registry confirm that at the 5-year follow-up, the revision rate of large-diameter COC articulations is not inferior to the revision rate of 32 mm heads.[143]

The superior wear resistance of ceramic materials can prolong the life of artificial joints, making the estimated life of ceramic and ceramic joints more than 20 years. Although COC hip joint has these advantages, they may crack and release millions of hard particles which cannot all be removed surgically. Moreover, noises such as clicking, grinding, clunking, scraping, and squeaking have been reported in the literature as adverse events after COC implantation, with squeaking being the most common.[2]

The best choice for ceramic hip joints is COC because ceramic particles are so hard that they can make metals or UHMWPE wear out quickly if they migrate onto the articulating surfaces. The improvement in material quality and processing technology, as well as the further development of ceramic design, make the second-generation alumina parts have better wear resistance. The superior wear resistance of ceramic materials can prolong the life of artificial joints, making the estimated life of ceramic and ceramic joints more than 20 years.

4.5 DIAMOND-LIKE CARBON (DLC) COATINGS FOR ARTIFICIAL HIP JOINT

As described above, to overcome the problem of wear particle generation in artificial implants, a new low wear material is required. The importance of the surface treatment was reported by Dowson in a comparative study of the performance of metallic and ceramic femoral heads. Therefore, the coating is applied to the hip joint replacement because the implant surface can be modified by deposition.

4.5.1 CLASSIFICATION AND DEPOSITION OF DLC COATINGS

DLC coatings is a metastable form of amorphous carbon containing both sp^2 (graphite-like) and sp^3 bonds (diamond-like) in its microstructure. DLC (at least 10% sp^3 content) is wildly used in mechanical fields due to excellent tribological properties, for example, high hardness and low friction coefficient. Moreover, DLC has good biocompatibility and no toxic effects on the human body.[144] DLC film, as a coating on the articular surface, can greatly improve the wear resistance of metal components and prevent metal ions from diffusing into the tissue fluid.

Figure 4.9 shows the ternary phase diagram for various DLC films concerning sp^3, sp^2, and H content. According to the hydrogen content in the DLC coating, it can be divided into two categories: hydrogenated amorphous carbon (a-C:H) and hydrogen-free amorphous carbon (a-C). Non-hydrogenated DLC coatings, with high sp^3 content of up to 80% and hardness of up to HV 80 GPa, can also be defined as tetrahedral amorphous carbon coatings (ta-C).[145] The structure of amorphous carbon depends on the carbon source and deposition method.

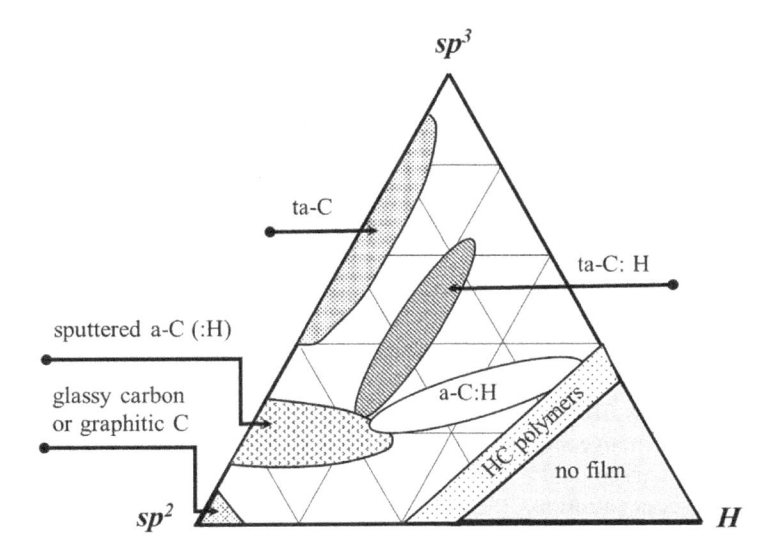

FIGURE 4.9 Ternary phase diagram for various DLC films with respect to sp^3, sp^2, and hydrogen contents [144,145]

The properties of DLC coatings depend on the deposition method which can be mainly classified into physical vapor deposition (PVD) and chemical vapor deposition (CVD), especially plasma-enhanced CVD (PECVD). Usually, a-C:H coatings are deposited using a hydrocarbon gas such as methane or acetylene as a precursor via PECVD, which can provide the required energy and the required deposition temperature. In contrast, a-C and ta-C coatings are prepared by evaporating carbon-containing materials to deposit carbon ions on the surface of the substrate. Common PVD methods include magnetron sputtering, pulsed laser, vacuum arc evaporation, and ion implantation.[35,146–148] Therefore, DLC surface modification for traditional artificial joints has become a research focus in the field of biomedical materials.

4.5.2 INTERNAL STRESS OF DLC COATINGS

The DLC coating is deposited in a non-thermal equilibrium state. Therefore, DLC coatings have high residual stress due to the violent deposition process, which results in poor adhesion of DLC coating and substrates and poor tribological properties. Residual stress is dominated by internal stress, and is mainly caused by impurity effects introduced during the film deposition process and lattice defects inside the film. For a-C film, the internal stress is related to the deformation of the carbon bond and the twist of the bond angle in the film. The higher the sp^3, the greater the internal stress. The internal stress of a-C:H film is related to the hydrogen content, the increase in hydrogen content, and the internal stress.[149] It was reported that the major shortcoming limiting the working life of DLC coatings in engine applications is high internal stress and insufficient coating thicknesses.[150]

At present, the internal stress of DLC films is mainly reduced by post-deposition thermal annealing[151] or by doping different elements during the deposition process using substrate biasing[152,153] or ion irradiation.[154] It was reported that a 10 µm thick high-quality DLC coating was successfully deposited with several steps of deposition and annealing.[155] Qiong et al. [149] reviewed the mechanism of different types of element doping to reduce the internal stress of DLC, mainly by forming nanocrystalline or amorphous embedded in the DLC amorphous matrix, changing the carbon bond and bond angle in the DLC film, and reducing its internal stress. Metal doping can also make DLC coatings have good tribological properties. The properties of DLC coatings are also different on adding different metal elements. For example, the hardness and adhesion of DLC coating-doped tungsten are significantly higher than of DLC coating-doped titanium. The coating hardness increased from 2,577 $HV_{0.025,15}$ to 3,550 $HV_{0.025,15}$, and the adhesion of coating increased from 44 N to 60 N.[155] However, not all doping improves wear resistance. For example, doping silver reduces hardness from 17 GPa to 7 GPa, and the ratio of sp^2 and sp^3 bond content (sp^2/sp^3) does not change significantly. When fetal bovine serum is lubricated with UHMWPE, the tribological behavior of DLC does not show a significant dependence on silver concentration.[156]

Anttila et al.[157] grew DLC coatings up to a thickness of 200 µm and reduced the wear of artificial hip joints by a factor of 10^6 in simulator experiments compared to other available materials. Earlier studies on DLC-coated Ti6Al4V implants sliding against PE showed that the failure rate of the DLC-coated femoral head was much higher than the alumina femoral head, which resulted from insufficient adhesion and thin coatings.

4.5.3 Adhesion of DLC Coatings

Due to poor adhesion, DLC coating delamination occurs under different conditions, which results in mechanical failure of DLC-coated implants. This mechanical failure is closely related to the residual stress of the DLC coating and the adhesion between the coating and substrate.[158,159] The main reason for the poor adhesion is the difference in the coefficient of thermal expansion and the lattice structure of the DLC coating and substrate. Therefore, long-term adhesion needs to be guaranteed to avoid premature replacements or revision of implants.

At present, adhesion was improved by preparing the interface layer on the substrate before depositing the DLC coating so that an interface layer (one or more layers) is formed between the DLC and the substrate.

The adhesion of DLC to a range of prosthetic materials including 316 stainless steel materials,[160,161] titanium,[162] and Ti6A14V[163] which is controlled by the interface is still an issue. Mainly adhesion failure at the interface needs to be attributed to the chemical stability of the interface. As described in the literature,[164] the approaches for improving the adhesion of DLC coatings include (1) forming an intermediate layer between the substrate and the DLC coating such as interfacial metal carbides;[3] (2) forming gradient composition coatings inclined from the base material through DLC coatings,[165] for example, silicon,[166] titanium,[167] chromium[168] which must be biocompatible and amorphous, as well as multilayers TiNx-TiCy;[162,169–171] and (3) using an ion-mixing process based on ion-implantation technology.[164,172] Actually, the problem of poor adhesion can, to an appreciable extent, be overcome by penetration of carbon atoms from the DLC coating to a substrate, as well as the reaction of the carbon atoms with the substrate metal atoms and the formation of carbide. The interface reaction layer may also consist of metal-oxycarbide which depends on the precleaning and the conditions at the beginning of the DLC deposition process.[40]

During 1993–1995, a series of DLC-coated Ti-Al-V femoral heads articulating against PE were studied in the clinic, and it was found that the coated implants had only a 54% survival rate due to the delamination of the coatings after 8.5 years causing severe wear of the PE counterpart.[173] Additionally, most delamination spots were round (more than 90%). Therefore, it is necessary to analyze the failure mechanism and to estimate the adhesion lifetime for DLC-coated implants. It was shown that mechanical failure is mainly caused by third body wear involving wear particles in simulator testing.[174] In addition to mechanical failure, other delayed interface crack growth mechanisms including hydrogen embrittlement, galvanic, pitting, and crevice corrosion (CC) as well as stress corrosion cracking (SCC) need to be considered, in which SCC and CC are related to the coating delamination as they depend on the stress and environment.[174–176] These studies have shown that one failure of DLC-CoCrMo tested in synovial testing fluid took place due to CC of the adhesion promoting interlayer or SCC which may occur in a few nanometers thin reactively formed interface layer such as carbides.

DLC coating should be the superior material for many biomedical applications, and there are already few companies that are realizing the potential of DLC as a hemocompatible material. For example, Phytis L.D.A. and KIST. J&L Tech MDMI Canada offer DLC-coated stents and Cardio Carbon Company Ltd is developing DLC-coated artificial heart valve applications.[177] However, after some clinical studies, it was found that there is still an apparent lack of commercially applied DLC coatings, especially for load-bearing medical applications. The main reasons for these failures have been insufficient coating thickness and bad material combinations.[177] Thin DLC coatings cannot be expected to survive when subjected to serious loads, as in artificial hip joints. According to the groundbreaking work by Paul, the peak load in human joints can be up to 3.9 times the body weight for hip joints.[178] Although *in-vivo* studies on DLC-coated implants are scarce, *in-vitro* experiments are essential and aim to simulate the *in-vivo* processes of wear and corrosion for a better understanding of related mechanisms and, ultimately, for improvements in clinical practice.

4.5.4 BIOCOMPATIBILITY OF DLC COATINGS

As is known, when one material is implanted into the human body, it has to be biocompatible. Therefore, DLC-coated implants used in biomedical applications need to withstand the corrosive environment and not cause any adverse effects on attached cells. Therefore, DLC coatings must be biocompatible, which has been confirmed *in vitro* and *in vivo* in many studies.[179–181] Additionally, the biocompatibility of DLC can be improved from the viewpoint of its atomic structure (by varying the sp^2/sp^3 ratio of carbon) and composition (by the introduction of heteroatoms such as Si, F, Ca, and P to DLC),[182,183] as well as introducing both anodic and cathodic functional group to a DLC surface.[184,185] The hemocompatible nature of DLC coating, not only its biocompatible property but is also reported in previous studies,[166,186,187] which makes DLC coatings available to be used for implants in direct contact with blood, for example, artificial heart valves, blood pumps, and stents. Moreover, due to outstanding tribological properties of DLC, it is also widely used to reduce wear in the load-bearing joints instead of the UHMWPE.

If one implant is in contact with blood directly, a key issue is to prevent thrombus formation which depends on the surface of the implant. Due to the good hemocompatibility and excellent tribological behavior of DLC coatings, several studies have reported *in vitro* that it may be a better coating for cardiovascular purposes because of the ability to suppress thrombus.[179,186] To adjust the surface chemical behavior of DLC, the different elements are introduced into the DLC coatings, for example, Si-DLC,[187] Ti-DLC,[166] and Cr-DLC.[188] These elements must also be biocompatible. Only a few studies *in vivo* have presented the results of DLC-coated implants: stainless steel stents[189,190] and blood pumps[191] (made by Sun Medical Technology Research Corporation, Nagano, Japan). In addition, a few companies have produced some DLC-coated implants and made them available commercially, for example, the Cardio Carbon Company, the Sorin Biomedica company, and the company PHYTLS. Up to now, the blood-contacted applications are still in the state of development.

4.5.5 DLC-Coated Artificial Joint Friction Pairs

DLC coatings, as the friction pair of the hip joints, are mainly deposited on polymer or metal substrates which abbreviated as DLC/P and DLC/M, respectively.[4] DLC can be used as a barrier to prevent the leaching of metallic ions into the body. Additionally, the adhesion of DLC coating to the substrate can be improved by the interface layer. Usually, there are three different DLC-coated hip joints: Metal femoral heads against DLC-coated UHMWPE implanted cups, DLC-coated metal femoral heads against UHMWPE implanted cups, DLC-coated femoral heads against metal cups, and DLC-coated femoral heads against metal DLC-coated cups, which can be abbreviated M-DLC/P, DLC/M-P, M-DLC/M, and DLC-DLC, respectively.

4.5.5.1 M-DLC/P Artificial Joint

The load-bearing implant matched with UHMWPE has poor wear resistance and ages easily, so that a large number of wear debris or polyethylene particles enter the joint and surrounding tissues, resulting in osteolysis and loosening of the prosthesis, which affects the lifetime of the prosthesis.

DLC film with a thickness of about 300 nm was deposited on the polymer substrate by ion bombardment to modify its surface leading to densification, which can cause hydrogen loss and cross-linking of the carbon network.[192–194] Additionally, the risk of delamination is strongly reduced due to a gradient in hardness and density of DLC film. A further benefit is that it is easy to introduce metal nanoparticles during deposition of DLC coatings to improve their antibacterial properties.[7] The conductive substrate is easily realized by plasma immersion ion implantation, but it is necessary to modify the surface of the flat insulating polymer substrate and add a cathode above the surface or at the substrate's backside, which can metallize polymers. In this manner, a layer of metal film on the surface of UHMWPE must be prepared.[195] If DLC coatings can be deposited uniformly on the complex-shaped UHMWPE as an implanted cup, the geometry of the electrode has to be optimized for each specific substrate geometry. Taiber et al. proposed the combination of finite element analysis and advanced optical examination to optimize the DLC modification of UHMWPE implants, and this method can also be used for DLC preparation of any non-planar and insulating materials such as UHMWPE joints.[196]

4.5.5.2 DLC/M-P Artificial Joint

Many studies have been reported on the friction and wear of UHMWPE and the friction pair with DLC film on the metal surface using a pin-on-disk or ball-on-disk device with hip joint simulators, and most reports about the tribological properties have been carried out *in vitro* with the saline solution or water as a lubricating fluid.[197,198] The results show that DLC film can improve the wear resistance and corrosion resistance of artificial joints. When the metal surface is coated with DLC film and slides against UHMWPE in 1% NaCl water, the wear of UHMWPE is reduced by 5–6 times or even 10–100 times.[176,199] Studies have also reported that UHMWPE is still a soft material compared to DLC-coated metal friction pairs, and the wear of UHMWPE cannot be reduced effectively by depositing DLC coatings on the metal surface for DLC/M-P artificial joints.[200] However, when the tribological test was simulated with body fluid and real loads, there was no significant improvement compared to uncoated samples.[176,201,202] According to the literature, a protective transfer layer is formed from DLC to the UHMWPE surface during tribological testing.[176,202] With protein-containing lubricants and real loads (the loads used in hip simulators can be up to 3 kN [203]), the formation of such transfer layers is inhibited.

Dorner-Reisel et al.[204] reported that DLC-coated femoral (Co28Cr6Mo) components articulated against UHMWPE inlays for knee joint protheses with the wear simulator in a bovine serum solution. It was found that compared with the uncoated Co28Cr6M, DLC coatings can reduce the release of metallic wear products, and the wear resistance was improved when DLC was coated with a thickness of 0.8 and 2.7 μm. Therefore, improved biocompatibility was expected. However, on increasing the thickness of DLC coatings, the wear of polymeric UHMWPE counter face was increasing. The femoral segment with a 4.5 μm thick DLC coating resulted in drastically increased wear and decreased wear resistance of the UHMWPE inlay in comparison with the material loss caused by the uncoated Co28Cr6M, which may result from the heat transfer. The tribological contact area may be heated up to higher temperatures with increasing DLC thickness. In 2017, researchers simulated artificial joints using a self-refit, multi-freedom degree friction tester to study the tribological behavior of DLC-coated Ti6Al4V swinging against UHMWPE in the 25% fetal bovine serum lubricating medium.[205] The results showed that with the increase of axial load and swing angular displacement, the friction coefficient and the wear loss increased, respectively. The swing angular displacement had a relatively great influence on the wear degree. The wear mechanisms of DLC coating involved a combination of fatigue, adhesive, and abrasive wear, while the main wear mechanisms of UHMWPE were abrasive wear and adhesive wear.[205]

4.5.5.3 M-DLC/M Artificial Joint

The M-DLC/M artificial joint is similar to the M-DLC/P artificial joint mentioned above, but the friction interface is metal and DLC coating. DLC coating in the M-DLC/M artificial joint is a modification of the MOM artificial joint, and only one side of the sliding surface is a DLC film. The friction coefficient and wear rate were greatly improved in NaCl solution and deionized water by depositing DLC coating on the stainless steel.[206,207] Azzi et al.[208] studied the friction and corrosion behavior of DLC film deposited on the 316 medical stainless steel, and found that the DLC coating with the interface layer of SiNx did not peel off during rubbing in sodium chloride solution to 1,800 revolutions. However, whether it is M-DLC/M artificial joint or M-DLC/P artificial joint, it is difficult to avoid the problem of metal ion allergy. Therefore, for MOM joints, both sliding surfaces need to be modified to reduce the release of metal ions.

4.5.5.4 DLC-DLC Artificial Joint

There are few studies on the DLC sliding against the DLC, and these results are particularly important. Table 4.5 shows the influence of thickness, hydrogen content, and sp^3 content of different DLC films on the wear rate when DLC and DLC are sliding and rubbing against each other. Comparing with a-C:H film, a-C film has a higher sp^3 content and a lower wear rate, as shown in Table 4.5. Moreover, the higher the thickness of the DLC film, the higher the corresponding sp^3 content, and the better the friction performance. The content of sp^3 was related to the hydrogen content in the DLC film. As the hydrogen content increases, the sp^3 content decreases, which resulted in a higher wear rate.

Sheeja et al.[200] used the same pin-disk friction device to study the influence of DLC coating and its thickness on MOP joints under the conditions of simulating the lubrication of human serum. The results show that, under the same conditions, the wear rate of DLC-DLC friction pair compared with the M-DLC/P or DLC/M-P friction pair was reduced by 104 times, which can significantly improve the friction and wear behavior of the joint, and indicated that thick DLC (2~6 μm) is more conducive to improving the

TABLE 4.5

Influence of Thickness and Hydrogen Content on the Properties of DLC Films[145]

DLC	H Content /%	Thickness/μm	sp^3 Content /%	Wear Rate
a-C[a]	–	40~100	80~85	$<10^{-4}$ mm^3/year
a-C	<1	0.2~1.0	70	4.6×10^{-19} m^3/(N·m)
			58	8.1×10^{-19} m^3/(N·m)
a-C	<1	2	85	0.02 mg/h
			80	5×10^{-20} m^3/(N·m)
a-C:H	20	2	48	0.11 mg/h
	30	1	45	0.05 mg/h

[a] ta-C

life of the prosthesis. The use of a thicker DLC coating (micron level) on the two sliding surfaces of the MOP implant can extend the life of the prosthesis. Subsequently, Reuter et al.[209] conducted a pin-on-disk friction experiment on five DLC coatings (13 μm) on the market, in which both the pin and the disk were coated with DLC films. It was found that high-quality ta-C coatings have the least wear. The two low-quality DLC coatings (such as metal-doped a-C and a-C:H) are also less wear-resistant.

The ta-C and ta-C films show excellent wear resistance when using the pin-disk device or hip joint simulation device for tribological tests.[210] Ren et al. [35] used a disk-on-disk tribological test and high-nitrogen austenitic stainless steel P2000 (made in Germany) as the disk material in which both sliding surfaces were coated with a-C film of 470 nm to study the influence of the substrate bias on the tribological properties. It has been shown that applying a high negative bias during DLC deposition can reduce the wear rate by 100 times. However, the best artificial joint materials are bound to dissolve or wear with long-term application. With artificial hip joints, the best materials will lose 0.02~0.06 mm (average linear wear rate) within 10 years.[157] Therefore, to improve the life of the DLC-DLC artificial joint, the DLC coating must first have enough thickness. When the thickness of ta-C coating is 60 μm, using the hip joint simulator and bovine serum as the lubricant, the wear of the prosthesis is reduced by 106 times compared with commercially available medical materials.[203]

Compared with other coatings, because of its outstanding properties DLC is a promising candidate in biomedical applications. Therefore, much research work about DLC coatings is needed, especially regarding DLC-coated load-bearing implants. The DLC-DLC artificial joint with thicker DLC coatings (micron level) deposited on the two sliding surfaces has the best wear resistance and good biocompatibility. Of course, a lot of experiments are required in the joint simulator, and the actual load and suitable lubricating medium must be considered.

REFERENCES

1. S. Kurtz, K. Ong, E. Lau, F. Mowat, M. Halpern. Projections of primary and revision hip and knee arthroplasty in the United States from 2005–2030. *J Bone Joint Surg Am.* 89(4) (2007) 780–785. doi:10.2106/JBJS.F.00222.
2. B.C. Rieker. Tribology of total hip arthroplasty prostheses: What an orthopaedic surgeon should know. *J EFORT Open Rev.* 1(2) (2016) 52–57. doi:10.1302/20585241.1.000004.
3. M.A.H. Gepreel, M. Niinomi. Biocompatibility of Ti-alloys for long-term implantation. *J Mech Behav Biomed Mater.* 20 (2013) 407–415. doi:10.1016/j.jmbbm.2012.11.014.
4. Q.Y. Deng, T.F. Zhang. B.J. Wu, S.S. Li, Y.X. Leng. N. Huang. Diamond-like carbon film and its application on articular surface of artificial joint for increasing wear resistance. *Surf Tech.* 45(5) (2016) 1–7. doi:10.16490/j.cnki.issn.1001-3660.2016.05.001. [Article in Chinese].
5. R. Hauert. A review of modified DLC coatings for biological applications. *Diam Relat Mater.* 12 (2003) 583–589. doi:10.1016/S0925-9635(03)00081-5.
6. L.C.L. Nguyen, M.S. Lehil, K.J. Bozic. Trends in total knee arthroplasty implant utilization. *J Arthroplasty.* 30(5) (2015) 739–742. doi:10.1016/j.arth.2014.12.009.
7. B.G. Xu, S.G. Yan. Progress of friction interface of artificial hip joints. *Chin J Bone Joint Surg.* 6(S1) (2013) 66–69. [Article in Chinese].
8. H.S. Dong, X.Y. Li. Surface engineering for joint prosthesis: State-of-the-art and future directions. *China Surf Eng.* 21(5) (2008) 1–14. [Article in Chinese].

9. B. Ben-Nissan, B.A. Latella, A. Bendavid. Biomedical thin films: Mechanical properties. in: P. Ducheyne (Ed.). *Comprehensive Biomaterials*. Elsevier Science, 2011, pp. 63–73.

10. G. Dearnaley, J.H. Arps. Biomedical applications of diamond-like carbon (DLC) coatings: A review. *Surf Coat Technol*. 200(7) (2005) 2518–2524.

11. S.B. Goodman, M. Lind, Y. Song, R.L. Smith. In vivo, in vitro, and tissue retrieval studies on particulate debris. *J Clin Orthop Relat Res*. 352 (1998) 25–34. doi:10.1097/00003086-199807000-00005.

12. K.J. Kim, J. Chiba, H.E. Rubash. In vivo and in vitro analysis of membranes from hip prostheses inserted without cement. *J Bone Joint Surg Am*. 76 (1994) 172–180. doi:10.2106/00004623-199402000-00002.

13. W.J. Maloney, R.L. Smith. Periprosthetic osteolysis in total hip arthroplasty: The role of particulate wear debris. *J Bone Joint Surg*. 77(9) (1995) 1448–1461. doi:10.1111/j.1365-2591.1995.tb00312.x.

14. M.D. Waters, D.E. Gardner, C. Aranyi, D.L. Coffin. Metal toxicity for rabbit alveolar macrophages in vitro. *J Environ Res*. 9(1) (1975) 32–47. doi:10.1016/001393-51(75)90047-x.

15. D.W. Murray, N. Rushton. Macrophages stimulate bone resorption when they phagocytose particles. *J Bone Joint Surg Br*. 72(6) (1990) 988–992. doi:10.1007/BF02471041.

16. D.R. Haynes, S.D. Rogers, S. Hay, M.J. Pearcy, D.W. Howie. The differences in toxicity and release of bone-resorbing mediators induced by titanium and cobalt-chromium-alloy wear particle. *J Bone Joint Surg Am*. 75 (1993) 825–834. doi:10.2106/00004623-199306000-00004.

17. Y. Kadoya, A. Kobayashi, H. Ohashi. Wear and osteolysis in total joint replacements. *J Acta Orthop Scand Suppl*. 278 (1998) 1–16. doi:10.1080/17453674.1998.11744778.

18. K.J. Kim, T. Itoh, M. Tanahashi, M. Kumeqawa. Activation of osteoclast-mediated bone resorption by the supernatant from a rabbit synovial cell line in response to polyethylene particles. *J Biomed Mater Res*. 32(1) (1996) 3–9. doi:10.1002/(SICI)1097-4636(199609)32:1<3::AID-JBM1>3.0.CO;2-O.

19. A.S. Shanbhag, J.J. Jacobs, J. Black, J.O. Galante, T.T. Glant. Macrophage/particle interactions: Effect of size, composition and surface area. *J Biomed Mater Res*. 28(1) (1994) 81–90. doi:10.1002/jbm.820280111.

20. A.S. Shanbhag, J.J. Jacobs, J. Black, J.O. Galante, T.T. Glant. Human monocytes response to particulate biomaterials generated in vivo and in vitro. *J. Orthop Res*. 13(5) (1995) 792–801. doi:10.1002/jor.1100130520.

21. T.R. Green, J. Fisher, M. Stone, B.M. Wroblewski, E. Ingham. Polyethylene particles of a "critical size" are necessary for the induction of cytokines by macrophages in vitro. *J Biomater*. 19 (1998) 2297–2302. doi:10.1016/s0142-9612(98)00140-9.

22. A.U. Daniels, F.H. Barnes, S.J. Charlebois, R.A. Smith. Macrophage cykokine response to particles and lipopolysaccharide in vitro. *J Biomed Mater Res*. 49(4) (2000) 469–478. doi:10.1002/(sici)1097-4636(20000315)49:4<469::aid-jbm5>3.0.co;2-a.

23. C. Brockett, S. Williams, Z.M. Jin, G. Isaac, J. Fisher. Friction of total hip replacements with different bearings and loading conditions. *J Biomed Mater Res B Appl Biomater*. (2006) 508–515. doi:10.1002/jbm.b.30691.

24. H.P. Sieber, C.B. Reiker, P. Köttig. Analysis of 118 second-generation metal-on-metal retrieved hip implants. *J Bone Joint Surg Br*. 81(1) (1999) 46–50. doi:10.1302/0301-620x.81b1.9047.

25. T. Hirayama, Y. Fujikawa, I. Itonaga, R. Torisu. Effect of particle size on macrophage-osteoclast differentiation in vitro. *J Orthop Sci*. 6 (2001) 53–58. doi:10.1007/s007760170025.

26. T.T. Glant, J.J. Jacobs, G. Molnar, A.S. Shanbhag, M. Valyon, J.O. Galante. Bone resorption activity of particulate-stimulated macrophages. *J. Bone Miner. Res*. 8(9) (1993) 1071–1079. doi:10.1002/jbmr.5650080907.

27. S.M. Horowitz, S.B. Doty, J.M. Lane, A.H. Burstein. Studies of the mechanism by which the mechanical failure of polymethylmethacrylate leads to bone resorption. *J Bone Joint Surg Am.* 75(6) (1993) 802–813. doi:10.1016/S0749-8063(05)80434-7.

28. R.M. Steinman, I.S. Mellman, W.A. Muller, Z.A. Cohn. Endocytosis and the recycling of plasma membrane. *J Cell Biol.* 96 (1983) 1–27. doi:10.1083/jcb.96.1.1.

29. M. Geetha, A.K. Singh, R. Asokamani, A.K. Gogia. Ti based biomaterials, the ultimate choice for orthopaedic implants-a review. *Prog Mater Sci.* 54(3) (2009) 397–425. doi:10.1016/j.pmatsci.2008.06.004.

30. G. Winters, M. Nutt. *Stainless Steels for Medical and Surgical Applications.* ASTM International, West Conshohocken, PA, 2003.

31. S. Koch, R. Buescher, I. Tikhovski, H. Brauer, A. Runiewicz, W. Dudzinski, et al. Mechanical, chemical and tribological properties of the nickel-free high-nitrogen steel X13CrMnMoN18-14-3 (1.4452). *J Matwiss u Werkstofftechn.* 33 (2002) 705–715. doi:10.1002/mawe.200290000.

32. M. Becerikli, H. Jaurich, C. Wallner, J.M. Wagner, M. Dadras, B. Jettkant, et al., 2019. P2000 – A high-nitrogen austenitic steel for application in bone surgery. *PLoS One.* 14(3), e0214384. doi:10.1371/journal.pone.0214384.

33. Y. Ren, H.K. Wang. Tribological properties of diamond-like carbon films deposited by vacuum arc. *J Mater Res.* 109(7) (2018) 654–660. doi:10.3139/146.111652.

34. S.G. Steineman, Corrosion of surgical implants-in vivo and in vitro tests, in: G.D. Winter, J.L. Leray, K.E. de Goot (Eds.). *Evaluation of biomaterials.* Wiley, New York, 1980, pp. 1–34.

35. S.G. Steinemann, S.M. Perren. Titanium alloys as metallic biomaterials. in *Proc. of the 5th International Conference on Titanium,* Munich, F.R.G., (1984) 1327–1334.

36. R. Hauert. DLC films in biomedical application, in: C. Donnet, A. Erdemir (Eds.). *Tribology of Diamond-like Carbon Films: Fundamentals and Applications.* Springer, Boston, MA, 2008, pp. 495–509.

37. R. Koster, D. Vieluf, M. Kiehn, M. Sommerauer, J. Khler, S. Baldus, T. Meinertz, C.W. Hamm. Nickel and molybdenum contact allergies in patients with coronary in-stent restenosis. *Lancet.* 356(9245) (2000), 1895–7–1897. doi:10.1016/S0140-6736(00)03262-1.

38. B.F. Boyce, J. Byars, S. McWilliams, M.Z. Mocan, H.Y. Elder, I.T. Boyle, B.J. Junor. Histological and electron microprobe studies of mineralization in aluminium-related osteomalacia. *J Clin Pathol.* 45 (1992) 502–508. doi:10.1136/jcp.45.6.502.

39. J.A. Davidson, A.K. Mishra, P. Kovacs, R.A. Poggie. New surface-hardened, low-modulus, corrosion-resistant Ti-13Nb-13Zr alloy for total hip arthroplasty. *J Biomed Mater Eng.* 4(3) (1994) 231–243. doi:10.3233/BME-1994-4310.

40. U.K. Mudali, T.M. Sridhar, B. Baldev. Corrosion of bio-implants. *Sadhana.* 28(3–4) (2003) 601–637. doi:10.1007/BF02706450.

41. M. Semlitsch, H.G. Willert. Properties of implant alloys for artificial hip joints. *Med Biol Eng Comput* 18 (1980) 511–520. doi:10.1007/BF02443329.

42. G. Ghalme Sachin, M. Ankush, B. Yogesh. Biomaterials in hip joint replacement. *Int J Mater Sci Eng.* 4(2) (2016) 113–125. doi:10.17706/ijmse.2016.4.2.113-125.

43. R. Singh, N.B. Dahotre. Corrosion degradation and prevention by surface modification of biometallic materials. *J Mater Sci Mater Med.* 18(5) (2007) 725–751. doi:10.1007/s10856-006-0016-y.

44. J.J. Ramsden, D.M. Allen, D.J. Stephenson, J.R. Alcock, G.N. Fuller, G.D. Goch. The design and manufacture of biomedical surfaces. *CIRP Ann-Manuf Tech.* 56(2) (2007) 687–711. doi:10.1016/j.cirp.2007.10.001.

45. N. Hallab, K. Merritt, J.J. Jacobs. Metal sensitivity in patients with orthopaedic implants. *J. Bone Joint Surg. Am.* 83-A(3) (2001) 428–436. doi:10.2106/00004623-200103000-00017.

46. H.J. Cooper, R.M. Urban, R.L. Wixson, R.M. Meneghini, J.J. Jacobs. Adverse local tissue reaction arising from corrosion at the femoral neck-body junction in a dualtaper stem with a cobalt-chromium modular neck. *J Bone Joint Surg Am.* 95(10) (2013) 865–872. doi:10.2106/JBJS.L.01042.

47. A.J. Hart, P.D. Quinn, F. Lali, B. Sampson, J.A. Skinner, J.J. Powell, J. Nolan, K. Tucker, S. Donell, A. Flanagan, J.F.W. Mosselmans. Cobalt from metal-on-metal hip replacements may be the clinically relevant active agent responsible for periprosthetic tissue reactions. *Acta Biomater.* 8(10) (2012) 3865–3873. doi:10.1016/j.actbio.2012.05.003.

48. G.A. Afolaranmi, J. Tettey, R.M. Meek, M.H. Grant. Release of chromium from orthopaedic arthroplasties. *Open Orthop J.* 2 (2008) 10–18. doi:10.2174/1874325000802010010.

49. K. Merritt, S.A. Brown. Distribution of cobalt chromium wear and corrosion products and biologic reactions. *Clin Orthop Relat Res.* 329(43) (1996) S233–S243. doi:10.1097/00003086-199608001-00020.

50. X.J. Tian, S.Q. Zhang, A. Li, H.M. Wang. Effect of annealing temperature on the notch impact toughness of a laser melting deposited titanium alloy Ti-4Al-1.5Mn. *Mater Sci Eng A.* 527 (2010) 1821–1827. doi:10.1016/j.msea.2009.11.014.

51. Y. Song, D.S. Xu, R. Yang, D. Li, W.T. Wu, Z.X. Guo. Theoretical study of the effects of alloying elements on the strength and modulus of beta-type bio-titanium alloys. *Mater Sci Eng A.* 260 (1–2) (1999) 269–274. doi:10.1016/S0921-5093(98)00886-7.

52. D. Kuroda, M. Niinomi, M. Morinaga, Y. Kato, T. Yashiro. Design and mechanical properties of new β type titanium alloys for implant materials. *Mater Sci Eng A.* 243(1–2) (1998) 244–249. doi:10.1016/s0921-5093(97)00808-3.

53. M. Niinomi, M. Nakai. Titanium-based biomaterials for preventing stress shielding between implant devices and bone. *Int J Biomater.* 2011 (2011) 1–10. doi:10.1155/2011/836587.

54. S. Nag, R. Banerjee. Fundamentals of medical implant materials, in: R.J. Narayan (Ed.). *Materials for Medical Devices.* ASM International, 2012, pp. 6–16. doi:10.31399/asm.hb.v23.a0005682.

55. W.F. Cui, A.H. Guo. Microstructures and properties of biomedical TiNbZrFe β-titanium alloy under aging conditions. *Mater Sci Eng A.* 527 (2009) 258–262. doi:10.1016/j.msea.2009.08.057.

56. M.F. Lopez, A. Gutierrez, J.A. Jimenez. Surface characterization of new non-toxic titanium alloys for use as biomaterials. *Surf Sci.* 482–485 (2001) 300–305. doi:10.1016/S0039-6028(00)01005-0.

57. Y. Oshida. *Bioscience and Bioengineering of Titanium Materials.* Elsevier Science, Oxford, 2007.

58. S. Radice, J. Westrick, K. Ebinger, T.M. Mathew, M.A. Wimmer. In-vitro studies on cells and tissues in tribocorrosion processes: A systematic scoping review. *Biotribology.* 24 (2020) 100145 1–10. doi:10.1016/j.biotri.2020.100145.

59. P. Ponthiaux, F. Wenger, J.P. Celis. Tribocorrosion: Material behavior under combined conditions of corrosion and mechanical loading, in: Dr Shih (Ed.). *Corrosion Resistance.* In Tech, Rijeka, 2012, pp. 81–106.

60. Y. Ren, R.J. Wang, Q.H. Cheng, Q.Q. Chen, Z.G. Xu. The effect of bias on properties of DLC coatings for artificial joints. *Adv Mater Lett.* 11(10) (2020) 1–5. doi:10.5185/amlett.2020.101568.

61. K. Merritt, L. Wenz, S.A. Brown. Cell association of fretting corrosion products generated in a cell culture. *J Orthop Res.* 9(2) (1991) 289–296. doi:10.1002/jor.1100090218.

62. A.M. Maurer, K. Merritt, S.A. Brown. Cellular uptake of titanium and vanadium from addition of salts or fretting corrosion in vitro. *J Biomed Mater Res.* 28(2) (1994) 241–246. doi:10.1002/jbm.820280215.

63. A. Impergre, A.M. Trunfio-Sfarghiu, C. Der-Loughian, L. Brizuela, S. Mebarek, B. Ter-Ovanessian, A. Bel-Brunon, Y. Berthier, B. Normand. Tribocorrosion of polyethylene/cobalt contact combined with real-time fluorescence assays on living macrophages: Development of a multidisciplinary Biotribocorrosion device. *Biotribology.* 18 (2019) 100091. doi:10.1016/j.biotri.2019.100091.

64. B. Shi, T.B. Kuhn, H. Liang. 2005. Tribochemical performance of cell-treated nickel matrix. *Proceedings of WTC 2005, World Tribology Congress IIII*, Washington, D.C., USA, WTC2005-63694. doi:10.1115/WTC2005-63694.

65. T. Hui, G.W. Kubacki, J.L. Gilbert. Voltage and wear debris from ti-6Al-4V interact to affect cell viability during in-vitro fretting corrosion. *J Biomed Mater Res A.* 106 (1) (2018) 160–167. doi:10.1002/jbm.a.36220.

66. H.P. Felgueiras, L. Castanheira, S. Changotade, F. Poirier, S. Oughlis, M. Henriques, C. Chakar, N. Naaman, R. Younes, V. Migonney, J.P. Celis, P. Ponthiaux, L.A. Rocha, D. Lutomski. Biotribocorrosion (tribo-electrochemical) characterization of anodized titanium biomaterial containing calcium and phosphorus before and after osteoblastic cell culture. *J Biomed Mater Res B Appl Biomater.* 103(3) (2014) 661–669. doi:10.1002/jbm.b.33236.

67. M.J. Runa, M.T. Mathew, M.H. Fernandes, L.A. Rocha. First insight on the impact of an osteoblastic layer on the bio-tribocorrosion performance of Ti6Al4V hip implants. *Acta Biomater.* 12 (2015) 341–351. doi:10.1016/j.actbio.2014.10.032.

68. M. Runa, E.L. Lau, C. Takoudis, C. Sukotjo, T. Shokuhfar, L. Rocha, M. Mathew. In vitro evaluation of tribocorrosion induced failure mechanisms at the cell-metal Interface for the hip implant application. *Adv Eng Mater.* 19(5) (2017). doi:10.1002/adem.201600797.

69. S. Ramakrishna, J. Mayer, E. Wintermantel, K.W. Leong. Biomedical applications of polymer- composite materials: A review. *Comp Sci Technol.* 61(9) (2001) 1189–1224. doi:10.1016/S0266-3538(00)00241-4.

70. W.S. Pietrzak, D.R. Sarver, M.L. Verstynen. Bioabsorbable polymer science for the practicing surgeon. *J Craniofac Surg.* 8(2) (1997) 87–91. doi:10.1097/00001665-199703000-00004.

71. D. Behrend, K.P. Schmitz, A. Haubold. Bioresorbable polymer materials for implant technology. *Adv Eng Mater.* 2(3) (2000) 123–125. doi:10.1002/(SICI)1527-2648(200003)2:3<123::AID-ADEM123>3.0.CO.

72. J. Park, R.S. Lakes, *Biomaterials: An Introduction.* Springer, New York, 2007.

73. J.J. Callaghan, E.E. Forest, J.P. Olejniczak, D.D. Goetz, R.C. Johnston. Charnley total hip arthroplasty in patients less than fifty years old: A twenty to twenty-five-year follow-up note. *J Bone Joint Surg.* 80(5) (1998) 704–714. doi:10.2106/00004623-199805000-00011.

74. J.K. Lancaster. Composites for aerospace dry bearing applications, in: K. Friedrich (Ed.). *Friction and Wear of Polymer Composites.* Elsevier, Amsterdam, 1986, pp. 363–396.

75. K. Friedrich, Z. Lu, A.M. Hager. Recent advance in polymer composites tribology. *Wear.* 190 (1995) 139–144. doi:10.1016/0043-1648(96)80012-3.

76. F.K. Chang, J.L. Perez, J.A. Davidson. Stiffness and strength tailoring of a hip prosthesis made of advanced composite materials. *J Biomed Res.* 24 (1990) 873–899. doi:10.1002/jbm.820240707.

77. M. Akay, N. Aslan. Numerical and experimental stress analysis of a polymeric composite hip joint prosthesis. *J Biomed Res.* 31 (1996) 167–182. doi:10.1002/(SICI)1097-4636(199606)31:23.0.CO;2-L.

78. S.L. Ruan, P. Gao, X.G. Yang, T.X. Yu. Toughening high performance ultrahigh molecular weight polyethylene using multiwalled carbon nanotubes. *Polymer.* 44(19) (2003) 5643–5654. doi:10.1016/S0032-3861(03)00628-1.

79. S. Kanagaraj, M.T. Mathew, A. Fonseca, M.S. Oliveira, J.A. Simoes, L.A. Rocha. Tribological characterization of carbon nanotubes/ultrahigh molecular weight polyethylene composites: The effect of sliding distance. *Int J Surf Sci Eng.* 4(4–6) (2010) 305–321. doi:10.1504/IJSURFSE.2010.035138.

80. O.K. Muratoglu, C.R. Bragdon, D.O. O'Connor, M. Jasty, W.H. Harris. A novel method of cross-linking ultra-high-molecular-weight polyethylene to improve wear, reduce oxidation, and retain mechanical properties. Recipient of the 1999 HAP Paul Award. *J Arthroplasty.* 16 (2001) 149–160. doi:10.1054/arth.2001.20540.

81. S.D. Reinitz, B.H. Currier, D.W Van Citters, R.A. Levine, J.P. Collier. Oxidation and other property changes of retrieved sequentially annealed UHMWPE acetabular and tibial bearings. *J Biomed Mater Res B Appl Biomater.* 103 (2015) 578–586. doi:10.1002/jbm.b.33240.

82. E. Oral, O.K. Muratoglu. Vitamin E diffused, highly crosslinked UHMWPE: A review. *Int Orthop.* 35 (2011) 215–223. doi:10.1007/s00264-010-1161-y.

83. B. Masson. Emergence of alumina matrix composite in total hip arthroplasty. *Int Orthopedic.* 33 (2009) 359–363. doi:10.1007/s00264-007-0484-9.

84. P. Boutin. Total arthroplasty of the hip by fritted aluminum prosthesis. Experimental study and 1st clinical applications. *J Rev Chir Orthop Reparatrice Appar Mot.* 58 (1972) 229–246. doi:10.1016/j.otsr.2013.12.004.

85. M. Al-Hajjar, J. Fisher, S. Williams, J.L. Tipper, L.M. Jennings. Effect of femoral head size on the wear of metal on metal bearings in total hip replacements under adverse edge-loading conditions. *J Biomed Mater Res B Appl Biomater.* 101 (2013) 213–222. doi:10.1002/jbm.b.32824.

86. J.A. D'Antonio, K. Sutton. Ceramic materials as bearing surfaces for total hip arthroplasty. *J Am Acad Orthop Surg.* 17 (2009) 63–68. doi:10.5435/00124635-200902000-00002.

87. M. Fenandez-Faire, A. Blanco, A. Murcia, P. Sevilla, F.J. Gil. Ageing of retrieved zirconia femoral heads. *Clin Orthopedic Relat Res.* 462 (2007) 122–129. doi:10.1021/cm9025057.

88. W. Wang, M. Hadfield, A.A. Wereszczak. Surface strength of silicon nitride in relation to rolling contact performance. *Cerma Int.* 35 (2009) 3339–3346. doi:10.1016/j.ceramint.2009.05.034.

89. J. Xu, K. Kato. Formation of a tribochemical layer of ceramics sliding in water and its role for low friction. *Wear.* 245 (2000) 61–75. doi:10.1016/S0043-1648(00)00466-X.

90. N.V. Boshitskaya, T.S. Bartnitskaya, G.N. Makareno, V.A. Lavrenkko, N.M. Danilenko, N.P. Tel'nikova. Chemical stability of silicon nitride powders in biochemical media. *Powder Metall Met Ceram.* 35 (1996) 497–500. doi:10.1007/BF01355964.

91. J. Olofsson, T.M. Grehk, B. Tourn, P. Cecilia, J. Staffan, E. Hakan. Evaluation of silicon nitride as a wear resistant and resorbable alternative for total hip joint replacement. *Biomatter.* 2(2) (2012) 94–102. doi:10.4161/biom.20710.

92. M.N. Rahaman, A. Yao, B.S. Bal, J.P. Garino, M.D. Ries. Ceramic for prosthetic hip and knee joint replacement. *Jr Am Ceramic Soc.* 90 (2007) 1965–1988. doi:10.1111/j.1551-2916.2007.01725.x.

93. M. Mazzocchi, A. Bellosi. On the possibility of silicon nitride as a ceramic for structural orthopedic implants. Part-I: Processing, microstructure, mechanical properties, cytotoxicity. *J Mater Sci: Mater Med.* 19 (2008) 2881–2887. doi:10.1007/s10856-008-3417-2.

94. B. Bal, M. Rahaman. Orthopedic application of silicon nitride ceramic. *Acta Biomater.* 8(8) (2012) 2889–2898. doi:10.1016/j.actbio.2012.04.031.

95. B. Cappie, S. Neuss, J. Salbe, R. Telle, F.H. Knuchel. Cytocompatibility of high strength non-oxide ceramics. *Jr Biomed Mater Res, A.* 93 (2010) 67–76. doi:10.1002/jbm.a.32527.

96. H.J. Cooper, C.J. Della Valle, R.A. Berger, M. Tetreault, W.G. Paprosky, S.M. Sporer, J.J. Jacobs. Corrosion at the head-neck taper as a cause for adverse local tissue reactions after total hip arthroplasty. *J Bone Jt Surg Am.* 94 (2012) 1655–1661. doi:10.2106/JBJS.K.01352.

97. M.R. Whitehouse, M. Endo, S. Zachara, T.O. Nielsen, N.V. Greidanus, B.A. Masri, D.S. Garbuz, C.P. Duncan. Adverse local tissue reactions in metal-on-polyethylene total hip arthroplasty due to trunnion corrosion: The risk of misdiagnosis. *Bone Joint J.* 97-B (2015) 1024–1030. doi:10.1302/0301-620X.97B8.34682.

98. H.G. Willert, M. Semlitsch. Reactions of the articular capsule to wear products of artificial joint prostheses. *J Biomed Mater Res.* 11 (1977) 157–164. doi:10.1002/jbm.820110202.

99. E. Ingham, J. Fisher. Biological reactions to wear debris in total joint replacement. *Proc Inst Mech Eng Part H: J Eng Med.* 214(1) (2000) 21–37. doi:10.1243/0954411001535219.

100. E. Ingham, J. Fisher. The role of macrophages in osteolysis of total joint replacement. *Biomaterials.* 26 (11) (2005) 1271–1286. doi:10.1016/j.biomaterials.2004.04.035.

101. J.L. Tipper, P.J. Firkins, A.A. Besong, P.S.M. Barbour, J. Nevelos, M.H. Stone, E. Ingham, J. Fisher. Characterisation of wear debris from UHMWPE on zirconia ceramic, metal-on-metal and alumina ceramic-on-ceramic hip prostheses generated in a physiological anatomical hip joint simulator. *Wear.* 250(1–12) (2001) 120–128. doi:10.1016/S0043-1648(01)00653-6.

102. T.R. Green, J. Fisher, J.B. Matthews, M.H. Stone, E. Ingham. Effect of size and dose on bone resorption activity of macrophages by in vitro clinically relevant ultra high molecular weight polyethylene particles. *J J Biomed Mater Res.* 53 (2000) 490–497. doi:10.1002/1097-4636(200009)53:5<490::AID-JBM7>3.0.CO;2-7.

103. H. Malchau, P. Herberts, T. Eisler, G. Garellick, P. Söderman. The Swedish total hip replacement Register. *J Bone Joint Surg Am.* 84 (2002) 2–20. doi:10.2106/00004623-200200002-00002.

104. M. Long, H.J. Rack. Titanium alloys in total joint replacement-A materials science perspective. *Biomaterials.* 19(18) (1998) 1621–1639. doi:10.1016/S0142-9612(97)00146-4.

105. M. Semlitsch, H.G. Willert. Clinical wear behaviour of ultra-high molecular weight polyethylene cups paired with metal and ceramic ball heads in comparison to metal-on-metal pairings of hip joint replacements. *J Proc Inst Mech Eng H.* 211(1997) 73–88. doi:10.1243/0954411971534700.

106. R.J.A, Bigsby, D.D. Auger, Z.M. Jin, D.Dowson, C.S. Hardaker, J. Fisher. A comparative tribological study of the wear of composite cushion cups in a physiological hip joint simulator. *J Biomech.* 31 (1998) 363–369. doi:10.1016/S0021-9290(98)00034-7.

107. J. Livermore, D Ilstrup, B. Morrey. Effect of femoral head size on wear of the polyethylene acetabular component. *J Bone Joint Surg Am.* 72(4) (1990) 518–528. doi:10.2106/00004623-199072040-00008.

108. G. Digas, J. Kärrholm, J. Thanner, P. Herberts. 5-year experience of highly cross-linked polyethylene in cemented and uncemented sockets: Two randomized studies using radiostereometric analysis. *Acta Orthop.* 78(6) (2007) 746–754. doi:10.1080/17453670710014518.

109. G.E. Thomas, D.J. Simpson, S. Mehmood, A. Taylor, P. M. Smith, H.S. Gill, D.W. Murray, S.G. Jones. The seven-year wear of highly cross-linked polyethylene in total hip arthroplasty: A double-blind, randomized controlled trial using radiostereometric analysis. *J Bone Join Surg Am.* 93(8) (2011) 716–722. doi:10.2106/JBJS.J.00287.

110. J.B. Stambough, G. Pashos, F.C. Bohnenkamp, W.J. Maloney, J.M. Martell, J.C. Clohisy. Long-term results of total hip arthroplasty with 28-millimeter cobalt-chromium femoral heads on highly cross-linked polyethylene in patients 50years and less. *J Arthroplasty.* 31(1) (2016) 162–167. doi:10.1016/j.arth.2015.07.025.

111. J.A. Keeney, J.M. Martell, G. Pashos, C.J. Nelson, W.J. Maloney, J.C. Clohisy. Highly cross-linked polyethylene improves wear and mid-term failure rates for young total hip arthroplasty patients. *Hip Int.* 25(5) (2015) 435–441. doi:10.5301/hipint.5000242.

112. H.C. Amstutz, P. Grigoris. Metal on metal bearings in hip arthroplasty. *Clin Orthop Relat Res* 329 (1996) S11–S34. doi:10.1097/00003086-199608001-00003.

113. S.A. Jacobsson, K. Djerf, O. Wahlstrom. Twenty-year results of McKee-Farrar versus Charnley prosthesis. *Clin Orthop Relat Res.* 329S (1996) S60–S68. doi:10.1097/00003086-199608001-00006.

114. F.S. Haddad, R.R. Thakrar, A.J. Hart, J.A. Skinner, A.V. Nargol, J.F. Nolan, H.S. Gill, D.W. Murray, A.W. Blom, C.P. Case. Metal-on-metal bearings: The evidence so far. *J Bone Joint Surg Br.* 93(5) (2011) 572–579. doi:10.1302/0301-620X.93B4.26429.

115. H.L. Anissian, A. Stark, A. Gustafson, V. Good, I.C. Clarke. Metal-on-metal bearing in hip prosthesis generate 100-fold less wear debris than metal-on-polyethylene. *Acta Orthop Scand.* 70(6) (1999) 578–582. doi:10.3109/17453679908997845.

116. J.P Collier, V.A. Surprenant, R.E. Jensen, M.B. Mayor. Corrosion at the interface of cobalt-alloy heads on titanium-alloy stems. *Clin Orthop Relat Res.* 271 (1991) 305–312. doi:10.1097/00003086-199110000-00042.

117. J.S. Kawalec, S.A. Brown, J.H. Payer, K. Merritt. Mixed-metal fretting corrosion of Ti6Al4V and wrought cobalt alloy. *J Biomed Mater Res.* 29(7) (1995) 867–873. doi:10.1002/jbm.820290712.

118. J.L. Gilbert, C.A. Buckley, J.J. Jacobs. In vivo corrosion of modular hip prosthesis components in mixed and similar metal combinations, the effect of crevice, stress, motion, and alloy coupling. *J Biomed Mater Res.* 27(12) (1993) 1533–1544. doi:10.1002/jbm.820271210.

119. J.R. Goldberg, J.L. Gilbert. In vitro corrosion testing of modular hip tapers. *J Biomed Mater Res Part B: Appl Biomater* 64B(2) (2003) 78–93. doi:10.1002/jbm.b.10526.

120. J.A. Browne, C.D. Bechtold, D.J. Berry, A.D. Hanssen, D.G. Lewallen. Failed metal-on-metal hip arthroplasties: A spectrum of clinical presentations and operative findings. *Clin Orthop Relat Res.* 468(9) (2010) 2313–2320. doi:10.1007/s11999-010-1419-0.

121. D.J. Langton, S.S. Jameson, T.J. Joyce, J.N. Gandhi, R. Sidaginamale, P. Mereddy, J. Lord, A.V. Nargol. Accelerating failure rate of the ASR total hip replacement. *J Bone Joint Surg Br.* 93(8) (2011) 1011–1016. doi:10.1302/0301-620X.93B8.26040.

122. B.M. Wroblewski, P.D. Siney, D. Dowson, S.N. Collins. Prospective clinical and joint simulator studies of a new total hip arthroplasty using alumina ceramic heads and cross-linked polyethylene cups. *J Bone Joint Surg.* 78-B (1996) 280–285. doi:10.1016/0020-1383(95)00199-9.

123. D. Dowson. A comparative study of the performance of metallic and ceramic femoral head components in total replacement hip joints. *Wear.* 190(2) (1995) 171–183. doi:10.1016/0043-1648(96)80015-9.

124. V. Saiko, T. Ahlroos, O. Calonius, J. Keranen. Wear simulation of total hip prostheses with polyethylene against CoCr, alumina and diamond-like carbon. *Biomaterials.* 22(12) (2001) 1507–1514. doi:10.1016/s0142-9612(00)00306-9.

125. I.C. Clarke, A. Gustaffson. Clinical and hip simulator comparisons of ceramic on polyethylene and metal on polyethylene wear. *Clin Orthop Relat Res.* 379 (2000) 34–40. doi:10.1097/00003086-200010000-00006.

126. A. Kusaba, Y. Kuroki, S. Kondo, I. Hirose, Y. Ito, Y. Shirasaki, T. Tateishi, J. Scholz. Frictional torque and wear of retrieved hip prostheses: A comparison between alumina/PE and CoCr-PE prostheses. *J Long Term Eff Med Implants.* 12(1) (2002) 53–62. doi:10.1615/JLongTermEffMedImplants.v12.i1.40.

127. K. Tanaka, J. Tamura, K. Kawanabe, M. Shimizu. Effect of alumina femoral heads on polyethylene wear in cemented total hip arthroplasty old versus current alumina. *Bone Joint J.* 85(5) (2003) 655–660. doi:10.1302/0301-620X.85B5.13923.

128. Y.H. Kim, Y.A. Choi, J.S. Kim. Cementless total hip arthroplasty with alumina-on-highly cross-linked polyethylene bearing in young patients with femoral head osteonecrosis. *J Arthroplasty.* 26(2) (2011) 218–223. doi:10.1016/j.arth.2010.03.010.

129. M. Ihle, S. Mai, W. Siebert. Ceramic versus metal femoral heads in combination with polyethylene cups: Long-term wear analysis at 20 years. *Semin Arthroplasty.* 22(4) (2011) 218–224. doi:10.1053/j.sart.2011.09.001.

130. K. Ise, K. Kawanabe, J. Tamura, H. Akiyama, K. Goto, T. Nakamura. Clinical results of the wear performance of cross linked polyethylene in total hip arthroplasty: Prospective randomised trial. *J Arthroplasty.* 24(8) (2009) 1216–1220. doi:10.1016/j.arth.2009.05.020.

131. N.H. Kelly, A.D. Rajadhyaksha, T.M. Wright, S.A. Maher, G.H. Westrich. High stress conditions do not increase wear of thin highly crosslinked UHMWPE. *Clin Orthop Relat Res.* 468(2) (2010) 418–423. doi:10.1007/s10776-007-0067-0.

132. P. Christel, A. Meunier, J.M. Dorlot, J.M. Crolet, J. Witvoet, L. Sedel, P. Boutin. Biomechanical compatibility and design of ceramic implants for orthopedic surgery. *Bioceram: Mater Charact Versus in Vivo Behav.* 523(1) (1988) 234–256. doi:10.1111/j.1749-6632.1988.tb38516.x.

133. J.W. David, D.J. Cash, V. Khanduj. The case for ceramic-on-polyethylene as the preferred bearing for a young adult hip replacement. *HIP Int.* 24(5) (2014) 421–427. doi:10.5301/hipint.5000138.

134. P. Griss, H.F. von Andrian-Werburg, G. Heimke, B. Krempien, S. Reipa, H.J. Hartung, H.J. Lauterbach. Results of experimental tests and clinical application possibilities of aluminum oxide ceramics in alloarthroplasty. *Z Orthop Ihre Grenzgeb.* 113(4) (1975) 756–759. [Article in German].

135. P. Massin, R. Lopes, B. Masson, D. Mainard. French Hip & Knee Society (SFHG), Does Biolox Delta ceramic reduce the rate of component fractures in total hip replacement? *Orthop Traumatol Surg Res.* 100(6) (2014) S317–S321. doi:10.1016/j.otsr.2014.05.010.

136. Y.K. Lee, Y.C. Ha, J.J. Yoo, K.H. Koo, H.J. Kim. Alumina-on-alumina total hip arthroplasty: A concise follow-up, at a minimum of ten years, of a previous report. *J Bone Joint Surg Am.* 92(8) (2010) 1715–1719. doi:10.2106/JBJS.I.01019.

137. J.A. D'Antonio, W.N. Capello, M. Naughton. Ceramic bearings for total hip arthroplasty have high survivorship at 10 years. *Clin Orthop Relat Res.* 470(2) (2012) 373–381. doi:10.1007/s11999-011-2076-7.

138. G.E. Petsatodis, P.P. Papadopoulos, K.A. Papavasiliou, I.G. Hatzokos. Primary cementless total hip arthroplasty with an alumina ceramic-on-ceramic bearing: Results after a minimum of twenty years of follow-up. *J Bone Joint Surg Am.* 92(3) (2010) 639–644. doi:10.2106/JBJS.H.01829.

139. P.R. Finkbone, E.P. Severson, M.E. Cabanela, R.T. Trousdale. Ceramic-on-ceramic total hip arthroplasty in patients younger than 20 years. *J Arthroplasty.* 27 (2012) 213–219. doi:10.1016/j.arth.2011.05.022.

140. J.W. Byun, T.R. Yoon, K.S. Park, J.K. Seon. Third-generation ceramic-on-ceramic total hip arthroplasty in patients younger than 30 years with osteonecrosis of femoral head. *J Arthroplasty.* 27(7) (2012) 1337–1343. doi:10.1016/j.arth.2011.07.004.

141. D. de Villiers, S. Collins. Wear of large diameter ceramic-on-ceramic hip bearings under standard and microseparation conditions. *Biotribology.* 21 (2020) 100117. doi:10.1016/j.biotri.2020.100117.

142. A.J. Smith, P. Dieppe, K. Vernon, P.W. Blom, A.W. Blom. National Joint Registry of England and Wales, Failure rates of stemmed metal-on-metal hip replacements: Analysis of data from the National Joint Registry of England and Wales. *Lancet.* 379 (2012) 1199–1204. doi:10.1016/S0140-6736(12)60353-5.

143. National Joint Replacement Registry annual report 2015. Adelaide. Australia: University of Adelaide; 2015. https://www.aoa.org.au/docs/default-source/annual-reports/annual-report-2014-2015_final-web.pdf?sfvrsn=4 (accessed 2 February 2020).

144. J. Roberston. Diamond-like amorphous carbon. *Mater Sci Eng R Rep.* 37(4/5/6) (2002) 129–281. doi:10.1016/S0927-796X(02)00005-0.

145. Y. Ren, R.J. Wang, Z.G. Xu. Progress on diamond-like carbon films in the surface modification of friction pairs of artificial joints. *Fine Chem.* 37(7) (2020) 1314–1319. doi:10.13550/j.jxhg.20200037. [Article in Chinese].

146. M. Bonelli, A.C. Farrari, A. Fooravanti, A.L. Bassi, P.M. Ossi. Structure and mechanical properties of low stress tetrahedral amorphous carbon films prepared by pulsed laser deposition. *Eur Phys J B-Conden Matter Complex Syst.* 25(3) (2002) 269–280. doi:10.1140/epjb/e20020031.

147. S. Chowdhury, M.T. Laugier, I.Z. Rahman. Characterization of DLC coatings deposited by rf magnetron sputtering. *J Mater Process Tech.* 153 (2004) 804–810. doi:10.1016/j.jmatprotec.2004.04.265.

148. T. Muguruma, M. Lijima, M. Kawaguchi, I. Mizoguchi. Effects of sp2/sp3 ratio and hydrogen content on in vitro bending and frictional performance of DLC-coated orthodontic stainless steels. *Surf Coat Technol.* 8(6) (2018) 199. doi:10.3390/coatings8060199.

149. Q. Zhou, B. Huang, E.G. Zhang, Z.F. Zhang. The research status on preparation of diamond-like carbon coating and measures to improve its internal stress and thermal stability. *J Ceram.* 40(5) (2019) 556–564. doi:10.13957/j.cnki.tcxb.2019.05.001. [Article in Chinese]

150. N.B. Dahotre, S. Nayak. Nanocoatings for engine application. *Surf Coat Technol.* 194(1) (2005) 58–67. doi:10.1016/j.surfcoat.2004.05.006.

151. T.A. Friedmann, J.P. Sullivan, J.A. Knapp, D.R. Tallant, D.M. Follstaedt, D.L. Medlin, P.B. Mirkarimi. Thick stress-free amorphous-tetrahedral carbon films with hardness near that of diamond. *Appl Phys Lett.* 71(26) (1997) 3820–3822. doi:10.1063/1.120515.

152. D. Sheeja, B.K. Tay, L. Yu, S.P. Lau. Low stress thick diamond-like carbon films prepared by filtered arc deposition for tribological applications. *Surf Coat Technol.* 154(2–3) (2002) 289–293. doi:10.1016/S0257-8972(02)00005-1.

153. M. Chhowalla, G.A.J. Amaratunga. Strongly adhering and thick highly tetrahedral amorphous carbon (ta-C) thin films via surface modification by implantation. *J Mater Res.* 16(1) (2001) 5–8. doi:10.1557/JMR.2001.0002.

154. D.H. Lee, S. Fayeulle, K.C. Walter, M. Nastasi. Internal stress reduction in diamond like carbon thin films by ion irradiation. *Nucl Instrum Methods Phys Res.* 148(1–4) (1999) 216–220. doi:10.1016/S0168-583X(98)00739-3.

155. S.S. Lin, K.S. Zhou, M.J. Dai. Preparation and microstructure of DLC/WC multilayer thin films. *Chin J Nonferrous Met.* 23(2) (2013) 434–438. [Article in Chinese].

156. S. Dominguez-Meister, T.C. Rojas, J.E. Frias, J.C. Sanchez-Lopez. Silver effect on the tribological and antibacterial properties of a-C: Ag coatings. *Tribol Int.* 140 (2019) 105837. doi:10.1016/j.triboint.2019.06.030.

157. A. Anttila, R. Lappalainen, H. Heinonen, S. Santavirta, Y.T. Konttinen. Superiority of diamondlike carbon coating on articulating surfaces of artificial hip joints. *New Diamond Frontier Carbon Technol.* 9(4) (1999) 283–288.

158. S. Wang, Z.H. Liao, W.Q. Liu. The application and research progress of diamond-like carbon films in the field of artificial joints. *J Funct Mater.* 45(5) (2014) 5008–5013. [Article in Chinese].

159. C. Donnet, A. Erdemir. *Tribology of Diamond-Like Carbon Films: Fundamentals and Applications.* Springer US, New York, 2008. doi:10.1016/S1369-7021(08)70060-9.

160. R.L.C. Wu. Synthesis and characterization of diamond-like carbon films for optical and mechanical applications. *Surf Coat Technol.* 51 (1992) 258–266. doi:10.1016/0257-8972(92)90249-A.

161. N. Yoshino, Y. Shibuya, K. Naoi, T. Nanya. Deposition of a diamond-like carbon film on a stainless steel substrate: Studies of intermediate layers. *Surf Coat Technol.* 47 (1991) 84–88. doi:10.1016/0257-8972(91)90270-7.

162. C. Dumkum, D.M. Grant, I.R. McColl. A multilayer approach to high adhesion diamond-like carbon coatings on titanium. *Diam Relat Mater.* 6 (1997) 802–806. doi:10.1016/S0925-9635(96)00762-5.

163. S.S. Perry, J.W. Ager, G.A. Somorjai, R.J. McClelland, M.D. Drory. Interface characterization of chemically vapor deposited diamond on titanium and Ti-6Al-4V. *J Appl Phys.* 74 (1993) 7542–7550. doi:10.1063/1.354980.

164. F. Kenji, W. Koichiro, U. Kazuo, S. Tadashi. Preparation of highly adhesive diamond-like carbon films by plasma CVD combined with ion implantation. *IHI Eng Rev.* 37(1) (2004) 30–34.

165. K. Miyoshi, B. Pohlchuck, K. W. Street, J. S. Zabinski, J. H. Sanders, A. A. Voevodin, R.L.C. Wu. Sliding wear and fretting wear of diamond-like carbon-based, functionally graded nanocomposite coatings. *Wear.* 225(1) (1999) 65–73. doi:10.1016/S0043-1648(98)00349-4.

166. R. Butter, M. Allen, L. Chendra, A.H. Lettington, N. Rushton. In vitro studies of DLC coatings with silicon intermediate layer. *Diam Relat Mater.* 4(5–6) (1995) 857–861. doi:10.1016/0925-9635(94)05280-8.

167. Y. Ren, I. Erdmann, B. Küzün, F. Deuerler, V. Buck. Effect of deposition parameters on wear particle size distribution of DLC coatings. *Diam Relat Mater.* 23 (2012) 184–188. doi:10.1016/j.diamond.2011.12.045.

168. B. Stamm, B. Küzün, O. Filipov, S. Reuter, I. Erdmann, F. Deuerler, D. Krix, K. Huba, H. Nienhaus, V. Buck. Adjustment of wear particle size distribution of DLC coatings for tribological metal-on-metal paring in artificial hip joints. *Materialwiss Werkstofftech.* 40(1–2) (2009) 98–100. doi:10.1002/mawe.200800374.

169. D.P. Monaghan, D.G. Teer, P.A. Logan, I. Efeoglu, R.D. Arnell. Deposition of wear resistant coatings based on diamond like carbon by unbalanced magnetron sputtering. *Surf Coat Technol.* 60 (1993) 525–530. doi:10.1016/0257-8972(93)90146-F.

170. J. Narayan, W.D. Fan, R.J. Narayan, P. Tiwari, H.H. Stadelmaier. Diamond, diamond-like and titanium nitride biocompatible coatings for human body parts. *Mater Sci Eng: B.* 25 (1) (1993) 5–10. doi:10.1016/0921-5107(94)90193-7.

171. L. Lu, M.W. Jones, R.L.C. Wu. Diamond-like carbon as biological compatible material for cell culture and medical application. *Biomed Mater Eng.* 3 (4) (1993) 223–228.

172. S. Miyake, T. Saitoh, S. Watanabe, M. Kanou, Y. Yasuda, Y. Mabuchi. Effects of ion implantation on scratching properties of diamond-Like carbon and boron carbide films. *Jap J Tribol.* 45(3) (2000) 283–296.

173. G. Taeger, L.E. Podleska, B. Schmidt, M. Ziegler, D. Nast-Kolb. Comparison of diamond-like-carbon and alumina-oxide articulating with polyethylene in total hip arthroplasty. *Materialwiss Werkstofftech.* 34(12) (2003) 1094–1100. doi:10.1002/mawe.200300717.

174. K. Thorwarth, U. Müller. G. Thorwarth, C.V. Falub, M. Stiefel, Ch. Affolter, B. Weisse, C. Voisard, R. Hauert. Failure mechanisms of DLC coated joint replacements. *Eur Cell Mater Suppl.* 19(2) (2010) 24.

175. U. Müller, C.V. Falub, G. Thorwarth, C. Voisard, R. Hauert. Diamond-like carbon coatings on a CoCrMo implant alloy: A detailed XPS analysis of the chemical states at the interface. *Acta Materialia.* 59 (2011) 1150–1161. doi:10.1016/j.actamat.2010.10.048.

176. E. Alakoski, V.M. Tiainen, A. Soinine, Y. Konttinen. Load-bearing biomedical applications of diamond-like carbon coatings-current status. *Open Orthop J.* 2 (2008) 43–50. doi:10.2174/1874325000802010043.

177. C.V. Falub, U. Mueller, G. Thorwarth, M. Parlinska-Wojtan, C. Voisard, R. Hauert. In vitro studies of the adhesion of diamond-like carbon thin films on CoCrMo biomedical implant alloy. *J Acta Mater.* 59 (2011) 4678–4689. doi:10.1016/j.actamat.2011.04.014.

178. J.P. Paul. Paper 8: Forces transmitted by joints in the human body. *J. Proc Inst Mech Eng.* 181 (1966) 8–15. doi:10.1243/PIME_CONF_1966_181_201_02.

179. E. Mitura, S. Mitura, P. Niedzielski, Z. Has, R. Wolowiec, A. Jakubowski, J. Szmidt, A. Sokołowska, P. Louda, J. Marciniak, B. Koczy. Diamond-like carbon for biomedical applications. *Diam Relat Mater.* 3(4–6) (1994) 896–898. doi:10.1016/0925-9635(94)90295-X.

180. M. Allen, B. Myer, N. Rushton. In vitro and in vivo investigations into the biocompatibility of diamond-like carbon (DLC) coatings for orthopedic applications. *J Biomed Mater Res.* 58(3) (2001) 319–328. doi:10.1002/1097-4636(2001)58:33.0.CO;2-F.

181. A. Singh, G. Ehteshami, S. Massia, J. He, R.G. Storer, G. Raupp. Glial cell and fibroblast cytotoxicity study on plasma-deposited diamond-like carbon coatings. *Biomaterials.* 24(28) (2003) 5083–5089. doi:10.1016/S0142-9612(03)00424-1.

182. T.I.T. Okpalugo, A.A. Ogwu, P.D. Maguire, J.A.D. McLaughlin, D.G. Hirst. In-vitro blood compatibility of a-C: H: Si and a-C: H thin films. *Diam Relat Mater.* 13 (2004) 1088–1092. doi:10.1016/j.diamond.2003.10.064.

183. T. Hasebe, S. Yohena, A. Kamijo, Y. Okazaki, A. Hotta, K. Takahashi, T. Suzuki. Fluorine doping into diamond-like carbon coatings inhibits protein adsorption and platelet activation. *J Biomed Mater Res A.* 83(4) (2007) 1192–1199. doi:10.1002/jbm.a.31340.

184. A. Mochizuki, T. Ogawa, K. Okamoto, T. Nakatani, Y. Nitta. Blood compatibility of gas plasma-treated diamond-like carbon surface-effect of physicochemical properties of DLC surface on blood compatibility. *Mat Sci Eng C.* 31(3) (2011) 567–573. doi:10.1016/j.msec.2010.11.019.

185. Y. Nitta, K. Okamoto, T. Nakatani, H. Hoshi, A. Homma, E. Tatsumi, Y. Taenaka. Diamond-like carbon thin film with controlled zeta potential for medical material application. *Diam Relat Mater.* 17(11) (2008) 1972–1976. doi:10.1016/j.diamond.2008.05.004.

186. M.I. Jones, I.R. Mccoll, D.M. Grant, K.G. Parker, T.L. Parker. Haemocompatibility of DLC and TiC/TiN interlayers on titanium. *Diam Relat Mater.* 8(2–5) (1999) 457–462. doi:10.1016/S0925-9635(98)00426-9.

187. Q. HuaFan, A. Fernandes, E. Pereira, J. Grácio. Adhesion of diamond to steel and copper with titanium interlayers. *Diam Relat Mater.* 8(8–9) (1999) 1549–1554. doi:10.1016/S0925-9635(99)00064-3.

188. N. All, Y. Kousar, J. Graclo, E. Titus, T.I. Okpalugo, V. Singh, M. Pease, A.A. Ogwu, E.I. Meletls, W. Ahmed, M.J. Jackson. Human microvascular endothelial cell seeding on Cr-DLC thin films for heart valve applications. *J Mater Eng Perform.* 15(2) (2006) 230–235. doi:10.1361/105994906X95931.

189. I.D. Scheerder, M. Szilard, H. Yanming, X.B. Ping, E. Verbeken, D. Neerinck, E. Demeyere, W. Coppens, F.V.D. Werf. Evaluation of the biocompatibility of two new diamond-like stent coatings (Dylyn) in a porcine coronary stent model. *J Invasive Cardiol.* 12(8) (2000) 389–394. doi:10.1017/S0266078413000369.

190. D. Antoniucci, A. Bartorelli, R. Valenti, P. Montorsi, G.M. Santoro, F. Fabbiocchi, L. Bolognese, A. Loaldi, M. Trapani, D. Trabattoni, G. Moschi, S. Galli. Clinical and angiographic outcome after coronary arterial stenting with the carbostent. *Am J Cardiol.* 85(7) (2000) 821–825. doi:10.1016/S0002-9149(99)00874-7.

191. K. Yamazaki, P. Litwak, O. Tagusari, T. Mori, K. Knon, M. Kameneva, M. Watach, L. Gordon, M. Miyaqishima, J. Tomioka, M. Umezu, F. Outa, J.F. Antaki, R.L. Kormos, H. Koyanaqi, B.P. Griffith. An implantable centrifugal blood pump with a recirculating purge system (Cool-Seal system). *Artif Organs.* 22(6) (1998) 466–474. https://doi.org/10.1046/j.1525-1594.1998.06156.x.

192. P.S. Florian, H.G. Irmgard, W. Tuomas, B. Stritzker. Antibacterial properties of silver containing diamond like carbon coatings produced by ion induced polymer densification. *Surf Coat Technol.* 205(20) (2011) 4850–4854. doi:10.1016/j.surfcoat.2011.04.078.

193. S. Buchegger, N. Schuster, B. Stritzker, A. Wixforth, C. Westerhausen. Multilayer diamond-like amorphous carbon coatings produced by ion irradiation of polymer films. *Surf Coat Technol.* 327 (2017) 42–47. doi:10.1016/j.surfcoat.2017.08.010.

194. F. Schwarz, G. Thorwarth, B. Stritzker. Synthesis of silver and copper nanoparticle containing a-C:H by ion irradiation of polymers. *Solid State Sci.* 11(10) (2009) 1819–1823. doi:10.1016/j.solidstatesciences.2009.05.012.

195. Y.N. Pei, D. Xie, X. Gui, H. Sun, N. Huang. The properties of the ultra-high molecular weight polyethylene (UHMWPE) modified by surface metallization and diamond-like carbon (DLC) film deposition duplex treatment. *J Funct Mater.* 42(3) (2011) 459–462. [Article in Chinese].

196. T. Jochen, B. Sascha, S. Bernd, W. Achim, W. Christoph. Optimizing lateral homogeneity of ion-induced surface modifications of non-planar dielectric polyethylene components employing ion fluence simulations and optical measurements of the sp2-dependent reflectivity. *Nucl Instrum Meth B.* 433 (2018) 98–105. doi:10.1016/j.nimb.2018.07.034.

197. Z.F. Shi, L.J. Hao, C.Y. Ning, Y.J. Wang. Tribological properties of diamond-like carbon and silicon-nitrogen bio-mechanical coatings on Co alloy. *J Chin Ceram Soc.* 47(4) (2019) 553–560. doi:10.14062/j.issn.0454-5648.2019.04.18. [Article in Chinese]

198. M. Madej, D. Ozimina, K.J. Kurzydtowski, T. Ptocinski. Diamond-like carbon coatings in biotribological applications. *Diamond.* 54(3) (2016) 185–194. doi:10.4149/km20163185.

199. H. Ronkainen, S. Varjus, K. Holmberg. Tribological performance of different DLC coatings in water-lubricated conditions. *Wear.* 249(3–4) (2001) 267–271. doi:10.1016/S0043-1648(01)00561-0.

200. D. Sheeja, B.K. Tay, L.N. Nung. Tribological characterization of surface modified UHMWPE against DLC-coated Co–Cr–Mo -ScienceDirect. *Surf Coat Technol.* 190(2–3) (2005) 231–237. doi:10.1016/j.surfcoat.2004.02.051.

201. S. Affatato, M. Frigo, A. Toni. Anin vitro investigation of diamond-like carbon as a femoral head coating. *J Biomed Mater Res.* 53(3) (2000) 221–226. doi:10.1002/(SICI)10974636(2000)53:33.0.CO;2-Z.

202. R. Hauert. An overview on the tribological behavior of diamond- like carbon in technical and medical applications. *Tribol Int.* 37(11–12) (2004) 991–1003. doi:10.1016/j.triboint.2004.07.017.

203. R. Lappalainen, M. Selenius, A. Anttila, Y.T. Konttinen, S.S. Santavirta. Reduction of wear in total hip replacement prostheses by amorphous diamond coatings. *J Biomed Mater Res B.* 66(1) (2003) 410–413. doi:10.1002/jbm.b.10026.

204. A. Dorner-Reisel, C. Schuerer, E. Mueller. The wear resistance of diamond-like carbon coated and uncoated Co28Cr6Mo knee prostheses. *Diam Relat Mater.* 13(4–8) (2004) 823–827. doi:10.1016/j.diamond.2003.11.080.

205. L. Xu, D. Zhang, K. Chen, X. Yang, Q. Wang, J. Qi. Tribological behavior of diamondlike carbon film-deposited Ti6Al4V alloy swinging against ultrahigh molecular weight polyethylene in fetal bovine serum. *J Tribol.* 139(3) (2017) 031301–031306. doi:10.1115/1.4034077.

206. A.H.S. Bueno, J. Solis, H. Zhao, C. Wang. Tribocorrosion evaluation of hydrogenated and silicon DLC coatings on carbon steel for use in valves, pistons and pumps in oil and gas industry. *Wear.* 394 (2018) 60–70. doi:10.1016/j.wear.2017.09.026.

207. C.X. Gou, S.H. Wang, L.L. Shang, G.A. Zhang, W.U. Zhi-Gou. Friction and wear behavior of diamond-like-carbon film in corrosive media. *Surf Tech.* 48(10) (2019) 172–179. doi:10.16490/j.cnki.issn.1001-3660.2019.10.021. [Article in Chinese]

208. M. Azzi, M. Paquette, J.A. Szpunar, J.E. Klemberg-Sapieha, L. Martinu. Tribocorrosion behaviour of DLC-coated 316L stainless steel. *Wear.* 267(5–8) (2009) 860–866. doi:10.1016/j.wear.2009.02.006.

209. S. Reuter, B. Wekamp, R. Buescher, A. Fischer, V. Buck. Correlation of structural properties of commercial DLC-coatings to their tribological performance in biomedical applications. *Wear.* 261(3–4) (2006) 419–425. doi:10.1016/j.wear.2005.12.009.

210. R. Lappalainen, H. Heinonen, A. Anttila, S. Santavirta. Some relevant issues related to the use of amorphous diamond coatings for medical applications. *Diam Relat Mater.* 7(2–5) (1998) 482–485. doi:10.1016/S0925-9635(98)80003-4.

5 Overview of Polymeric Biomaterials for Dental Applications

Zichen Wu, Xiaoxuan Lu, Xiaowei Wang, Xiangyang Li, and Jialong Chen
Anhui Medical University

CONTENTS

DOI: 10.1201/9781003161981-5

5.1 INTRODUCTION

Soft and hard tissues in human maxillofacial areas may be defective or lost due to a number of diseases, trauma, and biological degeneration, resulting in natural function and aesthetics of these tissues being diminished. Dental materials, including metals, ceramics, polymers, and composites, were developed to treat these defects. Metals and alloys have a long history in dentistry, starting with the Romans using gold to repair crowns and bridges, followed by stainless steel, cobalt-chrome alloys, nickel-chrome alloys, gold-based alloys, and dental amalgam. Their corrosion behavior, mismatched mechanical properties, high cost, low availability, and poor esthetics affect health, including local irritation, nausea, vomiting, and diarrhea [1]. However, numerous advancements within metal biomaterials have emerged over the last few decades and have revolutionized many materials for preventive, restorative, and regenerative treatments in dentistry such as titanium (Ti) and their alloys (nickel-titanium) [2]. Although dental metals are widely available, none of them has ideal physical, mechanical, biological, and surface properties.

With the increase in lifespan and the pursuit of high quality of life, the demands for improved function and esthetics of dental materials keep growing. Due to their excellent biocompatibility, satisfactory mechanical properties, and processability, polymers play an important role in different aspects of the biomedical field. Moreover, these materials can be tailored for specific requirements in regeneration or as advanced drug delivery systems, such as preventive, restorative, and regenerative therapies in dentistry [3]. Within dentistry, depending on their sources, polymers can be divided into natural and synthetic polymers. The most used natural polymers are chitosan, collagen, fibrin, and agar, while the most used synthetic polymers are polyetheretherketone, polyethylene, polycarbonate, polyethylene glycol, polyurethane, polymethyl methacrylate, and their derivatives. In addition, depending on their applications, polymers and polymer composites have been used as restorative materials such as direct or indirect restorations dental implants and surgical materials such as polyetheretherketone (PEEK), endodontic materials, periodontology materials, and devices such as orthodontic materials [4].

The basic principles of biomaterials include excellent biocompatibility and appropriate biomechanical and physicochemical properties, but specific requirements of polymer materials should be met in specific dental applications. Nowadays, new therapeutic concepts and higher clinical requirements are driving the research and development of new materials and techniques with excellent performance, high efficiency, and accuracy to the treatment of dental diseases. More than 700 pathogenic bacteria related to oral diseases (e.g., dental caries and denture stomatitis) exist in the oral environment [5], and therefore, antibacterial property is one of the most important for dental materials, such as acrylic resin-based dentures, composite resin, and adhesives. For enhancing the antibacterial properties, mixture or surface modification with antibacterial agents has been developed. In addition, the regeneration of hard/soft tissues has become another goal for dental materials, such as endodontic and periodontal treatment.

Although most polymers have been improved to meet the requirements of the oral environment, the longevity of these materials in clinical use faces challenges.

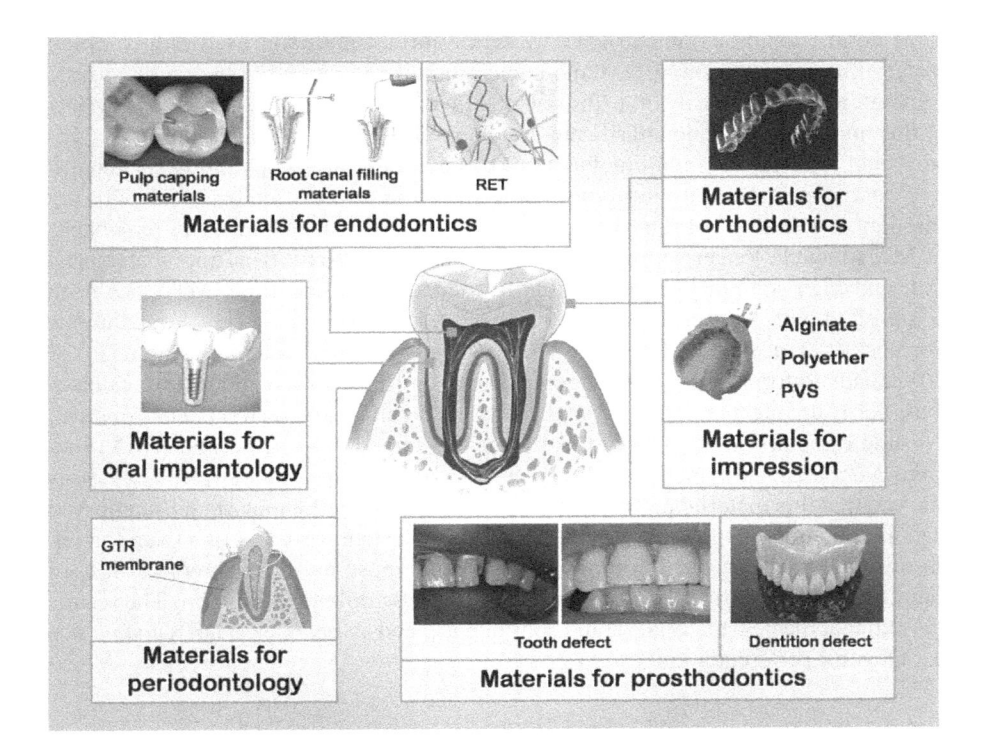

FIGURE 5.1 Schematic illustration of polymeric biomaterials in dental applications (endodontics, periodontology, impression, prosthodontics, impression and oral implantology).

In future, more clinical studies and strategies are needed to improve biomechanical properties, to develop antibacterial materials and bioactive materials for reducing failure rates and creating better treatment guidelines for practitioners. This chapter presents a brief overview of various polymers for different applications in dentistry (Figure 5.1).

5.2 ENDODONTIC MATERIALS

At present, there are three main types of endodontic materials: pulp capping materials, root canal filling materials, and materials for regenerative endodontic therapy (RET). In this section, we will introduce the applications of polymer materials in these three categories in detail.

5.2.1 PULP CAPPING MATERIALS

Pulp capping is used to cover the exposed pulp of carious teeth or the dentin close to the pulp to eliminate inflammation and protect the living pulp. Pulp capping materials should demonstrate strong permeability to form a seal with the dental tissues while also exhibiting excellent biocompatibility with the periodontal tissues [6].

Mineral trioxide aggregate (MTA), as the most commonly used pulp capping material, is derived from a Portland cement parent compound (a hydraulic silicate cement), relying primarily on hydration reactions for setting. The major constituents of this material are dicalcium silicate, tricalcium silicate, tricalcium aluminate, gypsum, and tetra-calcium aluminoferrite. It has excellent biocompatibility for reparative dentin formation in vital pulp therapies [7], as well as antibacterial property through its alkaline pH, and it regulates cytokine production [8]. The drawbacks of MTA include longer setting time (3–4 hours) [9], difficult handling characteristics, and high solubility in water [10]. To reduce the curing time, MTA has been composited with light-curing resin [11] or chemical curing resin [12]. For example, Formosa et al. used an LED curing wand to cure MTA with a light-curing resin for 20 seconds to form a new type of composite resin [13], and it could release calcium ions, form apatite precipitation, and build an alkaline antibacterial environment. To suppress pulp inflammation, the researchers mixed dexamethasone (DEX) in a chitosan/collagen polymeric porous sponge for direct pulp capping [14]. The results showed that this material promoted the differentiation of odontoblast and suppressed the inflammatory response in the pulp. Beta-cyclodextrins (β-CDs), as a drug carrier, are cyclic oligosaccharides composed of glucopyranose units. Daghrery et al. used electrospinning to load DEX into β-CDs to suppress inflammation [15]. The results showed that the new materials could continuously and stably release DEX and induce odontogenic differentiation.

5.2.2 ROOT CANAL FILLING MATERIALS

Caries and other hard tissue lesions of the teeth could cause dental pulp and periapical diseases, which are fundamentally and normally treated by root canal therapy (RCT). RCT aims to eliminate infected pulp and protect the decontaminated tooth from future invasion, including root canal preparation (opening, cleaning, and shaping), intracanal antisepsis, and root canal filling. The standard procedure for root canal filling is to fill the cleaned root canal with a solid core and seal it with a sealer.

5.2.2.1 Solid Core Filling Points

Gutta-percha (GP) is the preferred choice as a solid core filling material, which is a trans-1,4-polyisoprene-based nanocomposite, containing 20% GP (matrix), 66% zinc oxide (filler), 11% heavy metal sulfates (radiopacifier), and 3% waxes and/or resins (plasticizer) [16,17]. GP has been regarded as a gold standard material for root canal filling because no other material can replace it currently [18]. However, GP has no adhesive qualities, leading to apical or coronal leakage [19]. Attempts have been made to modify GP for optimal obturation and therapeutic effect, such as surface modifications and addition of medicine and nanoparticles [20–23].

To improve the adhesion of GP, Prado et al. used oxygen and argon plasma to treat GP surfaces for improving water wettability, forming highly reactive oxygen, and increasing the surface roughness [20]. The results showed that both treatments increased the surface free energy and had a positive effect on the adhesion to prevent leakage [20]. Cone-beam computed tomography (CBCT) and multijet printing technology were also combined to manufacture 3D printed teeth, which provided a matched working length and taper for a master GP, thus promoting the accuracy of root canal fillings [24].

Infection is another important cause of GP treatment failure. Alves et al. treated the surface of GP point with an argon plasma and deposited a layer of zinc oxide (ZnO) film on the surface to improve the antibacterial effect [23]. The results showed that the adhesion and proliferation of bacteria were significantly inhibited. Dong et al. filled GP point with ZnO bridged by carbon nanotubes to prepare a new type of GP composite with high thermal conductivity and low shear viscosity [25]. The results showed that the new material significantly increased the filling depth of lateral canal, inhibited bacterial proliferation, and had low cytotoxicity.

In addition to obturation and antibacterial effect, GP materials may also be appropriate scaffolds for pulp regeneration as the proliferation and differentiation of dental pulp stem cells were observed after 21-day incubation without soluble factors [26]. In addition to GP point, plastic point can also be used for filling, which has better elasticity and toughness, but needs to be used in combination with a methacrylate resin-based sealer.

5.2.2.2 Root Canal Sealer

Root canal sealers along with a solid core play an important role in achieving the tight seal of the root canal system [27], especially filling the accessory and lateral canals, voids, spaces, and irregularities among GP [28]. At present, sealers in clinical use contain zinc oxide-eugenol, resin, glass ionomer, silicone, and calcium hydroxide. Compared to conventional sealers with no adhesive qualities to dentin, polymeric root canal sealers have been introduced to solve the problem of poor adhesion between material and root canal [29]. Silicone and epoxy resin sealers polymerize by addition reaction while methacrylate-based resins via radical polymerization [30]. For example, AH Plus, existing in a paste-paste mixture, is an epoxy resin-based sealer and is widely acknowledged due to low solubility, good dimensional stability, and favorable infiltration into irregularities as a result of its creep property and long setting time. [30–32]. Methacrylate resin-based sealer could provide a monoblock, a single unit in which the root becomes a perfectly sealed and stable solid mass without gaps, thus mechanically reinforcing the root structure and obstructing bacteria ingress pathways [29, 33].

Recently, bioactive sealers have been the focus of endodontic biomaterials, and multiple bioactive additives have been used for ideal antibacterial ability, biocompatibility, and remineralization. Studies have proven that biofilms are vital predisposing factors to persistent infections and can lead to the failure of root canal treatment [34]. Wang et al. prepared a novel resin-based endodontic sealer incorporating dimethylaminohexadecyl methacrylate (DMAHDM), 2-methacryloyloxyethyl phosphorylcholine (MPC), and nanoparticles of amorphous calcium phosphate (NACP). The results showed that this bioactive sealer could substantially suppress endodontic biofilm formation by reducing CFU by three log at both early and mature stages. Large amounts of calcium and phosphate ions were released for a long period from NACP, inducing root dentin remineralization and potentially root structure reinforcement [35]. Bashayer et al. also developed a resin-based sealer containing DMAHDM and NACP and additionally incorporated silver nanoparticles (NAg) in another experiment. The results showed that both sealers exhibited considerable anti-biofilm and remineralization properties without compromising flow and sealing properties [36,37]. In addition, AH Plus integrated with DMAHDM and NAg showed excellent antibacterial properties, and the physical properties did not decrease [38].

Because of close contact between the root-end filling material and periapical tissues, the biocompatibility of these sealers is also one of the most important properties closely associated with the composition of the materials [39,40]. Methacrylate resin-based sealers contain ingredients toxic to periapical tissue, while epoxy resin-based sealers are cytotoxic, causing inflammation and releasing chemicals known as mutagens, such as bisphenol diglycidyl ether, formaldehyde, and potentially carcinogens [41–46]. The addition of N-Acetylcysteine (NAC) or beta-tricalcium phosphate nanoparticles (β-TCP) into epoxy resin-based sealer (AH Plus) can reduce the cytotoxicity of these sealers because NAC or β-TCP is a stimulus for healing of periapical tissues and performs better therapeutic effect by achieving a hermetic seal [47]. Nano-magnesium hydroxide (NMH) was also added to AH Plus to improve biocompatibility. The study proved that NMH was biocompatible to MC3T3-E1 cells, and AH Plus mixed with 3%w/w of NMH promoted cell proliferation and osteogenic differentiation [48]. Furthermore, the addition of calcium methacrylate or dibutyltin methacrylate to sealers (Real Seal) showed increased resistance to *Enterococcus faecalis*, but only low concentrations of calcium methacrylate (0.5%, 1%, and 2%) showed lower cytotoxicity than commercial Real Seal [49].

5.2.3 MATERIALS FOR ENDODONTIC REGENERATION

RET is a treatment in which dental stem cells are delivered to the root canal space for replacing damaged tooth tissue and regenerating the root canal. Apical papilla stem cells (SCAP) are mesenchymal stem cells from the peri-root tips of immature teeth that can differentiate into dentin cells, and thus SCAPs are often used as a candidate for pulp-dentin complex regeneration in infected periodontal tissue [50]. However, some studies demonstrated that in the absence of scaffolds, exogenous SCAPs were difficult to adhere to the root canal wall, leading to failure of regeneration. Therefore, scaffolds as templates for tissue growth are required to provide SCAPs with growth adhesion sites and support sites [51, 52].

5.2.3.1 Naturally-Derived Polymeric Scaffolds

The main materials that can be used as naturally derived polymer scaffolds are alginate, hyaluronic acid (HA) and derivatives, as well as chitosan derivatives. Alginate and HA scaffolds are in the form of hydrogels, into which cells could be mixed. The advantages of alginates are their good biocompatibility, lack of immunogenicity, and porous structure that facilitates the exchange of substance and solute diffusion [53]. Atreasala et al. mixed alginate with synthetic dentin extract in equal mass ratios to form a highly stable bioink, which provided nutritional support to dentin cells [54]. However, pathogen transmission and insufficient mechanical strength restrict its use.

HA, as a ubiquitous component of the extracellular matrix (ECM), is a non-sulfated glycosaminoglycan. Due to its excellent biocompatibility, biodegradability, and hygroscopic property, HA plays an important role in cell migration, proliferation, differentiation, wound healing, and inflammation [50]. Lambricht et al. evaluated the influence of the ratio of sodium alginate and HA on the bioactivity of hydrogels [55]. The results showed that compared to sodium alginate, the hydrogel with a high proportion of HA had better mechanical strength and microenvironment, leading to high proliferative activity and low apoptosis rate of cells in this hydrogel.

Chitosan, as an amino polysaccharide biopolymer, has a unique chemical structure of linear polycation, possessing high charge density and a large number of reactive hydroxyl and amino groups. Due to its excellent biocompatibility, biodegradability, and low toxicity, chitosan is one of the most widely used biomaterials in tissue engineering. Shrestha et al. prepared two variants of dexamethasone (DEX) releasing chitosan nanoparticles (DEX-CSnpI and DEX-CSnpII) to evaluate the influence of DEX release rate on SCAP adhesion, proliferation, and odontogenic differentiation in regenerative endodontics [56]. The results showed that DEX-CSnpI and DEX-CSnpII enhanced SCAP adherence and viability on conditioned dentin and led to a well developed cytoplasmic matrix and lower circularity. In addition, SCAPs cultured in DEX-CSnpII group (rapid releasing) expressed higher levels for DSPP and DMP-1 than in other groups, indicating that rapid release of DEX from DEX-CSnpII enhanced odontogenic differentiation of SCAP and improved the local environment in regenerative endodontics.

5.2.3.2 Synthetic Scaffolds

By properly designing of the functional groups of the polymer, scaffolds prepared by synthesized polymer present tailored structure and controlled properties [57]. These advantages guarantee predictable, reproducible, and tunable features that can change depending on the specific application. Poly(L-lactic acid) (PLLA), as the most used aliphatic polyester, has been widely used in the field of tissue regeneration. Due to injectability and biodegradability, PLLA nanofibrous microsphere (PLLA NF-MS) is often used for drug delivery to load with BMP-2, miRNA, and growth factors to promote tissue regeneration. Wang et al. prepared BMP-2-loaded PLLA NF-MS to induce odontogenic differentiation of SCAP [58]. The results demonstrated that this material induced SCAP to odontogenic differentiation and then regenerated mineralized tissues. PLGA-PEG, as the most widespread synthetic polymer material, has already reached clinical application due to the high tunability of its degradation rate, ranging from weeks to months. Compared to naturally derived polymeric scaffolds, PLGA-PEG nanoparticles are more conducive to the proliferation of dental pulp fibroblasts [59] and have anti-fouling properties to inhibit bacterial adhesion [60]

5.3 MATERIALS FOR PERIODONTOLOGY

Teeth are held by the surrounding gums, bones, and other tissues. Periodontal disease, or periodontitis, is a process in which bacteria get trapped under the gums leading to chronic infection, followed by the rupture of hard and soft tissues that support the teeth [61]. Because the damaged periodontal tissue can hardly return to normal, some techniques, known as regenerative procedures, can be used to stimulate the growth of new bone and to achieve the formation of periodontal tissue. This growth increases the height of the bone around the tooth, giving more support to the tooth, and increases the amount of attachment around the root. Getting back even half the lost bone height can prolong the life of the tooth.

One type of regenerative surgery is called guided tissue regeneration (GTR), which has been used to repair periodontal defects to give a tooth or a set of teeth more support and stability. These gaps or bone defects usually require a separate, specialized operation called a bone graft. This is the placement of a special material into the defect to promote the growth of new bone. GTR must use an absorbable or non-absorbable artificial membrane to prevent soft tissue growth (e.g., epithelial and connective tissue cells of the gingiva from the wound) into the gaps or the bone defects. This membrane is critical because it prevents rapidly migrating soft tissue cells from the growing site, while providing space for slow-migrating bone-producing cells to grow at the site [62].

An ideal GTR film possesses anti-inflammatory, anti-infective, and appropriate mechanical properties, including permeability, stability, elasticity, flexibility, plasticity, and resorbability [63]. In the past decade, many new biomaterials have been developed for periodontal regeneration. There is also no shortage of polymer materials containing gelatin, collagen, polycaprolactone (PCL), poly(lactic-co-glycolic acid) (PLGA), polytetrafluoroethylene (PTFE), etc. Because of the predictability of its performance, PTFE has advantages in clinical management and reduces the risk of long-term complications [64]. However, due to non-absorbable property, it requires second-stage surgical extraction, and exposure of the membrane in the air increases the risk of infection [65]. Therefore, the GTR membrane constructed by biodegradable materials has a wide application prospect. PCL has excellent mechanical properties, but with slow degradation [66], so researchers mixed PCL with gelatin by electrospinning for increasing the degradation rate. The results demonstrated that the membrane could be degraded rapidly but with poor mechanical properties. Zhang et al. prepared chitosan/polycaprolactone/gelatin scaffolds with sandwich-like structure. The results showed that the scaffolds possessed appropriate porosity (<50%), pore size (about 10 μm), mechanical stability, good swelling, hydrophilicity, and appropriate degradation rates. Meanwhile, subcutaneous implantation revealed that the scaffolds offered strong cell barrier effects and protection from external cell invasion [67].

Furthermore, researchers often combine GTR membrane with different components to form a suitable microenvironment for promoting periodontal regeneration [68]. The oral environment contains more than 700 pathogenic bacteria related to oral diseases [5]. While the GTR membrane is conducive to the adhesion of host cells, it also attracts the colonization of bacteria such as *A. actinomycetemcomitans* and *P. gingivalis* [69]. A clinical study reported that the GTR membrane was contaminated with bacteria within 3 minutes after surgery [70], and then caused infection and inflammatory response, thereby interfering with tissue regeneration. To inhibit local infection and inflammation, tetracycline or amoxicillin, as effective antibiotics against most periodontal pathogens, were loaded onto the GTR membranes to reduce bacterial adhesion and kill pathogens [71]. Shi et al. grafted the esterified antibacterial drug metronidazole (MNA) onto PCL-gelatin polymer matrix to construct drug-loaded electrospun nanofiber membranes [72]. When infection occurs, the cholesterol esterase released by a large number of macrophages can mediate the on-demand release of MNA containing ester bonds, giving the GTR membrane certain antibacterial activity. Limoee et al. loaded ibuprofen (IBU) on GTR membrane with controlled-release and slow-release ability to prevent inflammation [73].

For enhancing osteoblast adhesion, proliferation, differentiation, and new tissue formation, bioactive molecules were integrated into the GTR membrane. Heparin and heparin sulfate glycosaminoglycans can protect bioactive molecules from denaturation and proteolysis, as well as prolong the sustained release of bioactive molecules [74]. Ma et al. combined BMP-2 with heparin and then immobilized onto nanofiber microspheres. The nanofibrous microsphere could self-assemble to form a layered structure with superior surface area, high porosity, low density, and support of cell adhesion and tissue growth [75,76].

5.4 MATERIALS FOR IMPRESSION

Dental impression materials, as negative reproduction or molds, are used to record or reproduce the shape and relationship of the teeth and oral tissues. A replica (positive reproduction) of the oral tissues from the impression is obtained by pouring gypsum or epoxy materials into the impression. These reproductions can be utilized as study models for disease assessing, treatment planning and casts, or as a working model to fabricate dentures, crowns, orthodontic appliances, and other devices [77]. The quality of replication of the oral environment which reflects the accuracy of the impression heavily affects the success of the product. The accuracy of the impression is influenced by the operator's understanding of the impression material's properties and practical experience [78]. Existing impression materials with different properties and indications range from natural compounds to polymers, but none of them meets the requirements of an ideal impression material. Usually, choosing an impression material depends on the operator's empirical or preferred consideration. However, using an impression material without a complete understanding of its properties may lead to a failed outcome. Impression materials are liquid or semi-liquid when initially prepared, while after being set in the mouth for some time, they solidify rapidly. Ideal properties for impression materials include accuracy, elastic recovery, dimensional stability, flow, flexibility, workability, hydrophilicity, a long shelf-life, patient comfort, and economics [79]. Impression materials vary considerably concerning these desirable properties, which are the foundation of selecting specific materials in different clinical cases. Currently, most chosen impression materials include alginate hydrocolloids, addition silicones, polyether, and polysulfides. Some of the older impression materials (e.g., zinc oxide-eugenol impression paste, impression plaster, and impression compound) are still used on certain occasions, but are limited in use as they cannot be removed past undercuts without destroying the impression [80].

5.4.1 ALGINATE

Alginate, one of the most popularly used dental materials, is an irreversible hydrocolloid produced by sol-gel transition and has been applied in acquiring impressions before dental prosthesis due to its low cost and good hydrophilicity. A moderate capacity of reproducing details is displayed in the presence of saliva and blood on account of the hydrophilic nature of the material. If poured for more than 10 minutes, distortion and shrinkage occur due to poor dimensional stability after losing water [81]. At the same time, it cannot be poured one more time after failure because of distortion and low tear strength. This material is flexible and easy to remove from the mouth compared to other materials if they flow into undercuts. The material is also easy to use and easy to mix with sufficient setting time to be handled and placed in the oral cavity [78]. Alginate impression materials comprise fine diatomaceous earth fillers particles. However, in practical applications, these particles may disperse in the air as dust due to lack of density. Dimensional changes occur because of highly hydrophilic alginates absorbing water. Further, low viscosity may result in gag reflex among patients. Perforated trays should be equipped when making impressions with alginate materials as they do not adhere well to the impression trays [82]. Therefore, evolutionary changes have come up in the alginate impression material to meet various needs, including dustless alginate, chromatic alginate, self-disinfected alginate, etc. [83].

5.4.2 POLYETHER

Polyether consists of a base paste comprising a long-chain polyether copolymer with alternating oxygen atoms and methylene groups ($O\text{-}[CH_2]_n$) and reactive terminal groups, which was first introduced in the late 1960s. The setting reaction for these materials is via cationic polymerization by opening the reactive ethylene imine terminal rings to unite molecules with no by-product formation [81]. Polyether impression materials are moderately hydrophilic and get accurate impressions in the presence of some saliva or blood. Because of its hydrophilic nature, it is easier to capture a full arch impression and to fabricate gypsum casts than polyvinyl siloxanes. Provided there is no tearing of the impression, pouring of accurate casts can be repeatedly accomplished within 1–2 weeks owing to the exceptional capacity of detailed reproduction and dimensional stability [84]. These materials are available in low, medium, and high viscosities and can be used as a single-phase material or using a syringe-and-tray technique [80]. The most popular method of dispensing this material is via a motorized mixing unit.

However, the disadvantages of polyether are obvious, such as rigid, susceptibility to moisture absorption, and potential for allergic reactions. Newer polyether impression materials are slightly more flexible, which makes them easier to remove from the mouth. Owing to the nature of the material absorbing water, the impression should not be immersed in water for a long time to avoid distortion [85].

5.4.3 POLYVINYL SILOXANES

Polysiloxane (PVS), usually called addition silicone, has been widely utilized in advanced restorative dentistry because of its excellent properties and availability in different viscosities, ranging from the extra light body to putty by altering filler usage [86]. The most well-known forms are extra light-bodied (low filler content), light-bodied, universal or medium-bodied, heavy-bodied, and putty (high filler content) [85]. PVS impressions, as the preferred material for fixed prosthodontics, could achieve great detailed reproduction and can be poured multiple times due to outstanding tearing strength and elastic recovery abilities [87,88]. PVS are more accurate and stable than the condensation reaction silicones because they do not release any by-product upon setting [89]. However, attention should be taken to avoid contact with latex rubber dams or latex gloves, which may inhibit polymerization of the material due to a left sulfur or sulfur compound [90]. PVS materials are inherently hydrophobic, which makes impression capturing and cast manufacturing challenging. Surfactants are often added to improve the wettability of oral tissue during impression and gypsum during pouring of the cast. "Hybrid" impression materials have also been developed to overcome these problems. A representative material is vinyl siloxanether (VPS), which combines the properties of both polyether and additional silicones. Due to hydrophilicity, ease of removal, and high elastic recovery, VPS promises the reflection of some structures which have unclear moisture, such as narrow gingival crevice, thus further improving the imprint accuracy [91,92].

5.5 MATERIALS FOR PROSTHODONTICS

5.5.1 Restorative Material for Tooth Defect

5.5.1.1 Resin Composite

Dental caries, as one of the most prevalent chronic diseases worldwide, is the main cause of tooth defect, followed by tooth injury, abrasion, acid etching, and odontogenic malformation. Once tooth defects occur, restorative treatment is the most commonly used clinical technique. Due to their esthetic appearance and direct-filling competence, resin composites are becoming the dominant choice for tooth defect patients and have been increasingly chosen as the material of restorations such as inlay, crown, and laminate [4]. Compared to previous materials (such as amalgam), resin composites for restorative treatment can better protect natural tooth tissue through a strong chemical combination with enamel and dentin and low modulus of elasticity. However, due to several inherent physical and chemical property drawbacks including polymerization shrinkage, a relatively high coefficient of thermal expansion, and a relatively low wear resistance, the long-term durability in clinical application faces challenges, with potential failures resulting from secondary caries and bulk fractures. Half of all dental restorations by resin composites fail within 10 years [93].

A resin composite is composed of monomer, inorganic filler, coupling agent, and initiating system along with other materials such as colorant, catalyst, and stabilizer system [94]. The most commonly used monomers in dental materials are methacrylate monomers and their derivatives containing bisphenol A-diglycidyl methacrylate (Bis-GMA), hydroxyethyl methacrylate (HEMA), triethylene glycol dimethacrylate (TEGDMA), and urethane dimethacrylate (UDMA). During the polymerization process, the monomers are transformed into a three-dimensional cross-linked network structure with close packing of molecules, resulting in volumetric shrinkage and weakening of the bonds between the tooth and the prosthesis, which cause marginal cracks, discoloration, postoperative sensitivity, recurrence of dental caries, and fracture and failure of the prosthesis.

Recently, novel monomer combinations and alterations of the resin composite formulation have been developed and evaluated to decrease polymerization shrinkage stress [95], such as monomer with high molecular weight, low concentration of reactive functional group (C=C) [96], and ringing-opening polymerization (e.g., Filtek LS, 3M-ESPE) [97]. However, due to the high molecular weight and low double-bond concentration of monomers, the cross-linking density of the final polymer network diminishes and leads to low mechanical properties. Therefore, it is essential to increase the double-bond conversion for reducing the unreacted monomers and elevating the cross-linking density [98]. Bis-GMA, most widely used in commercial composites, has high viscosity restricting the double-bond conversion, which necessitates copolymerization with other monomers with lower molecular weight for increasing conversion and obtaining suitable viscosity to add fillers [99]. The most common comonomer system is based on Bis-GMA and TEGDMA. Because TEGDMA has deficiencies related to its relatively high polymerization shrinkage, susceptibility to cyclization, and cytotoxic effects [100,101], the replacement of TEGDMA with other comonomer as diluents has been continually explored. Tay et al. substituted partial TEGDMA with 2,2,2-trifluoroethyl methacrylate (TFEMA) in the experiment. The Bis-GMA/TEGDMA/UDMA dental composite after substitution exhibited lower water solubility, lower polymerization shrinkage, and sustainable release of fluoride ions [102]. Allycarbonate monomers have also been studied to substitute TEGDMA. González-López et al. synthesized allyl(2(2-(((allyloxy)carbonyl)oxy)benzoyl)-5-methoxyphenyl) carbonate (BZ-AL) as a diluent monomer for Bis-GMA. Compared to Bis-GMA/TEGDMA, Bis-GMA/BZ-AL enhanced flexural strength and reduced polymerization stress [103]. Diallyl (propane-2,2-diylbis (1,4-phenylene)) biscarbonatemonomer (BPhADAC), as diallyl carbonate monomer, contributed to not only low volumetric shrinkage but high double-bond conversion and hydrophobicity correlating the stability after aging [104].

Furthermore, due to Bis-GMA and/or bisphenol A inducing changes in estrogen-sensitive organs or cells [105,106], Bis-GMA free composite resins have been invented. Urethane-dimethacrylates (UDMA) is currently the only commercial alternative to the Bis-GMA [107]. The trimethacrylate tris(4-hydroxyphenyl)methanetriglycidyl methacrylate (TTM) monomer, which is used as a base monomer in photopolymerizable composite resins, had similar values of flexural strength, elastic modulus, degree of conversion, and polymerization shrinkage compared to Bis-GMA [108].

Inorganic fillers include colloidal silica, quartz, silica glass-containing barium, strontium, zirconium, and ceramic powder. Their morphology, sizes, and contents have a great impact on the mechanical, operating, transparent, and polishing performances of resin composites. The fillers can increase the elasticity and strength while reducing the shrinkage of the composite during polymerization [109]. The composites are most commonly classified as macrofilled, microfilled, hybrid, modern hybrid, and nanofilled composites based on the average size of filler particles and their distribution [110,111]. The early composite had macrofillers ranging from 10 to 50 μm in size, but with bad polishing performance and low wear resistance [112]. Later, microfilled composites were formulated by incorporating amorphous spherical silica with an average size of approximately 40–50 nm, which is included in the scale of nanoparticles (1–100 nm) [113]. Both macrofillers and microfillers are contained in a typical hybrid composite. Even if acceptable smoothness and better surface morphology are achieved, the conventional hybrid composite still displays longevity problems due to the intrinsic wear pattern of the resin system containing macrofillers [114]. Modern hybrid composites include microhybrid composites (0.6–1μm and ~40 nm) and nanohybrid composites that contain more nanoparticles based on the modification of microhybrids. They are universally applied to anterior and posterior restoration because of a combination of superior strength and polishing performance [113]. The latest innovation is nanofilled composites with totally nanoscale particles. Nanoparticles can increase the surface area of fillers and the overall filler level of composites due to small sizes and great quantities, leading to lower shrinkage and higher esthetics and strength [109].

A silane coupling agent commercially available in dentistry is trialkoxysilane, such as 3-methacryloxypropyl trimethoxysilane (MPS). A silane coupling agent has two functional groups at the end of the molecular backbone chemically linking the inorganic fillers and unpolymerized resin matrix. The bonding of fillers with resin matrix is formed through two essential steps: (1) silane is activated by an acid to generate silanol groups which react with hydroxyl groups on the filler surface by condensation reaction. (2) Another functional group of silane reacts with resin monomers to form new C-C single bonds by free radicals [115]. The silane coupling agent can improve the mechanical and physical properties of resin composite [116]. A latest meta-analysis suggested that the application of silane coupling could improve the repair bond strength of methacrylate-based resin composites [117].

Most resin composites cure via free radical chain polymerization, which is initiated by various cure methods to generate free reactive radicals. Upon the cure modes or initiating systems, the resin composites can also be classified into four types: self-cured, heat-cured, light-cured, and dual-cured composites. Self-cured composites, also called chemically cured composites, are used as resin-based luting cement or core materials instead of direct restorations. The self-cured composite is a paste-paste or powder-liquid mixture containing initiators (e.g., benzoyl peroxide, BPO) and accelerators (e.g., tertiary amines) such as N, N-dimethyl-p-toluidine (DMPT) and N, N-dihydroxyethyl-p-toluidine (DHPT). The heat-curing method is still applied in PMMA-based restorations and utilizes BPO as initiators; however, the method is not effective for intraoral treatment due to the needed temperature above 60°C [118]. When the powder and liquid are mixed, the redox reaction between BPO and amine accelerators produces an intermediate molecule, which then decomposes into the benzoyl radical and amine-derived radical [119]. The initiating system of the paste-paste self-cured composite differs slightly from the powder-liquid. Because BPO mixed with the demethacrylate monomer is sensitive to heat decomposition, inhibitors are added to the system for a stable catalyst. Phenolic compounds, such as butylated hydroxytoluene (BHT) and monomethyl ether of hydroquinone (MEHQ), are commonly used as dental inhibitors. These inhibitors react with active radicals to reduce reactive sites, thus preventing spontaneous initiation and suppressing premature polymerization [118,120]. For light-cured composites, camphorquinone (CQ) is a common photoinitiator and amines are co-initiators or accelerators. Currently, the majority of clinical resin composites are light-cured, and the CQ/amines initiating system with visible light curing is nearly used in all dental restorative composites because of better safety than UV-curing and one-component systems [4]. The CQ molecule attains an excited triplet state by visible light absorption, and then promptly interacts with amine reductant via electron transfer, forming a new excited complex (exciplex) which abstracts hydrogen from the amine and finally generates radicals for rapid polymerization of monomers [118,121]. Photoinitiators influence mechanical properties, color, and translucency of resin-based composites [122,123]. The dual-cured composites constitute two pastes, including both chemical initiating system and photoinitiation system. As soon as the two parts are mixed, the chemical curing begins, and during the process of chemical polymerization, the composites can be light-cured at any time [124]. Dual-cured composites are comprehensively used for manufacturing core buildups and cementing endodontic posts [4]. However, the major disadvantage of CQ/amines initiating system is the negative effect on color stability of the restoration. CQ is a kind of yellow powder that gives a yellow tint to uncured composite [125]. The color should be bleached after irradiation, but CQ has poor bleaching due to its chromophore groups [126]. Tertiary amines are also responsible for the long-term darkening of the composites to some extent [127,128]. Furthermore, CQ is considered to be toxic to pulp cells and potentially genetically toxic as well [129,130]. 2,4,6-trimethylbenzoyl-diphenylphosphine oxide (TPO) can be utilized solely as a photoinitiator system or collaboratively with CQ with no requirement of co-initiators [129,131]. Bisacylphosphine oxide (BAPO) is a photosensitizer with no need for co-initiators. Extensive researches have been done to compare TPO, BAPO, and CQ. Both TPO and BAPO have superior properties to CQ. Materials containing TPO and BAPO have a higher conversion rate and faster polymerization [132–135]. TPO and BAPO both exerted less cytotoxic effect in cell culture, and TPO had no genotoxicity while BAPO had a weak genotoxic effect [136]. In terms of color stability, they also exhibited better performances as the optical characteristics of TPO-based materials were comparable to those of teeth, and yellow staining did not occur when BAPO was applied [134]. Novel initiators have been discovered and are being evaluated experimentally, among which germanium compounds are the most promising, such as benzoyltrimethylgermane (BTMGe) and dibenzoyldiethyl-germane (DBDEGe) [137]. Co-initiator is not required to start the polymerization process when the germanium photoinitiator is applied to the composite. Compared to CQ, they also displayed good solubility in most monomers, high photocuring reactivity, and slight yellowing which could be diminished by suitable stabilizers [127,137].

5.5.1.2 Adhesive Materials

Direct and indirect composite resin restorations containing inlays, onlays, and veneers require dental adhesives for bonding, and endodontic posts and cores also benefit from the use of dental adhesives in conjunction with resin luting materials. Furthermore, adhesive materials have been widely used in pit-and-fissure sealers, endodontic obturation, fixed orthodontic devices, and dentinal hypersensitivity treatments. Therefore, the advancement of the science of dental adhesions has an important influence on modern clinical prosthodontics [138].

The procedures for resin composite restoration include enamel etching, dentin conditioning, adhesive application (dentin priming and application of a dentin bonding agent), and resin composite filling. The most important component of the adhesive is the functional monomers, which give adhesive system formulations the capacity to interact with dental substrates to provide the promise of a specific chemical interaction capable of achieving more stable and long-lasting adhesion. Functional monomers have at least an acrylic group (especially methacrylates) for polymerization with resin composite and a functional group that wets and demineralizes the substrate/or bonds to the tooth substrate [139]. The functional group usually contains one or more carboxylic acid groups, carboxylic acid anhydrides, or phosphoric acid groups, such as 2-hydroxyethyl methacrylate (HEMA) and 10-methacryloyloxydecyl dihydrogen phosphate (10-MDP), which perform various functions, such as etching tooth substrates (partially dissolving the smear layer and demineralizing hydroxyapatite), enhancing monomer penetration, and imparting the adhesives with potential for chemical interactions with dental substrates [140]. The low molar mass allows functional monomers to infiltrate into dentin, but their chain structure restricts the formation of a strong polymer network. Song et al. synthesized silyl-functionalized Bis-GMA via reaction between isocyanate and the hydroxyl group of Bis-GMA. Compared to HEMA/Bis-GMA adhesive, the incorporation of silyl-Bis-GMA accessed not only higher conversion, lower viscosity, and self-strengthening property but a higher cross-linked network without compromising the homogenous structure. The leaching ratio of HEMA was also reduced to approximately 1% when silyl-Bis-GMA entirely replaced Bis-GMA [141]. Methacrylates have desirable reactivity and mechanical properties but display a tendency to hydrolytic and enzymatic degradation by esterase from microorganisms [142]. Relatively hydrophobic monomers such as Bis-GMA and TEGDMA are preferred for the prevention of hydrolytic degradation, but hydrophobic monomers are unfavorable for the infiltration of adhesives into hydrophilic dentin. A preliminary attempt to create functional monomers with hydrolytic and enzymatic stability has been made. Difunctional and hybrid methacrylate-methacrylamide monomers showed remarkably decreased water sorption and bonding stability to dentin, suggesting the potential to be further studied as an alternative functional monomer [143]. A new methacrylamide-based monomer HMTAF was synthesized and proven to be hydrolytically resistant, polymerizable, and non-toxic to Vero cell lines [144].

As an unconventional component of the adhesive, the filler has recently been added to the adhesive because it could fortify the adhesive layer, modulate the viscosity of adhesives, and relieve contraction stresses from resin composite restoration [120]. The studies showed that small amounts of fillers were appropriate for adhesives without compromising the wetting of bonding substrate, and appropriate size (preferably less than 20 nm) was essential to the penetration of the adhesive resin into dentin tubes and even collagen network. Normally, silane coupling agents are also utilized to silanize the fillers for the chemical bonding of the resin matrix and fillers, which not only benefits the stress transmission between the resin and filler but also prevents the adhesive from premature degrading [145]. Solvents, such as water, ethanol, and acetone, serving as diluting agents of the resin mixture, are an indispensable component of adhesives, especially for dentin bonding due to the wet nature of dentin [146]. The dissolution of the monomers in the solvent partly results in the low viscosity of primers and adhesive resin, and the diffusion ability of the adhesive is also promoted by solvents [147].

Adhesives are designed to bond resin composites to enamel and dentin, possessing the ability to withstand mechanical forces and prevent microleakage [3]. Adhesives for restorative filling are mainly applicable to direct resin composite filling of the tooth defect, pit-and-fissure sealing, and dentin desensitizing. They can be classified based on their objects as enamel adhesive and dentin adhesive. Enamel adhesive is responsible for bonding enamel, while dentin adhesive can bond both enamel and dentin with an emphasis on dentin bonding. The structural characteristics of enamel and dentin make two adhesives differ in many aspects. As enamel is a relatively dry substrate containing 92% (by vol) hydroxyapatite, the enamel adhesive is hydrophobic and is applied with phosphoric acid etching, which is efficient on enamel and is fundamental for the durability of adhesion [148]. The acid chemically dissolves the enamel causing the diffusion and interlocking of resin monomers into an array of micropores. After curing, plenty of resin tags form and produce micromechanical interaction between enamel and adhesives [149]. As opposed to enamel adhesion, dentin adhesion remains challengeable in adhesive dentistry. In addition to the unique structure that contains more organic matter and vital constituents from dentinal tubules to odontoblasts, biological factors such as pulpal fluid flow, dentin depth, and permeability, etc. also add complexity to the dentin adhesion [150,151]. Dentin adhesives/dental adhesives can be divided into etch rinse (ER) and self-etch (SE). Original components of the adhesive system are etchant, primer, and bonding resin, the three separate procedures can be merged in two or one steps. The two types of ER adhesives are "three-step" and "two-step" ER adhesives, while primer and bonding resin are combined for the "two-step". As for the self-etch, the etchant is removed. The first type of self-etch adhesives is "two-step" SE adhesive with acidic primer and hydrophobic bonding resin included, and the other is "one-step" SE adhesive which combines the acidic primer and hydrophobic resin. In ER adhesives, etching completely removes the smear layer, demineralizes the surface layer of dentin, exposes the microporous collagen-fiber network, allows the resin to flow and diffuse, and finally forms micromechanical interlocks with dentin structure [152]. SE adhesives use acidic monomers rather than etchant to demineralize enamel with lower depth than ER adhesives [153].

In addition to the exploration of novel components and mechanical properties of resin composites and adhesives, antibacterial properties, biocompatibility, and remineralization have also been studied widely. Almeida et al. evaluated the biocompatibility of different initiating systems and proved that the pair of CQ and 1,3-diethyl-2-thiobarbituric acid (TBA) presented higher cell viability among the tested systems [134]. The respective and combinatorial effects of monomers and photoinitiators on cells and genes have also been studied. A novel urethane-based monomer FIT-852 possessed less cytotoxic and genotoxic properties than Bis-GMA, suggesting great biocompatibility and potential use in resin composites, while the monoacylphosphine oxide photoinitiator (Lucirin TPO) showed more cytotoxicity and genotoxicity than CQ and 2-(N, N-dimethylamino)ethyl methacrylate (DMAEMA). In terms of interaction between tested monomers and initiators, TPO increased the overall toxicity in Bis-GMA-based mixture but decreased it in FIT-based mixture [154].

The introduction of nanoparticles is a vital advancement in improving the biological properties of dental resin. Nanoparticles are capable of enhancing mechanical strength and adhesion to tissues, as well as polishing and improving aesthetic properties [112]. The mechanical property of resin composites was assessed to be improved with no cytotoxicity after adding nanozirconia fillers, which also achieved a better opacity effect for possible use as resin cement when the content was conditioned to 55 wt% [155]. The incorporation of nitrogen-doped titanium dioxide nanoparticles (N-TiO$_2$) to adhesive resin contributed to greater antibacterial behaviors and maintained similar wettability to the unmodified resin [156]. The combination of graphene and Ag nanoparticles (G-AgNp) added to an auto-polymerizing resin was also studied, which presented better flexural properties as well as favorable antibacterial activity, with no significant decrease in cell viability [157].

The addition of multiple bioactive agents is comprehensively studied. The dental composite and adhesive combined with methacryloyloxyethyl phosphorylcholine (MPC) and quaternary ammonium dimethylaminohexadecyl methacrylate (DMAHDM) are reported to possess both antibacterial and protein-repellent properties, and can be considered to be promising for inhibition of biofilm formation and secondary caries [158,159]. In another study, magnetic nanoparticles with an iron core and a silica coating were combined with dimethylaminohexadecyl methacrylate (DMAHDM) and amorphous calcium phosphate (NACP) in an adhesive system. The novel adhesive considerably enhanced the dentin bond strength and exhibited satisfactory antibacterial performance. The amount and activity of biofilm were decreased and the pH of biofilm was raised to over 6.5, indicating promising application for inhibiting secondary caries [160]. The produced polyHEMA/TMPT(trimethylolpropane trimethacrylate) particles carrying fibroblast growth factor-2 (FGF-2) were incorporated into 4-[2-(methacryloyloxy)ethoxycarbonyl] phthalic anhydride/methyl methacrylate-tri-n-butylborane (4-META/MMA-TBB) resin, and the novel resin was demonstrated to promote cell proliferation without adverse impact on bonding and mechanical properties [161]. Song et al. designed a hybrid network of adhesive with the incorporation of two synthesized amino-functional alkoxysilanes to attain buffering and self-strengthening capabilities. The copolymers showed promising neutralization capacity, which provided a new approach for creating dental adhesive that could autonomously undermine the damage from cariogenic and aciduric bacteria [162].

5.5.2 RESTORATIVE MATERIAL FOR DENTITION DEFECT

Dentition defect, namely missing tooth, is not only detrimental to oral health because of series of structural and functional problems but also to the psychological status and social interactions [163]. The dominant treatment for dentition defect is making prostheses, including conventional dentures and implants.

Conventional dentures are basically of three types: removable partial dentures, complete dentures, and fixed partial dentures. Removable partial dentures are regularly used as a conservative and cheap option and are preferred under certain circumstances such as poor oral tissue, deep undercuts, inadequate bone density, and systemic health problems such as diabetes [164]. Acrylic resin and its composites are the most common removable denture fabricating material. As for fixed prostheses, ceramic is the most commonly used crown and bridge material [92].

Denture base, one of the significant components of removable partial denture, covers the alveolar ridge and related labial and lingual sides as well as hard palate to provide adhesion for artificial tooth, conduct and disperse occlusal force, and unify the whole denture. Polymethyl methacrylate (PMMA) was introduced as a denture base material in 1937 and retains its popularity and significance in prosthodontic practice [147,165].

PMMA possess virtues such as aesthetics, clinical and laboratory operability, adjustability, and stability in the oral cavity except for undesirable mechanical properties [166,167]. Consequently, numerous researches into the modification of denture material have been conducted. Main strategies include optimizing the chemical structure of polymers, seeking alternatives, and introducing reinforcement additives.

Polyamide and acetals materials can be considered as alternatives for PMMA. Ensuring the color matching of gingiva and tooth tissues, they also have greater flexibility to improve patients' comfort of use, but probably expedite alveolar resorption [79]. Recently, high-performance thermoplastic polyaryletherketone (PAEK) groups have entered the research of PMMA alternatives. PAEK exhibits better stability to discoloration, low solubility, and water sorption [168]. PAEK-based prostheses also reveal positive appearance, fit, and retention from a clinical perspective [169,170]. A novel aryl-ketone-polymer (UAKP) was developed to balance flexibility and rigidity [164]. The elastic properties were also testified to be suitable for the indication of removable partial dentures [171].

Inorganic fillers, fibers, and nanoparticles are frequently introduced. Metal oxides, noble metals, and minerals can be used as fillers, and, notably, metal oxides enhance the mechanical and physical properties of PMMA, as well as boost patients' oral rhigosis and thalposis [172]. The fibers include glass fibers, polyethylene fibers, rayon fibers, polyester fibers, and nylon fibers, which are all reported to have reinforcing effects [173]. The incorporation of nanoparticles often improves antibacterial property in addition to mechanical properties. The addition of titanium dioxide (TiO_2) to PMMA improves the stiffness, creep recovery and relaxation behaviors, as well as antibacterial ability through reduction of bacteria adherence [174]. Low concentrations of nano-silicon dioxides (nano-SiO_2) decrease the adhesion of *Candida albicans* to PMMA denture base resin showing anti-fungal efficacy, as well as improve wettability and hardness, while having an adverse effect on surface roughness and translucency [175].

The latest reinforcement system are hybrid fillers which substantially promoting properties of PMMA [172]. Cheng et al. prepared PMMA-based resin combined with TiO_2 nanofillers and PEEK microfillers and demonstrated that the addition of 1% of TiO_w and 1% of PEEK achieved optimal mechanical and antibacterial properties. The prepared resin also showed smooth surface and high resolution after 3D printing, indicating the potential to be a restorative material for the 3D industry [176]. Zirconium dioxide nanoparticles (ZrO_2-NPs) and silver nanoparticles (AgNPs) were simultaneously used to modify double-layered acrylic resin denture base, which displayed promising results for fabricating antimicrobial dentures [177].

Denture liners provide a soft cushion or a fitting surface on tissues to protect edentulous patients from injury caused by bone resorption [178]. Soft liners and resilient liners are both auto-polymerizing and light-cured liners based on plasticized acrylic resin and silicone [179]. Because materials of denture liners are primarily PMMA-based, susceptible to microbial adhesion, infiltration, and proliferation [92], inhibition of microbes for liners is necessary. Polyhexamethylene guanidine hydrochloride (PHMGH) is an effective antimicrobial agent of the guanidine family, and protects against G^+ and G^- bacteria, fungi, virus, and even highly antibiotic-resistant microbes, while having great water solubility [180–182]. A PHGMH-water solution, prepared as an antiseptic, was able to eliminate the biofilm of *Candida albicans* after 72-hour growth within 5 minutes, and the liners preserved mechanical properties [183].

5.6 MATERIALS FOR ORTHODONTICS

Clear orthodontic aligners were first introduced by Kesling in 1984 for minor tooth corrections [74]. With the introduction and advancement of computer-aided design/computer-aided manufacturing (CAD/CAM), the indications of clear aligner treatment have enlarged from mild to severe malocclusions [184–188]. Compared to fixed appliances, the current prevalence of aligners is derived from numerous advantages such as being removable, esthetic, more hygienic, fewer appointments, less chair time, and tailor-made in sequence on specific malocclusion setups of patients [189,190]. The material structure also strongly influences the prominence of aligners [190]. Polyester, polyurethane, and polypropylene are the three predominant kinds of thermoplastic materials for the fabrication of clear aligners [191]. Polyethylene terephthalate (PET) and poly(ethylene terephthalate)-glycol (PET-G), a non-crystallizing amorphous copolymer of PET, have good mechanical properties, dimensional stability, and fatigue resistance, which make them widely applicable as raw materials of aligners [191–194]. Polycarbonate (PC) not only has high strength, impact resilience, durability, and dimensional stability but also has higher transparency to visible light than many types of glass, thus appearing to be more esthetic in related orthodontic devices [191,195]. Thermoplastic polyurethane (TPU) possesses both mechanical properties of vulcanized rubber and processability of thermoplastic polymers. Without the existence of chemical networks in normal rubber, TPU can be repeatedly melted and processed [196,197]. Polymer blending is an efficient and inexpensive approach to diversify polymer properties through an appropriate blend of different materials [198]. It is commonly utilized in the engineering of aligners, some commercial aligners consisting of more than one material, such as Erkoloc-Pro (PET-G/TPU) and Durasoft (TPU/PC). Several studies have concentrated on evaluating the physical and mechanical properties and comparing present aligners [199,200]. According to a comprehensive comparison, thermoplastic material is more suitable to manufacture aligners [201]. Ahn et al. developed a new orthodontic retainer incorporating hybrid materials of three layers: the outer PET-G, the middle TPU, and the inner reinforced resin. Each layer plays a certain role: the PET-G layer dominantly maintains the arch form, TPU buffers the impact effect, and the resin core enhances the mechanical strength and wear resistance [202].

5.7 MATERIALS FOR ORAL IMPLANTOLOGY

Dental implants increase the quality of life for many patients with tooth loss and have been widely utilized in patients. Therefore, implant restoration has become an effective restoration method for dentition defect and missing dentition. The materials used for medical applications, especially for dental and orthopedic implants, should possess excellent biocompatibility, corrosion resistance in the body environment, and superior mechanical properties, wear resistance, and non-toxicity. Titanium and its alloys are expected to be ideal materials for dental application on account of higher resistance to corrosion, good biocompatibility, and repassivation along with excellent mechanical properties. However, due to hypersensitivity to titanium, poor distribution of forces to bone because of the mismatched elastic modulus, and poor esthetics in thin gingival biotypes, PEEK as a new implant material has been widely studied.

PEEK is a high-performance thermoplastic polymer consisting of an aromatic molecular backbone chain with combination of ketone and ether functional groups between the aryl rings. This special structure determines PEEK's excellent inherent performance considering its environmental stability and a broad range of mechanical behaviors. The major attractive property of PEEK for dental implant application relies on its Young's (elastic) modulus (3–4 GPa) which is relatively close to human bone, enamel, and dentin. For further improving its mechanical properties to endow PEEK with broader adaptability, the addition of reinforcing agents like carbon fibers can increase the elastic modulus of PEEK up to 14 GPa, which approaches the elastic modulus of human cortical bone (18 Gpa). Compared to the elastic modulus of titanium (>100 GPa), we assume theoretically that PEEK could induce less stress shielding than titanium. Yet, it is unknown if there is a difference between bone resorption around PEEK and titanium implants in human bodies as PEEK dental implants have not been used widely in clinical practice. Apart from that, PEEK could avoid artifacts during imageological examination due to radiolucency. However, due to hydrophobicity, biological inertness, and inferior osteoconduction of PEEK, it is necessary to endow PEEK with bioactive properties for improving cell interaction. Stubinger et al. coated PEEK with hydroxyapatite (HA), and the results showed that the surface possessed excellent osteoconductive or osteoinductive properties [203]. Wang et al. prepared PEEK/HA binary mixtures, which showed better biocompatibility. However, ultimate tensile strength and fatigue limit reduced [204]. Hence, a new ternary composite may be beneficial to improve mechanical properties and biological activity. Deng et al. fabricated a PEEK/nano-HA/carbon fiber (PEEK/n-HA/CF) composite, and the results showed that the new material possessed better mechanical properties and better cytocompatibility for osteogenic differentiation than pure PEEK [205]. Furthermore, a considerable amount of researches, including nano-modification of surfaces and incorporation of bioactive inorganic particles, have been carried out to improve its bioactivity for enhanced osseointegration. A randomized controlled clinical trial reported that PEEK and titanium abutments exhibited no significant difference in bone loss and soft tissue inflammation. Moreover, compared to titanium, zirconia, and PMMA, the oral microbial biofilm formation around PEEK abutments was not getting more severe. Hence, PEEK could be an ideal alternative to titanium in implant abutments.

Up to now, in addition to the existing applications in dentistry, the study of PMMA used for dental implants has been implemented [206], suggesting that the graphene doped PMMA has a superior performance in low cytotoxicity, inflammatory reaction after implantation, and biocompatibility than titanium. PMMA deserves further investigation in oral implant application.

In summary, this chapter reviewed the application of various polymers in dentistry. All polymeric biomaterials must meet basic requirements, such as good biocompatibility, appropriate biomechanical properties, and special functions for clinical purposes like excellent antimicrobial properties. In addition, bioactivity is considered to be an important property of dental materials. For example, the traditional treatments for root canal diseases are limited to root canal obturation, but the new materials make treatment not only seal root canal but also control infection, promote root formation, and prevent external root absorption. Recently, 3D printing technology provided a more convenient method for fabricating dental prostheses or scaffolds. With advances in therapeutic techniques and updating of materials, the requirement of patients and simplification of dental operations will be better satisfied. Polymer materials have great potential in dentistry, which opens up broad prospects for the new field of dentistry.

ACKNOWLEDGEMENTS

This work was supported by the National Natural Science Foundation of China (no. 31670967 and 32000932), the Scientific Research Foundation of the Institute for Translational Medicine of Anhui Province (no. 2017zhyx19), University Outstanding Youth Talent Support Program of Anhui Province (no.gxyq2018007) and Postdoctoral Science Foundation of Anhui Province (No. 2018B264).

AUTHOR CONTRIBUTIONS

Zichen Wu, Xiaoxuan Lu, Xiaowei Wang contributed equally to this work.

REFERENCES

1. M. Saini, Y. Singh, P. Arora, V. Arora, K. Jain. Implant biomaterials: A comprehensive review. *World J. Clin. Cases* 3(1) (2015) 52–57.
2. M. Navarro, A. Michiardi, O. Castano, J.A. Planell. Biomaterials in orthopaedics. *J. R. Soc., Interface* 5(27) (2008) 1137–1158.
3. X.Y. Xu, L.B. He, B.G. Zhu, J.Y. Li, J.S. Li. Advances in polymeric materials for dental applications. *Polym. Chem.* 8(5) (2017) 807–823.
4. X.X. Zhou, X.Y. Huang, M.Y. Li, X. Peng, S.P. Wang, X.D. Zhou, L. Cheng. Development and status of resin composite as dental restorative materials. *J. Appl. Polym. Sci.* 136(44) (2019) 48180.
5. J.A. Aas, B.J. Paster, L.N. Stokes, I. Olsen, F.E. Dewhirst. Defining the normal bacterial flora of the oral cavity. *J. Clin. Microbiol.* 43(11) (2005) 5721–5732.
6. Y.L. Lee, B.S. Lee, F.H. Lin, A. Yun Lin, W.H. Lan, C.P. Lin. Effects of physiological environments on the hydration behavior of mineral trioxide aggregate. *Biomaterials* 25(5) (2004) 787–793.
7. H.W. Roberts, J.M. Toth, D.W. Berzins, D.G. Charlton. Mineral trioxide aggregate material use in endodontic treatment: A review of the literature. *Dent. Mater.* 24(2) (2008) 149–164.

8. G. Cervino, L. Laino, C. D'Amico, D. Russo, L. Nucci, G. Amoroso, F. Gorassini, M. Tepedino, A. Terranova, D. Gambino, R. Mastroeni, M.D. Tozum, L. Fiorillo. Mineral trioxide aggregate applications in endodontics: A review. *Eur. J. Dent.* 14(4) (2020) 683–691.

9. T. Dammaschke, H.U. Gerth, H. Zuchner, E. Schafer. Chemical and physical surface and bulk material characterization of white ProRoot MTA and two Portland cements. *Dent. Mater.* 21(8) (2005) 731–738.

10. T.J. Hilton. Keys to clinical success with pulp capping: A review of the literature. *Oper. Dent.* 34(5) (2009) 615–625.

11. M.G. Gandolfi, P. Taddei, F. Siboni, E. Modena, G. Ciapetti, C. Prati. Development of the foremost light-curable calcium-silicate MTA cement as root-end in oral surgery. Chemical-physical properties, bioactivity and biological behavior. *Dent. Mater.* 27(7) (2011) e134–e157.

12. H. Chung, M. Kim, H. Ko, W. Yang. Evaluation of physical and biologic properties of the mixture of mineral trioxide aggregate and 4-META/MMA-TBB resin. *Oral Surg. Oral Med. Oral Pathol. Oral Radiol. Endod.* 112(5) (2011) e6–e11.

13. L.M. Formosa, B. Mallia, J. Camilleri, The chemical properties of light- and chemical-curing composites with mineral trioxide aggregate filler. *Dent. Mater.* 29(2) (2013) e11–e19.

14. A. Alagha, A. Nourallah, S. Alhariri. Dexamethasone- loaded polymeric porous sponge as a direct pulp capping agent. *J. Biomater. Sci. Polym. Ed.* 31(13) (2020) 1689–1705.

15. A. Daghrery, Z. Aytac, N. Dubey, L. Mei, A. Schwendeman, M.C. Bottino. Electrospinning of dexamethasone/cyclodextrin inclusion complex polymer fibers for dental pulp therapy. *Colloids Surf. B. Biointerfaces* 191 (2020) 111011.

16. A.R. Kemp, H. Peters. Fractionation and molecular weight of rubber and gutta-percha. *Ind. Eng. Chem.* 33(11) (1941) 1391–1398.

17. C.M. Friedman, J.L. Sandrik, M.A. Heuer, G.W. Rapp. Composition and mechanical properties of gutta-percha endodontic points. *J. Dent. Res.* 54(5) (1975) 921–925.

18. V. Vishwanath, H.M. Rao. Gutta-percha in endodontics - A comprehensive review of material science. *J Conserv. Dent.* 22(3) (2019) 216–222.

19. P.R. Pradeep, K.J. Kasti, S. Ananthakrishna, T.N. Raghu, R. Vikram. Evaluation of different dentin adhesive systems and its effect on apical microleakage: An in vitro study. *J. Int. Oral Health* 7(5) (2015) 44–48.

20. M. Prado, M.S.O. Menezes, B. Gomes, C.A.M. Barbosa, L. Athias, R.A. Simao. Surface modification of gutta-percha cones by non-thermal plasma. *Mater. Sci. Eng. C Mater. Biol. Appl.* 68 (2016) 343–349.

21. M. Tomino, K. Nagano, T. Hayashi, K. Kuroki, T. Kawai. Antimicrobial efficacy of gutta-percha supplemented with cetylpyridinium chloride. *J. Oral Sci.* 58(2) (2016) 277–282.

22. D.K. Lee, S.V. Kim, A.N. Limansubroto, A. Yen, A. Soundia, C.Y. Wang, W. Shi, C. Hong, S. Tetradis, Y. Kim, N.H. Park, M.K. Kang, D. Ho. Nanodiamond-gutta percha composite biomaterials for root canal therapy. *ACS Nano* 9(11) (2015) 11490–11501.

23. M.J. Alves, L. Grenho, C. Lopes, J. Borges, F. Vaz, I.P. Vaz, M.H. Fernandes. Antibacterial effect and biocompatibility of a novel nanostructured ZnO-coated gutta-percha cone for improved endodontic treatment. *Mater. Sci. Eng. C Mater. Biol. Appl.* 92 (2018) 840–848.

24. X. Liang, W. Liao, H. Cai, S. Jiang, S. Chen. 3D-printed artificial teeth: Accuracy and application in root canal therapy. *J. Biomed. Nanotechnol.* 14(8) (2018) 1477–1485.

25. M.J. Dong, J.C. Zhang, L. Liu, G.Y. Hou, Y. Yu, C.Y. Yuan, X.Y. Wang. New gutta percha composite with high thermal conductivity and low shear viscosity contributed by the bridging fillers containing ZnO and CNTs. *Compos. B. Eng.* 173 (2019) 106903.

26. L. Zhang, Y. Yu, C. Joubert, G. Bruder, Y. Liu, C.C. Chang, M. Simon, S.G. Walker. M. Rafailovich. Differentiation of dental pulp stem cells on gutta-percha scaffolds. *Polymers (Basel)* 8(5) (2016) 193.

27. A. Washio, T. Morotomi, S. Yoshii, C. Kitamura. Bioactive glass-based endodontic sealer as a promising root canal filling material without semisolid core materials. *Materials (Basel)* 12(23) (2019) 3967.

28. G.H. Li, L.N. Niu, W. Zhang, M. Olsen, G. De-Deus, A.A. Eid, J.H. Chen. D.H. Pashley, F.R. Tay. Ability of new obturation materials to improve the seal of the root canal system: A review. *Acta Biomater.* 10(3) (2014) 1050–1063.

29. B.H. Baras, M.A.S. Melo, V. Thumbigere-Math, F.R. Tay, A.F. Fouad, T.W. Oates, M.D. Weir, L. Cheng, H.H.K. Xu. Novel bioactive and therapeutic root canal sealers with antibacterial and remineralization properties. *Materials (Basel)* 13(5) (2020) 1096.

30. T. Komabayashi, D. Colmenar, N. Cvach, A. Bhat, C. Primus, Y. Imai. Comprehensive review of current endodontic sealers. *Dent. Mater. J.* 39(5) (2020) 703–720.

31. S. Tyagi, P. Tyagi, P. Mishra. Evolution of root canal sealers: An insight story. *Eur. J. Gen. Dent.* 2(3) (2013) 199–218.

32. M.A. Marciano, B.M. Guimaraes, R. Ordinola-Zapata, C.M. Bramante, B.C. Cavenago, R.B. Garcia, N. Bernardineli, F.B. Andrade, I.G. Moraes, M.A. Duarte. Physical properties and interfacial adaptation of three epoxy resin-based sealers. *J. Endod.* 37(10) (2011) 1417–1421.

33. R.S. Schwartz. Adhesive dentistry and endodontics. Part 2: Bonding in the root canal system-the promise and the problems: A review. *J. Endod.* 32(12) (2006) 1125–1134.

34. R.C.D. Swimberghe, T. Coenye, R.J.G. De Moor, M.A. Meire. Biofilm model systems for root canal disinfection: A literature review. *Int. Endod. J.* 52(5) (2019) 604–628.

35. L. Wang, X. Xie, C. Li, H. Liu, K. Zhang, Y. Zhou, X. Chang, H.H.K. Xu. Novel bioactive root canal sealer to inhibit endodontic multispecies biofilms with remineralizing calcium phosphate ions. *J. Dent.* 60 (2017) 25–35.

36. B.H. Baras, J. Sun, M.A.S. Melo, F.R. Tay, T.W. Oates, K. Zhang, M.D. Weir, H.H.K. Xu. Novel root canal sealer with dimethylaminohexadecyl methacrylate, nano-silver and nano-calcium phosphate to kill bacteria inside root dentin and increase dentin hardness. *Dent. Mater.* 35(10) (2019) 1479–1489.

37. B.H. Baras, S. Wang, M.A.S. Melo, F. Tay, A.F. Fouad, D.D. Arola, M.D. Weir, H.H.K. Xu. Novel bioactive root canal sealer with antibiofilm and remineralization properties. *J. Dent.* 83 (2019) 67–76.

38. J. Seung, M.D. Weir, M.A.S. Melo, E. Romberg, A. Nosrat, H.H.K. Xu, P.A. Tordik. A modified resin sealer: Physical and antibacterial properties. *J. Endod.* 44(10) (2018) 1553–1557.

39. R.K. Scarparo, F.S. Grecca, E.V. Fachin. Analysis of tissue reactions to methacrylate resin-based, epoxy resin-based, and zinc oxide-eugenol endodontic sealers. *J. Endod.* 35(2) (2009) 229–232.

40. L.T. Cintra, P.F. Bernabe, I.G. de Moraes, J.E. Gomes-Filho, T. Okamoto, A. Consolaro, T.N. Pinheiro. Evaluation of subcutaneous and alveolar implantation surgical sites in the study of the biological properties of root-end filling endodontic materials. *J. Appl. Oral Sci.* 18(1) (2010) 75–82.

41. R.A. Augsburger, D.D. Peters. Radiographic evaluation of extruded obturation materials. *J. Endod.* 16(10) (1990) 492–497.

42. T.H. Huang, J.J. Yang, H. Li, C.T. Kao. The biocompatibility evaluation of epoxy resin-based root canal sealers in vitro. *Biomaterials* 23(1) (2002) 77–83.

43. A.U. Eldeniz, K. Mustafa, D. Orstavik, J.E. Dahl. Cytotoxicity of new resin-, calcium hydroxide- and silicone-based root canal sealers on fibroblasts derived from human gingiva and L929 cell lines. *Int. Endod. J.* 40(5) (2007) 329–337.

44. R. Holland, V. de Souza. Ability of a new calcium hydroxide root canal filling material to induce hard tissue formation. *J. Endod.* 11(12) (1985) 535–543.

45. F.M. Huang, M.Y. Chou, Y.C. Chang. Induction of cyclooxygenase-2 mRNA and protein expression by epoxy resin and zinc oxide-eugenol based root canal sealers in human osteoblastic cells. *Biomaterials* 24(11) (2003) 1869–1875.

46. C.H. Camargo, S.E. Camargo, M.C. Valera, K.A. Hiller, G. Schmalz, H. Schweikl. The induction of cytotoxicity, oxidative stress, and genotoxicity by root canal sealers in mammalian cells. *Oral Surg. Oral Med. Oral Pathol. Oral Radiol. Endod.* 108(6) (2009) 952–960.

47. C.H.R. Camargo, L.C.L. Gomes, M.C.M. Franca, T.S. Bittencourt, M.C. Valera, S.E.A. Camargo, M.C. Bottino. Incorporating N-acetylcysteine and tricalcium phosphate into epoxy resin-based sealer improved its biocompatibility and adhesiveness to radicular dentine. *Dent. Mater.* 35(12) (2019) 1750–1756.

48. X. Sun, A. Sun, X. Jia, S. Jin, D. Zhang, K. Xiao, Q. Wang. In vitro bioactivity of AH plus with the addition of nano-magnesium hydroxide. *Ann. Transl. Med.* 8(6) (2020) 313.

49. T.C.A. Rossato, J.A. Gallas, W.L.O. da Rosa, A.F. da Silva, E. Piva, S.L. Peralta, R.G. Lund. Experimental sealers containing metal methacrylates: Physical and biological properties. *J. Endod.* 43(10) (2017) 1725–1729.

50. G. Raddall, I. Mello, B.M. Leung. Biomaterials and scaffold design strategies for regenerative endodontic therapy. *Front Bioeng. Biotechnol.* 7 (2019) 317.

51. E.G. Trevino, A.N. Patwardhan, M.A. Henry, G. Perry, N. Dybdal-Hargreaves, K.M. Hargreaves. A. diogenes, effect of irrigants on the survival of human stem cells of the apical papilla in a platelet-rich plasma scaffold in human root tips. *J. Endod.* 37(8) (2011) 1109–1115.

52. G. Jadhav, N. Shah, A. Logani. Revascularization with and without platelet-rich plasma in nonvital, immature, anterior teeth: A pilot clinical study. *J. Endod.* 38(12) (2012) 1581–1587.

53. L.Z. A, Y.M. B, Y.W. A, Y.L. A, S.R. C. Review scaffold design and stem cells for tooth regeneration. *Jpn. Dent. Sci. Rev.* 49 (2013) 14–26.

54. A. Athirasala, A. Tahayeri, G. Thrivikraman, C.M. Franca, N. Monteiro, V. Tran, J. Ferracane, L.E. Bertassoni. A dentin-derived hydrogel bioink for 3D bioprinting of cell laden scaffolds for regenerative dentistry. *Biofabrication* 10(2) (2018) 024101.

55. L. Lambricht, P. De Berdt, J. Vanacker, J. Leprince, A. Diogenes, H. Goldansaz, C. Bouzin, V. Preat, C. Dupont-Gillain, A. des Rieux. The type and composition of alginate and hyaluronic-based hydrogels influence the viability of stem cells of the apical papilla. *Dent. Mater.* 30(12) (2014) e349–e361.

56. S. Shrestha, C.D. Torneck, A. Kishen. Dentin conditioning with bioactive molecule releasing nanoparticle system enhances adherence, viability, and differentiation of stem cells from apical papilla. *J. Endod.* 42(5) (2016) 717–723.

57. G. Ceccarelli, R. Presta, L. Benedetti, M.G. Cusella De Angelis, S.M. Lupi. Y.B.R. Rodriguez, emerging perspectives in scaffold for tissue engineering in oral surgery. *Stem Cells Int.* 2017 (2017) 4585401.

58. W. Wang, M. Dang, Z. Zhang, J. Hu, T.W. Eyster, L. Ni, P.X. Ma. Dentin regeneration by stem cells of apical papilla on injectable nanofibrous microspheres and stimulated by controlled BMP-2 release. *Acta Biomater.* 36 (2016) 63–72.

59. V. Shiehzadeh, F. Aghmasheh, F. Shiehzadeh, M. Joulae, E. Kosarieh, F. Shiehzadeh. Healing of large periapical lesions following delivery of dental stem cells with an injectable scaffold: New method and three case reports. *Indian J. Dent. Res.* 25(2) (2014) 248–253.

60. B. Chang, N. Ahuja, C. Ma, X. Liu. Injectable scaffolds: Preparation and application in dental and craniofacial regeneration. *Mater. Sci. Eng. R Rep.* 111 (2017) 1–26.

61. U.S. Department of Health and Human Services. Oral health in America: A report of the Surgeon General. *J. Calif. Dent. Assoc.* 28(9) (2000) 685–695.

62. J. Gottlow, S. Nyman, T. Karring, J. Lindhe. New attachment formation as the result of controlled tissue regeneration. *J. Clin. Periodontol.* 11(8) (1984) 494–503.

63. A. Kumar, R.V. Chandra, A.A. Reddy, B.H. Reddy, C. Reddy, A. Naveen. Evaluation of clinical, anti-inflammatory and anti-infective properties of amniotic membrane used for guided tissue regeneration: A randomized controlled trial. *Dent. Res. J. (Isfahan)* 12(2) (2015) 127–135.

64. J. Zhang, Q. Xu, C. Huang, A. Mo, J. Li, Y. Zuo. Biological properties of an anti-bacterial membrane for guided bone regeneration: An experimental study in rats. *Clin. Oral Implants Res.* 21(3) (2010) 321–327.

65. Y.D. Rakhmatia, Y. Ayukawa, A. Furuhashi, K. Koyano. Current barrier membranes: Titanium mesh and other membranes for guided bone regeneration in dental applications. *J. Prosthodont Res.* 57(1) (2013) 3–14.

66. A. Hamlekhan, F. Moztarzadeh, M. Mozafari, M. Azami, N. Nezafati. Preparation of laminated poly(epsilon-caprolactone)-gelatin-hydroxyapatite nanocomposite scaffold bioengineered via compound techniques for bone substitution. *Biomatter* 1(1) (2011) 91–101.

67. L. Zhang, Y. Dong, N. Zhang, J. Shi, X. Zhang, C. Qi, A.C. Midgley, S. Wang. Potentials of sandwich-like chitosan/polycaprolactone/gelatin scaffolds for guided tissue regeneration membrane *Mater. Sci. Eng. C Mater. Biol. Appl.* 109 (2020) 110618.

68. Y. Liang, X. Luan, X. Liu. Recent advances in periodontal regeneration: A biomaterial perspective. *Bioact Mater* 5(2) (2020) 297–308.

69. E.E. Machtei, M.I. Cho, R. Dunford, J. Norderyd, J.J. Zambon, R.J. Genco. Clinical, microbiological, and histological factors which influence the success of regenerative periodontal therapy. *J. Periodontol.* 65(2) (1994) 154–161.

70. H. Nowzari, E.S. MacDonald, J. Flynn, R.M. London, J.L. Morrison, J. Slots. The dynamics of microbial colonization of barrier membranes for guided tissue regeneration. *J. Periodontol.* 67(7) (1996) 694–702.

71. G. Sam, B.R. Pillai. Evolution of barrier membranes in periodontal regeneration-"are the third generation membranes really here?". *J. Clin. Diagn. Res.* 8(12) (2014) ZE14–ZE17.

72. R. Shi, J. Ye, W. Li, J. Zhang, J. Li, C. Wu, J. Xue, L. Zhang, Infection-responsive electrospun nanofiber mat for antibacterial guided tissue regeneration membrane. *Mater. Sci. Eng. C Mater. Biol. Appl.* 100 (2019) 523–534.

73. M. Limoee, P. Moradipour, M. Godarzi, E. Arkan, L. Behbood. Fabrication and invitro investigation of polycaprolactone - (polyvinyl alcohol/collagen) hybrid nanofiber as anti-inflammatory guided tissue regeneration membrane. *Curr. Pharm. Biotechnol.* 20(13) (2019) 1122–1133.

74. H.D. Kesling. The philosophy of the tooth positioning appliance. *Am. J. Orthod. Oral Surg.* 31(6) (1945) 297–304.

75. C. Ma, X. Liu. Formation of nanofibrous matrices, three-dimensional scaffolds, and microspheres: From theory to practice. *Tissue Eng. Part C Methods* 23(1) (2017) 50–59.

76. B. Chang, C. Ma, X. Liu. Nanofibers regulate single bone marrow stem cell osteogenesis via FAK/RhoA/YAP1 Pathway. *ACS Appl. Mater. Interfaces* 10(39) (2018) 33022–33031.

77. R. Perry. Dental impression materials. *J. Vet. Dent.* 30(2) (2013) 116–124.

78. T.E. Donovan, W.W. Chee. A review of contemporary impression materials and techniques. *Dent. Clin. North Am.* 48(2) (2004) vi-vii, 445–470.

79. M. Kawala, J. Smardz, L. Adamczyk, N. Grychowska, M. Wieckiewicz. Selected applications for current polymers in prosthetic dentistry - state of the art. *Curr. Med. Chem.* 25(42) (2018) 6002–6012.

80. B.S. Rubel. Impression materials: A comparative review of impression materials most commonly used in restorative dentistry. *Dent. Clin. North Am.* 51(3) (2007) 629–642.

81. A. Punj, D. Bompolaki, J. Garaicoa. Dental impression materials and techniques. *Dent. Clin. North Am.* 61(4) (2017) 779–796.

82. A. Srivastava, J. Aaisa, T. Kumar T.A., K. Ginjupalli, N. Upadhya P. Alginates: A review of compositional aspects for dental applications. *Trends Biomater. Artif. Organs* 26(1) (2012) 31–36.

83. S. Alaghari, S. Velagala, R.K. Alla, A. Ramaraju. Advances in alginate impression materials: A review. *Int. J. Dent. Mater.* 1(2) (2019) 55–59.

84. R. Mehta, S. Wadhwa, N. Duggal, A. Kumar, M. Goel, S. Pande. Influence of repeat pours of addition silicone impressions on the dimensional accuracy of casts. *J. Interdiscipl. Med. Dent. Sci.* 2(1) (2014) 1000108

85. P. Zarrintaj, S. Rezaei, S.H. Jafari, M.R. Saeb, S. Ghalami, M. Roshandel, B.M. Peiman, D.A. Ehsaneh, F. Sefat, M. Mozafari. Impression materials for dental prosthesis, in: Z. Khurshid, S. Najeeb, M.S. Zafar, F. Sefat (Eds.), *Advanced Dental Biomaterials.* Woodhead Publishing Inc., Duxford, 2019, pp. 197–215.

86. Z. Wang. Comparison of dimensional accuracies using two elastomeric impression materials in casting three-dimensional tool marks. *J. Forensic Sci.* 61(3) (2016) 792–797.

87. H. Rudolph, M.R. Graf, K. Kuhn, S. Rupf-Kohler, A. Eirich, C. Edelmann, S. Quaas, R.G. Luthardt. Performance of dental impression materials: Benchmarking of materials and techniques by three-dimensional analysis. *Dent. Mater. J.* 34(5) (2015) 572–584.

88. M. Kawara, M. Iwasaki, Y. Iwata, Y. Komoda, S. Inoue, O. Komiyama, H. Suzuki, T. Kuroki, K. Hashizaki. Rheological properties of elastomeric impression materials for selective pressure impression technique. *J. Prosthodont. Res.* 59(4) (2015) 254–261.

89. M.B. Blatz, A. Sadan, J.O. Burgess, D. Mercante, S. Hoist. Selected characteristics of a new polyvinyl siloxane impression material--a randomized clinical trial. *Quintessence Int.* 36(2) (2005) 97–104.

90. C.D. Reitz, N.P. Clark. The setting of vinyl polysiloxane and condensation silicone putties when mixed with gloved hands. *J. Am. Dent. Assoc.* 116(3) (1988) 371–375.

91. N. Enkling, S. Bayer, P. Johren, R. Mericske-Stern. Vinylsiloxanether: A new impression material. Clinical study of implant impressions with vinylsiloxanether versus polyether materials. *Clin. Implant Dent. Relat. Res.* 14(1) (2012) 144–151.

92. F. Saeed, N. Muhammad, A.S. Khan, F. Sharif, A. Rahim, P. Ahmad, M. Irfan. Prosthodontics dental materials: From conventional to unconventional. *Mater. Sci. Eng., C* 106 (2020) 110167.

93. J.L. Drummond. Degradation, fatigue, and failure of resin dental composite materials. *J. Dent. Res.* 87(8) (2008) 710–719.

94. P. Makvandi, R. Jamaledin, M. Jabbari, N. Nikfarjam, A. Borzacchiello. Antibacterial quaternary ammonium compounds in dental materials: A systematic review. *Dent. Mater.* 34(6) (2018) 851–867.

95. H. Alzraikat, M.F. Burrow, G.A. Maghaireh, N.A. Taha. Nanofilled resin composite properties and clinical performance: A review. *Oper. Dent.* 43(4) (2018) E173–E190.

96. C.S. Pfeifer. Polymer-based direct filling materials. *Dent. Clin. North Am.* 61(4) (2017) 733–750.

97. A.P.P. Fugolin, C.S. Pfeifer. New resins for dental composites. *J. Dent. Res.* 96(10) (2017) 1085–1091.

98. K.S. Anseth, M.D. Goodner, M.A. Reil, A.R. Kannurpatti, S.M. Newman, C.N. Bowman. The influence of comonomer composition on dimethacrylate resin properties for dental composites. *J. Dent. Res.* 75(8) (1996) 1607–1612.

99. E. Asmussen, A. Peutzfeldt. Influence of UEDMA BisGMA and TEGDMA on selected mechanical properties of experimental resin composites. *Dent. Mater.* 14(1) (1998) 51–56.

100. J.E. Elliott, L.G. Lovell, C.N. Bowman. Primary cyclization in the polymerization of bis-GMA and TEGDMA: A modeling approach to understanding the cure of dental resins. *Dent. Mater.* 17(3) (2001) 221–229.

101. W. Geurtsen, G. Leyhausen. Chemical-biological interactions of the resin monomer triethyleneglycol-dimethacrylate (TEGDMA). *J. Dent. Res.* 80(12) (2001) 2046–2050.

102. J.S. Tay, B.B.L. Choong, I.H. Ooi, B.S. Tan. Effect of trifluoroethyl methacrylate comonomer on physical properties of Bis-GMA based dental composites. *Dent. Mater. J.* 38(2) (2019) 226–232.

103. J.A. Gonzalez-Lopez, A.A. Perez-Mondragon, C.E. Cuevas-Suarez, S.C. Esparza Gonzalez, A.M. Herrera-Gonzalez. Dental composite resins with low polymerization stress based on a new allyl carbonate monomer. *J. Mech. Behav. Biomed. Mater.* 110 (2020) 103955.

104. C.E. Cuevas-Suárez, J.A. González-López, A.F. Da Silva, E. Piva, A.M. Herrera-González. Synthesis of an allyl carbonate monomer as alternative to TEGDMA in the formulation of dental composite resins. *J. Mech. Behav. Biomed. Mater.* 87 (2018) 148–154.

105. R. Becher, H. Wellendorf, A.K. Sakhi, J.T. Samuelsen, C. Thomsen, A.K. Bolling, H.M. Kopperud. Presence and leaching of bisphenol a (BPA) from dental materials. *Acta Biomater. Odontol. Scand.* 4(1) (2018) 56–62.

106. T. Marzouk, S. Sathyanarayana, A.S. Kim, A.L. Seminario, C.M. McKinney. A systematic review of exposure to bisphenol a from dental treatment. *JDR Clin. Trans. Res.* 4(2) (2019) 106–115.

107. I.M. Barszczewska-Rybarek. A guide through the dental dimethacrylate polymer network structural characterization and interpretation of physico-mechanical properties. *Materials (Basel)* 12(24) (2019) 4057.

108. A.A. Perez-Mondragon, C.E. Cuevas-Suarez, J.A. Gonzalez-Lopez, N. Trejo-Carbajal, M. Melendez-Rodriguez, A.M. Herrera-Gonzalez. Preparation and evaluation of a BisGMA-free dental composite resin based on a novel trimethacrylate monomer. *Dent. Mater.* 36(4) (2020) 542–550.

109. M.H. Chen. Update on dental nanocomposites. *J. Dent. Res.* 89(6) (2010) 549–560.

110. L.D. Randolph, W.M. Palin, G. Leloup, J.G. Leprince. Filler characteristics of modern dental resin composites and their influence on physico-mechanical properties. *Dent. Mater.* 32(12) (2016) 1586–1599.

111. R. Wang, E. Habib, X.X. Zhu. Evaluation of the filler packing structures in dental resin composites: From theory to practice. *Dent. Mater.* 34(7) (2018) 1014–1023.

112. B. Pratap, R.K. Gupta, B. Bhardwaj, M. Nag. Resin based restorative dental materials: Characteristics and future perspectives. *Jpn. Dent. Sci. Rev.* 55(1) (2019) 126–138.

113. J.L. Ferracane. Resin composite--state of the art. *Dent. Mater.* 27(1) (2011) 29–38.

114. F. Lutz, R.W. Phillips. A classification and evaluation of composite resin systems. *J. Prosthet. Dent.* 50(4) (1983) 480–488.

115. J.P. Matinlinna, C.Y.K. Lung, J.K.H. Tsoi. Silane adhesion mechanism in dental applications and surface treatments: A review. *Dent. Mater.* 34(1) (2018) 13–28.

116. C.Y. Lung, Z. Sarfraz, A. Habib, A.S. Khan, J.P. Matinlinna. Effect of silanization of hydroxyapatite fillers on physical and mechanical properties of a bis-GMA based resin composite. *J. Mech. Behav. Biomed. Mater.* 54 (2016) 283–294.

117. L.T. Mendes, B.A.C. Loomans, N.J.M. Opdam, C.L.D. Silva, L. Casagrande, T.L. Lenzi. Silane coupling agents are beneficial for resin composite repair: A systematic review and meta-analysis of in vitro studies. *J. Adhes. Dent.* 22(5) (2020) 443–453.

118. T.Y. Kwon, R. Bagheri, Y.K. Kim, K.H. Kim, M.F. Burrow. Cure mechanisms in materials for use in esthetic dentistry. *J. Investig. Clin. Dent.* 3(1) (2012) 3–16.

119. I.D. Sideridou, D.S. Achilias, O. Karava. Reactivity of benzoyl peroxide/amine system as an initiator for the free radical polymerization of dental and orthopaedic dimethacrylate monomers: Effect of the amine and monomer chemical structure. *Macromolecules* 39(6) (2006) 2072–2080.

120. K.L. Van Landuyt, J. Snauwaert, J. De Munck, M. Peumans, Y. Yoshida, A. Poitevin, E. Coutinho, K. Suzuki, P. Lambrechts, B. Van Meerbeek. Systematic review of the chemical composition of contemporary dental adhesives. *Biomaterials* 28(26) (2007) 3757–3785.

121. J. Jakubiak, X. Allonas, J.P. Fouassier, A. Sionkowska, J.F. Rabek. Camphorquinone–amines photoinitating systems for the initiation of free radical polymerization. *Polymer* 44(18) (2003) 5219–5226.

122. D.C. de Oliveira, M.G. Rocha, A. Gatti, A.B. Correr, J.L. Ferracane, M.A. Sinhore. Effect of different photoinitiators and reducing agents on cure efficiency and color stability of resin-based composites using different LED wavelengths. *J. Dent.* 43(12) (2015) 1565–1572.

123. D. Manojlovic, M.D. Dramicanin, M. Lezaja, P. Pongprueksa, B. Van Meerbeek, V. Miletic. Effect of resin and photoinitiator on color, translucency and color stability of conventional and low-shrinkage model composites. *Dent. Mater.* 32(2) (2016) 183–191.

124. L. Feng, B.I. Suh. The effect of curing modes on polymerization contraction stress of a dual cured composite. *J. Biomed. Mater. Res., Part B* 76(1) (2006) 196–202.

125. F.A. Rueggeberg, M. Giannini, C.A.G. Arrais, R.B.T. Price. Light curing in dentistry and clinical implications: A literature review. *Braz. Oral Res.* 31(suppl 1) (2017) e61.

126. H.H. Alvim, A.C. Alecio, W.A. Vasconcellos, M. Furlan, J.E. de Oliveira, J.R. Saad. Analysis of camphorquinone in composite resins as a function of shade. *Dent. Mater.* 23(10) (2007) 1245–1249.

127. N. Moszner, U.K. Fischer, B. Ganster, R. Liska, V. Rheinberger. Benzoyl germanium derivatives as novel visible light photoinitiators for dental materials. *Dent. Mater.* 24(7) (2008) 901–907.

128. Y.J. Park, K.H. Chae, H.R. Rawls. Development of a new photoinitiation system for dental light-cure composite resins. *Dent. Mater.* 15(2) (1999) 120–127.

129. D. Maciel, A.B. Caires-Filho, M. Fernandez-Garcia, C. Anauate-Netto, R.C.B. Alonso. Effect of camphorquinone concentration in physical-mechanical properties of experimental flowable resin composites. *Biomed. Res. Int.* 2018 (2018) 7921247.

130. S. Wang, Y. Xiong, J. Lalevee, P. Xiao, J. Liu, F. Xing. Biocompatibility and cytotoxicity of novel photoinitiator pi-conjugated dithienophosphole derivatives and their triggered polymers. *Toxicol. In Vitro* 63 (2020) 104720.

131. H.C. Georg, K. Coutinho, S. Canuto. Solvent effects on the UV-visible absorption spectrum of benzophenone in water: A combined Monte Carlo quantum mechanics study including solute polarization. *J. Chem. Phys.* 126(3) (2007) 034507.

132. G. Conte, M. Panetta, M. Mancini, A. Fabianelli, A. Brotzu, R. Sorge, L. Cianconi. Curing effectiveness of single-peak and multi-peak led light curing units on tpo-containing resin composites with different chromatic characteristics. *Oral Implantol. (Rome)* 10(2) (2017) 140–150.

133. L.F. Schneider, L.M. Cavalcante, S.A. Prahl, C.S. Pfeifer, J.L. Ferracane. Curing efficiency of dental resin composites formulated with camphorquinone or trimethylbenzoyl-diphenyl-phosphine oxide. *Dent. Mater.* 28(4) (2012) 392–397.

134. S.M. Almeida, C.T.W. Meereis, F.B. Leal, R.V. Carvalho, P.O. Boeira, L.A. Chisini, C.E. Cuevas-Suarez, G.S. Lima, E. Piva. Evaluation of alternative photoinitiator systems in two-step self-etch adhesive systems. *Dent. Mater.* 36(2) (2020) e29–e37.

135. L.D. Randolph, W.M. Palin, D.C. Watts, M. Genet, J. Devaux, G. Leloup, J.G. Leprince. The effect of ultra-fast photopolymerisation of experimental composites on shrinkage stress, network formation and pulpal temperature rise. *Dent. Mater.* 30(11) (2014) 1280–1289.

136. M. Popal, J. Volk, G. Leyhausen, W. Geurtsen. Cytotoxic and genotoxic potential of the type I photoinitiators BAPO and TPO on human oral keratinocytes and V79 fibroblasts. *Dent. Mater.* 34(12) (2018) 1783–1796.

137. A. Kowalska, J. Sokolowski, K. Bociong. The photoinitiators used in resin based dental composite-a review and future perspectives. *Polymers (Basel)* 13(3) (2021) 470.

138. E. Carrilho, M. Cardoso, M. Marques Ferreira, C.M. Marto, A. Paula, A.S. Coelho. 10-MDP based dental adhesives: Adhesive interface characterization and adhesive stability-a systematic review. *Materials (Basel)* 12(5) (2019) 790.

139. M. Cadenaro, T. Maravic, A. Comba, A. Mazzoni, L. Fanfoni, T. Hilton, J. Ferracane, L. Breschi. The role of polymerization in adhesive dentistry. *Dent. Mater.* 35(1) (2019) e1–e22.

140. K. Yoshihara, N. Nagaoka, T. Okihara, M. Kuroboshi, S. Hayakawa, Y. Maruo, G. Nishigawa, J. De Munck, Y. Yoshida, B. Van Meerbeek. Functional monomer impurity affects adhesive performance. *Dent. Mater.* 31(12) (2015) 1493–1501.

141. L. Song, Q. Ye, X. Ge, A. Misra, C. Tamerler, P. Spencer. New silyl-functionalized BisGMA provides autonomous strengthening without leaching for dental adhesives. *Acta Biomater.* 83 (2019) 130–139.

142. B. Huang, W.L. Siqueira, D.G. Cvitkovitch, Y. Finer. Esterase from a cariogenic bacterium hydrolyzes dental resins. *Acta Biomater.* 71 (2018) 330–338.

143. A.P. Fugolin, S. Lewis, M.G. Logan, J.L. Ferracane, C.S. Pfeifer. Methacrylamide-methacrylate hybrid monomers for dental applications. *Dent. Mater.* 36(8) (2020) 1028–1037.

144. N. Decha, S. Talungchit, P. Iawsipo, A. Pikulngam, P. Saiprasert, C. Tansakul. Synthesis and characterization of new hydrolytic-resistant dental resin adhesive monomer HMTAF. *Des. Monomers Polym.* 22(1) (2019) 106–113.

145. Y. Yoshida, K. Shirai, Y. Nakayama, M. Itoh, M. Okazaki, H. Shintani, S. Inoue, P. Lambrechts, G. Vanherle, B. Van Meerbeek. Improved filler-matrix coupling in resin composites. *J. Dent. Res.* 81(4) (2002) 270–273.

146. L. Breschi, A. Mazzoni, A. Ruggeri, M. Cadenaro, R. Di Lenarda, E. De Stefano Dorigo. Dental adhesion review: Aging and stability of the bonded interface. *Dent. Mater.* 24(1) (2008) 90–101.

147. M. Gundogdu, N. Yanikoglu, F. Bayindir, H. Ciftci. Effect of repair resin type and surface treatment on the repair strength of polyamide denture base resin. *Dent. Mater. J.* 34(4) (2015) 485–489.

148. J. Perdigão. Current perspectives on dental adhesion:(1) Dentin adhesion–not there yet. *Jpn. Dent. Sci. Rev.* 56(1) (2020) 190–207.

149. B. Van Meerbeek, J. De Munck, Y. Yoshida, S. Inoue, M. Vargas, P. Vijay, K. Van Landuyt, P. Lambrechts, G. Vanherle. Buonocore memorial lecture. Adhesion to enamel and dentin: Current status and future challenges. *Oper. Dent.* 28(3) (2003) 215–235.

150. N. Manuja, R. Nagpal, I.K. Pandit. Dental adhesion: Mechanism, techniques and durability. *J. Clin. Pediatr. Dent.* 36(3) (2012) 223–234.

151. G.C. Lopes, L.N. Baratieri, M.A. de Andrada, L.C. Vieira. Dental adhesion: Present state of the art and future perspectives. *Quintessence Int.* 33(3) (2002) 213–224.

152. B. Van Meerbeek, K. Yoshihara, K. Van Landuyt, Y. Yoshida, M. Peumans. From Buonocore's Pioneering acid-etch technique to self-adhering restoratives. A status perspective of rapidly advancing dental adhesive technology. *J. Adhes. Dent.* 22(1) (2020) 7–34.

153. M. Hannig, H. Bock, B. Bott, W. Hoth-Hannig. Inter-crystallite nanoretention of self-etching adhesives at enamel imaged by transmission electron microscopy. *Eur. J. Oral Sci.* 110(6) (2002) 464–470.

154. D. Manojlovic, M.D. Dramićanin, V. Miletic, D. Mitić-Ćulafić, B. Jovanović, B. Nikolić. Cytotoxicity and genotoxicity of a low-shrinkage monomer and monoacylphosphine oxide photoinitiator: Comparative analyses of individual toxicity and combination effects in mixtures. *Dent. Mater.* 33(4) (2017) 454–466.

155. G. Hong, J. Yang, X. Jin, T. Wu, S. Dai, H. Xie, C. Chen. Mechanical properties of nanohybrid resin composites containing various mass fractions of modified zirconia particles. *Int. J. Nanomed.* 15 (2020) 9891–9907.

156. F.L. Esteban Florez, R.D. Hiers, P. Larson, M. Johnson, E. O'Rear, A.J. Rondinone, S.S. Khajotia. Antibacterial dental adhesive resins containing nitrogen-doped titanium dioxide nanoparticles. *Mater. Sci. Eng. C Mater. Biol. Appl.* 93 (2018) 931–943.

157. C. Bacali, I. Baldea, M. Moldovan, R. Carpa, D.E. Olteanu, G.A. Filip, V. Nastase, L. Lascu, M. Badea, M. Constantiniuc, F. Badea. Flexural strength, biocompatibility, and antimicrobial activity of a polymethyl methacrylate denture resin enhanced with graphene and silver nanoparticles. *Clin. Oral Investig.* 24(8) (2020) 2713–2725.

158. N. Zhang, J. Ma, M.A. Melo, M.D. Weir, Y. Bai, H.H. Xu. Protein-repellent and antibacterial dental composite to inhibit biofilms and caries. *J. Dent.* 43(2) (2015) 225–234.

159. N. Zhang, M.D. Weir, E. Romberg, Y. Bai, H.H. Xu. Development of novel dental adhesive with double benefits of protein-repellent and antibacterial capabilities. *Dent. Mater.* 31(7) (2015) 845–854.

160. Y. Li, X. Hu, Y. Xia, Y. Ji, J. Ruan, M.D. Weir, X. Lin, Z. Nie, N. Gu, R. Masri, X. Chang, H.H.K. Xu. Novel magnetic nanoparticle-containing adhesive with greater dentin bond strength and antibacterial and remineralizing capabilities. *Dent. Mater.* 34(9) (2018) 1310–1322.

161. R. Tsuboi, H. Kitagawa, S. Imazato. FGF-2 release and bonding/physical properties of 4-META/MMA-based adhesive resins incorporating small FGF-2-loaded polymer particles. *Dent. Mater.* 36(12) (2020) 1586–1594.

162. L. Song, Q. Ye, X. Ge, A. Misra, C. Tamerler, P. Spencer. Fabrication of hybrid cross-linked network with buffering capabilities and autonomous strengthening characteristics for dental adhesives. *Acta Biomater.* 67 (2018) 111–121.

163. S. Kisely. No mental health without oral health. *Can. J. Psychiatry.* 61(5) (2016) 277–282.

164. S.D. Campbell, L. Cooper, H. Craddock, T.P. Hyde, B. Nattress, S.H. Pavitt, D.W. Seymour. Removable partial dentures: The clinical need for innovation. *J. Prosthet. Dent.* 118(3) (2017) 273–280.

165. M. Alkurt, Z. Yesil Duymus, M. Gundogdu. Effect of repair resin type and surface treatment on the repair strength of heat-polymerized denture base resin. *J. Prosthet. Dent.* 111(1) (2014) 71–78.

166. P. Spasojevic, M. Zrilic, V. Panic, D. Stamenkovic, S. Seslija, S. Velickovic. The mechanical properties of a poly(methyl methacrylate) denture base material modified with dimethyl itaconate and di-n-butyl Itaconate. *Int. J. Polym. Sci.* 2015 (2015) 1–9.

167. D.C. Jagger, A. Harrison, K.D. Jandt. The reinforcement of dentures. *J. Oral Rehabil.* 26(3) (1999) 185–194.

168. A. Liebermann, T. Wimmer, P.R. Schmidlin, H. Scherer, P. Loffler, M. Roos, B. Stawarczyk. Physicomechanical characterization of polyetheretherketone and current esthetic dental CAD/CAM polymers after aging in different storage media. *J. Prosthet. Dent.* 115(3) (2016) 321–328 e322.

169. C. Arnold, J. Hey, R. Schweyen, J.M. Setz. Accuracy of CAD-CAM-fabricated removable partial dentures. *J. Prosthet. Dent.* 119(4) (2018) 586–592.

170. H. Ye, X. Li, G. Wang, J. Kang, Y. Liu, Y. Sun, Y. Zhou. A novel computer-aided design/computer-assisted manufacture method for one-piece removable partial denture and evaluation of fit. *Int. J. Prosthodont.* 31(2) (2018) 149–151.

171. N. Lumkemann, M. Eichberger, R.J. Murphy, B. Stawarczyk. Suitability of the new Aryl-Ketone-Polymer indicated for removable partial dentures: Analysis of elastic properties and bond strength to denture resin. *Dent. Mater. J.* 39(4) (2020) 539–546.

172. M.M. Gad, S.M. Fouda, F.A. Al-Harbi, R. Napankangas. A. Raustia. PMMA denture base material enhancement: A review of fiber, filler, and nanofiller addition. *Int. J. Nanomed.* 12 (2017) 3801–3812.

173. T. Takahashi, T. Gonda, Y. Mizuno, Y. Fujinami, Y. Maeda. Reinforcement in removable prosthodontics: A literature review. *J. Oral Rehabil.* 44(2) (2017) 133–143.

174. A. Alrahlah, H. Fouad, M. Hashem, A.A. Niazy, A. AlBadah. Titanium Oxide (TiO(2))/Polymethylmethacrylate (PMMA) denture base nanocomposites: Mechanical, viscoelastic and antibacterial behavior. *Materials (Basel)* 11(7) (2018) 1096.

175. S.T. Alzayyat, G.A. Almutiri, J.K. Aljandan, R.M. Algarzai, S.Q. Khan, S. Akhtar. A. Matin, M.M. Gad. Antifungal efficacy and physical properties of poly(methylmethacrylate) denture base material reinforced with SiO_2 nanoparticles. *J. Prosthodont.* (2021). doi:10.1111/jopr.13271.

176. S.G. Chen, J. Yang, Y.G. Jia, B. Lu, L. Ren. TiO_2 and PEEK reinforced 3D printing PMMA composite resin for dental denture base applications. *Nanomaterials (Basel)* 9(7) (2019) 1049.

177. M.M. Gad, R. Abualsaud, A. Rahoma, A.M. Al-Thobity, S. Akhtar, S.M. Fouda. Double-layered acrylic resin denture base with nanoparticle additions: An in vitro study. *J. Prosthet. Dent.* 3913(20) (2020) 30555–30552.

178. M. Lau, G.S. Amarnath, B.C. Muddugangadhar, M.U. Swetha, K.A. Das. Tensile and shear bond strength of hard and soft denture relining materials to the conventional heat cured acrylic denture base resin: An In-vitro study. *J. Int. Oral Health* 6(2) (2014) 55–61.

179. M.I. Hashem. Advances in soft denture liners: An update. *J. Contemp. Dent. Pract.* 16(4) (2015) 314–318.

180. O. Aviv, N. Amir, N. Laout, S. Ratner, A. Basu, A.J. Domb. Poly(hexamethylene guanidine)-poly(ethylene glycol) solid blend for water microbial deactivation. *Polym. Degrad. Stab.* 129 (2016) 239–245.

181. H. Choi, K.J. Kim, D.G. Lee. Antifungal activity of the cationic antimicrobial polymer-polyhexamethylene guanidine hydrochloride and its mode of action. *Fungal Biol.* 121(1) (2017) 53–60.

182. Z. Zhou, D. Wei, Y. Lu. Polyhexamethylene guanidine hydrochloride shows bactericidal advantages over chlorhexidine digluconate against ESKAPE bacteria. *Biotechnol. Appl. Biochem.* 62(2) (2015) 268–274.

183. I.M. Garcia, S.B. Rodrigues, M.E. Rodrigues Gama, V.C. Branco Leitune, M.A. Melo, F.M. Collares. Guanidine derivative inhibits C. albicans biofilm growth on denture liner without promote loss of materials' resistance. *Bioact. Mater.* 5(2) (2020) 228–232.

184. R. Khosravi, B. Cohanim, P. Hujoel, S. Daher, M. Neal, W. Liu, G. Huang. Management of overbite with the Invisalign appliance. *Am. J. Orthod. Dentofacial Orthop.* 151(4) (2017) 691–699 e692.

185. F. Elkholy, F. Schmidt, R. Jager, B.G. Lapatki. Forces and moments delivered by novel, thinner PET-G aligners during labiopalatal bodily movement of a maxillary central incisor: An in vitro study. *Angle Orthod.* 86(6) (2016) 883–890.

186. F. Elkholy, T. Panchaphongsaphak, F. Kilic, F. Schmidt, B.G. Lapatki. Forces and moments delivered by PET-G aligners to an upper central incisor for labial and palatal translation. *J. Orofac. Orthop.* 76(6) (2015) 460–475.

187. J.P. Gomez, F.M. Pena, V. Martinez, D.C. Giraldo, C.I. Cardona. Initial force systems during bodily tooth movement with plastic aligners and composite attachments: A three-dimensional finite element analysis. *Angle Orthod.* 85(3) (2015) 454–460.

188. M. Simon, L. Keilig, J. Schwarze, B.A. Jung, C. Bourauel. Forces and moments generated by removable thermoplastic aligners: Incisor torque, premolar derotation, and molar distalization, *Am. J. Orthod. Dentofacial Orthop.* 145(6) (2014) 728–736.

189. F. Celenza. Clear aligner therapy, in: J.B. Levine (Ed.), *Smile Design Integrating Esthetics and Function (1st Edition)*. Mosby Ltd., Saint Louis, 2016, pp. 183–212.

190. L. Lombardo, E. Martines, V. Mazzanti, A. Arreghini, F. Mollica, G. Siciliani. Stress relaxation properties of four orthodontic aligner materials: A 24-hour in vitro study. *Angle Orthod.* 87(1) (2017) 11–18.

191. N. Zhang, Y. Bai, X. Ding, Y. Zhang. Preparation and characterization of thermoplastic materials for invisible orthodontics. *Dent. Mater. J.* 30(6) (2011) 954–959.

192. T.A. Raja, S.J. Littlewood, T. Munyombwe, N.L. Bubb. Wear resistance of four types of vacuum-formed retainer materials: A laboratory study. *Angle Orthod.* 84(4) (2014) 656–664.

193. W. Hahn, H. Dathe, J. Fialka-Fricke, S. Fricke-Zech, A. Zapf, D. Kubein-Meesenburg, R. Sadat-Khonsari. Influence of thermoplastic appliance thickness on the magnitude of force delivered to a maxillary central incisor during tipping. *Am. J. Orthod. Dentofacial Orthop.* 136(1) (2009) 12 e11–e17; discussion 12–13.

194. R.B. Dupaix, M.C. Boyce. Finite strain behavior of poly(ethylene terephthalate) (PET) and poly(ethylene terephthalate)-glycol (PETG). *Polymer* 46(13) (2005) 4827–4838.

195. Y.S. Ma, D.Y. Fang, N. Zhang, X.J. Ding, K.Y. Zhang, Y.X. Bai. Mechanical properties of orthodontic thermoplastics PETG/PC2858 after blending. *Chin. J. Dent. Res.* 19(1) (2016) 43–48.

196. Q.W. Lu, C.W. Macosko. Comparing the compatibility of various functionalized polypropylenes with thermoplastic polyurethane (TPU). *Polymer* 45(6) (2004) 1981–1991.

197. A. Frick, A. Rochman. Characterization of TPU-elastomers by thermal analysis (DSC). *Polym. Test.* 23(4) (2004) 413–417.

198. D.R. Paul, J.W. Barlow. Polymer blends. *J. Macromol. Sci., Polym. Rev.* 18(1) (2007) 109–168.

199. F. Jaggy, S. Zinelis, G. Polychronis, R. Patcas, M. Schatzle, G. Eliades, T. Eliades. ATR-FTIR analysis and one-week stress relaxation of four orthodontic aligner materials. *Materials (Basel)* 13(8) (2020) 1868.

200. F. Tamburrino, V. D'Anto, R. Bucci, G. Alessandri-Bonetti, S. Barone, A.V. Razionale. Mechanical properties of thermoplastic polymers for aligner manufacturing: In vitro study. *Dent. J. (Basel)* 8(2) (2020) 47.

201. W. Ruyi, Z. Zhihe, L. Yu. [Current situation and prospect for orthodontic thermoplastic materials]. *Hua Xi Kou Qiang Yi Xue Za Zhi* 36(1) (2018) 87–91.

202. H.W. Ahn, K.A. Kim, S.H. Kim. A new type of clear orthodontic retainer incorporating multi-layer hybrid materials. *Korean J. Orthod.* 45(5) (2015) 268–272.

203. S. Stubinger, A. Drechsler, A. Burki, K. Klein, P. Kronen, B. von Rechenberg. Titanium and hydroxyapatite coating of polyetheretherketone and carbon fiber-reinforced polyetheretherketone: A pilot study in sheep. *J. Biomed. Mater. Res., Part B* 104(6) (2016) 1182–1191.

204. L. Wang, S. He, X. Wu, S. Liang, Z. Mu, J. Wei, F. Deng, Y. Deng, S. Wei. Polyetheretherketone/nano-fluorohydroxyapatite composite with antimicrobial activity and osseointegration properties. *Biomaterials* 35(25) (2014) 6758–6775.

205. Y. Deng, P. Zhou, X. Liu, L. Wang, X. Xiong, Z. Tang, J. Wei, S. Wei. Preparation, characterization, cellular response and in vivo osseointegration of polyetheretherketone/nano-hydroxyapatite/carbon fiber ternary biocomposite. *Colloids Surf. B. Biointerfaces* 136 (2015) 64–73.

206. A. Scarano, T. Orsini, F. Di Carlo, L. Valbonetti, F. Lorusso. Graphene-doped poly (methyl-methacrylate) (Pmma) implants: A micro-CT and histomorphometrical study in rabbits. *Int. J. Mol. Sci.* 22(3) (2021) 1441. doi:10.3390/ijms22031441.

6 Recent Progress of Hydrogel in Skin Tissue Engineering

Kun Zhang, Shuaimeng Guan, Longlong Cui, Jiankang Li, Jiaheng Liang, and Jingjing Su
Zhengzhou University

CONTENTS

6.1 INTRODUCTION

Wounds are one of the major health problems caused by complications such as diabetes or infection. According to the World Health Organization, 58 million people are directly or indirectly affected by wounds each year, with the mortality rate close to 10%, and the remaining require proper treatment and care [1]. This not only places a significant burden on the health system in terms of expensive treatment and long hospital stay but also places a heavy financial and psychological burden on families and patients themselves [2]. Wound healing is a complex, continuous, and dynamic process. It is usually divided into four stages, hemostasis, inflammation, proliferation, and remodeling [3]. These phases have no clearly defined corresponding periods, and each phase overlaps to a certain extent. The healing of chronic wounds may

DOI: 10.1201/9781003161981-6

be impeded at any of these four stages. For large burn wounds, natural healing is also affected due to the loss of large amounts of skin tissue.

Although various products and skin grafting technology have been developed to treat wounds, there are still many shortcomings to overcome. The rapid development of tissue engineering and regenerative medicine has provided new therapeutic strategies for wound healing [4]. Skin tissue engineering plays an important role in the treatment of large burns and other skin defects. The goal is to effectively heal wounds, completely mimic physiological skin, close to normal skin, and eliminate host toxicity and immune rejection. In skin tissue engineering, common seed cells include keratinocytes, fibroblasts, melanocytes, hair follicle-related cells, etc. Growth factors include epidermal growth factor, blood vessel growth factor, and fibroblast growth factor. Scaffold materials include natural and artificial biomaterials.

The selection of suitable scaffold material is the key to successful treatment of skin injury. The requirements of skin tissue engineering scaffolds are good biocompatibility, biodegradability, maneuverability, wound healing promotion. Several studies have found that appropriate pore structure and water retention rates are necessary for cell adhesion, growth, migration, and new tissue formation. Interlinked three-dimensional pore structures enhance matrix permeability, facilitate diffusion of nutrients and wastes, as well as cellular signaling within the scaffold. Good water retention of the scaffold, keeping the wound moist, and the shape of the scaffold are essential for cell adhesion, differentiation, and proliferation.

Hydrogels are polymer networks formed by chemical or physical cross-linking. As scaffold materials, they can meet most requirements. Hydrogels have been used in tissue engineering and regenerative medicine for decades due to their good biocompatibility and similarity to the structure of the natural extracellular matrix (ECM). Hydrogels are clinically easy to operate and widely used in skin tissue engineering. They not only provide a moisturizing environment for the wound surface but also serve as a supporting structure for cell growth, contributing to wound regeneration. The environmental responsive hydrogels (such as temperature-responsive and pH-responsive gels) usually behave like a solution forming gels at near-physiological conditions. This facilitates in situ cross-linking within the biopolymer and with natural wound edge tissue. Another advantage of this strategy is that it is easier to use and more intelligent. With the development of this technology and further research, hydrogels can be modified to obtain several properties, for example, physical and chemical properties such as hardness, porosity, degradability, and cargo release. Other functions can also be achieved such as adhesion, hemostasis, antioxidant, and antibacterial. The more advanced multifunctional materials are more effective, sensitive to patients, and economical than existing treatments.

For hydrogels in the field of skin tissue engineering, the commonly used natural biological materials mainly include collagen, gelatin, silk fibroin, fibrinogen, chitosan, alginate, hyaluronic acid (HA), and so on [5]. In addition, more and more researchers have paid attention to artificial polymer biomaterials, such as polycaprolactone (PCL) and polyethylene glycol (PEG) [6]. Synthetic materials have advantages in terms of source and cost, and they are very effective in improving the strength of scaffold materials. These synthetic polymers have also contributed significantly to the development of a new generation of wound dressings.

Therefore, in this chapter, complicated structure and functions of the skin and the repair mechanism after skin injury are introduced. The application of skin tissue engineering, especially the important role of hydrogels in wound healing, is described. Natural and synthetic polymer hydrogel scaffolds in skin tissue engineering are reviewed.

6.2 COMPLICATED STRUCTURE AND FUNCTIONS OF SKIN

Skin is one of the largest organs in the human body, with a surface area of about $1.8\,m^2$, an average thickness of about 2.5 mm, an average density of 1.1, and a total mass of about 5–6 kg, which is about 6% of the total body weight. The skin acts as a huge physical barrier between the body and the environment, protecting us from external mechanical, chemical, and microbial damage [7]. When talking about skin, some people describe it as a "coat" because it is exposed to the environment and is the body's outermost barrier. Its appearance also conveys something about the body [8]. Some believe that it is the external "brain" of the human body because of its innervation, immune regulation, ultraviolet radiation sensing, pigment deposition, and endocrine functions [9]. It also keeps the body hydrated, synthesizes vitamins and hormones, protects against UV damage, and interacts with the outside world through its sensory ability. In addition, its complex immune network provides further protection to the deeper tissues [10]. Overall, as a complex organ, the skin is very important to human beings.

The skin has a multilayer structure and can be roughly divided into the epidermis, dermis and subcutaneous tissue from the outside to the inside (Figure 6.1). The

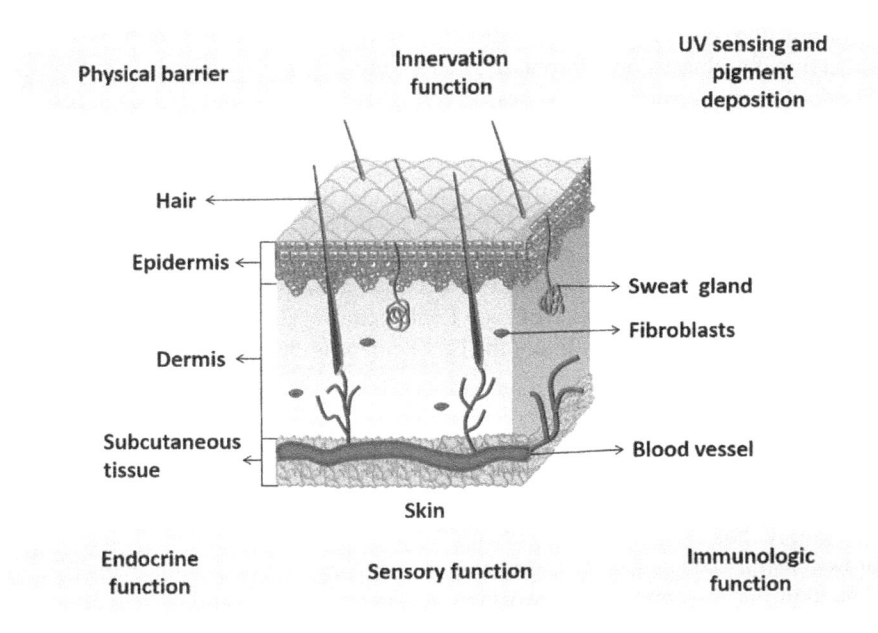

FIGURE 6.1 The structure and functions of the skin.

epidermis is a layered epithelium with continuous keratinization [11]. The outermost to innermost layers are the cornified layer, the granular layer, the spiny layer, and the basal layer. The cornified layer is composed of dead keratinocytes. The granular layer is made up of undivided keratinocytes, which produce a protein particle called keratohyalin. The spiny layer consists of keratinocytes, which have a limited ability to divide, as well as Langerhans cells, which are involved in the skin's immune response [12]. The basal layer contains differentiated keratinocytes and keratinocytes capable of division. There are also Merkle cells and melanocytes [13]. Merkle cells are associated with sensory function. Melanocytes secrete melanin, the deposition of which helps protect against ultraviolet radiation. Keratinocytes contain keratin intermediate filaments, and different layers of the epidermis contain varying amounts of keratin, ranging 30%–80%. The barrier function of the epidermis depends on transglutaminase-mediated cross-linking of structural proteins and lipids at the final stage of keratinocyte differentiation. In addition, the corneous barrier function depends on ceramides, cholesterol, and free fatty acids. Changes in the concentration of these substances can affect barrier function. Inhibition of key enzymes involved in the synthesis of these lipids can interfere with barrier permeability. Ca^+, K^+, and pH are also important for barrier regulation [14].

The dermis is a type of connective tissue rich in collagen that is usually less than 2 mm thick, but can be as thick as 4 mm in some areas (e.g., the back of adults). Structurally, it can be divided into the papillary layer with thin collagen fiber and a thick collagen fiber reticular layer [15]. In the human body, the papillary dermis extends to the portion of the epidermis and contains capillaries that facilitate the transport of nutrients. The reticular dermis contains skin appendages such as hair follicles, sebaceous glands, and sweat glands. It is noticeably thicker than the papillary dermis due to the high concentration of collagen and reticular fibers. Both dermis contains fibroblasts, myofibroblasts, and immune cells. The dermis is composed of ECM, fibroblasts, nerves, blood vessels, lymphatic system, and various accessory elements (such as excretory glands, sebaceous glands, exocrine glands, apocrine glands, hair follicles, nerve receptors, and baroreceptors). Collagen fibers provide the mechanical barrier and structural framework that houses blood vessels and many immune cells, such as dermal dendritic cells, T cells, natural killer cells, B cells, mast cells, and macrophages. About 90% of the total skin protein is composed of collagen macromolecules, accounting for about 75% of the total dry weight of the skin. Mainly there are 85%–90% of type I collagen, 8%–11% type III collagen, and 2%–4% type V collagen. In addition, the ECM contains elastin, which provides elasticity to the skin [16].

Underlying the dermis is the subcutaneous tissue, which consists mainly of fibroblasts and adipocytes and is rich in proteoglycans and glycosaminoglycans. Skin adipose tissue stores energy in the form of fatty acids and plays an important role in glucose homeostasis and lipid metabolism. Also, because fat is a poor conductor of heat, this layer has a good insulating effect. Subcutaneous tissue can produce a variety of growth factors and cytokines and contains a large number of immune cells [17].

The skin and its appendages have neuroendocrine functions that help keep the body's internal environment stable. The cutaneous neuroendocrine system operates in a way that is not controlled by the traditional central nervous system. It has a center equivalent to "hypothalamic-pituitary-adrenal". Although this "stress system" in the skin may not be found in the structure of the specific tissue, it still exists widely. Its main constituent activities include the production of adrenocorticotropin-releasing hormone and the downstream precancertin peptide; synthesis, metabolism, and targeting of androgens and estrogens; and the synthesis of serotonin and melatonin promotes inflammation, edema, vasodilation, and pigmentation [18]. Almost all cell types present in the skin can show immune function. The most obvious cells include keratinocytes, lymphocytes, Langerhans cells, monocytes and macrophages, vascular and lymphatic endothelial cells, mast cells, neutrophils, eosinophils, and basophils. In addition, free radicals, antimicrobial peptides (including defensins and Kathleen), cytokines, chemokines, neuropeptides, adhesion molecules, various pro-inflammatory and anti-inflammatory mediators, and immunoglobulins secreted by lymphocytes can promote the expression of skin immune function.

6.3 TYPES AND TREATMENT OF SKIN DISEASES

Skin diseases are one of the leading causes of the global burden of disease, affecting millions of people worldwide. It was reported that skin conditions accounted for 1.79% of the global disease burden of 306 diseases and injuries in 2013 [19]. Skin diseases are the fourth leading cause of disability worldwide. Age, environmental, and genetic factors, as well as trauma, can contribute to the development of various skin diseases, over 3,000 of which have been identified in the literature. According to a survey, nearly 85 million Americans were treated by a doctor for at least one skin condition in 2013. This resulted in $75 billion in direct healthcare costs and $11 billion in indirect opportunity cost losses. In addition, death has occurred in several patients with skin diseases. The cost and prevalence of skin diseases are comparable to or exceeds that of other diseases with major public health problems, such as cardiovascular disease and diabetes. Here, we focus on acute or chronic skin injuries caused by various conditions, which account for a large proportion of skin diseases and are an important problem to be solved clinically [20].

Skin injuries can be acute or chronic. An acute wound progresses through stages of healing in an orderly manner and tends to heal faster. Acute wounds include mechanical injuries such as sharp and blunt injuries, mild scalds, and postoperative wounds. A chronic wound is stagnant in the healing process for more than 3–4 weeks. Because of excessive and long-term inflammation and ischemia, the wound does not heal properly and is prone to infection, requiring long-term care. Chronic wounds include diabetic foot ulcers, bedsores, and ulcers in the veins and arteries of the legs. According to the data, about 8 million people in Europe suffered chronic trauma out of an estimated 830 million people in 2009 [21]. In addition to the enormous impact on patients' quality of life, chronic wounds impose a huge economic burden on the society. Nearly 2% of the European health budget is spent on the wound healing of chronic wounds, and about one-third of the skin health budget in the United States is spent on chronic wounds. Chronic wound care alone is estimated to cost more than $25 billion a year. The lifetime probability of chronic foot ulcers in diabetics is estimated to be between 10% and 25% and is the leading cause of non-traumatic amputation in the United States. In addition, pressure sores in intensive care patients are also on the rise [22].

Wound healing time depends on several factors, including wound size, depth, location, age of the patients, and local and systemic diseases. Acute trauma can proceed through the traditional four stages of wound healing, but chronic trauma cannot proceed through the normal orderly and timely sequence of repair, or the restoration of normal anatomy and function. Chronic wounds have elevated levels of cytokines and proteases that destroy essential ECM components, growth factors, and growth factor receptors. Acute wound fibroblasts show high mitotic activity, but chronic wound fibroblasts show low mitotic activity due to senescence. In addition, matrix metalloproteinases (MMPs) are overactive in chronic wounds, and the levels of tissue inhibitors of metalloproteinases were reduced [23].

Acute wounds are much more numerous than chronic wounds. The superficial wound injury of the skin extends to the superficial portion of the epidermis and dermis. Deep wounds involve a larger portion of the dermis and the whole layer of the wound, even the subcutaneous tissue layer. It is thought that in these wounds there should be no problems with wound healing and that skin barrier function and normal anatomical structure can be effectively restored, although scarring is possible. However, these wounds still require proper care to prevent complications, especially infection. Acute wound care includes thorough cleaning with potable tap water or saline, followed by appropriate dressing in accordance with the principles of wet wound treatment [24]. There is evidence in the literature that good hydration is the most important external factor leading to optimal wound healing. Healing in wet conditions not only speeds up the healing process and reduces pain, but may have a beneficial effect on reducing scarring [25].

There are three main causes of chronic trauma: venous ulcers, diabetic ulcers, and pressure ulcers. Venous ulcers occur mainly in the legs and are caused by a malfunctioning valve. Diabetic ulcers can start with minor bruising, often go unnoticed due to nerve damage, especially in the lower extremities, and can become severely infected due to a compromised immune system, poor circulation, and damaged capillaries. People who are bedridden or have limited mobility may develop pressure ulcers. Although the mechanism of chronic wound healing is unclear, it is closely related to dysfunctional inflammation and macrophage behavior. In addition, chronic wounds are associated with increased production of MMPs and decreased tissue inhibitors of metalloproteinases (TIMPs) [26]. Vascular disease is also a major cause of poor healing of chronic wounds, and its mechanisms include reduced bioavailability of growth factors and receptors, destruction of matrix proteins, reduced proliferation of resident cells, and insufficient recruitment of progenitor cells. Chronic wounds are consistently alkaline in pH (pH: 7.2–8.9) compared to acute wounds, which are characterized as neutral or alkaline (pH: 6.5–8.5). Acidification of the initial wound is essential for fibroblast proliferation, oxygenation, collagen formation, angiogenesis, and macrophage activity [27]. These critical processes are jeopardized by the alkaline environment of chronic wounds and are more likely to cause bacterial infection. There is a wide variety of approaches to chronic wound care in the extensive literature. Some biological agents with biological activity were introduced into chronic wounds to induce vascular remodeling and re-epithelialization to guide wound healing. Some use cell therapy, introducing stem cells to help heal wounds, but more are looking to new bioactive wound dressings or tissue-engineered scaffolds and skin substitutes

TABLE 6.1
The Types of Skin Injuries

Acute Wounds	Chronic Wounds
It can be recovered by the wound healing process in a short time	It cannot be recovered through the normal orderly process in more than 3–4 weeks
Low levels of bacteria	High levels of bacteria, susceptible to infection
Low levels of inflammatory cytokines and proteases	High levels of inflammatory cytokines and proteases
The fibroblasts have high mitotic activity	The fibroblasts are senescent and have low mitotic activity
pH 6.5–8.5	pH 7.2–8.9
Matrix metalloproteinase activity was normal	Matrix metalloproteinases are overactive

TABLE 6.2
The Treatments of Skin Injuries

Approaches	Features
Wound cleansing and debridement	Debris, exudate, and deactivated tissue are removed from the wound using four methods: surgery, autolysis, enzyme, and mechanical debridement
Biologic therapy	Biologics, which play a key role in wound healing, were introduced to guide wound healing by inducing vascular remodeling and re-epithelialization. One example is the commercially approved Regranex
Cell therapy	Use bone marrow MSCs, disaccharide-derived cells, epidermal cells, amniotic fluid stem cells, umbilical cord Wharton tissue stem cells, and macrophages to help treat skin injuries
Tissue engineering therapy	Skin injuries are treated with bioactive wound dressings, skin substitutes, and a variety of tissue-engineered scaffolds including electrospun fibers and three-dimensional printing

for chronic wounds. These new tissue engineering products have different advantages and disadvantages, but they have great potential and are an important direction for the development of wound care in the future [28] (Tables 6.1 and 6.2).

6.4 WOUND HEALING MECHANISM

Wound healing mainly consists of four overlapping stages: hemostasis, inflammation, proliferation, and remodeling (Figure 6.2) [29,30]. The body should stop bleeding immediately after injury. Hemostasis refers to the process of preventing bleeding at the site of wound injury and maintaining the integrity of blood vessels through platelet aggregation and activation of thrombin [31]. During hemostasis, fibrinogen first forms fibrin, thus providing a skeleton for cell migration and platelet aggregation to form a thrombus [32]. Cells migration near the wound secrete growth factors

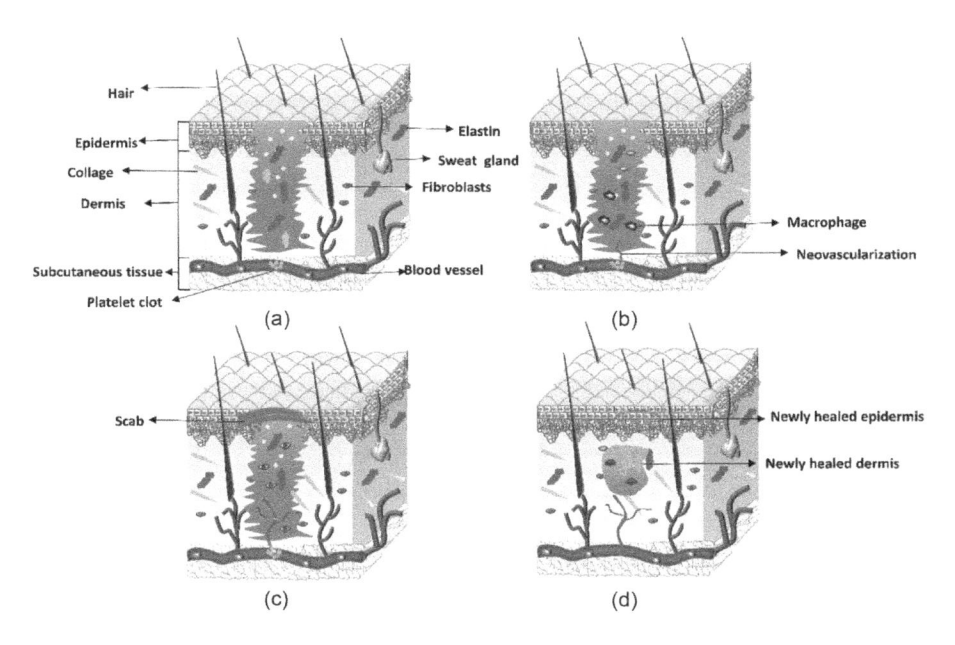

FIGURE 6.2   Four overlapping stages of the wound healing process (a. Hemostasis, b. Inflammation, c. Proliferation, d. Remodeling).

and cytokines to attract fibroblasts, immune cells, and endothelial cells to activate the healing cascade [33]. Inflammation is a defensive response of tissues to biofeedback against a pathogen or irritant. It starts immediately or within minutes after the injury, lasts hours to days in acute wounds, and can last for weeks or even months in chronic wounds (lower limb ulcers, pressure sores, diabetic foot ulcers, etc.). After inflammation occurs, a large number of neutrophils phagocytose and kill bacteria, monocytes differentiate into macrophages, remove surrounding pathogens or cell debris, and promote cell proliferation by releasing a large number of growth factors and cytokines [34,35]. During the proliferation stage, the proliferation of fibroblasts and endothelial cells promotes the formation of new blood vessels and the formation of ECM, the wound contracts, and re-epithelialization begins [36]. During the remodeling stage, the proportion of different types of collagen begins to change: the proportion of type I collagen increases, the proportion of type III collagen decreases, myofibroblast level decreases, fibroblast density increases, the ECM is further strengthened, and mechanical strength increases [37].

6.4.1 Hemostasis

Severe bleeding can lead to serious injury and even death. Therefore, it is important to stop bleeding quickly and promptly in patients [38,39]. Hemostasis can be divided into three types (Table 6.3): primary hemostasis, secondary hemostasis, and tertiary hemostasis. Blood vessel constriction, platelet blockage to form platelet thrombus, and coagulation together constitute the main process of hemostasis. After the blood vessel ruptures, noxious stimuli are transmitted through sympathetic nerves to cause

TABLE 6.3
The Mechanical Pathway of Three Different Types of Hemostasis

Type of Hemostasis	Mechanism
Primary hemostasis	Vascular contraction, platelet adhesion, and aggregation to form platelet plugs in the wound
Secondary hemostasis	Activation of the coagulation cascade, deposition and stabilization of fibrin
Tertiary hemostasis	Plasminogen is activated, fibrin clot is dissolved

reflex vasoconstriction. During the vasoconstriction, the collagen exposed to the damaged surface promotes the adhesion, activation, and aggregation of platelets to form platelet blockage and seal the damaged area. Collagen binds to the platelet GPVI receptor to promote the interaction between VWF and GPIBα, thereby stimulating platelet activation [40,41]. A strong signal pathway is induced by FcRγ, tyrosine-based immune receptor activation motif, Src kinase, and Syk tyrosine kinase, leading to activation of PLCγ. Subsequently, PLCγ hydrolyzes phosphatidylinositol-4,5-diphosphate in inositol triphosphate (IP3) and 1,2-diacylglycerol (DAG). IP3 binds to the dense tubular system (DTS) and allows Ca^{2+} to escape from DTS to the cytoplasm. Membrane-bound DAG and Ca^{2+} activate protein kinase C (PKC), leading to integrin activation, platelet diffusion, and granule secretion. The P2Y1 receptor helps to stimulate the initial changes in platelet shape and platelet aggregation. The activated platelets release thromboxane A2 (TXA2) to increase the number of platelets at the wound site [42]. However, when blood is exposed to subcutaneous tissue or ECM which express tissue factor (TF), TF forms FVIIA-TF complex with activated FVIIA, which then activates FIX and FX. FXa has the following functions: (1) activate FV and FVIII; (2) activate FXI to cut FIX into FIXa; (3) activate platelets through PAR-1 and PAR-4; and (4) promote the rapid generation of thrombin. After activation of FIX and FVIII, the formed FIXa-FVIIIa complex converts FX to FXa. Subsequently, the formation of the prothrombin complex (FXa-FVa) leads to the burst of thrombin, which can cleave fibrinogen into fibrin, which then stabilizes the thrombus [43,44].

6.4.2 INFLAMMATION

In the inflammatory stage, the main cells involved in the inflammatory response are mast cells, neutrophils, and macrophages. Normally, as the wound begins to clot, neutrophils and macrophages are aggregated into the wound and the inflammatory phase begins [45]. The activation of various endogenous inflammatory mediators, such as pro-inflammatory cytokines (TNF-α, IL-1), prostaglandins, leukotrienes, and histamine, promote the aggregation and activation of inflammatory cells. Platelet-activating factor, while aggregating and activating platelets, releases active amines, activates neutrophils and eosinophils, and promotes inflammation. Neutrophils are the first cells to recruit to the site of injury. Neutrophils have the following functions: (1) Phagocytosis. After the neutrophils are in contact with the foreign body that produces chemokines, the surrounding cytoplasm will bulge to form pseudopods, surrounding the invading stimulus in the local area. Because neutrophils contain a large amount of lysosomal enzymes, they can initiate rapid and non-specific phagocytosis; (2) Degranulation. When neutrophils aggregate to the corresponding tissue sites and are activated, they will increase the number of neutrophils and change their appearance, resulting in the degranulation effect, the release of superoxide and lysosomal enzymes, and then clear the invading pathogens; (3) Neutrophil trapping net. They can capture, neutralize, and kill various microorganisms [46,47]. Macrophages remove bacteria-filled neutrophils, foreign bodies, and pathogens through phagocytosis. Macrophages also secrete a large number of cytokines, pro-angiogenic factors, and fibrogenic factors, attracting cells into the proliferation stage of wound healing [48]. At the end of the inflammatory period, they turn to a repair phenotype and secrete anti-inflammatory mediators (IL-4/10/13) to promote tissue repair. However, in chronic wounds, neutrophil infiltration will release a large amount of Ca^{2+}-dependent protease MMPs. MMPs can degrade growth factors such as transforming growth factor β (TGF-β) [49] and PDGF, inhibit the production of TIMPs, and cause ECM degradation. Cell migration is lost and collagen synthesis is insufficient. In chronic wounds, the inflammation phase lasts longer.

6.4.3 PROLIFERATION

This process mainly involves neovascularization, fibroblast proliferation, and re-epithelialization. Many growth factors, such as fibroblast growth factor (FGF), TGF-β, vascular endothelial cell growth factor (VEGF), epidermal growth factor (EGF), and BMPs, play an important role in promoting cell proliferation and migration. FGF1/ FGF 2/ FGF 7/ FGF 10/ FGF 22 are expressed during dermal injury, and the FGF-FGFR-mediated signaling pathway enhances cell migration, proliferation, and growth factor production and epithelial formation [50]. VEGF binds to tyrosine kinase receptors on various cell surfaces to mediate angiogenesis, promote fibroblast proliferation, and keratinization, Fibroblasts proliferate rapidly in the low oxygen environment of the wound and promote the production of myofibroblasts [51]. Myofibroblasts build-up structures to synthesize fibronectin and collagen. A network of new blood vessels, fibroblasts, and a matrix of cells work together to form granulation tissue to fill a damaged wound. With the gradual formation of granulation tissue, the wound heals slowly. The superficial wound (superficial dermis) after healing is the same as normal skin. The deep wound (the middle and lower dermis) is gradually replaced by fibroblasts to form fibrous tissue, which replaces the original normal skin to form a scar. TGF-β [52], BMPs, and activin are the main members of the wound healing process. They induce the rearrangement of the cytoskeleton, promote the migration of keratinocytes, re-epithelialization, ECM formation, and remodeling [53,54].

6.4.4 REMODELING

Collagen plays a key role in this process [55]. Collagen from the initial disorder gradually arranged into an orderly structure to achieve the purpose of forming enough tension against external tension. The ratio of different types of collagen begins to change:

the ratio of type I collagen increases, the ratio of type III collagen decreases, the level of myofibroblasts decreases, the density of fibroblasts increases, the ECM is further strengthened, and the mechanical strength is increased. Then new skin is formed.

6.5 SKIN TISSUE ENGINEERING

The field of tissue engineering was originally established by Langer and Vacanti to combine the principles of engineering design with the understanding of biological mechanisms to replace or regenerate damaged tissue, which has been used for various biomedical applications, including disease modeling, resource sustainability, novel clinical treatments, and has facilitated the development of powerful technologies such as gene editing, bioreactor culture, and three-dimensional bioprinting [56,57]. One of the main goals of tissue engineering and regenerative medicine is to develop skin substitutes for the treatment of deep dermal and full-thickness wounds [58]. For centuries, advances have been made in the field of regenerative skin tissue engineering to promote faster wound healing and skin restoration. Many of the challenges in skin grafting for wound healing have attracted researchers to focus on skin tissue engineering in the 1980s.

The core idea of tissue engineering is to use scaffolds, cells, and/or bioactive molecules to help the skin recover properly from injury (Figure 6.3) [59,60]. Skin tissue engineering uses biological and engineering principles to construct tissue replacements that repair and improve damaged skin, which has made a significant contribution to reconstructive surgery as well as burn management [61,62]. Three-dimensional scaffolds and hydrogels alone or combined with bioactive molecules, genes, and cells can guide the development of functional engineering tissues and provide mechanical support during implantation *in vivo*. Biomaterials for skin tissue

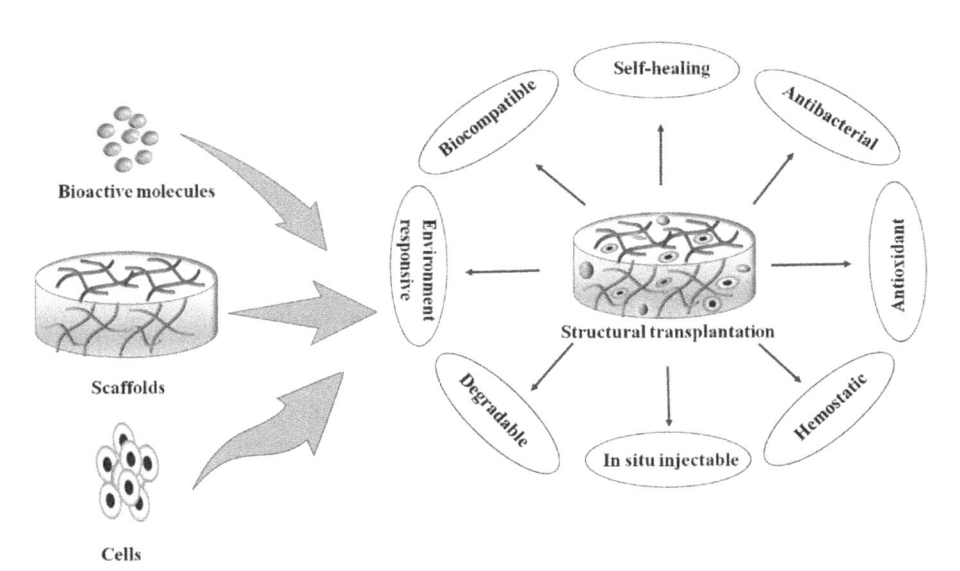

FIGURE 6.3 The properties of hydrogels for skin tissue engineering.

repair include several scaffold types, synthetic or natural, absorbable, degradable or nondegradable polymers, porous or dense scaffolds, and cells encapsulated in hydrogels or globular bodies. As a scaffold in tissue engineering, hydrogels have many attractive characteristics. They are biocompatible and biodegradable and have specific cell-binding sites suitable for cell attachment, growth, and differentiation [63]. Skin tissue engineering substitutes and scaffolds need to be biocompatible to overcome immune rejection and inflammation [64]. In addition, an appropriate hydrophilic interface is needed between tissue and biomaterials to effectively promote cell adhesion and proliferation. In addition, the structure needs to be lightweight to minimize foreign body sensation, biodegradable, and promote construction, allowing proper water retention, nutrient transport, air permeability, and structural stability, providing the best regeneration niche [65,66].

Stem cells are recognized as the best seed cells for tissue-engineered skin due to their self-renewal and multi-differentiation potential, as well as their ability to secrete various cytokines to promote wound healing. At present, the most studied stem cells are epidermal stem cells, bone marrow mesenchymal stem cells (MSCs), adipose-derived stem cells (ASCs), and umbilical cord MSCs [67]. Epidermal stem cells in the skin and its appendages (such as sweat glands and hair balls) are proliferative units, showing slow and limited division, self-renewal, and responsible for the generation of various lineages in mature skin, which are suitable for tissue engineering research and play an important role in wound repair [68]. MSCs can differentiate into epithelial cells and can be used as an alternative source to produce heterotypic artificial skin substitutes [69]. Compared with bone marrow-derived stem cells, ASCs are easier to obtain, and their isolation produces a higher number of stem cells. Therefore, ASCs have a high interest in stem cell-based therapy and skin tissue engineering [70]. The results of the skin injured mice with ASCs showed that the macroscopic aspect was better, the incidence of epidermolysis was lower, the hair follicle loss was less, and the wound healing was effectively promoted [71]. According to the complex definition of tissue engineering in the National Science Foundation symposium, a scaffold is the best material to restore, maintain, and improve tissue function [72], which can be made of synthetic or absorbable, naturally occurring, biological, degradable, or non-degradable polymeric materials [73]. Currently, there are four main scaffolding methods [74], including decellularized ECM scaffolds [75], cells entrapped in hydrogels [76], ECM secreted cell sheets [77], and prefabricated porous scaffolds made of synthetic, natural, and biodegradable materials [78].

Due to the lack of skin donors after extensive skin damage, new sources of cells have been used for skin tissue regeneration [70]. It is difficult to replicate multilayer anisotropic structures in vitro using traditional tissue engineering techniques. Three-dimensional bioprinting techniques include computer-controlled deposition of cells and scaffolds into spatially controlled patterns that can control not only macroscopic structures but also micro and nanostructures and offer the potential to replicate natural skin more faithfully [79,80]. The process of three-dimensional bioprinting of human skin tissue can be divided into four steps: (1) pretreatment, including cell selection, biomaterial selection, and skin tissue blueprint design; (2) processing or actual printing process; (3) post-processing, including cell proliferation, tissue remodeling, and maturation after printing skin constructs; and (4) functionality, including biochemical and biological properties of printed skin tissue physiological characteristics [81]. Pourchet et al. developed alginate, gelatin, and fibrinogen-mixed biological links for three-dimensional bioprinting of dermis with higher fidelity and stability [82]. Recently, Huang et al. proposed a three-dimensional cell printing method using a skin-derived ECM. They successfully used acellular pigskin as a new biological link, which contains the intrinsic factors required for cell proliferation, and showed that the new construct was highly stable within 2 weeks and had significant wound healing performance *in vivo* [83].

6.6 STRUCTURE AND PROPERTIES OF HYDROGELS

Hydrogels are a group of materials with a three-dimensional polymer network, which can hold a large amount of water. They have good biocompatibility, predictable degradation rate, adjustable mechanical properties, and good elasticity, and are ideal materials for biomedical applications [84,85]. Hydrogels are degradable polymer networks, and cross-linking plays a crucial role in the structure formation and degradation of hydrogels which can be divided into two categories based on the type of cross-linking connection: chemical cross-linking and physical cross-linking [86,87]. Networks are formed by covalent or non-covalent cross-linked polymers, and then their structures can be designed to suit the final application [88]. Hydrogels often have many properties that make them an interesting object of study: they are highly versatile as their chemical and physical properties can be manipulated to design gels that are best suited to the desired application. The unique ability of hydrogels to form swollen three-dimensional networks makes it possible for them to diffuse molecules and cells, although their similarity to natural soft tissues is also of great interest for biomedical applications [89]. For example, the water content of the double enzyme-catalyzed HA hydrogel prepared is as high as 98%, which can maintain the survival of bone marrow MSCs for up to 20 days [90]. Biodegradable biomaterials are designed to reproduce the dynamic microenvironment of natural cell exposure [91]. D.L. Gan et al. have designed a hydrogel with high cell affinity, toughness, and recoverability through mussel inspiration, which can effectively promote wound healing [92]. Jing Chen reported a new type of hydrogels with intrinsic adhesiveness for sustained release of drugs and cells [93]. Hydrogels have been investigated as potential candidates for ECM replacement and have recently emerged as promising platforms for studying stem cell migration and proliferation [85,94].

Due to various properties of hydrogels such as ROS scavenging, inflammation, and antibacterial property, they have been used in a wide range of areas of biomedical science (Table 6.4) since their first practical application in the 1960s [110,111]. Their final properties can be easily adjusted to contain cues and triggers for cell adhesion and cell function (including migration, proliferation and differentiation), as well as adjusting the mechanical and degradation properties of the material [112,113]. Many of the key properties of hydrogels, such as mechanical stiffness, elasticity, water content, bioactivity, and degradability, can be rationally designed and easily regulated by the appropriate choice of materials and chemical composition [114].

TABLE 6.4

Major Properties of Hydrogel

Materials	Property	Application	Reference
Polyvinyl alcohol	ROS scavenging	Wound healing	[95]
Gallic acid, gelatin	ROS scavenging	Wound healing	[96]
Methacrylate hyaluronic acid	ROS scavenging and O_2 generating	Myocardial infarction	[97]
Polymer	ROS scavenging, injectable and responsive	Soft tissue injection	[98]
N-isopropyl acrylamide, methoxy poly(ethylene glycol) methacrylate	ROS scavenging and thermosensitive	Myocardial infarction	[99]
Poly(acrylic acid), PArg-PEG-PArg	Redox and injectable	Cardiovascular therapy	[100]
Gelatin, β-cyclodextrin and adamantane	Self-healing and injectable	Localized therapeutic cell delivery	[101]
Chitosan, sodium alginate	Injectable self-healing	Wound healing	[102]
Alginate, DNA network	Injectable self-healing	Drug delivery	[103]
Polyaniline nanofibers, glycerol	Injectable self-healing	Strain and temperature sensor	[104]
Dextran phosphate	pH-sensitive	Tumor therapy	[105]
Propylmalonate, NIPAAm, PAA, HEMA-oTMC, and MA-PEG	pH-sensitive and thermosensitive	Cardiac therapy	[106]
Chitosan-g-polyaniline, poly(ethylene glycol)-co-poly(glycerol sebacate)	Antibacterial antioxidant electroactive injectable, self-healing, hemostatic and adherent	Wound healing	[107]
Porphyrin photosensitizer sinoporphyrin sodium, PLGA, carboxymethyl chitosan	Antibacterial phototherapy	Wound healing	[108]
Poly-tetrahydropyrimidine, poly-tetrahydropyrimidine, vanillin polymer P	Antibacterial and self-healing	Wound healing	[109]

Among them, injectable hydrogel has attracted much attention in wound repair. It can be injected into skin defect with irregular shape and form contours with different sizes *in situ* [115]. In general, there are two main mechanisms, physical cross-linking and chemical (covalent) cross-linking, which result in hydrogels with different structures and properties. Physical cross-linking is usually induced by changes in environmental factors, including temperature, pH, force, concentration, and ions. Typical methods to induce physical cross-linking include cooling, lyophilization, presence of acids, dehydrating agents, and cation exchange. Typical methods of chemical cross-linking include ultraviolet irradiation, dehydrogenation heat treatment, and addition of cross-linking agent [116].

Recently, hydrogels mainly have self-healing, antibacterial, hemostatic, antioxidant, adhesiveness, originally injectable, electrical conductivity, and other properties in skin treatment [117,118] (Figure 6.3). Liang et al. used glycidyl methacrylate functionalized quaternized chitosan, gelatin methacrylate, and graphene oxide as the main raw materials to prepare a series of injectable antibacterial conductive hydrogels for antibacterial disinfection and infectious wound healing [119]. A wet environment plays an important role in accelerating wound healing management. Compared with other scaffold forms, hydrogel can keep the moist environment of the wound area. Oxidized hydroxyethyl starch and modified carboxymethyl chitosan were used to produce an *in situ* hydrogel with excellent scalability, biocompatibility, biodegradability, and transparency, which can accelerate wound healing [120].

To accelerate chronic wound healing, many hydrogel dressings with antioxidant function have appeared, which have been proven to accelerate wound healing, especially for chronic wound repair [121]. Zhu et al. described the development of an antioxidant shape-consistent hydrogel, which uses laminin-derived dodecapeptide A5G81 as effective tethered cell adhesion, proliferation, and mononucleosis-inducing ligand to locally promote wound closure [122]. Zhang et al. cross-linked poly(vinyl alcohol) with polypyrrole or Zn-functionalized chitosan molecules to form an antibacterial and conductive hydrogel, which can promote the healing of infected chronic wounds [123].

In addition, some hydrogels have environmental responsiveness, such as temperature-responsiveness, pH-responsiveness, enzyme-responsiveness and so on, which has aroused great interest [124]. In recent years, thermal/pH-responsive soft polymers have attracted great interest due to their softness, biocompatibility, response to stimuli, excellent solubility, and biodegradability [125]. Stimulus-responsive matrix has potential application prospects in tissue engineering, cell culture, and innovative drug delivery system technology, which can release active substances under the control of internal and external stimuli [126]. β-glucan methacrylate (MA-β- glucan) was used as a biodegradable and biocompatible cross-linking agent to prepare β-glucan-poly(N-isopropyl acrylamide)-based, temperature-responsive hydrogel, which was used as a sustained-release carrier of 5-ASA [127]. Compared with synthetic materials, natural polymers have better biocompatibility and are widely used in the preparation of thermosensitive/acid-base hydrogels. Chitosan is a natural polymer. Because of its advantages compared with other natural polymers, chitosan is widely recommended for the synthesis of injectable hydrogels [128]. Natnicha Jommanee et al. synthesized a series of temperature-responsive diblock copolymers based on polyethylene glycol methyl ether (mPEG) and ε -caprolactone (CL) and then grafted the diblock copolymers onto chitosan to form chitosan graft-(mPEG-block-PCL) (Chitosan-g-(mPEG-b-PCL)). Chitosan is pH-responsive and mPEG-b-PCL is temperature-sensitive in this hydrogel [129]. Photosensitive hydrogels can be divided into ultraviolet-sensitive hydrogels and visible light sensitive hydrogels. Unlike ultraviolet rays, visible light is easy to obtain, cheap, safe, clean, and easy to operate [130]. Photo-responsive hybrid sodium alginate hydrogel was prepared from β-cyclodextrin-grafted sodium alginate (β-CD-Alg) and diazobenzene-modified polyethylene glycol (az2peg) through Ca(2+)-mediated cross-linking reaction. High-power incident light and mild acid environment can accelerate light-triggered release, so it has potential application prospect in acute wound healing [131].

6.7 APPLICATION OF NATURAL POLYMER HYDROGEL SCAFFOLD IN SKIN TISSUE ENGINEERING

Natural polymers are organic molecules synthesized from natural resources such as animals, plants, and microorganisms. Structurally, they are composed of repeating units of amino acids, monosaccharides, nucleotides, or esters, which are then covalently bonded to form polymers such as peptides, polysaccharides, polyphenols, or polyesters [5,132]. Natural polymer hydrogels consisting of proteins or polysaccharides, such as collagen, gelatin, sericin, sodium alginate, hyaluronic acid, chitosan, and cellulose, which are very biocompatible, biodegradable, and promote cell adhesion and growth [133]. However, natural polymer hydrogels tend to have poor mechanical properties and are prone to degradation, and are often cross-linked/blended with other polymers or modified to maintain good biocompatibility and enhance the mechanical properties of the hydrogel [134,135]. The following focuses on the hydrogel formed by HA, sodium alginate, chitosan, collagen, and gelatin (Figure 6.4).

Glucosaminoglycan, such as HA, heparin, and chondroitin sulfate, are essential for skin regeneration because they are the most important components of the ECM [136]. HA is a non-sulfated glycosaminoglycan composed of disaccharide units of D-glucuronic acid-N-acetylglucosamine and is an important component of the ECM [137,138]. The structural and biological properties of HA determine its important role in cell signaling, wound repair, and tissue formation. HA and its derivatives have been used clinically for over 30 years as medical products [139]. HA's good biocompatibility, biodegradability, anti-adhesion, non-immunogenicity, and high hydrophilicity ensure that it is a good material for physical and chemical hydrogels [140,141]. HA-based hydrogels are widely used as effective engineering scaffolds for bone [142], cartilage [143], nerve [144], and skin tissue engineering. More specifically, HA has been found to play a key role in all stages of wound healing. During the inflammatory phase, HA promotes neutrophil recruitment, removal of necrotic tissue, and subsequent release of tumor necrosis factor-α (TNF-α), IL-1β, and IL-8, which regulate the inflammatory response [145]. During the proliferative phase, HA also promotes collagen deposition, fibroblast differentiation [146], formation of new ECM, and regulates epithelial regeneration, thus promoting wound healing more effectively [147]. When HA hydrogels are used as wound dressings, their weak mechanical properties and rapid biodegradability make it difficult for the hydrogel to adhere to the wound surface, making it difficult to promote wound healing. It needs to be combined with other macromolecules to regulate mechanical strength [148]. Wu et al. used HA hydrogel as a matrix and loaded it with a pH-controllable H$_2$S donor, JK1, to form a novel HA-JK1 hybrid system. The hydrogel achieved long-term H$_2$S release. In addition, the authors demonstrated *in vivo* that HA-JK1 hydrogel enhances re-epithelialization, collagen deposition, angiogenesis, and cell proliferation, and contributes to the polarization of M2 phenotype to reduce inflammation and ultimately promote wound healing.

Alginate is a natural polymer derived from brown algae *Phaeophyta*, composed of two types of uronic acid monomers distributed as blocks of 1→4 linked α-l-guluronic acid(G) or β-d-mannuronic acid(M), as well as heteropolymeric mixed sequences

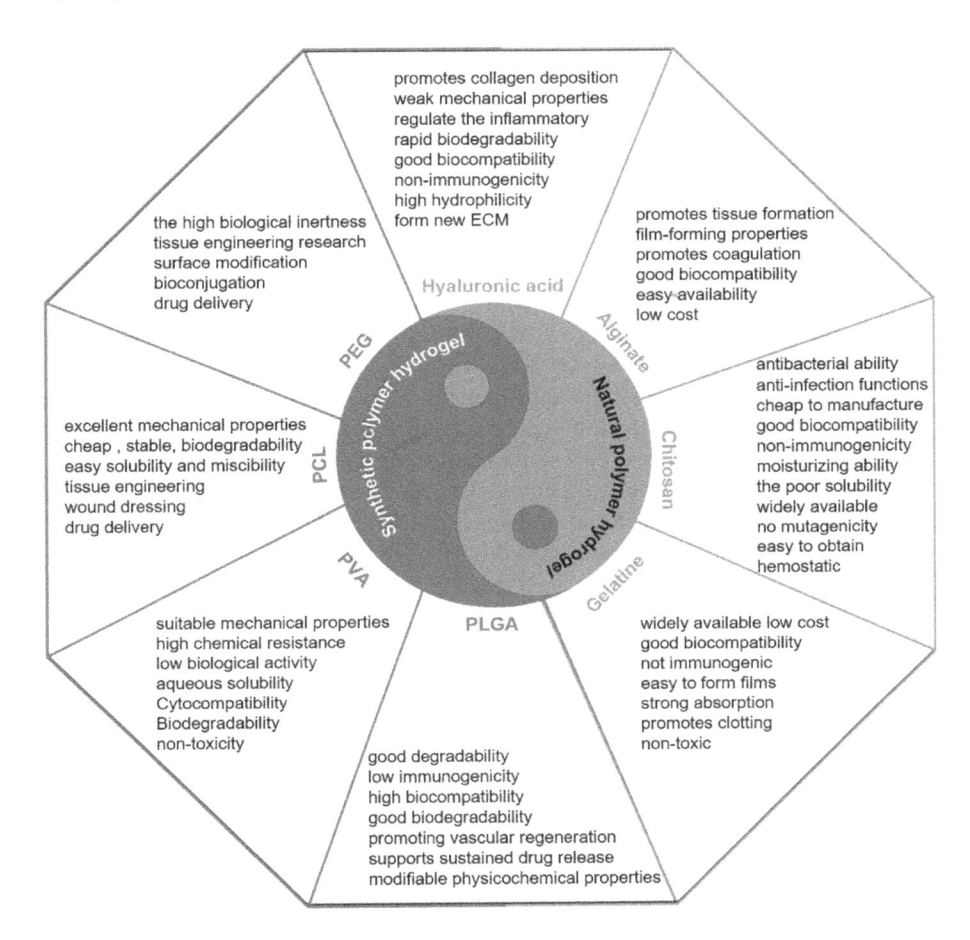

FIGURE 6.4   Hydrogels composed of natural/synthetic polymers and their properties.

[149]. Alginate is widely used in tissue engineering for its low cost, easy availability, good biocompatibility and biodegradability, excellent film-forming properties, and ease of forming hydrogels [150,151]. The alginate is a good absorber of wound exudate and keeps the wound moist [152]. Alginate also acts as a matrix for platelet and red blood cell adhesion, stimulating the clotting mechanism and promoting coagulation [153]. Alginate hydrogel dressings maintain a moist microenvironment at the wound site to promote healing and granulation tissue formation. In addition, alginate hydrogel absorbs wound exudate from the wound site and can be used for a wide range of wound types [154]. Thomas confirmed that some dressings containing alginate activate human macrophages to secrete pro-inflammatory cytokines and regulate the expression of IL-6 and TNF-α to promote wound healing [155]. Alginate promotes the proliferation of fibroblasts and the formation of granulation tissue, thereby promoting wound healing [156].

Chitosan comprises randomly distributed β (1–4)-linked D-glucosamine and N-acetyl-D-glucosamine units and it is obtained by deacetylation of chitin [156,157].

Chitin, a structural component in the exoskeleton of crustaceans and insects, is the second most abundant natural biopolymer on earth. Chitosan is therefore widely available, easy to obtain, and cheap to manufacture [158]. Chitosan and its derivatives are active in tissue engineering because of its many advantages such as good biocompatibility, biodegradability, non-immunogenicity, broad-spectrum antibacterial ability, moisturizing ability, and no mutagenicity [159,160]. However, the poor solubility of chitosan in physiological pH environments has limited its application [161]. This has led to the development of a range of derivatives with superior properties to chitosan, such as trimethyl chitosan, carboxymethyl chitosan (CMC), and carboxymethyl-trimethyl-chitosan (CMTMC). Chitosan and its derivatives are rich in amine groups, which can enrich and activate negatively charged red blood cells and platelets, thereby causing blood coagulation. In addition, the presence of amine groups also gives chitosan the inherent broad-spectrum antibacterial properties. As a wound dressing, chitosan hydrogels have hemostatic, antibacterial, and anti-infection functions [162,163]. Chitosan has been widely used in the treatment of burn wounds due to its hemostasis, antibacterial, and antifungal properties [164]. X.Zhao et al. prepared an injectable multifunctional hydrogel using chitosan-g-polyaniline (QCSP) and benzaldehyde group functionalized poly(ethylene glycol)-co-poly(glycerol sebacate). The hydrogel presented good self-healing, free radical scavenging capacity, electroactivity, adhesiveness, antibacterial activity, blood clotting capacity, conductivity, and biocompatibility. In a full-thickness skin defect model, compared with commercial dressing (Tegaderm™ film), hydrogel can promote granulation tissue thickness and collagen deposition, and upregulating the gene expression of growth factors, including VEGF, EGF and TGF-β, and promote wound healing [107].

Collagen gels are a perfect example of the hydration network, which shows great potential for developing functional living skin *in vitro*. Collagen, a component of the ECM produced by fibroblasts, promotes faster wound healing. It is the most abundant biological substance of natural proteins. Gelatin is a partially hydrolyzed form of collagen that has low immunogenicity and enhances cell adhesion due to the presence of arginine, glycine, and aspartic acid sequences. Silk fibroin proteins are useful in wound dressings and skin grafts due to their high biocompatibility, flexibility, and minimal inflammatory response. Gelatin is a natural product derived from animal skin and bone, derived from collagen, and has a similar structure to collagen. Compared to collagen, gelatin overcomes the deficiencies of collagen's environmental PH solubility and is not immunogenic [165,166]. Gelatin has been used in food for a long time and has been used in medicine for decades. Gelatin has many excellent properties, such as being widely available, low cost, non-toxic, easy to form films, strong absorption, good biocompatibility, biodegradable, and completely absorbed by the body without harmful by-products, improving its utilization in drug delivery and tissue engineering [167,168]. Gelatin has been shown to have hemostatic properties since the 19th century [169], then gelatin-based hemostatic hydrogel has been widely used for wound healing [170]. Assmann et al. used gelatin methacryloyl (GelMA) to form a photopolymeric hydrogel with excellent mechanical properties and tissue adhesion, good biocompatibility and biodegradability, and effective in reducing the inflammatory response to promote wound healing [171].

6.8 APPLICATION OF SYNTHETIC POLYMER HYDROGEL SCAFFOLD IN SKIN TISSUE ENGINEERING

Compared with natural polymers, synthetic polymers such as poly(vinyl alcohol), poly(ethylene oxide), poly(ethyleneimine), poly(vinyl pyrrolidone), and poly-N iso-propylacrylamide are generally approved by the market, easier to process, and better mechanical properties, adjustable physical and chemical properties, and controllable degradation rate [172]. However, the biocompatibility of synthetic polymers is lower than that of natural polymers, they have no biological activity, and cannot support cell adhesion and growth. In most cases, neither natural nor synthetic polymers provide the desired properties when formed alone as a hydrogel. In contrast, however, synthetic and natural polymer hydrogels have well-defined structures with more controllable physicochemical properties [173,174]. Therefore, it is common to polymerize different synthetic polymers or natural and synthetic polymers to form composite hydrogels [175]. The following focuses on the hydrogel formed by PEG, PCL, PVA, and PLGA (as shown in Figure 6.4).

In the 1970s, PEG was approved as a pharmaceutical excipient by the US Food and Drug Administration for its biosafety and biocompatibility [176]. Since then, PEG has been widely used for biomedical applications, including surface modification, bioconjugation, drug delivery, and tissue engineering research [177]. The basic structure of PEG is a PEG diol with two hydroxyl end groups [178], which can be modified to give PEG more reactive groups so that it can react with other polymers by Michael-type addition [179], Click chemistry [180], enzymatic reaction [181], and native chemical ligation[182] into hydrogels. Because of the high biological inertness of PEG, PEG hydrogels cannot support cell growth and have biological activity [183], and this has greatly limited their development in skin tissue engineering. Therefore, PEG hydrogels are often loaded with drug, peptides, growth factors, and other bioactive ingredients that act together to engineer skin tissue [184]. Chen et al. constructed a double network hydrogel using a covalent polyethylene glycol diacrylate (PEGDA) network in combination with a non-covalent network of PEG chains, which has good adhesion, is highly stretchable, and has self-healing ability. In *in vivo* experiments, the authors found that the hydrogel was effective in promoting wound healing and reducing scar formation and inflammation compared to commercially available dressings [185]. Mao et al. prepared injectable PEG hydrogel loaded with mangiferin liposomes (MF-Lip). The hydrogel was cross-linked by four-armed PEG with Ag by Ag-s coordination. The hydrogel can continuously release Ag and MF, resist infection, protect cells, and promote angiogenesis under a hypoxic environment. The hydrogel can match the renewal of random skin flap regeneration progress and promote skin flap survival [186].

PCL is a semi-crystalline hydrophobic aliphatic polyester composed of repeating units of caproate [187]. It can be digested by many microorganisms in nature, but it cannot be degraded in the body. Because of its cheap, stable, excellent mechanical properties, biodegradability, easy solubility, and miscibility, it is FDA-approved and widely used in drug delivery, wound dressing, tissue engineering, and skin regeneration [188]. Bae et al. first synthesized PEO/PLLA multiblock copolymer and insoluble PEO/PLLA copolymer and then mixed the two with bFGF to prepare a hydrogel with drug retardation, which could effectively improve wound healing [189]. Liao et al. first synthesized a kind of porous microsphere made of poly(εcaprolactone)-b-poly(ethylene glycol)-b-poly(ε-caprolactone) (PCL-PEG-PCL, abbreviated as PCEC) copolymer. The porous microspheres are hydrophilic and promote cell adhesion and growth, followed by the deposition of calcium gluconate crystals in the microspheres, and finally cross-linking with sodium alginate to form a hydrogel, which significantly improved the inflammatory response, promoted collagen deposition, reduced scar formation, and promoted wound healing *in vivo* experiments [190].

PVA is a linear synthetic polymer formed by the partial or complete hydrolysis of polyvinyl acetate. The use of PVA hydrogels as biomaterials was explored in the 1970s [191]. For the past 30 years, PVA hydrogels have been used in industrial applications, contact lenses, cartilage implants, drug delivery systems, wound dressings, and medical applications for their high chemical resistance, aqueous solubility, non-toxicity, cytocompatibility, suitable mechanical properties, and biodegradability [192]. However, compared with other polymers, the biological activity of PVA is relatively low, and it is difficult for PVA hydrogel alone to effectively promote wound healing [193]. Therefore, it is common to add other active factors to PVA hydrogels or to polymerize PVA with other active ingredients to form a composite hydrogel to promote wound healing more effectively [194]. Zhao et al. developed a PVA hydrogel loaded with mupirocin and GM-CSF that responds to and scavenges ROS signals. The hydrogel responded to and scavenged ROS in the wound, reduced the release of pro-inflammatory factors, and promoted the conversion of macrophages to M2 type to reduce the inflammatory response, while effectively killing bacteria, promoting vascular regeneration and collagen deposition, and ultimately promoting diabetic wound healing [97]. Chen et al. constructed a multifunctional hydrogel by adding the active ingredient novel tea polyphenol nanospheres to a PVA/alginate hydrogel. In a diabetic rat skin injury model, the hydrogel reduced the inflammatory response by activating the PI3K/AKT pathway, effectively promoted collagen deposition, reduced scar formation, and accelerated wound healing [195].

PLGA, one of the widely used biodegradable polymers in medical applications, is composed of lactic acid and glycolic acid monomers [196], and it is approved by the FDA and EMA for parenteral administration because of its high biocompatibility [197]. PLGA possesses good degradability under physiological conditions, modifiable physicochemical properties, has good biodegradability and low immunogenicity, and supports sustained drug release, making it a widely used clinical drug carrier and tissue engineering [198]. PLGA is hydrolyzed in the body to form lactic acid and glycolic acid monomers, and these metabolites can enter the Krebs cycle and be completely metabolized [199]. In addition, studies have shown that lactic acid stimulates endothelial cell proliferation, migration, and capillary formation, thereby promoting vascular regeneration [200,201]. Therefore, PLGA hydrogels as donors of lactic acid have also attracted a great deal of interest from researchers for their application in skin tissue engineering [202]. Ma et al. synthesized an injectable SA/BG-SACM-PLGAPFD hydrogel with sequential delivery of bioactive molecules to meet the bioactivity requirements of different stages of wound healing. The researchers first synthesized PLGA microspheres loaded with pirfenidone (PFD), then embedded them in SA microspheres containing conditioned medium (CM) of cells, and finally formed composite hydrogels using sodium alginate/bioglass (SA/BG). The hydrogel first modulates the inflammatory response by releasing BG and then releases CM to promote the formation of the vascularized granulation tissue. Finally, release the PFD to prevent fibrosis and scar formation in the regenerated skin. The hydrogel can release active molecules according to the needs of regenerating tissues to promote wound healing, and has wide application potential in the regenerative medicine field [203].

6.9 SUMMARY AND OUTLOOK

The skin is the largest organ of the body and performs important functions such as regulation of body temperature, excretion, absorption, pigmentation, and physical and immune barrier functions. The loss of just 15% of the total body surface area is enough to be life-threatening [204,205]. The skin has multiple layers, which can be divided into the epidermis, dermis, and hypodermis [206]. The epidermis is the outermost layer of mammalian skin and provides an important barrier to sustain life [207]. Keratinocytes, formed by the division of germ cells (basal cells) in the basal cell layer, while migrating through the granular layer to the upper epidermis, are the most abundant cells in the epidermis (about 90%), while the remaining are melanocytes, Langham's cells, and Merkel's cells [208,209]. The dermis is a connective tissue consisting of ECM, vascular endothelial cells, fibroblasts, adipose glands, sweat glands, hair follicles, blood vessels, and nerve endings [210]. The subcutaneous tissue is the deepest layer of the skin and consists of loose connective tissue, cells that store fat (half of the body fat is stored in this area), blood vessels, and nerves [211]. Despite the significant contribution to clinical and dermatological research, traditional manufacturing strategies require post-processing, with several disadvantages such as inadequate bionics, high production costs, fixed dimensions, and time consumption [212]. Some factors, such as diabetes, kidney infections, the presence of foreign bodies, malnutrition, immune deficiency, and aging, affect the normal healing process of the wound and thus the recovery of the tissue [213,214]. When the skin is extensively injured, it loses its ability to prevent bacterial infection and regulate temperature or fluid transport [215,216]. This tissueless collection of tissues leads to scar fibrosis and is often accompanied by a lack of sensation and elasticity as well as defective features. In practice, healing does not restore natural skin function, tissue structure, or aesthetics.

In the application of wound treatment, hydrogel is a very promising material. Whether used as a scaffold material for skin tissue engineering or simple cell-free hydrogel dressing, it has incomparable advantages over other scaffold materials. In general, there are three main advantages. First, hydrogel materials come from a wide range of sources. Whether its natural biomaterials like proteins or polysaccharides, artificial synthetic biological materials, as mentioned above, PLA, PEG, polyacrylamide, etc. These materials are widely distributed and easy to obtain, and most of them are very cheap. Second, hydrogels are highly functional. Hydrogel is similar to the three-dimensional network structure of the ECM and can provide a good microecology for cell growth. It is conducive to cell attachment, proliferation, and migration, as well as intercellular signal transduction and metabolism. Lastly, hydrogels also have good biocompatibility, degradability, modifiability, ultra-high moisture content, and versatility. With the deepening of the research on the properties of hydrogel materials, as well as the exchange and cooperation in the interdisciplinary field, the specific microscopic modification and modification of hydrogel materials can give hydrogels a lot of functionality. For example, some catechuic acid substances (such as dopamine and tannin) can be grafted into hydrogels to give them special wet adhesion, oxidation resistance, and greatly improve the mechanical properties of hydrogels [217].

However, the application of hydrogels in tissue engineering and wound dressings also has some problems. For example, limited supply, high production costs, inflammation, disease risk, repair effectiveness, and treatment costs. This requires the development of more advanced skin substitutes for clinical use. Multifunctional composite scaffolds are made of natural or synthetic biological materials. An appropriate understanding of the characteristics, advantages, and disadvantages of various biological materials and scaffolds, followed by the modification and composite of the materials will help to prepare scaffolds suitable for skin tissue regeneration, which may be a development trend in the future. At the same time, some of the major challenges facing the field of skin tissue engineering are inevitable, such as cell-scaffold interaction, faster cell proliferation and differentiation, vascularization of engineered tissue, and recovery and reconstruction of skin function after healing.

With the development of the technology, a cellular scaffold for skin regeneration was developed that has a three-dimensional structure similar to the real ECM, and there is evidence that a cellular scaffold prepared by the cell sheet technique is biocompatible. In addition, researchers have developed a double-layer wound dressing. The outer layer acts as a barrier to protect bacteria, while the inner layer guides cell growth, thus speeding up wound healing. Over the past few years, scaffold design considerations have changed significantly with the introduction of electrospinning and three-dimensional bioprinting. Nanofiber substrates are suitable candidates for the delivery of bioactive molecules such as growth factors, antibiotics, and other small molecules. In one study, nanofilament matrix composed of SF biopolymer showed significantly higher cell recruitment and potential to accelerate wound healing compared to flat film. This significant difference is attributed to the nanostructure provided by the electrospinning pad, which improves cell adhesion and migration. The advent of three-dimensional bioprinting, an innovative approach to skin treatment based on intelligent technology, has revolutionized the field of tissue engineering. Technological advances in recent years have led to the development of hand-held skin printers, which could be revolutionary in the current medical market as patients do not have to wait for a lab-grown cell skin graft. The technology could also be used in emergencies such as burn injuries and provide immediate treatment. SiRNA-based and miRNA-based trauma repair strategies have gained momentum over the past few years. Both siRNA and miRNA are short fragments of nucleotide double-strand RNA and have the potential to inhibit mRNA translation in various ways [218]. In these wound repair therapies, siRNA is particularly noteworthy because of the complex interactions between the myriad cellular pathways that dominate the four stages of the process. Various miRNAs have been shown to modulate angiogenesis, fibroblast, and keratinocyte proliferation by participating in major wound healing pathways in various wound bed environments. The specificity and effectiveness of this strategy are promising in the field of wound healing. However, the safety of gene editing is also a concern.

In summary, each method, technique, and material has its advantages and disadvantages. Compared with these emerging technologies, hydrogels may have a lot to improve on. Combining innovative technologies with traditional methods has great potential in the future. Developments in tissue engineering and regenerative medicine may further open the door to new treatments for skin wounds that can heal painlessly, more quickly, and without scars.

REFERENCES

1. J.L. Soriano-Ruiz, A.C. Calpena-Campmany, M. Silva-Abreu, L. Halbout-Bellowa, N. Bozal-de Febrer, M.J. Rodríguez-Lagunas, B. Clares-Naveros. Design and evaluation of a multifunctional thermosensitive poloxamer-chitosan-hyaluronic acid gel for the treatment of skin burns. *Int. J. Biol. Macromol.* 142 (2020) 412–422.
2. D. Chouhan, N. Dey, N. Bhardwaj, B.B. Mandal. Emerging and innovative approaches for wound healing and skin regeneration: Current status and advances. *Biomaterials.* 216 (2019) 119267.
3. S.A. Castleberry, B.D. Almquist, W. Li, T. Reis, J. Chow, S. Mayner, P.T. Hammond. Self-assembled wound dressings silence MMP-9 and improve diabetic wound healing in vivo. *Adv. Mater.* 28(9) (2016) 1809–1817.
4. M. Movahedi, A. Asefnejad, M. Rafienia, M.T. Khorasani. Potential of novel electrospun core-shell structured polyurethane/starch (hyaluronic acid) nanofibers for skin tissue engineering: In vitro and in vivo evaluation. *Int. J. Biol. Macromol.* 146 (2020) 627–637.
5. T.G. Sahana, P.D. Rekha. Biopolymers: Applications in wound healing and skin tissue engineering. *Mol. Biol. Rep.* 45(6) (2018) 2857–2867.
6. D. Gan, L. Han, M. Wang, W. Xing, T. Xu, H. Zhang, K. Wang, L. Fang, X. Lu. Conductive and tough hydrogels based on biopolymer molecular templates for controlling in situ formation of polypyrrole nanorods. *ACS. Appl. Mater. Interfaces.* 10(42) (2018) 36218–36228.
7. G.E. Costin, V.J. Hearing. Human skin pigmentation: Melanocytes modulate skin color in response to stress. *FASEB. J.* 21(4) (2007) 976–94.
8. N. Ali, M.D. Rosenblum. Regulatory T cells in skin. *Immunology.* 152(3) (2017) 372–381.
9. E. Berardesca, H. Maibach. Ethnic skin: Overview of structure and function. *J. Am. Acad. Dermatol.* 48(6 Suppl) (2003) S139–S142.
10. P. Di Meglio, G.K. Perera, F.O. Nestle. The multitasking organ: Recent insights into skin immune function. *Immunity.* 35(6) (2011) 857–869.
11. K.C. Madison. Barrier function of the skin: "la raison d'etre" of the epidermis. *J. Invest. Dermatol.* 121(2) (2003) 231–241.
12. A.V. Nguyen, A.M. Soulika. The dynamics of the skin's immune system. *Int. J. Mol. Sci.* 20(8) (2019) 1811.
13. L. Norlen. Skin barrier structure and function: The single gel phase model. *J. Invest. Dermatol.* 117(4) (2001) 830–836.
14. J.M. Pullar, A. C. Carr, M.C.M. Vissers. The roles of vitamin C in skin health. *Nutrients.* 9(8) (2017) 866.
15. N.N. Schommer, R.L. Gallo. Structure and function of the human skin microbiome. *Trends. Microbiol.* 21(12) (2013) 660–668.

16. M. Takeo, W. Lee, M. Ito. Wound healing and skin regeneration. *Cold. Spring. Harb. Perspect. Med.* 5(1) (2015) a023267.

17. D.J. Tobin. Biochemistry of human skin--our brain on the outside. *Chem. Soc. Rev.* 35(1) (2006) 52–67.

18. J.A. Bouwstra, P.L. Honeywell-Nguyen. Skin structure and mode of action of vesicles. *Adv. Drug. Deliv. Rev.* 54 (2002) S41–S55.

19. L.M. Morton, T.J. Phillips. Wound healing and treating wounds: Differential diagnosis and evaluation of chronic wounds. *J. Am. Acad. Dermatol.* 74(4) (2016) 589–606.

20. J.A. Molnar, L.G. Vlad, T. Gumus. Nutrition and chronic wounds: Improving clinical outcomes. *Plast. Reconstr. Surg.* 138 (2016) 71S–81S.

21. P. Martin, R. Nunan. Cellular and molecular mechanisms of repair in acute and chronic wound healing. *Br. J. Dermatol.* 173(2) (2015) 370–378.

22. M.B. Dreifke, A.A. Jayasuriya, A.C. Jayasuriya. Current wound healing procedures and potential care. *Mater. Sci. Eng. C. Mater. Biol. Appl.* 48(2015) 651–662.

23. C. Karimkhani, R.P. Dellavalle, L.E. Coffeng, C. Flohr, R.J. Hay, S.M. Langan, E.O. Nsoesie, A.J. Ferrari, H.E. Erskine, J.I. Silverberg, T. Vos, M. Naghavi. Global skin disease morbidity and mortality: An update from the global burden of disease study 2013. *JAMA. Dermatol.* 153(5) (2017) 406–412.

24. M.H. Kathawala, W.L. Ng, D. Liu, M.W. Naing, W.Y. Yeong, K.L. Spiller, M. Van Dyke, K.W. Ng. Healing of chronic wounds: An update of recent developments and future possibilities. *Tissue. Eng. Part. B. Rev.* 25(5) (2019) 429–444.

25. G. Valacchi, I. Zanardi, C. Sticozzi, V. Bocci, V. Travagli. Emerging topics in cutaneous wound repair. *Ann. N. Y. Acad. Sci.* 1259 (2012) 136–144.

26. H.C. Korting, C. Schollmann, R.J. White. Management of minor acute cutaneous wounds: Importance of wound healing in a moist environment. *J. Eur. Acad. Dermatol. Venereol.* 25(2) (2011) 130–137.

27. S. Schreml, R.M. Szeimies, L. Prantl, S. Karrer, M. Landthaler, P. Babilas. Oxygen in acute and chronic wound healing. *Br. J Dermatol.* 163(2) (2010) 257–268.

28. H.W. Lim, S.A.B. Collins, J.S. Resneck, J.L. Bolognia, J.A. Hodge, T.A. Rohrer, M.J. Van Beek, D.J. Margolis, A.J. Sober, M.A. Weinstock, D.R. Nerenz, W. Smith Begolka, J.V. Moyano. The burden of skin disease in the United States. *J. Am. Acad. Dermatol.* 76(5) (2017) 958–972 e2.

29. K. Chen. Injectable melatonin-loaded carboxymethyl chitosan (CMCS)-based hydrogel accelerates wound healing by reducing inflammation and promoting angiogenesis and collagen deposition. *J. Mater. Sci. Technol.* 63 (2021) 236–245.

30. S. Homaeigohar, A.R. Boccaccini. Antibacterial biohybrid nanofibers for wound dressings. *Acta. Biomater.* 107 (2020) 25–49.

31. J.S. Chin, L. Madden, S.Y. Chew, D.L. Becker. Drug therapies and delivery mechanisms to treat perturbed skin wound healing. *Adv. Drug Deliv. Rev.* 149 (2019) 2–18.

32. Y. Sang, M. Roest, B. de Laat, P.G. de Groot, D. Huskens. Interplay between platelets and coagulation. *Blood Rev.* (2020) 100733.

33. P. Victor, D. Sarada, K.M. Ramkumar. Pharmacological activation of Nrf2 promotes wound healing. *Eur. J. Pharmacol.* 886 (2020) 173395.

34. M. Mollaei, A. Abbasi, Z.M. Hassan, N. Pakravan. The intrinsic and extrinsic elements regulating inflammation. *Life Sci.* 260 (2020) 118258.

35. P. Govindaraju, L. Todd, S. Shetye, J. Monslow, E. Puré. CD44-dependent inflammation, fibrogenesis, and collagenolysis regulates extracellular matrix remodeling and tensile strength during cutaneous wound healing. *Matrix Biol.* 75 (2019) 314–330.

36. Y. Li, J. Zhang, J. Yue, X. Gou, X. Wu. Epidermal stem cells in skin wound healing. *Adv. Wound Care.* 6 (2017) 297–307.

37. W. Han. Biofilm-inspired adhesive and antibacterial hydrogel with tough tissue integration performance for sealing hemostasis and wound healing. *Bioact. Mater.* 5 (2020) 768–778.

38. S. Zhang, J. Li, S. Chen, X. Zhang, J. Ma, J. He. Oxidized cellulose-based hemostatic materials. *Carbohydr. Polym.* 230 (2020) 115585.
39. S.A. Shah. Biopolymer-based biomaterials for accelerated diabetic wound healing: A critical review. *Int. J. Biol. Macromol.* 139 (2019) 975–993.
40. J. Ishihara. The heparin binding domain of von Willebrand factor binds to growth factors and promotes angiogenesis in wound healing. *Blood.* 133 (2019) 2559–2569.
41. A.V.S. Faria, S.S. Andrade, M.P. Peppelenbosch, C.V. Ferreira-Halder, G.M. Fuhler. The role of phospho-tyrosine signaling in platelet biology and hemostasis. *Biochimica et Biophysica Acta (BBA) – Mol. Cell Res.* 1868 (2021) 118927.
42. G.S. Nam, K.-S. Lee, K.-S. Nam. Morin hydrate inhibits platelet activation and clot retraction by regulating integrin $\alpha IIb\beta 3$, TXA2, and cAMP levels. *Eur. J. Pharmacol.* 865 (2019) 172734.
43. M. López, S. Heitmeier, V. Laux, G. Nowak. The dual FXa/thrombin inhibitor SATI prevents fibrin and platelet deposition in hypercoagulant rats. *Thromb. Res.* 193 (2020) 15–21.
44. J.P. Wood, H.H. Petersen, B. Yu, X. Wu, I. Hilden, A.E. Mast. TFPIα interacts with FVa and FXa to inhibit prothrombinase during the initiation of coagulation. *Blood Adv.* 1 (2017) 2692–2702.
45. A.M. Boniakowski. SIRT3 regulates macrophage-mediated inflammation in diabetic wound repair. *J. Investig. Dermatol.* 139 (2019) 528–537.e2.
46. P. Sadiku, J. A. Willson, E. M. Ryan, D. Sammut, P. Coelho. Neutrophils fuel effective immune responses through gluconeogenesis and glycogenesis. *Cell. Metab.* 33 (2) (2020) 411–423.e4.
47. C.K. Postnikoff, K. Held, V. Viswanath, K.K. Nichols. Enhanced closed eye neutrophil degranulation in dry eye disease. *The. Ocular. Surface.* 18 (2020) 841–851.
48. W. Liu, M. Wang, W. Cheng, W. Niu, M. Chen, M. Luo, C. Xie, T. Leng, L. Zhang, B. Lei. Bioactive antiinflammatory antibacterial hemostatic citrate-based dressing with macrophage polarization regulation for accelerating wound healing and hair follicle neogenesis. *Bioact. Mater.* 6 (2021) 721–728.
49. Y. Zhang. P. B. Alexander, X. F. Wang. TGF-β family signaling in the control of cell proliferation and survival. *Cold Spring Harb. Perspect. Biol.* 9 (2016) a022145.
50. Y. Zhao. Kanglexin accelerates diabetic wound healing by promoting angiogenesis via FGFR1/ERK signaling. *Biomed. Pharmacother.* 132 (2020) 110933.
51. L. Chen. Adipose-derived stem cells promote diabetic wound healing via the recruitment and differentiation of endothelial progenitor cells into endothelial cells mediated by the VEGF-PLCγ-ERK pathway. *Arch. Biochem. Biophys.* 692 (2020) 108531.
52. D. Mokoena, S.S. Dhilip Kumar, N.N. Houreld, H. Abrahamse. Role of photobiomodulation on the activation of the Smad pathway via TGF-β in wound healing. *J. Photochem. Photobiol. B: Biol.* 189 (2018) 138–144.
53. B.J. Peiffer. Activation of BMP signaling by FKBP12 ligands synergizes with inhibition of CXCR4 to accelerate wound healing. *Cell Chem. Biol.* 26 (2019) 652–661.e4.
54. L. Zhang. Activin B regulates adipose-derived mesenchymal stem cells to promote skin wound healing via activation of the MAPK signaling pathway. *Int. J. Biochem. Cell Biol.* 87 (2017) 69–76.
55. R. Lakra, M.S. Kiran, P.S. Korrapati. Effect of magnesium ascorbyl phosphate on collagen stabilization for wound healing application. *Int. J. Biol. Macromol.* 166 (2021) 333–341.
56. R. Langer, J.P. Vacanti. Tissue engineering. *Science* 260(5110) (1993) 920–926.
57. A. Khademhosseini, R. Langer. A decade of progress in tissue engineering. *Nat. Protoc.* 11(10) (2016) 1775–1781.
58. B. Farhadihosseinabadi, M. Farahani, T. Tayebi, A. Jafari, F. Biniazan, K. Modaresifar, H. Moravvej, S. Bahrami, H. Redl, L. Tayebi, H. Niknejad. Amniotic membrane and its epithelial and mesenchymal stem cells as an appropriate source for skin tissue engineering and regenerative medicine. *Artif. Cell Nanomed. B.* 46 (2018) 431–440.

59. A. Amirsadeghi, A. Jafari, L.J. Eggermont, S.S. Hashemi, S.A. Bencherif, M. Khorram. Vascularization strategies for skin tissue engineering. *Biomater. Sci.* 8(15) (2020) 4073–4094.
60. H. Green, O. Kehinde, J. Thomas. Growth of cultured human epidermal cells into multiple epithelia suitable for grafting. *Proc. Natl. Acad. Sci. U. S. A.* 76(11) (1979) 5665–5668.
61. L. Cui, J. Liang, H. Liu, K. Zhang, J. Li. Nanomaterials for angiogenesis in skin tissue engineering. *Tissue Eng. Part B. Rev.* 26(3) (2020) 203–216.
62. S. MacNeil. Progress and opportunities for tissue-engineered skin. *Nature.* 445(7130) (2007) 874–880.
63. S.J. Lee, J.H. Lee, J. Park, W.D. Kim, S.A. Park. Fabrication of 3D printing scaffold with porcine skin decellularized bio-ink for soft tissue engineering. *Materials (Basel)* 13(16) (2020)3522.
64. M.F. Zhu, W. Li, X.H. Dong, X.Y. Yuan, A.C. Midgley, H. Chang, Y.H. Wang, H.Y. Wang, K. Wang, P.X. Ma, H.J. Wang, D.L. Kong. In vivo engineered extracellular matrix scaffolds with instructive niches for oriented tissue regeneration. *Nat Commun.* 10 (1) (2019) 4620.
65. J.R. Dias, P.L. Granja, P.J. Bartolo. Advances in electrospun skin substitutes. *Prog Mater Sci.* 84 (2016) 314–334.
66. C. Cleeton, A. Keirouz, X.F. Chen, N. Radacsi. Electrospun nanofibers for drug delivery and biosensing. *ACS Biomater Sci Eng.* 5(9) (2019) 4183–4205.
67. C.X. Wu, T. Chen, Y.J. Xin, Z. Zhang, Z. Ren, J. Lei, B. Chu, Y.F. Wang, S.Q. Tang. Nanofibrous asymmetric membranes self-organized from chemically heterogeneous electrospun mats for skin tissue engineering. *Biomed Mater.* 11(3) (2016) 035019.
68. N.K. Cankirili, O. Altundag, B. Celebi-Saltik. Skin stem cells, their niche and tissue engineering approach for skin regeneration. *Cell Biol. Trans. Med.,* 6 (2020) 107–126.
69. M.A. Martin-Piedra, C.A. Alfonso-Rodriguez, A. Zapater, D. Durand-Herrera, J. Chato-Astrain, F. Campos, M.C. Sanchez-Quevedo, M. Alaminos, I. Garzon. Effective use of mesenchymal stem cells in human skin substitutes generated by tissue engineering. *Eur Cell Mater.* 37 (2019) 233–249.
70. A.S. Klar, J. Zimoch, T. Biedermann. Skin tissue engineering: Application of adipose-derived stem cells. *Biomed Res Int* 2017 (2017) 1–12.
71. S.B. Vidor, P.B. Terraciano, F.S. Valente, V.M. Rolim, C.P. Kuhl, L.S. Ayres, T.N.A. Garcez, N.E. Lemos, C.E. Kipper, S.B. Pizzato, D. Driemeier, E.O. Cirne-Lima, E.A. Contesini. Adipose-derived stem cells improve full-thickness skin grafts in a rat model. *Res. Vet. Sci.* 118 (2018) 336–344.
72. F.J. O'Brien. Biomaterials & scaffolds for tissue engineering. *Mater Today.* 14(3) (2011) 88–95.
73. M.G. Cascone, N. Barbani, C. Cristallini, P. Giusti, G. Ciardelli, L. Lazzeri. Bioartificial polymeric materials based on polysaccharides. *J Biomater Sci Polym Ed.* 12(3) (2001) 267–281.
74. L.J. Chen, M. Wang. Production and evaluation of biodegradable composites based on PHB-PHV copolymer. *Biomaterials.* 23(13) (2002) 2631–2639.
75. R.L. Knight, H.E. Wilcox, S.A. Korossis, J. Fisher, E. Ingham. The use of acellular matrices for the tissue engineering of cardiac valves. *Proc Inst Mech Eng H.* 222(H1) (2008) 129–143.
76. G.H. Borschel, Y.C. Huang, S. Calve, E.M. Arruda, J.B. Lynch, D.E. Dow, W.M. Kuzon, R.G. Dennis, D.L. Brown. Tissue engineering of recellularized small-diameter vascular grafts. *Tissue Eng.* 11(5–6) (2005) 778–786.
77. T. Takezawa, Y. Mori, K. Yoshizato. Cell culture on a thermo-responsive polymer surface. *Biotechnology (N Y).* 8(9) (1990) 854–856.

78. A.R. Boccaccini, J.J. Blaker. Bioactive composite materials for tissue engineering scaffolds. *Expert Rev. Med. Devices* 2(3) (2005) 303–317.
79. S.P. Tarassoli, Z.M. Jessop, A. Al-Sabah, N. Gao, S. Whitaker, S. Doak, I.S. Whitaker. Skin tissue engineering using 3D bioprinting: An evolving research field. *J Plast Reconstr Aesthet Surg.* 71(5) (2018) 615–623.
80. B.S. Kim, Y.W. Kwon, J.S. Kong, G.T. Park, G. Gao, W. Han, M.B. Kim, H. Lee, J.H. Kim, D.W. Cho. 3D cell printing of in vitro stabilized skin model and in vivo pre-vascularized skin patch using tissue-specific extracellular matrix bioink: A step towards advanced skin tissue engineering. *Biomaterials.* 168 (2018) 38–53.
81. W.C. Yan, P. Davoodi, S. Vijayavenkataraman, Y. Tian, W.C. Ng, J.Y.H. Fuh, K.S. Robinson, C.H. Wang. 3D bioprinting of skin tissue: From pre-processing to final product evaluation. *Adv. Drug Del. Rev.* 132 (2018) 270–295.
82. L.J. Pourchet, A. Thepot, M. Albouy, E.J. Courtial, A. Boher, L.J. Blum, C.A. Marquette. Human skin 3D bioprinting using scaffold-free approach. *Adv Healthc Mater.* 6(4) (2017).
83. Q. Huang, Y. Zou, M.C. Arno, S. Chen, T. Wang, J. Gao, A.P. Dove, J. Du. Hydrogel scaffolds for differentiation of adipose-derived stem cells. *Chem. Soc. Rev.* 46(20) (2017) 6255–6275.
84. D. Seliktar. Designing cell-compatible hydrogels for biomedical applications. *Science (New York, N.Y.).* 336(6085) (2012) 1124–1128.
85. B.V. Slaughter, S.S. Khurshid, O.Z. Fisher, A. Khademhosseini, N.A. Peppas. Hydrogels in regenerative medicine. *Adv. Mater. (Deerfield Beach, Fla.)* 21(32–33) (2009) 3307–3329.
86. L.Y. Lu, S.L. Yuan, J. Wang, Y. Shen, S.W. Deng, L.Y. Xie, Q.X. Yang. The formation mechanism of hydrogels. *Curr. Stem Cell Res. Ther.* 13(7) (2018) 490–496.
87. Y.S. Zhang, A. Khademhosseini. Advances in engineering hydrogels. *Science.* 356(6337) (2017).
88. M.C. Catoira, L. Fusaro, D. Di Francesco, M. Ramella, F. Boccafoschi. Overview of natural hydrogels for regenerative medicine applications. *J. Mater. Sci. Mater. Med.* 30(10) (2019) 115.
89. L. Francis, K.V. Greco, A.R. Boccaccini, J.J. Roether, N.R. English, H. Huang, R. Ploeg, T. Ansari. Development of a novel hybrid bioactive hydrogel for future clinical applications. *J. Biomater. Appl.* 33(3) (2018) 447–465.
90. F. Gao, J. Li, L. Wang, D. Zhang, J. Zhang, F. Guan, M. Yao. Dual-enzymatically cross-linked hyaluronic acid hydrogel as a long-time 3D stem cell culture system. *Biomed. Mater.* 15(4) (2020) 045013.
91. A. Lueckgen, D.S. Garske, A. Ellinghaus, R.M. Desai, A.G. Stafford, D.J. Mooney, G.N. Duda, A. Cipitria. Hydrolytically-degradable click-crosslinked alginate hydrogels. *Biomaterials.* 181 (2018) 189–198.
92. D.L. Gan, T. Xu, W.S. Xing, X. Ge, L.M. Fang, K.F. Wang, F.Z. Ren, X. Lu. Mussel-inspired contact-active antibacterial hydrogel with high cell affinity, toughness, and recoverability. *Adv Funct Mater.* 29(1) (2019) 1805964.
93. J. Chen, D. Wang, L.H. Wang, W.J. Liu, A. Chiu, K. Shariati, Q.S. Liu, X. Wang, Z. Zhong, J. Webb, R.E. Schwartz, N. Bouklas, M.L. Ma. An adhesive hydrogel with "load-sharing" effect as tissue bandages for drug and cell delivery. *Adv Mater.* 32(43) (2020) 2001628.
94. C. Merceron, S. Portron, M. Masson, J. Lesoeur, B.H. Fellah, O. Gauthier, O. Geffroy, P. Weiss, J. Guicheux, C. Vinatier. The effect of two- and three-dimensional cell culture on the chondrogenic potential of human adipose-derived mesenchymal stem cells after subcutaneous transplantation with an injectable hydrogel. *Cell Transplant.* 20(10) (2011) 1575–1588.
95. H. Zhao, J. Huang, Y. Li, X. Lv, H. Zhou, H. Wang, Y. Xu, C. Wang, J. Wang, Z. Liu. ROS-scavenging hydrogel to promote healing of bacteria infected diabetic wounds. *Biomaterials.* 258 (2020) 120286.

96. P.L. Thi, Y. Lee, D.L. Tran, T.T.H. Thi, J.I. Kang, K.M. Park, K.D. Park. In situ forming and reactive oxygen species-scavenging gelatin hydrogels for enhancing wound healing efficacy. *Acta Biomater.* 103 (2020) 142–152.

97. J. Ding, Y.J. Yao, J.W. Li, Y.Y. Duan, J.R. Nakkala, X. Feng, W.B. Cao, Y.C. Wang, L.J. Hong, L.Y. Shen, Z.W. Mao, Y. Zhu, C.Y. Gao. A reactive oxygen species scavenging and O-2 generating injectable hydrogel for myocardial infarction treatment in vivo. *Small.* 16(48) (2020) 2005038.

98. Y. Zhu, Y. Matsumura, M. Velayutham, L.M. Foley, T.K. Hitchens, W.R. Wagner. Reactive oxygen species scavenging with a biodegradable, thermally responsive hydrogel compatible with soft tissue injection. *Biomaterials.* 177 (2018) 98–112.

99. K.A. Spaulding, Y. Zhu, K. Takaba, A. Ramasubramanian, A. Badathala, H. Haraldsson, A. Collins, E. Aguayo, C.R. Shah, A.W. Wallace, N.P. Ziats, D.H. Lovett, A.J. Baker, K.E. Healy, M.B. Ratcliffe. Myocardial injection of a thermoresponsive hydrogel with reactive oxygen species scavenger properties improves border zone contractility. *J Biomed Mater Res A.* 108(8) (2020) 1736–1746.

100. L.B. Vong, T.Q. Bui, T. Tomita, H. Sakamoto, Y. Hiramatsu, Y. Nagasaki. Novel angiogenesis therapeutics by redox injectable hydrogel - Regulation of local nitric oxide generation for effective cardiovascular therapy. *Biomaterials.* 167 (2018) 143–152.

101. A.M. Sisso, M.O. Boit, C.A. DeForest. Self-healing injectable gelatin hydrogels for localized therapeutic cell delivery. *J Biomed Mater Res A.* 108(5) (2020) 1112–1121.

102. Y. Kong, Z. Hou, L. Zhou, P. Zhang, Y. Ouyang, P. Wang, Y. Chen, X. Luo. Injectable self-healing hydrogels containing CuS nanoparticles with abilities of hemostasis, antibacterial activity, and promoting wound healing. *ACS Biomater Sci Eng* 7 (1) (2020) 335–349.

103. S. Basu, S. Pacelli, A. Paul. Self-healing DNA-based injectable hydrogels with reversible covalent linkages for controlled drug delivery. *Acta Biomater.* 105 (2020) 159–169.

104. G. Ge, Y. Lu, X. Qu, W. Zhao, Y. Ren, W. Wang, Q. Wang, W. Huang, X. Dong. Muscle-inspired self-healing hydrogels for strain and temperature sensor. *ACS Nano.* 14(1) (2020) 218–228.

105. S.O. Solomevich, P.M. Bychkovsky, T.L. Yurkshtovich, N.V. Golub, P.Y. Mirchuk, M.Y. Revtovich, A.I. Shmak. Biodegradable pH-sensitive prospidine-loaded dextran phosphate based hydrogels for local tumor therapy. *Carbohydr. Polym.* 226 (2019) 115308.

106. Z.Q. Li, Z.B. Fan, Y.Y. Xu, W.S. Lo, X. Wang, H. Niu, X.F. Li, X.Y. Xie, M. Khan, J.J. Guan. pH-sensitive and thermosensitive hydrogels as stem-cell carriers for cardiac therapy. *ACS Appl Mater Interfaces.* 8(17) (2016) 10752–10760.

107. X. Zhao, H. Wu, B.L. Guo, R.N. Dong, Y.S. Qiu, P.X. Ma. Antibacterial anti-oxidant electroactive injectable hydrogel as self-healing wound dressing with hemostasis and adhesiveness for cutaneous wound healing. *Biomaterials.* 122 (2017) 34–47.

108. B.J. Mai, M.Q. Jia, S.P. Liu, Z.H. Sheng, M. Li, Y.R. Gao, X.B. Wang, Q.H. Liu, P. Wang. Smart hydrogel-based DVDMS/bFGF nanohybrids for antibacterial phototherapy with multiple damaging sites and accelerated wound healing. *ACS Appl Mater Interfaces.* 12(9) (2020) 10156–10169.

109. Y. Tian, L. Pang, R. Zhang, T. Xu, S. Wang, B. Yu, L. Gao, H. Cong, Y. Shen. Polytetrahydropyrimidine antibacterial hydrogel with injectability and self-healing ability for curing the purulent subcutaneous infection. *ACS Appl Mater Interfaces.* 12(45) (2020) 50236–50247.

110. S. Crunkhorn. Hydrogel fights infection and inflammation. *Nat. Rev. Drug Discov.* 19(2) (2020) 92.

111. S. Cascone, G. Lamberti. Hydrogel-based commercial products for biomedical applications: A review. *Int. J. Pharm.* 573 (2020) 118803.

112. K. Chwalek, K.R. Levental, M.V. Tsurkan, A. Zieris, U. Freudenberg, C. Werner. Two-tier hydrogel degradation to boost endothelial cell morphogenesis. *Biomaterials.* 32(36) (2011) 9649–9657.

113. F. Lin, J. Yu, W. Tang, J. Zheng, A. Defante, K. Guo, C. Wesdemiotis, M.L. Becker. Peptide-functionalized oxime hydrogels with tunable mechanical properties and gelation behavior. *Biomacromolecules.* 14(10) (2013) 3749–58.

114. J. Yang, Y.S. Zhang, K. Yue, A. Khademhosseini. Cell-laden hydrogels for osteochondral and cartilage tissue engineering. *Acta Biomater.* 57 (2017) 1–25.

115. Y. Zhang, D. An, Y. Pardo, A. Chiu, W. Song, Q.S. Liu, F. Zhou, S.P. McDonough, M.L. Ma. High-water-content and resilient PEG-containing hydrogels with low fibrotic response. *Acta Biomater.* 53 (2017) 100–108.

116. W. Zhao, X. Jin, Y. Cong, Y.Y. Liu, J. Fu. Degradable natural polymer hydrogels for articular cartilage tissue engineering. *J. Chem. Technol. Biotechnol.* 88(3) (2013) 327–339.

117. N. Asadi, H. Pazoki-Toroudi, A.R. Del Bakhshayesh, A. Akbarzadeh, S. Davaran, N. Annabi, Multifunctional hydrogels for wound healing: Special focus on biomacromolecular based hydrogels. *Int. J. Biol. Macromol.* 170 (2020) 728–750.

118. Z. Deng, H. Wang, P.X. Ma, B. Guo. Self-healing conductive hydrogels: Preparation, properties and applications. *Nanoscale.* 12(3) (2020) 1224–1246.

119. Y. Liang, B. Chen, M. Li, J. He, Z. Yin, B. Guo. Injectable antimicrobial conductive hydrogels for wound disinfection and infectious wound healing. *Biomacromolecules.* 21(5) (2020) 1841–1852.

120. J. Li, F. Yu, G. Chen, J. Liu, X.L. Li, B. Cheng, X.M. Mo, C. Chen, J.F. Pan. Moist-retaining, self-recoverable, bioadhesive, and transparent in situ forming hydrogels to accelerate wound healing. *ACS Appl. Mater. Interfaces.* 12(2) (2020) 2023–2038.

121. Z. Xu, S. Han, Z. Gu, J. Wu. Advances and impact of antioxidant hydrogel in chronic wound healing. *Adv. Healthcare Mater.* 9(5) (2020) e1901502.

122. Y. Zhu, Z. Cankova, M. Iwanaszko, S. Lichtor, M. Mrksich, G.A. Ameer. Potent laminin-inspired antioxidant regenerative dressing accelerates wound healing in diabetes. *Proc. Natl. Acad. Sci. U. S. A.* 115(26) (2018) 6816–6821.

123. J.Y. Zhang, C. Wu, Y.Y. Xu, J.L. Chen, N. Ning, Z.Y. Yang, Y. Guo, X.F. Hu, Y.B. Wang. Highly stretchable and conductive self-healing hydrogels for temperature and strain sensing and chronic wound treatment. *ACS Appl. Mater. Interfaces.* 12(37) (2020) 40990–40999.

124. M. Prabaharan, J.F. Mano. Stimuli-responsive hydrogels based on polysaccharides incorporated with thermo-responsive polymers as novel biomaterials. *Macromol. Biosci.* 6(12) (2006) 991–1008.

125. M.E. Harmon, M. Tang, C.W. Frank. A microfluidic actuator based on thermoresponsive hydrogels. *Polymer.* 44(16) (2003) 4547–4556.

126. A. Kasinski, M. Zielinska-Pisklak, E. Oledzka, M. Sobczak. Smart hydrogels - synthetic stimuli-responsive antitumor drug release systems. *Int J Nanomedicine.* 15 (2020) 4541–4572.

127. A. Eyigor, F. Bahadori, V.B. Yenigun, M.S. Eroglu. Beta-Glucan based temperature responsive hydrogels for 5-ASA delivery. *Carbohydr Polym.* 201 (2018) 454–463.

128. K. Lavanya, S.V. Chandran, K. Balagangadharan, N. Selvamurugan. Temperature- and pH-responsive chitosan-based injectable hydrogels for bone tissue engineering. *Mater Sci Eng C Mater Biol Appl.* 111 (2020) 110862.

129. N. Jommanee, C. Chanthad, K. Manokruang. Preparation of injectable hydrogels from temperature and pH responsive grafted chitosan with tuned gelation temperature suitable for tumor acidic environment. *Carbohydr Polym.* 198 (2018) 486–494.

130. J.E.S. Shay, M.C. Simon. Hypoxia-inducible factors: Crosstalk between inflammation and metabolism. *Semin. Cell Dev. Biol.* 23(4) (2012) 389–394.

131. C.Y. Chiang, C.C. Chu. Synthesis of photoresponsive hybrid alginate hydrogel with photo-controlled release behavior. *Carbohydr Polym.* 119 (2015) 18–25.

132. P.B. Malafaya, G.A. Silva, R.L. Reis. Natural-origin polymers as carriers and scaffolds for biomolecules and cell delivery in tissue engineering applications. *Adv. Drug. Deliv. Rev.* 59 (2007) 207–233.

133. M. Mahinroosta, Z. Jomeh Farsangi, A. Allahverdi, Z. Shakoori. Hydrogels as intelligent materials: A brief review of synthesis, properties and applications. *Mater. Today Chem.* 8 (2018) 42–55.

134. S. Bashir, M. Hina, J. Iqbal, A.H. Rajpar, M.A. Mujtaba, N.A. Alghamdi, S. Wageh, K. Ramesh, S. Ramesh. Fundamental concepts of hydrogels: Synthesis, properties, and their applications. *Polymers (Basel).* 12 (2020) 2702.

135. N. Ghane, M.H. Beigi, S. Labbaf, M.H. Nasr-Esfahani, A. Kiani. Design of hydrogel-based scaffolds for the treatment of spinal cord injuries. *J. Mater. Chem. B.* 8 (2020) 10712–10738.

136. G. Eke, N. Mangir, N. Hasirci, S. MacNeil, V. Hasirci. Development of a UV cross-linked biodegradable hydrogel containing adipose derived stem cells to promote vascularization for skin wounds and tissue engineering. *Biomaterials.* 129 (2017) 188–198.

137. X. Li, A. Li, F. Feng, Q. Jiang, H. Sun, Y. Chai, R. Yang, Z. Wang, J. Hou, R. Li. Effect of the hyaluronic acid-poloxamer hydrogel on skin-wound healing: In vitro and in vivo studies. *Animal. Model. Exp. Med.* 2 (2019) 107–113.

138. R. Xu, K. Zhang, J. Liang, F. Gao, J. Li, F. Guan. Hyaluronic acid/polyethyleneimine nanoparticles loaded with copper ion and disulfiram for esophageal cancer. *Carbohydr. Polym.* 261(2021) 117846.

139. S. Liu, X. Liu, Y. Ren, P. Wang, Y. Pu, R. Yang, X. Wang, X. Tan, Z. Ye, V. Maurizot, B. Chi. Mussel-inspired dual-cross-linking hyaluronic acid/ε-polylysine hydrogel with self-healing and antibacterial properties for wound healing. *ACS. Appl. Mater. Interfaces.* 12 (2020) 27876–27888.

140. J.E. Rayahin, J.S. Buhrman, Y. Zhang, T.J. Koh, R.A. Gemeinhart. High and low molecular weight hyaluronic acid differentially influence macrophage activation *ACS. Biomater. Sci. Eng.* 1 (2015) 481–493.

141. Y.S. Jung, W. Park, H. Park, D.K. Lee, K. Na. Thermo-sensitive injectable hydrogel based on the physical mixing of hyaluronic acid and Pluronic F-127 for sustained NSAID delivery. *Carbohydr. Polym.* 156 (2017) 403–408.

142. J. Patterson, R. Siew, S.W. Herring, A.S.P. Lin, R. Guldberg, P.S. Stayton. Hyaluronic acid hydrogels with controlled degradation properties for oriented bone regeneration. *Biomaterials.* 31 (2010) 6772–6781.

143. I.L. Kim, R.L. Mauck, J.A. Burdick. Hydrogel design for cartilage tissue engineering: A case study with hyaluronic acid. *Biomaterials.* 32 (2011) 8771–8782.

144. N. Broguiere, L. Isenmann, M. Zenobi-Wong. Novel enzymatically cross-linked hyaluronan hydrogels support the formation of 3D neuronal networks. *Biomaterials.* 99 (2016) 47–55.

145. A.G. Tavianatou, I. Caon, M. Franchi, Z. Piperigkou, D. Galesso, N.K. Karamanos. Hyaluronan: Molecular size-dependent signaling and biological functions in inflammation and cancer. *FEBS. J.* 286 (2019) 2883–2908.

146. J. Webber, R.H. Jenkins, S. Meran, A. Phillips, R. Steadman. Modulation of TGFbeta1-dependent myofibroblast differentiation by hyaluronan. *Am. J. Pathol.* 175 (2009) 148–160.

147. R. Stern, A.A. Asari, K.N. Sugahara. Hyaluronan fragments: An information-rich system. *Eur. J. Cell. Biol.* 85 (2006) 699–715.

148. J. Wu, A. Chen, Y. Zhou, S. Zheng, Y. Yang, Y. An, K. Xu, H. He, J. Kang, J.A. Luckanagul, M. Xian, J. Xiao, Q. Wang. Novel H2S-Releasing hydrogel for wound repair via in situ polarization of M2 macrophages. *Biomaterials.* 222 (2019) 119398.

149. E. Ruvinov, S. Cohen. Alginate biomaterial for the treatment of myocardial infarction: Progress, translational strategies, and clinical outlook: From ocean algae to patient bedside. *Adv. Drug. Deliv. Rev.* 96 (2016) 54–76.

150. Lee, K.Y., Mooney, D.J. Alginate: Properties and biomedical applications. *Prog. Polym. Sci.* 37 (2012) 106–126.

151. K. Zhang, Z. Shi, J. Zhou, Q. Xing, S. Ma, Q. Li, Y. Zhang, M. Yao, X. Wang, Q. Li, J. Li, F. Guan. Potential application of an injectable hydrogel scaffold loaded with mesenchymal stem cells for treating traumatic brain injury. *J. Mater. Chem. B.* 6 (2018) 2982–2992.

152. W. Yang, H. Xu, Y. Lan, Q. Zhu, Y. Liu, S. Huang, S. Shi, A. Hancharou, B. Tang, R. Guo. Preparation and characterisation of a novel silk fibroin/hyaluronic acid/sodium alginate scaffold for skin repair. *Int. J. Biol. Macromol.* 130 (2019) 58–67.

153. Y. Fan, W. Wu, Y. Lei, C. Gaucher, S. Pei, J. Zhang, X. Xia. Edaravone-loaded alginate-based nanocomposite hydrogel accelerated chronic wound healing in diabetic mice. *Mar. Drugs.* 17 (2019) 285.

154. O. Catanzano, V. D'Esposito, S. Acierno, M. R. Ambrosio, C. De. Caro, C. Avagliano, P. Russo, R. Russo, A. Miro, F. Ungaro, A. Calignano, P. Formisano, F. Quaglia. Alginate-hyaluronan composite hydrogels accelerate wound healing process. *Carbohydr. Polym.* 131 (2015) 407–414.

155. A. Thomas. Alginates from wound dressings activate human macrophages to secrete tumour necrosis factor-α. *Biomaterials.* 21 (2000) 1797–802.

156. N. Golafshan, R. Rezahasani, M. Tarkesh Esfahani, M. Kharaziha, S.N. Khorasani. Nanohybrid hydrogels of laponite: PVA-Alginate as a potential wound healing material. *Carbohydr. Polym.* 176 (2017) 392–401.

157. H.S. Koh, K. Kazazian, M.S. Shoichet. Controlling cell adhesion and degradation of chitosan films by N-acetylation. *Biomaterials.* 26 (2005) 5872–5878.

158. R. Jayakumar, M. Prabaharan, P.T. Sudheesh Kumar, S.V. Nair, H. Tamura. Biomaterials based on chitin and chitosan in wound dressing applications. *Biotechnol. Adv.* 29 (2011) 322–337.

159. M. Rinaudo. Chitin and chitosan: Properties and applications. *Prog. Polym. Sci.* 31 (2006) 603–632.

160. J. Xu, S. Strandman, J.X.X. Zhu, J. Barralet, M. Cerruti. Genipin-crosslinked catechol-chitosan mucoadhesive hydrogels for buccal drug delivery. *Biomaterials.* 37 (2015) 395–404.

161. A.B. Sieval, M. Thanou, A.F. Kotze´, J.C. Verhoef, J. Brussee, H.E. Junginger. Preparation and NMR characterization of highly substituted N-trimethyl chitosan chloride. *Carbohydr. Polym.* 36 (1998) 157–165.

162. Z. Wu, W. Zhou, W. Deng, C. Xu, Y. Cai, X. Wang. Antibacterial and hemostatic thiol-modified chitosan-immobilized AgNPs composite sponges. *ACS. Appl. Mater. Interfaces.* 12 (2020) 20307–20320.

163. M. Li, Z. Zhang, Y. Liang, J. He, B. Guo. Multifunctional tissue-adhesive cryogel wound dressing for rapid nonpressing surface hemorrhage and wound repair. *ACS. Appl. Mater. Interfaces.* 12 (2020) 35856–35872.

164. B. Vigani, S. Rossi, G. Sandri, M.C. Bonferoni, C.M. Caramella, F. Ferrari. Hyaluronic acid and chitosan-based nanosystems: A new dressing generation for wound care. *Expert. Opin. Drug. Deliv.* 16(7) (2019) 715–740.

165. S. Pourshahrestani, E. Zeimaran, N.A. Kadri, N. Mutlu, A.R. Boccaccini. Polymeric hydrogel systems as emerging biomaterial platforms to enable hemostasis and wound healing. *Adv. Healthc. Mater.* 9 (2020) e2000905.

166. M.C. Echave, L. Saenz del Burgo, J.L. Pedraz, G. Orive. Gelatin as biomaterial for tissue engineering. *Curr. Pharm. Des.* 23 (2017) 3567–3584.

167. B.J. Klotz, D. Gawlitta, A.J.W.P. Rosenberg, J. Malda, F.P.W. Melchels. Gelatin-methacryloyl hydrogels: Towards biofabrication-based tissue repair. *Trends. Biotechnol.* 34 (2016) 394–407.

168. S. Huang, X. Fu. Naturally derived materials-based cell and drug delivery systems in skin regeneration. *J. Control. Release.* 142 (2010) 149–159.

169. M.R. Hait. Microcrystalline collagen. A new hemostatic agent. *Am. J. Surg.* 120 (1970) 330.

170. D.A. Hickman, C.L. Pawlowski, U.D.S. Sekhon, J. Marks, A.S. Gupta. Biomaterials and advanced technologies for hemostatic management of bleeding. *Adv. Mater.* 30 (2018) 1700859.

171. A. Assmann, A. Vegh, M. Ghasemi-Rad, S. Bagherifard, G. Cheng, E. S. Sani, G. U. Ruiz-Esparza, I. Noshadi, A. D. Lassaletta, S. Gangadharan, A. Tamayol, A. Khademhosseini, N. Annabi. A highly adhesive and naturally derived sealant. *Biomaterials.* 140 (2017) 115–127.

172. M. Hamidi, A. Azadi, P. Rafiei. Hydrogel nanoparticles in drug delivery. *Adv. Drug. Deliv. Rev.* 60 (2008) 1638–1649.

173. S. Naahidi, M. Jafari, M. Logan, Y. Wang, Y. Yuan, H. Bae, B. Dixon, P. Chen. Biocompatibility of hydrogel-based scaffolds for tissue engineering applications. *Biotechnol. Adv.* 35 (2017) 530–544.

174. L.F. Santos, I.J. Correia, A.S. Silva, J.F. Mano. Biomaterials for drug delivery patches. *Eur. J. Pharm. Sci.* 118 (2018) 49–66.

175. M. Sohail, M.U. Minhas, S. Khan, Z. Hussain, M. De. Matas, S.A. Shah, S. Khan, M. Kousar, K. Ullah. Natural and synthetic polymer-based smart biomaterials for management of ulcerative colitis: A review of recent developments and future prospects. *Drug. Deliv. Transl. Res.* 9 (2019) 595–614.

176. X. Zhao, J. Si, D. Huang, K. Li, Y. Xin, M. Sui. Application of star poly(ethylene glycol) derivatives in drug delivery and controlled release. *J. Control. Release.* 323 (2020) 565–577.

177. Harris, J.M., and Zalipsky, S. eds., *Poly(ethylene glycol).* Washington. DC: American Chemical Society, (1997).

178. N.A. Alcantar, E.S. Aydil, J.N. Israelachvili. Polyethylene glycol-coated biocompatible surfaces. *J. Biomed. Mater. Res.* 51 (2000) 343–351.

179. Y. Park, M.P. Lutolf, J.A. Hubbell, E.B. Hunziker, M. Wong. Bovine primary chondrocyte culture in synthetic matrix metalloproteinase-sensitive poly(ethylene glycol)-based hydrogels as a scaffold for cartilage repair. *Tissue. Eng.* 10 (2004) 515–522.

180. B.D. Polizzotti, B.D. Fairbanks, K.S. Anseth. Three-dimensional biochemical patterning of click-based composite hydrogels via thiolene photopolymerization. *Biomacromolecules.* 9 (2008) 1084–1087.

181. M. Ehrbar, S.C. Rizzi, R. Hlushchuk, V. Djonov, A.H. Zisch, J.A. Hubbell, F.E. Weber, M.P. Lutolf. Enzymatic formation of modular cell-instructive fibrin analogs for tissue engineering. *Biomaterials.* 28 (2007) 3856–3866.

182. B.H. Hu, J. Su, P.B. Messersmith. Hydrogels cross-linked by native chemical ligation. *Biomacromolecules.* 10 (2009) 2194–2200.

183. C.R. Nuttelman, M.A. Rice, A.E. Rydholm, C.N. Salinas, D.N. Shah, K.S. Anseth. Macromolecular monomers for the synthesis of hydrogel niches and their application in cell encapsulation and tissue engineering. *Prog. Polym. Sci.* 33 (2008) 167–179.

184. F. Zhang, C. Hu, Q. Kong, R. Luo, Y. Wang. Peptide-/drug-directed self-assembly of hybrid polyurethane hydrogels for wound healing. *ACS. Appl. Mater. Interfaces.* 11 (2019) 37147–37155.

185. K. Chen, Y. Feng, Y. Zhang, L. Yu, X. Hao, F. Shao, Z. Dou, C. An, Z. Zhuang, Y. Luo, Y. Wang, J. Wu, P. Ji, T. Chen, H. Wang. Entanglement-driven adhesion, self-healing, and high stretchability of double-network PEG-based hydrogels. *ACS. Appl. Mater. Interfaces.* 11 (2019) 36458–36468.

186. X. Mao, R. Cheng, H. Zhang, J. Bae, L. Cheng, L. Zhang, L. Deng, W. Cui, Y. Zhang, H.A. Santos, X. Sun. Self-healing and injectable hydrogel for matching skin flap regeneration. *Adv. Sci. (Weinh).* 6 (2019) 1801555.

187. D.M. Dos Santos, I.S. Leite. A.d.L. Bukzem, R.P. De. Oliveira Santos, E. Frollini, N.M. Inada, S.P. Campana-Filho. Nanostructured electrospun nonwovens of poly(ε-caprolactone)/quaternized chitosan for potential biomedical applications. *Carbohydr. Polym.* 186 (2018) 110–121.

188. M. Jikei, Y. Yamadoi, T. Suga, K. Matsumoto. Stereocomplex formation of poly(l-lactide)-poly(ε-caprolactone) multiblock copolymers with Poly(d-lactide). *Polymer.* 123 (2017) 73–80.

189. Y.H. Bae, K.M. Huh, Y. Kim, K.H. Park. Biodegradable amphiphilic multiblock copolymers and their implications for biomedical applications. *J. Control Release.* 64 (2000) 3–13.

190. J. Liao, Y. Jia, B. Wang, K. Shi, Z. Qian. Injectable hybrid poly(ε-caprolactone)-b-poly(ethylene glycol)-b-poly(ε-caprolactone) porous microspheres/alginate hydrogel cross-linked by calcium gluconate crystals deposited in the pores of microspheres improved skin wound healing. *ACS. Biomater. Sci. Eng.* 4 (2018) 1029–1036.

191. N.A. Peppas, E.W. Merrill. Crosslinked poly(vinyl alcohol) hydrogels as swollen elastic networks. *J. Appl. Polym. Sci.* 21 (1977) 1763–1770.

192. M.I. Baker, S.P. Walsh, Z. Schwartz, B.D. Boyan. A review of polyvinyl alcohol and its uses in cartilage and orthopedic applications. *J. Biomed. Mater. Res. B. Appl. Biomater.* 100 (2012) 1451–1457.

193. W.C. Lin, C.M. Tang. Evaluation of polyvinyl alcohol/cobalt substituted hydroxyapatite nanocomposite as a potential wound dressing for diabetic foot ulcers. *Int. J. Mol. Sci.* 21 (2020) 8831.

194. Y. Li, J. Wang, Y. Yang, J. Shi, H. Zhang, X. Yao, W. Chen, X. Zhang. A rose bengal/graphene oxide/PVA hybrid hydrogel with enhanced mechanical properties and light-triggered antibacterial activity for wound treatment. *Mater. Sci. Eng. C. Mater. Biol. Appl.* 118 (2021) 111447.

195. G. Chen, L. He, P. Zhang, J. Zhang, X. Mei, D. Wang, Y. Zhang, X. Ren, Z. Chen. Encapsulation of green tea polyphenol nanospheres in PVA/alginate hydrogel for promoting wound healing of diabetic rats by regulating PI3K/AKT pathway. *Mater. Sci. Eng. C. Mater. Biol. Appl.* 110 (2020) 110686.

196. E. Ranucci, G. Capuano, A. Manfredi, P. Ferruti. One-step synthesis of poly(lactic-co-glycolic acid)- g -poly-1-vinylpyrrolidin-2-one copolymers. *J. Polym. Sci. Part A: Polym. Chem.* 54 (2016) 1919.

197. N. Vázquez, F. Sánchez-Arévalo, A. Maciel-Cerda, I. Garnica-Palafox, R. Ontiveros-Tlachi, C. Chaires-Rosas, G. Piñón-Zarate, M. Herrera-Enríquez, M. Hautefeuille, R. Vera-Graziano, A. Castell-Rodríguez. Influence of the PLGA/gelatin ratio on the physical, chemical and biological properties of electrospun scaffolds for wound dressings. *Biomed. Mater.* 14(4) (2019) 045006.

198. R.C. Mundargi, V.R. Babu, V. Rangaswamy, P. Patel, T.M. Aminabhavi. Nano/micro technologies for delivering macromolecular therapeutics using poly(D, L-lactide-co-glycolide) and its derivatives. *J. Control. Release.* 125(3) (2008) 193–209.

199. A. Shenderova, T.G. Burke, S.P. Schwendeman. The acidic microclimate in poly(lactide-co-glycolide) microspheres stabilizes camptothecins. *Pharm. Res.* 16(2) (1999) 241–248.

200. B. Murray, D.J. Wilson. A study of metabolites as intermediate effectors in angiogenesis. *Angiogenesis.* 4(1) (2001) 71–77.

201. T.N. Milovanova, V.M. Bhopale, E.M. Sorokina, J.S. Moore, T.K. Hunt, M. Hauer-Jensen, O.C. Velazquez, S.R. Thom. Lactate stimulates vasculogenic stem cells via the thioredoxin system and engages an autocrine activation loop involving hypoxia-inducible factor 1. *Mol. Cell. Biol.* 28(20) (2008) 6248–6261.

202. R.A. Jain. The manufacturing techniques of various drug loaded biodegradable poly(lactide-co-glycolide) (PLGA) devices. *Biomaterials.* 21(23) (2000) 2475–2490.

203. Z. Ma, W. Song, Y. He, H. Li. Multilayer injectable hydrogel system sequentially delivers bioactive substances for each wound healing stage. *ACS. Appl. Mater. Interfaces.* 12(26) (2020) 29787–29806.

204. S. Choudhury, A. Das. Advances in generation of three-dimensional skin equivalents: Pre-clinical studies to clinical therapies. *Cytotherapy* 23(1) (2021) 1–9.

205. H. Shahin, M. Elmasry, I. Steinvall, F. Soberg, A. El-Serafi. Vascularization is the next challenge for skin tissue engineering as a solution for burn management. *Burns. Trauma* 8 (2020)tkaa022.

206. C. Pailler-Mattei, S. Nicoli, F. Pirot, R. Vargiolu, H. Zahouani. A new approach to describe the skin surface physical properties in vivo. *Colloids. Surf B. Biointerfaces.* 68(2) (2009) 200–206.

207. R.H. Yang, S. Yang, J.L. Zhao, X.M. Hu, X.D. Chen, J.R. Wang, J.L. Xie, K. Xiong. Progress in studies of epidermal stem cells and their application in skin tissue engineering. *Stem Cell. Res. Ther.* 11(1) (2020) 303.

208. M. Pasparakis, I. Haase, F.O. Nestle. Mechanisms regulating skin immunity and inflammation. *Nat Rev Immunol.* 14(5) (2014) 289–301.

209. E. Candi, R. Schmidt, G. Melino. The cornified envelope: A model of cell death in the skin. *Nat. Rev. Mol. Cell. Biol.* 6(4) (2005) 328–340.

210. K. Vig, A. Chaudhari, S. Tripathi, S. Dixit, R. Sahu, S. Pillai, V.A. Dennis, S.R. Singh. Advances in skin regeneration using tissue engineering. *Int. J. Mol. Sci.* 18(4) (2017) 789.

211. R. Wong, S. Geyer, W. Weninger, J.C. Guimberteau, J.K. Wong. The dynamic anatomy and patterning of skin. *Exp. Dermatol.* 25(2) (2016) 92–98.

212. W.L. Ng, S. Wang, W.Y. Yeong, M.W. Naing. Skin bioprinting: Impending reality or fantasy?, *Trends. Biotechnol.* 34(9) (2016) 689–699.

213. G.D. Mogosanu, A.M. Grumezescu. Natural and synthetic polymers for wounds and burns dressing. *Int. J. Pharm.* 463(2) (2014) 127–136.

214. H. Debels, M. Hamdi, K. Abberton, W. Morrison. Dermal matrices and bioengineered skin substitutes: A critical review of current options. *Plast. Reconstr. Surg. Glob. Open.* 3(1) (2015) e284.

215. M. Peck, J. Molnar, D. Swart. A global plan for burn prevention and care. *Bull. W.H.O.* 87(10) (2009) 802–803.

216. D. Markeson, J.M. Pleat, J.R. Sharpe, A.L. Harris, A.M. Seifalian, S.M. Watt. Scarring, stem cells, scaffolds and skin repair. *J. Tissue. Eng. Regen. Med.* 9(6) (2015) 649–668.

217. T. Chen, Y. Chen, H.U. Rehman, Z. Chen, Z. Yang, M. Wang, H. Li, H. Liu. Ultratough, self-healing, and tissue-adhesive hydrogel for wound dressing. *ACS. Appl. Mater. Interfaces.* 10(39) (2018) 33523–33531.

218. B.P. O'Rourke, A.H. Kramer, L.L. Cao, M. Inayathullah, H. Guzik, J. Rajadas, J.D. Nosanchuk, D.J. Sharp. Fidgetin-like 2 siRNA enhances the wound healing capability of a surfactant polymer dressing. *Adv. Wound. Care. (New Rochelle).* 8 (2019) 91–100.

7 3D Printing in Nerve Regeneration

Guicai Li[1,2,3] and Liling Zhang[1]

[1]Key laboratory of Neuroregeneration of Jiangsu and Ministry of Education, Nantong University, 226001, Nantong, P.R. China

[2]Co-innovation Center of Neuroregeneration, Nantong University, 226001, Nantong, P.R. China

[3]NMPA Key Laboratory for Research and Evaluation of Tissue Engineering Technology Products, Nantong University, 226001, Nantong, P.R. China

CONTENTS

7.1 INTRODUCTION: NERVE SYSTEM

7.1.1 CENTRAL NERVE SYSTEM

The nervous system is mainly composed of two parts: the central nervous system (CNS) and the peripheral nervous system (PNS) [1,2]. The CNS consists of the brain located in the cranial cavity and spinal cord located in the spinal canal, which are the central parts

DOI: 10.1201/9781003161981-7

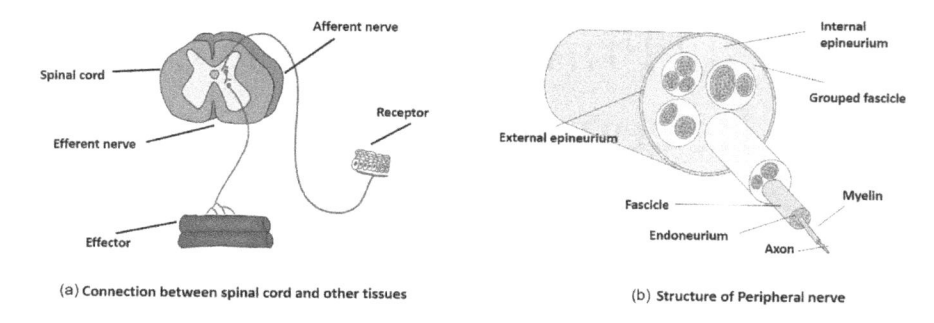

FIGURE 7.1 (a) Connection between the spinal cord and other tissues, (b) The structure of a peripheral nerve bundle.

of various reflex arcs (Figure 7.1a). The location of the CNS is often on the central axis of the animal body, consisting of cranial ganglia, nerve cords, brain, and spinal cord, as well as the connections between them. The brain and spinal cord are the main components of the human nervous system. In the CNS, a large number of nerve cells together form a network or circuit organically. Its main function is to transmit, store, and process information, produce various mental activities, and dominate and control all animal behaviors. The CNS accepts the information from the left and right of the entire body, and after its integration and processing, it becomes a coordinated motor transmission, or it is stored in the CNS to become the neural basis of learning and memory.

In the CNS, the brain can be divided into six parts, namely, the telencephalon, diencephalon, cerebellum, midbrain, pons, and medulla oblongata. The telencephalon and diencephalon are collectively called the forebrain, and the pons and medulla oblongata are collectively called the hindbrain [3]. Telencephalon refers to the two hemispheres of the brain, the oblongata or medulla oblongata. The midbrain, pons, and medulla oblongata form the brainstem, and there is a brainstem network structure composed of nerve cell clusters and nerve fibers that are intertwined. The two hemispheres of the brain are mainly composed of gray matter surface layer, white matter, and subcutaneous ganglia, that is, cerebral cortex, nerve fiber medulla, and basal ganglia. The two hemispheres of the brain, which are connected by joint nerve fibers (mainly the corpus callosum), are divided into the frontal lobe, parietal lobe, occipital lobe, temporal lobe, and insula, with each having a certain division of functions. The basic building units of the brain are nerve cells (neurons) and glial cells.

The spinal cord is a slightly flattened cylinder with full length ranging in thickness. It is located in the spinal canal. The upper end is connected to the medulla oblongata at the foramen magnum, and the lower end is tapered to form a cone [4]. The silk ends down through the sacral canal to the back of the second coccyx. The adult spinal cord is about 42–45 cm in length. The spinal cord has two enlargements. The upper one is called cervical enlargement, which spans from the third segment of the cervical spinal cord to the second segment of the thoracic spinal cord, and is the thickest at the sixth segment of the cervical spinal cord; the lower one is called lumbar enlargement, starting from the ninth segment of the thoracic spinal cord to the spinal cord cone. The cone is the thickest at the 12th thoracic vertebra. The formation of these two swellings is related to the appearance of limbs and is caused by the increase in neurons inside the spinal cord. There are six longitudinal grooves parallel to each other on the surface of the spinal cord. The deep sulcus in the middle of the front is called the anterior (ventral) median fissure. There is an anterior (ventral) lateral sulcus on the anterolateral side, and the anterior root goes out between them. There is a shallow groove in the middle of the back, called the posterior (dorsal) median sulcus, and its posterolateral (dorsal) lateral sulcus, from which the posterior root fibers enter the spinal cord. Between the posterior median sulcus and the posterolateral sulcus, there is also the posterior median sulcus. The anterior and posterior root fibers converge at the intervertebral foramen to form spinal nerves. Before confluence, an enlarged spinal ganglion is formed at the posterior root, which contains pseudo-unipolar sensory neurons. In total, spinal cord comprises 31 pairs of spinal nerves. The part of the spinal cord corresponding to each pair of spinal nerves is called the spinal cord. There are 31 segments, including 8 cervical segments, 12 thoracic segments, 5 lumbar segments, 5 sacral segments, and 1 tail section.

7.1.2 PERIPHERAL NERVE SYSTEM

The PNS is composed of nerve fibers and neuron cell bodies outside the CNS [5] (Figure 7.1b). There is a reciprocating fiber connection between the PNS and the CNS. The neurons of the PNS form a bridge connecting the CNS and the peripheral structures. Bundles of nerve fibers (axons) in the PNS are enveloped by connective tissue, forming a single peripheral nerve. When observed in vivo, it appears as a strong and whitish cord-like structure. Neurons outside the CNS gather in ganglia, such as spinal ganglia. PNS consists of three parts: (1) axon, (2) myelin sheath, and (3) endoneurium composed of connective tissue. There are two forms of myelin sheath based on the two types of nerve fibers. The myelin sheath of myelinated nerve fibers is formed by continuous Schwann cells arranged in order and enveloping a single axon. Myelin cells do not produce sphingomyelin. Most of the nerve fibers located in the skin are unmyelinated. Since the nerve fibers are supported and protected by three layers of connective tissue membranes, the peripheral nerves are relatively strong and flexible. The three-layered film includes a thin layer of loose connective tissue membrane surrounding myelin cells and axons in the endoneurium. The perineurium wraps the connective tissue membrane of each bundle of nerve fibers, which has a barrier effect on substances entering and exiting the peripheral nerve fibers. The epineurium is a thick and loose connective tissue membrane surrounding multiple nerve bundles, which constitutes the outermost layer of the nerve and contains adipose tissue, blood vessels, and lymphatic vessels.

7.2 INJURY IN NERVE SYSTEM

In the CNS, the global prevalence of neurodegenerative diseases is increasing every year due to the increase in the proportion of the aging population and the incidence of CNS damage [6]. Typical examples of neurological disorders include acute trauma (such as brain trauma, spinal cord injury (SCI)), neurodegenerative diseases (such as Alzheimer's disease, Huntington's disease, Parkinson's disease), or neurodevelopmental disorders (such as autism and microcephaly) [7,8]. Brain injuries can be caused by stroke and craniocerebral injury. A stroke is a group of diseases whose main clinical manifestations are cerebral ischemia and hemorrhagic injury. It is also called a stroke or cerebrovascular accident. It has very high mortality and disability rate. Stroke is mainly divided into hemorrhagic stroke (cerebral hemorrhage or subarachnoid hemorrhage) and ischemic stroke (cerebral infarction, cerebral thrombosis). Cerebral infarction is the most common type of stroke. Stroke is acute and has a high mortality rate, making it one of the most important fatal diseases in the world. Craniocerebral injury can easily lead to neurological deficits, which is the main cause of disability or death in patients [9,10]. After the patient's cranial nerves are injured, serious problems such as blood–brain barrier damage, cerebral ischemia and hypoxia, cerebral edema, local circulatory disorders, or intracranial pressure surges can occur. Cranial nerve damage is mainly ascribed to trauma, tumor, vascular disease, surgical damage, and the invasive injury of surgery. Brain injury can lead to hemiplegia, aphasia, difficulty in movement, numbness, and other symptoms in patients.

SCI often leads to paralysis of the limbs below the injury level, incontinence, and sexual dysfunction [11]. Due to the different stages of injury, SCI can be divided into primary and secondary SCI. Primary SCI is directly caused by the immediate injury, and the magnitude of the violence is closely related to the severity of the SCI. Pathologically, extensive edema can appear in the spinal cord after injury [12,13]. Due to the bony limitation of the spinal canal, the dura mater and pia mater, nerve compression, and intramedullary edema can be further aggravated, leading to spinal cord and spinal canal. The circulatory disturbances of the epidural veins and spinal cord arteries and veins cause spinal cord ischemia, edema, hemorrhage, and necrosis.

In PNS, peripheral nerve injuries (PNIs) caused by traffic accidents, work-related injuries, wars, earthquakes, and clinical surgical accidents seriously impact patient's life and health [14]. PNIs can be divided into open injury and non-open injury. The former is generally accompanied by open injury of soft tissues, causing partial or full amputation of nerves; the latter is complicated by blunt non-open injuries of soft tissues, causing contusion, compression or stretching of nerve trunks, and small occurrences in nerves hemorrhage and edema, myelin edema, and degeneration. The result of PNI is mainly clinically manifested as nerve paralysis. The symptoms of PNI mainly include (1) sensory dysfunction: weakened or lost sensation manifested as a weakened or disappeared pain response during skin injury; (2) motor dysfunction: the motor function of the muscles and tendons innervated by the nerves is weakened or lost, which is manifested by the weakness of muscles and tendons, and the loss of the ability to fix the limbs and automatically stretch; (3) muscle atrophy: neurotrophic disorders and inadequate movement of the affected limb cause the muscles to atrophy for some time after the disease, which is manifested as muscle depression and shrinkage [15,16].

7.3 TREATMENT OF SCI AND PNI USING TISSUE ENGINEERING METHODS

7.3.1 TREATMENT OF SCI

Rehabilitation of the injured spinal cord is an unsolved medical problem today [17,18]. The reason is that the human CNS only has extremely weak viability, and various pathophysiological activities and metabolites are involved in causing the microenvironmental changes, which are not conducive to the regeneration of nerve axons. In recent years, cell transplantation, tissue engineering, transfer gene technology, and other treatment methods have been used to repair SCI [19–23]. Among these, nerve tissue engineering technology has made great progress in repairing SCI and promoting functional rehabilitation. Biomaterials scaffold can effectively reduce the injury reaction in the early stage of SCI, inhibit the inflammatory response and the formation of glial scars in the injured area, and improve the spinal cord [24,25]. Implantation of biomaterials scaffolds can induce regeneration of endogenous neural stem cells. It can also be used as a support matrix for inducing cell migration, proliferation, and differentiation after implantation at the injured site, while isolating or reducing local glial scar invasion, as well as promoting and guiding the regeneration of axons. Using biomaterials scaffolds as drug carriers can control the release of drugs longer and is more accessible, which is conducive to the long-term nutrition and functional recovery of the spinal cord [26]. The ideal spinal cord scaffold material needs to have the following characteristics [27,28]: good tissue biocompatibility, reduced transplantation failure caused by rejection, specific mechanics, easy to process with plasticity, appropriate degradation rate, non-reducible, three-dimensional configuration with appropriate pore size and porosity, good for mass exchange, cell adhesion growth, high surface area to volume ratio, facilitating cell adhesion, and growth and cell-specific gene expression. Until now, various natural biological scaffolds including natural fibers, biological tissues, structural proteins and biominerals, and artificial synthetic scaffold (as opposed to "natural materials") have been used for preparing scaffolds in SCI treatment. Natural biological scaffolds with good biocompatibility, non-toxicity, good degradation products, and good adhesion have become a research focus [29–31].

7.3.2 TREATMENT OF PNI

Currently, autologous nerve transplantation is considered a gold standard for PNI. However, long-segment (>30 mm) nerve defects is one of the urgent problems in the medical field [32]. Studies have shown that although the peripheral nerve has a certain regeneration ability, due to the low efficiency of this regeneration ability, it is easily blocked by the surrounding scars, which disperses the regenerated axons and forms neuroma, as well as further hinders nerve repair [33,34]. With the development of tissue engineering in recent years, tissue-engineered nerve scaffolds containing seed cells and growth factors, as important components of the microenvironment, play a huge role in the treatment of PNI [35]. Implanting functional seed cells into nerve scaffolds to repair nerve defects can often achieve a good repair effect similar to autologous nerve transplantation [36,37]. Nerve grafts mainly include autologous non-neural materials such as blood vessels and muscles, naturally degradable macromolecular materials including collagen, chitosan, hyaluronic acid, and artificial synthetic materials including polylactic acid-polyglycolic acid copolymer (PLGA), polycaprolactone (PCL), polyglycolic acid (PGA), etc. [38,39]. The functional seed cells implanted in the nerve scaffold can secrete growth factors and extracellular matrix molecules [40], provide a favorable microenvironment for nerve regeneration, and further accelerate nerve regeneration. These cells mainly include olfactory

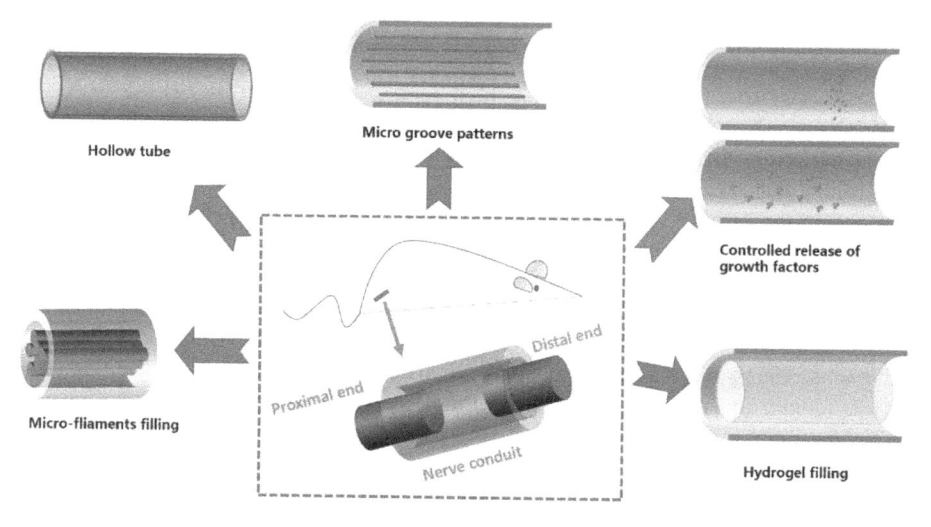

FIGURE 7.2   Nerve conduit with various inner structures for peripheral nerve regeneration.

ensheathing cells, embryonic stem cells, neural stem cells, and Schwann cells. In addition, previous studies have shown that, when peripheral nerves are injured, various growth factors secreted by distal nerve cells support the regeneration of axons [41,42]; however, the level of growth factors secreted by cells decreases over time. Therefore, controlling the release of growth factors has become the focus of current research. Until now, various growth factors including nerve growth factor, neurotrophins-3 (NT-3), glial-derived neurotrophic factor, brain-derived neurotrophic factor, vascular endothelial growth factor, and fibroblast growth factor have been combined into nerve grafts for peripheral nerve regeneration (Figure 7.2) [43–45].

7.4   DEVELOPMENT OF NERVE IMPLANTS: PREPARATION METHODS

The ideal nerve conduit must first meet the basic requirements for nerve cell growth [46]: (1) conduit degradation can be synchronized with nerve recovery, and complete degradation; (2) good histocompatibility and non-toxicity; (3) the inner surface should promote the growth of regenerative nerves and should be prone to cell growth and adhesion; (4) the wall needs to have selective permeability and can absorb nutrients from external tissues; (5) good physical and mechanical properties and flexibility; and (6) easy to process and plasticize [47]. For natural or synthetic materials with good thermal stability, a single-channel nerve conduit can be directly prepared by melt casting. For polymers with poor thermal stability, a suitable solvent should be selected, and a spinning coating method combined with air drying can be used to prepare a single sheet or channeled nerve conduits. In addition, nerve conduits can be prepared by conventional methods such as electrospinning and phase separation (Figure 7.3) [48–50]. Single-channel hollow nerve conduits are commonly used

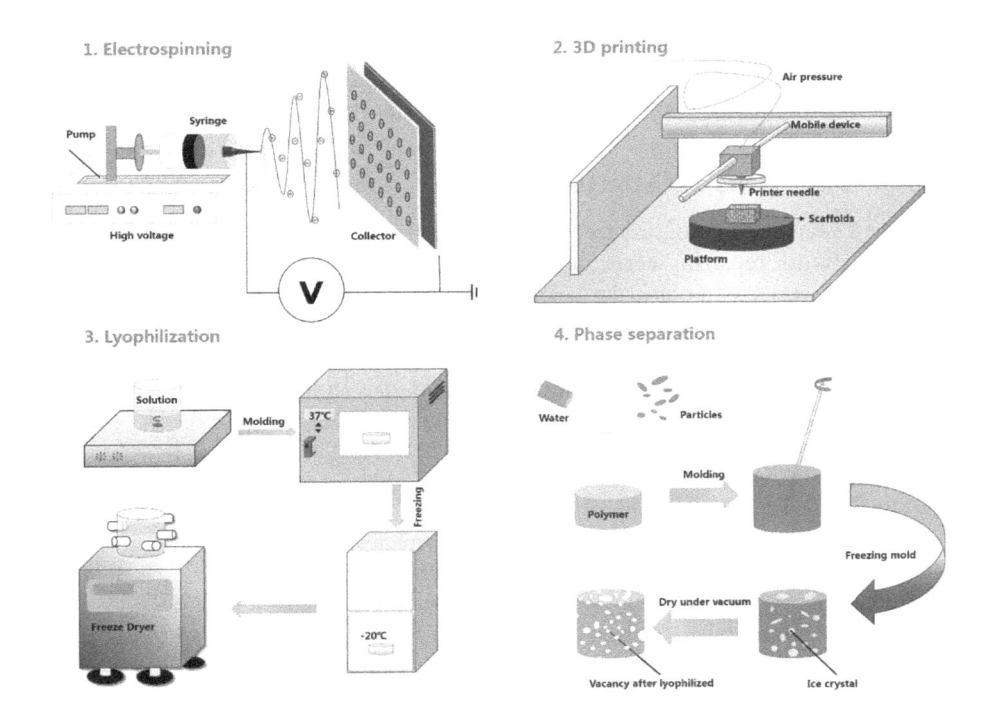

FIGURE 7.3 Commonly used preparation methods of artificial nerve implants.

for short-term nerve injury treatments of less than 30 mm. To treat long-term nerve defects, it is necessary to improve the structural and functional design of the nerve conduit [51]. Multichannel nerve conduits have multiple smaller diameter channels, which can mimic the structure of the nerve bundle and provide guidance for nerve growth. Multichannel nerve conduits can reduce the dispersion of regenerative nerves to some extent [52]. However, multichannel nerve conduits do not exhibit significant neurorestorative advantages over single-channel nerve conduits. This indicates that the number of channels and the diameter of the multichannel nerve conduit need to be further designed to be similar to the size of the actual nerve bundle [53]. Compared with single-channel nerve conduits, multichannel nerve conduits have a higher specific surface area, which facilitates cell adhesion, nutrient adsorption, and transport, as well as enhances axonal regeneration [54]. However, it cannot be ignored that multiple channels with more channel walls may reduce the permeability of the conduit to some extent. Therefore, the influence of the number of channels and the diameter of the channel on nerve regeneration need to be studied [55]. The defect is that in the absence of exogenous support, the formation of fibrin bundles and Büngner bands becomes difficult, which makes it difficult for the regenerative nerve bundle to grow to the distal end of the fracture. Therefore, filling the biological material inside the nerve conduit tube, such as fiber and gel, can facilitate the adhesion, proliferation, and migration of Schwann cells inside the tube cavity, as well as promote axonal regeneration [56,57]. However, filling the material in the lumen inevitably reduces the volume in the lumen. If the density of the filling material is large or the degradation time of the filling material does not match the rate of nerve regeneration, the filling material hinders nerve regeneration to a certain extent [58,59].

7.5 3D PRINTING TECHNOLOGY

In recent years, great progress has been made in the fabrication of tissue-engineered nerve grafts for repairing nerve defects. 3D printing is a kind of rapid prototyping technology, which can construct objects by layer-by-layer printing based on digital model files and using adhesive materials such as powder metal or plastic [60,61]. 3D bioprinting is a family of enabling technologies that can be used to manufacture human organs with predefined hierarchical structures, material constituents, and physiological functions [62]. 3D in vitro neural tissue models provide a better recapitulation in vivo cell-cell and cell-extracellular matrix interactions than conventional two-dimensional (2D) cultures [63,64]. Different 3D culture systems, such as cell biology-based models (spheroids and organoids) and engineering-based models (scaffold and microfluidic platforms), have been widely explored for their ability to generate more faithful neural tissue-like structures that incorporate diverse cell types and materials, as well as both physical and biochemical signals [65–67].

The application of 3D printing technology in the field of biomedicine has been rapidly developed in recent years, with good development prospects and great social value [68–70]. Until now, various types of 3D printing techniques have been developed [71], including (1) fused deposition technology: the filamentous material is heated and melted in the nozzle, and then solidified using the extrusion nozzle to form a cross-section [72]; (2) liquid phase in combination with inkjet technology: the nozzle squeezes out the liquid binder to bond the powder material of the stage to form a cross-section; (3) selective laser curing technology: the laser selectively cures the powder material or the photosensitive material to form a cross-section; (4) bioprinting technology: the nozzle pushes the cell and liquid material composites under high pressure to form a cross-section. The use of 3D printing technology requires the construction of models (biological structures), preparation of materials (bio-ink), and selection of suitable printers. For example, Mouser et al. [73] showed that low polymer concentrations are too high to form defined filaments at 15°C–37°C using fused deposition techniques; the material exhibited shear thinning behavior. On the other hand, high polymer concentration formed a too hard hydrogel at 37°C and could not be mixed with the cells. Zheng et al. [74] used a 3D bioprinter to prepare a hydrogel using silk/polyethylene glycol (PEG) as a 3D-printed self-standing bio-ink. The "bio-ink" they used was biocompatible and could directly mix with cells, and the filled mesh cylinder structure printed by this technology retained its original shape after being implanted in mice for 6 weeks, and the cells grew well in the material. Extrusion-based bioprinting can fabricate 2D and 3D structures by continuous dispersion of a hydrogel containing cells through a micronozzle [75]. Marga et al. [76] introduced a bioprinting technique based on a decellularized organ matrix. The self-assembly of agarose, BMSCs, and SCs has been discussed in detail, and the bio-ink made of SC (10%) and BMSC (90%) has been bio-assembled and bio-printed to form a 2-mm diameter conduit. Zhu et al. [77] introduced a circular porous network support structure with the help of stereolithography-based 3D bioprinting technology. The print of the support was nano-bio-ink, which was made of gelatin methacrylamide (GelMA), containing neural stem cells and bioactive graphene nanoplatelets. The scaffolds could target nerve tissue regeneration. After 2 weeks of culture, neural stem cells showed neuronal differentiation and neurite elongation in the printed construct. Sarig-Nadir et al. [78] used laser light-emitting 3D printing technology to prepare 3D tissue engineering scaffolds based on the micropatterning method. They proved that focused laser ablation caused by pulsed laser could produce guiding structures in transparent hydrogels, which could direct the orientation growth of dorsal root ganglion neurites.

7.6 MODELS FOR 3D PRINTING

Tissue engineering aims at creating bioactive constructs to replace damaged or diseased tissue and rehabilitate the complex function of natural human tissue [79]. The design principle of the models of 3D printed neural structures is usually determined by basic principles, including easy to print, cell types [80], mechanical properties [81–84], porosity [85], tissue characteristics [86,87], and biochemical and physical gradients. Until now, various designed models have been used for 3D printing, including hollow cylindrical structure and cube structure. Wang et al. [88] successfully combined the MoS2 nanosheets with 3D printing technology and hydrothermal method to prepare a hollow cylindrical stent for tumor treatment and tissue regeneration. This scaffold was designed to facilitate the attachment, proliferation, and osteogenic differentiation of bone mesenchymal stem cells and induce bone regeneration in vivo. They demonstrated that this versatile biomaterial could be used in a variety of tissue engineering methods for treatment and tissue regeneration. Akkineni et al. [89] used a composite of 16.7% by weight of alginate and 2% or 3% by weight of gellan gum (GG) as bio-ink and used 3D mapping method based on extrusion-based multi-functional AM technology to successfully prepare a 25-layer height cube structure composite. The scaffold showed improved stiffness and cell attachment compared to the pure alginate scaffold, and the composite scaffolds showed support for hMSC proliferation and early osteogenic differentiation, making it attractive for tissue engineering applications. Wu et al. [90] formulated 1.5% GG and 10% poly(ethylene glycol) diacrylate (PEGDA) composite biomaterial for printing double-network hydrogels based on extruded cell 3D bios structure. They printed five-pointed stars, even human ears and noses, which had high fidelity and could be UV cross-linked to improve mechanical properties, and ultimately achieved permanent stability. BMSCs and MC3T3-E1 cells encapsulated in GG/PEGDA hydrogels showed a higher percentage of viable cells above 87% during the 21-day 3D culture. The study demonstrated that GG/PEGDA dual-network hydrogels had significant print potential for human-scale biological tissues and organs. Ning et al. [91] bioprinted Schwann cell-encapsulated scaffolds using alginate, fibrin, hyaluronic acid, and/or RGD peptide composite hydrogels to obtain spliced multi-network structures, cubes, and cylinder at different angles. The distribution of Schwann cells and the concentration of fibrin were regulated to obtain a suitable hydrogel combination. The results showed that the printed scaffold could promote the arrangement of Schwann cells in the scaffold, thus providing tactile cues to guide the extension of the dorsal root ganglion neurites along the printed scaffolds, indicating great potential for application in the field of neural tissue engineering. Akkineni et al. [92] used a 3D printed coaxial needle to print a mechanically stable and robust hydrogel 3D core/shell (c/s) stent using a high concentration (16.7 wt%) of alginate as a hard shell and low concentration, soft biopolymer as the core. The scaffold had open pores connected, and both the core and the shell could be loaded with growth factors, and the living cells could be wrapped in the core material. Visser et al. [93–95] used additive manufacturing technology (AM) to prepare several complex anatomies by composite deposition of polyvinyl alcohol, poly-ε-caprolactone, gelatin methacrylamide/GG, and alginate hydrogel. The prepared scaffolds were porous and could encapsulate living cells for use in tissue regeneration. Ahlfeld et al. [96] used 3D drawing technology to prepare scaffolds containing calcium phosphate cement (CPC) [97,98], alginate, and GG. The printed model was designed as a cylinder with a double layer, and alternate corner replacement was formed. Such a structural design allowed the hydrogel to swell without closing the large pores. Costa printed [98] a crescent-shaped structural scaffold by 3D bioprinting fast-curing enzyme cross-linked silk fibroin (SF), which had good mechanical properties, facilitated adhesion of living cells, and could be degraded in vivo. Moreover, the scaffolds could be adjusted to meet the pore structure for cell growth.

7.7 MATERIALS AS "BIO-INK" FOR 3D PRINTING

Bio-inks are biomaterial solutions containing living cells and are key components in 3D printing. Generally, various biocompatible and cell-friendly natural or synthetic biomaterials can be used as "bio-ink" for 3D printing [99–101]. The materials present in the biomaterial solution must protect the cells against stress during the printing process. In addition, bio-ink should provide a stable 3D structure for cell adhesion and growth during tissue development. Due to the above properties, the requirements for bio-ink are also very high. Bio-ink must have printability, shear-thinning behavior, swelling ratio, in vivo degradation, surface tension, and gelation kinetics [101–103]. The four main types of bio-ink materials are hydrogels, microcarriers, cell aggregates, and decellularized matrix components [104]. In addition to the bioprinting techniques chosen for the targeted tissue requirements, appropriate bio-ink selection, including cells, biomaterials, and biochemical signals, is necessary for the successful fabrication [105]. For example, Zheng et al. [74] used silk/PEG hydrogel as bio-ink for tissue engineering 3D printing. Mixing PEG with silk led to the formation of a silk β-sheet structure, which led to gelation and water insolubility through physical cross-linking. This biocompatible hybrid bio-ink could be used to print various constructs with high resolution, high shape fidelity, and a uniform gel matrix. Because the material is cell-friendly, it could also pre-mix human cells with silk solution before printing, and then form the ideal 3D structure to provide a suitable microenvironment for cell growth [74,106,107]. Zhang et al. [108] used PCL and PLCL as bio-inks and used 3D bioprinting technology to fabricate cell-wrapped urethral scaffolds in vitro. This spiral scaffold exhibited the same mechanical properties as the natural scaffold, and the cells could survive 7 days after printing. These results laid the foundation for further research on 3D bioprinting of urethral structure. Costa

TABLE 7.1

A Summary of the Basic Conditions Including Models and "Bio-ink" for 3D Printing Applied in the Field of Tissue Engineering

Materials "Bio-ink"	Cell Type	Models	Culture Period	Functional Evaluation	Ref
Gelatin methacrylate (GelMA) and poly(ethyleneglycol) diacrylate (PEGDA)	Schwann cells platelet	Cylinder tube	6 weeks	Nerve regeneration	[110]
PCL/rGO	PC12 cells	Cuboid scaffold	7 days	Sciatic nerve regeneration	[111]
Silk fibroin	Human adipose-derived stem cells (hASCs)	Cuboid Half moon	7 days	Nerve Regeneration	[109]
Poly(2-hydroxyethyl) methacrylate (pHEMA)	Dorsal root ganglion (DRG)	Cuboid	14 days	Nerve Regeneration	[112]
PCL/PAA	PC12 cells	Cylinder tube	7 days	Neural differentiation	[113]
GelMa/LAP	PC12 cells Schwann cells	Tube	12 weeks	Nerve regeneration	[114]
PPy and Polycaprolactone (PPy-b-PCL)	Human embryonic stem cell-derived neural crest stem cells (hESC-NCSCs)	Cuboid scaffold	5 days	Neural differentiation	[115]
Alginate, fibrin, hyaluronic acid	Schwann cells	Star cuboid	10 days	Nerve tissue engineering	[91]
Gelatin and graphene	Mesenchymal stem cell (MSCs)	Cuboid scaffold	7 days	Neural differentiation	[116]

et al. [109] developed a fast-curing enzyme cross-linked SF bio-ink for 3D bioprinting. The bio-ink after enzyme cross-linking exhibited a unique ability to produce a hydrogel with good resolution, repeatability, and mechanical strength following tissue engineering and nerve regeneration. This bio-ink was environmentally friendly and simple to be constructed and was proven to be suitable for nerve regeneration. A summary of the basic conditions including models and "bio-ink" for 3D printing applied in the field of tissue engineering is shown in Table 7.1.

7.8 APPLICATION OF 3D PRINTING IN NERVE REGENERATION

Globally, the prevalence of neurodegenerative diseases caused by CNS damage is increasing, and many CNS diseases such as Parkinson's syndrome and Alzheimer's disease are caused by neurodegenerative processes [117,118]. However, there is currently no effective way to treat these neurodegenerative diseases. Cell transplantation therapy provides a new approach to the treatment of neurodegenerative diseases

[119]. However, the limitation is that cells may be easily released from the lesion site. As a powerful tool, 3D bioprinting technology could be used to deliver cells in scaffolds for long-term treatment of CNS diseases [120,121]. The scaffolds encapsulated with cells could not only support tissue growth but also provide cell transplantation therapy for a long time. Hsieh et al. [122] successfully prepared a thermostable and biodegradable polyurethane hydrogel with neural stem cells loading by 3D bioprinting. The two thermally responsive hydrogels they synthesized were biodegradable polyurethane dispersions (PU1 and PU2) that could be gelled at around 37°C without the need for any cross-linkers. Interestingly, the stiffness of this hydrogel could be easily fine-tuned by increasing or decreasing the solid content of the dispersion. NSC in 25%–30% PU2 hydrogel (680–2,400 Pa) had excellent proliferation and differentiation ability, while not in 25%–30% PU1 hydrogel. Finally, after implantation of a 3D-printed 25% PU2 construct carrying NSC to zebrafish, the function of the adult zebrafish with brain injury was restored. In addition, 3D printing can be tailored to realize personalized treatment according to the patient's needs [123]. Lee et al. [124] combined stereolithography and electrospinning using synthetic materials and natural materials as bio-inks to create new 3D biomimetic nerve scaffolds with adjustable porous structure and embedded array fibers. The scaffold was embedded in a 3D-printed hydrogel scaffold by a microfiber composed of a PCL polymer and PCL mixed with gelatin. The results showed that the electrospun 3D-printed stent significantly improved the adhesion of neural stem cells compared to the unspun 3D printed stent, and the PCL/gelatin fiber scaffold greatly increased the primary cortical neurons. Gu et al. [125] used direct writing 3D printing technology to print polysaccharide-based bio-inks (alginate, agarose, and carboxymethyl chitosan), which supported in situ hNSC expansion and differentiation. After cross-linking, it rapidly gelled to form a porous 3D scaffold with a network structure inside. The scaffold was proven to be suitable for neuronal and non-neuronal structures. Lozano et al. [105, 126] used a simple hand-printed bioprinting 3D device to print brain-like structures. It is worth mentioning that the brain-like structure was composed of discrete layers of primary nerve cells wrapped in a hydrogel. The biological ink used in this experiment was an RGD gel (RGD-GG) composed of a novel peptide-modified biopolymer GG. This experiment proved that the neuron cells encapsulated in the hydrogel were not significantly different from hydrogel without the printing step after being molded by 3D printing technology. However, the application of 3D printing in the treatment of CNS diseases is still under development. More work needs to be done in this field to realize the advantages and disadvantages of 3D printing for patients with Parkinson's syndrome and Alzheimer's disease.

In contrast, 3D printing has been widely applied in the field of peripheral nerve regeneration [127,128]. The GelMA hydrogel was used to print a multichannel hydrogel conduit with an outer diameter of 6mm and a length of 5mm, aiming for repairing large gap nerve injury [129]. Zhu et al. [130] prepared the prepolymer solution by dissolving GelMA, poly(ethyleneglycol)diacrylate (PEGDA), and phenyl-2,4,6-trimethylbenzoylphosphinate (LAP) in different ratios in phosphate-buffered saline. The prepared prepolymer solution was printed through a digital light processing-based fast continuous 3D printing platform to print NGC with microchannels and cannulas, which were highly emulated human-sized branch facial nerves. Subsequently, a complete transection of the sciatic nerve by implanting NGC into a mouse model in vivo showed that the sciatic nerve could be effectively regenerated by branching into the microchannel and extending to the distal end of the injury site. Evangelista et al. [131] used 3D printing methods of stereolithography to create a new type of PEG conduit. The conduit is divided into two groups, one is a single cavity and the other is a multi-lumen. This compares the ability of the conduit to promote peripheral nerve regeneration. The sciatic nerve trauma of 10 mm in Sprague Dawley rats showed that the PEG nerve conduit produced by single-chamber stereolithography promoted nerve regeneration, and the number of regenerating axons was close to normal nerves. A composite hydrogel containing fibrin, alginate, and hyaluronic acid/RGD peptide was prepared using 3D printing technology. The effect of the scaffold on the Schwann cells was evaluated after wrapping cells in the composite hydrogel. The results showed that the alignment of cells in the scaffold could be promoted, indicating potential application in neural tissue engineering [91].

7.9 FURTHER CONSIDERATION BEYOND 3D PRINTING IN NERVE REGENERATION

Successful 3D bioprinting must overcome the following specific technical problems [132]. (1) Cell selection. What type of cells to choose is very important when 3D bioprinting related biological tissues or organs. Different tissues of the human body are made of a combination of unique cells. The liver mainly contains hepatocytes and the heart mainly contains cardiomyocytes. Therefore, not all tissue-specific cells can be isolated and cultured in vitro, and not all cells can maintain their biological activity after the 3D bioprinting process. So, how to optimize cell separation, culture, and value-added technology is the predetermined condition to ensure the success of 3D bioprinting. (2) Biomaterials. Different tissues and organs of the human body have their own physical and mechanical properties. The softness of the skin and the rigidity of the bone tissue make it necessary to use suitable biomaterials corresponding to the characteristics of the tissues during the 3D printing process of different tissues, and these materials need to maintain the biological activity and function of the selected cells to the greatest extent [133]. More importantly, the selected material must be able to be manipulated by the 3D printing system. This makes the selection of biomaterials very challenging and requires continuous optimization and improvement during the printing process. (3) Manufacturing platform. Currently used in 3D bioprinting platforms are mainly including laser-based injection, inkjet-based printing, and extrusion-based extrusion [134]. Each of the three platforms has its advantages and disadvantages and different special functions, as well as the demand for hardware technology. How to choose the platform reasonably according to the different tissues and organs that need to be manufactured is also key to the success of 3D bioprinting [135]. These three platforms have been used in traditional printing or 3D manufacturing systems, so it is more critical to understand how to integrate them with the bio-manufacturing system to maximize its effectiveness while maintaining the biological activity of cells and the physical properties of biomaterials, as well as ensuring that the products meet the standards of medical applications, which must be overcome and continuously optimized.

In addition, most human tissues and organs have a vascular system, and sufficient blood supply is needed to maintain biological activity [136]. However, the current 3D bioprinting technology is not yet fully capable of producing substitutes with functions equivalent to the human vascular system, let alone fusing the vascular system into 3D-printed tissue. If there is no corresponding vascular system, even if similar organ replacements can be made, they cannot survive for a long time [137]. Therefore, the use of organ transplantation to rescue patients with organ failure can only be an illusion. In the opinion of the respondent, 3D bioprinting of tissues and organs with the vascular system and being able to integrate with the entire blood circulation system of the human body is the biggest challenge and difficulty in achieving the ultimate goal [138].

7.10 FUTURE REMARKS

In this chapter, we have briefly summarized the injuries in the nerve system, including CNS and PNS, and the bio-engineering methods for treating these injuries. Among these, the development and application of 3D printing were mainly introduced for nerve regeneration. Initially, in the field of nerve regeneration, the application of 3D printing was limited to the PNS for constructing nerve conduits. With the development of biomaterials science in recent years, such as new generation of a type of bio-ink, 3D printing has been gradually applied in the treatment of SCI and traumatic brain injury. From growing literature in this field, it is clear that researchers in academic and industrial areas are interested in the advantages and challenges of 3D printing for the treatment of nerve system diseases. As a newly developed technique, 3D printing is still in its infancy, though significant progress has been made in recent years [139]. Due to the complexity, functionality, and variety in the nerve system, 3D-printed constructs for the treatment of nerve system diseases is still a major challenge. For example, different tissues (PNS, brain, spinal cord) are composed of multiple types of cells located inside with complex biochemistries and geometries of the extracellular matrix. Thus, the accurate reconstruction of the tissue structure with suitable cell location using 3D printing technology is very important for tissue regeneration and functional recovery. 3D printing can construct some sophisticated structures that better mimic in vivo microenvironment [86,105,140]. Overall, for better scaffolds printing using 3D printing technique in nerve regeneration, the scaffold design, preparation of bio-ink, and precise printing should be considered thoroughly and comprehensively. For better functional recovery of the nerve system, printing with growth factors, cells, chemical functionalization, and conductivity with suitable mechanical properties leading to printable and cell-friendly systems will pave the way for much better treatment of nerve system diseases.

AUTHOR CONTRIBUTIONS

Guicai Li conceived the idea and planned the text content. Guicai Li, Liling Zhang wrote the chapter.

FUNDING

The authors gratefully acknowledge assistance from Tiantian Zheng, Linliang Wu, and Jiawei Xu, and the financial support of the National Natural Science Foundation of China (31771054), Natural Key Science Research Program of Jiangsu Education Department (19KJA320006).

CONFLICTS OF INTEREST

The authors declare no conflict of interest.

REFERENCES

1. Ghosh, S.K. and R.K. Narayan, Anatomy of nervous system and emergence of neuroscience: A chronological journey across centuries. *Morphologie*, 2020. **104**(347): pp. 267–79.
2. Illustrations of the comparative anatomy of the nervous system. *British and Foreign Medical Review*, 1839. **8**(15): pp. 226–29.
3. Messe, A., et al., Relating structure and function in the human brain: Relative contributions of anatomy, stationary dynamics, and non-stationarities. *PLoS Computational Biology*, 2014. **10**(3): p. e1003530.
4. Sheerin, F., Spinal cord injury: Anatomy and physiology of the spinal cord. *Emergency Nurse*, 2004. **12**(8): pp. 30–6.
5. Goldstein, B., Anatomy of the peripheral nervous system. *Physical Medicine and Rehabilitation Clinics of North America*, 2001. **12**(2): pp. 207–36.
6. Katzman, R., The prevalence and malignancy of alzheimer disease a major killer. *Alzheimers & Dementia*, 2008. **4**(6): pp. 378–80.
7. Akhtar, A., et al., Neurodegenerative diseases and effective drug delivery: A review of challenges and novel therapeutics. *Journal of Controlled Release*, 2021. **330**: pp. 1152–1167.
8. Emard, J.F., J.P. Thouez, and D. Gauvreau, Neurodegenerative diseases and risk factors: A literature review. *Social Science & Medicine*, 1995. **40**(6): pp. 847–58.
9. Brawanski, N., et al., Cerebral foreign body granuloma in brain triggering generalized seizures without obvious craniocerebral injury: A case report and review of the literature. *Surgical Neurology International*, 2016. **7**(Suppl 29): pp. S775–8.
10. Manifold, S.L., Craniocerebral trauma. A review of primary and secondary injury and therapeutic modalities. *Focus on Critical Care*, 1986. **13**(2): pp. 22–35.
11. Gorman, P.H., The review of systems in spinal cord injury and dysfunction. *Continuum (Minneap Minn)*, 2011. **17**(3 Neurorehabilitation): pp. 630–4.
12. He, B. and G. Nan, Pulmonary edema and hemorrhage after acute spinal cord injury in rats. *Spine Journal*, 2016. **16**(4): pp. 547–51.
13. Kobrine, A.I., T.F. Doyle, and H.V. Rizzoli, A method for estimating edema in experimental traumatic spinal cord injury. *Experimental Neurology*, 1976. **50**(1): pp. 240–5.
14. Zhu, W., et al., 3D nano/microfabrication techniques and nanobiomaterials for neural tissue regeneration, *Nanomedicine*, 2014. **9**(6): pp. 859–75.
15. Lim, T.K., et al., Peripheral nerve injury induces persistent vascular dysfunction and endoneurial hypoxia, contributing to the genesis of neuropathic pain. *Journal of Neuroscience*, 2015. **35**(8): pp. 3346–59.
16. Kraft, G.H., Fibrillation potential amplitude and muscle atrophy following peripheral nerve injury. *Muscle Nerve*, 1990. **13**(9): pp. 814–21.

17. Christodoulou, V.N., et al., Rehabilitation of the multiple injured patient with spinal cord injury: A systematic review of the literature. *Injury*, 2019. **50**(11): pp. 1847–52.

18. Stover, S.L., Review of forty years of rehabilitation issues in spinal cord injury. *Journal of Spinal Cord Medicine*, 1995. **18**(3): pp. 175–82.

19. Hodgetts, S.I., et al., Cortical AAV-CNTF gene therapy combined with intraspinal mesenchymal precursor cell transplantation promotes functional and morphological outcomes after spinal cord injury in adult rats. *Neural Plasticity*, 2018. **2018**: p. 9828725.

20. Blesch, A. and M.H. Tuszynski, Gene therapy and cell transplantation for Alzheimer's disease and spinal cord injury. *Yonsei Medical Journal*, 2004. **45 Suppl**: pp. 28–31.

21. Bedir, T., et al., 3D bioprinting applications in neural tissue engineering for spinal cord injury repair. *Materials Science & Engineering C-Materials for Biological Applications*, 2020. **110**: p. 110741.

22. Dumont, C.M., D.J. Margul, and L.D. Shea, Tissue engineering approaches to modulate the inflammatory milieu following spinal cord injury. *Cells Tissues Organs*, 2016. **202**(1–2): pp. 52–66.

23. Talac, R., et al., Animal models of spinal cord injury for evaluation of tissue engineering treatment strategies. *Biomaterials*, 2004. **25**(9): pp. 1505–10.

24. Guo, S., et al., Prevascularized scaffolds bearing human dental pulp stem cells for treating complete spinal cord injury. *Advanced Healthcare Materials*, 2020. **9**(20): p. e2000974.

25. Li, X., et al., Promotion of neuronal differentiation of neural progenitor cells by using EGFR antibody functionalized collagen scaffolds for spinal cord injury repair. *Biomaterials*, 2013. **34**(21): pp. 5107–16.

26. Faccendini, A., et al., Nanofiber scaffolds as drug delivery systems to bridge spinal cord injury. *Pharmaceuticals (Basel)*, 2017. **10**(3): pp. 63-93.

27. Shi, B., et al., Multifunctional three-dimensional scaffolds for treatment of spinal cord injury. *Journal of Controlled Release*, 2015. **213**: pp. e12–e23.

28. Kim, M., S.R. Park, and B.H. Choi, Biomaterial scaffolds used for the regeneration of spinal cord injury (SCI). *Histology and Histopathology*, 2014. **29**(11): pp. 1395–408.

29. Papa, S., et al., Regenerative medicine for spinal cord injury: Focus on stem cells and biomaterials. *Expert Opinion on Biological Therapy*, 2020. **20**(10): pp. 1203–13.

30. Haggerty, A.E., I. Maldonado-Lasuncion, and M. Oudega, Biomaterials for revascularization and immunomodulation after spinal cord injury. *Biomedical Materials*, 2018. **13**(4): p. 044105.

31. Tsintou, M., K. Dalamagkas, and A.M. Seifalian, Advances in regenerative therapies for spinal cord injury: A biomaterials approach. *Neural Regeneration Research*, 2015. **10**(5): pp. 726–42.

32. Colsa Gutierrez, P., et al., Intraoperative peripheral nerve injury in colorectal surgery. An update. *Cirugía Española*, 2016. **94**(3): pp. 125–36.

33. Li, R., et al., Chitosan conduit combined with hyaluronic acid prevent sciatic nerve scar in a rat model of peripheral nerve crush injury. *Molecular Medicine Reports*, 2018. **17**(3): pp. 4360–8.

34. Pasterkamp, R.J., P.N. Anderson, and J. Verhaagen, Peripheral nerve injury fails to induce growth of lesioned ascending dorsal column axons into spinal cord scar tissue expressing the axon repellent Semaphorin3A. *European Journal of Neuroscience*, 2001. **13**(3): pp. 457–71.

35. Zhang, P.X., et al., Tissue engineering for the repair of peripheral nerve injury. *Neural Regeneration Research*, 2019. **14**(1): pp. 51–8.

36. Jones, I., et al., Regenerative effects of human embryonic stem cell-derived neural crest cells for treatment of peripheral nerve injury. *Journal of Tissue Engineering and Regenerative Medicine*, 2018. **12**(4): pp. e2099–109.

37. Craff, M.N., et al., Embryonic stem cell-derived motor neurons preserve muscle after peripheral nerve injury. *Plastic and Reconstructive Surgery*, 2007. **119**(1): pp. 235–45.

38. Daly, W., et al., A biomaterials approach to peripheral nerve regeneration: Bridging the peripheral nerve gap and enhancing functional recovery. *Journal of the Royal Society Interface*, 2012. **9**(67): pp. 202–21.

39. Nectow, A.R., K.G. Marra, and D.L. Kaplan, Biomaterials for the development of peripheral nerve guidance conduits. *Tissue Engineering Part B Reviews*, 2012. **18**(1): pp. 40–50.

40. Grochmal, J. and R. Midha, Recent advances in stem cell-mediated peripheral nerve repair. *Cells Tissues Organs*, 2014. **200**(1): pp. 13–22.

41. Li, R., et al., Growth factors-based therapeutic strategies and their underlying signaling mechanisms for peripheral nerve regeneration. *Acta Pharmacologica Sinica*, 2020. **41**(10): pp. 1289–300.

42. Sarker, M.D., et al., Regeneration of peripheral nerves by nerve guidance conduits: Influence of design, biopolymers, cells, growth factors, and physical stimuli. *Progress in Neurobiology*, 2018. **171**: pp. 125–50.

43. Liu, H.M., Growth factors and extracellular matrix in peripheral nerve regeneration, studied with a nerve chamber. *Journal of the Peripheral Nervous System*, 1996. **1**(2): pp. 97–110.

44. Raivich, G. and G.W. Kreutzberg, Peripheral nerve regeneration: Role of growth factors and their receptors. *International Journal of Developmental Neuroscience*, 1993. **11**(3): pp. 311–24.

45. Lien, B.V., et al., Enhancing peripheral nerve regeneration with neurotrophic factors and bioengineered scaffolds: A basic science and clinical perspective. *Journal of the Peripheral Nervous System*, 2020. **25**(4): pp. 320–34.

46. Hsueh, Y.S., et al., Design and synthesis of elastin-like polypeptides for an ideal nerve conduit in peripheral nerve regeneration. Mater Sci Eng C Mater Biol Appl, 2014. **38**: pp. 119–26.

47. Ji, S. and M. Guvendiren. Recent advances in bioink design for 3D bioprinting of tissues and organs. *Frontiers in Bioengineering and Biotechnology*, 2017. **5**: p. 23.

48. Freier, T., et al., Controlling cell adhesion and degradation of chitosan films by N-acetylation. *Biomaterials*, 2005. **26**(29): pp. 5872–8.

49. Wang, H.B., et al., Creation of highly aligned electrospun poly-L-lactic acid fibers for nerve regeneration applications. *Journal of Neural Engineering*, 2009. **6**(1): p. 016001.

50. Chiono, V., et al., Enzymatically-modified melt-extruded guides for peripheral nerve repair. *Engineering in Life Sciences*, 2008. **8**(3): pp. 226–37.

51. Brushart, T.M., et al., Joseph H. Boyes Award. Dispersion of regenerating axons across enclosed neural gaps. *Journal of Hand Surgery (American Volume)*, 1995. **20**(4): pp. 557–64.

52. Chang, C.J. and S.H. Hsu, The effect of high outflow permeability in asymmetric poly(dl-lactic acid-co-glycolic acid) conduits for peripheral nerve regeneration. *Biomaterials*, 2006. **27**(7): pp. 1035–42.

53. Hoppen, H.J., et al., Two-ply biodegradable nerve guide: Basic aspects of design, construction and biological performance. *Biomaterials*, 1990. **11**(4): pp. 286–90.

54. Groves, M.L., et al., Axon regeneration in peripheral nerves is enhanced by proteoglycan degradation. *Experimental Neurology*, 2005. **195**(2): pp. 278–92.

55. Koh, H.S., et al., In vivo study of novel nanofibrous intra-luminal guidance channels to promote nerve regeneration. *Journal of Neural Engineering*, 2010. **7**(4): p. 046003.

56. Chen, S., et al., Characterization of topographical effects on macrophage behavior in a foreign body response model. Biomaterials, 2010. **31**(13): pp. 3479–91.

57. Yoshii, S., et al. Bridging a 30-mm nerve defect using collagen filaments. *Journal of Biomedical Materials Research Part A*, 2003. **67A**(2): pp. 467–74.

58. Ngo, T.T.B., et al., Poly(L-lactide) microfilaments enhance peripheral nerve regeneration across extended nerve lesions. *Journal of Neuroscience Research*, 2003. **72**(2): pp. 227–38.

59. Wang, X.D., et al., Dog sciatic nerve regeneration across a 30-mm defect bridged by a chitosan/PGA artificial nerve graft. *Brain*, 2005. **128**: pp. 1897–910.

60. Brivio, D., et al., 3D printing for rapid prototyping of low-Z/density ionization chamber arrays. *Medical Physics*, 2019. **46**(12): pp. 5770–79.

61. He, H.Y., et al., Rapid prototyping for tissue-engineered bone scaffold by 3D printing and biocompatibility study. *International Journal of Clinical and Experimental Medicine*, 2015. **8**(7): pp. 11777–85.

62. Wang, X.H., et al., Gelatin-based hydrogels for organ 3D bioprinting. *Polymers*, 2017. **9**(9): p. 401.

63. Bangaru, M.L.Y., et al., Growth suppression of mouse pituitary corticotroph tumor AtT20 cells by curcumin: A model for treating cushing's disease. *PLoS One*, 2010. **5**(4): pp. e9893–9.

64. Zhuang, P., et al., 3D neural tissue models: From spheroids to bioprinting. *Biomaterials*, 2018. **154**: pp. 113–33.

65. Haring, A.P., H. Sontheimer, and B.N. Johnson, Microphysiological human brain and neural systems-on-a-chip: Potential alternatives to small animal models and emerging platforms for drug discovery and personalized medicine. *Stem Cell Reviews and Reports*, 2017. **13**(3): pp. 381–406.

66. Kato-Negishi, M., et al., Millimeter-sized neural building blocks for 3D heterogeneous neural network assembly. *Advanced Healthcare Materials*, 2013. **2**(12): pp. 1564–70.

67. Jo, J., et al., Midbrain-like organoids from human pluripotent stem cells contain functional dopaminergic and neuromelanin-producing neurons. *Cell Stem Cell*, 2016. **19**(2): pp. 248–57.

68. Antman-Passig, M. and O. Shefi, Remote magnetic orientation of 3D collagen hydrogels for directed neuronal regeneration. *Nano Letters*, 2016. **16**(4): p. 2567–73.

69. Naghieh, S., et al., Combinational processing of 3D printing and electrospinning of hierarchical poly(lactic acid)/gelatin-forsterite scaffolds as a biocomposite: Mechanical and biological assessment. *Materials & Design*, 2017. **133**: pp. 128–35.

70. Naghieh, S., et al., Numerical investigation of the mechanical properties of the additive manufactured bone scaffolds fabricated by FDM: The effect of layer penetration and post-heating. *Journal of the Mechanical Behavior of Biomedical Materials*, 2016. **59**: pp. 241–50.

71. Tack, P., et al., 3D-printing techniques in a medical setting: A systematic literature review. *Biomedical Engineering Online*, 2016. **15**(1): p. 115.

72. Kim, H., et al., Gelatin/PVA scaffolds fabricated using a 3D-printing process employed with a low-temperature plate for hard tissue regeneration: Fabrication and characterizations. *International Journal of Biological Macromolecules*, 2018. **120**: pp. 119–27.

73. Mouser, V.H.M., et al., Yield stress determines bioprintability of hydrogels based on gelatin-methacryloyl and gellan gum for cartilage bioprinting. *Biofabrication*, 2016. **8**(3): p. 035003.

74. Zheng, Z.Z., et al., 3D bioprinting of self-standing silk-based bioink. *Advanced Healthcare Materials*, 2018. **7**(6): p. 1701026.

75. Seol, Y.J., et al., Bioprinting technology and its applications. *European Journal of Cardio-Thoracic Surgery*, 2014. **46**(3): pp. 342–8.

76. Marga, F., et al., Toward engineering functional organ modules by additive manufacturing. *Biofabrication*, 2012. **4**(2): p. 022001.

77. Zhu, W., B.T. Harris, and L.J.G. Zhang. Gelatin methacrylamide hydrogel with graphene nanoplatelets for neural cell-laden 3D bioprinting. *2016 38th Annual International Conference of the IEEE Engineering in Medicine and Biology Society (EMBC)*, 2016: pp. 4185–88. Florida, USA.

78. Sarig-Nadir, O., et al., Laser photoablation of guidance microchannels into hydrogels directs cell growth in three dimensions. *Biophysical Journal*, 2009. **96**(11): pp. 4743–52.

79. Lazaro, B.C.R. and J.A. Landeiro, Tectal plate tumors. *Arquivos De Neuro-Psiquiatria*, 2006. **64**(2B): pp. 432–36.

80. Benam, K.H., et al., Engineered in vitro disease models. *Annual Review of Pathology: Mechanisms of Disease*, 2015. **10**: pp. 195–262.

81. Hopkins, A.M., et al., 3D in vitro modeling of the central nervous system. *Progress in Neurobiology*, 2015. **125**: pp. 1–25.

82. Wang, C., X.M. Tong, and F. Yang, Bioengineered 3D brain tumor model to elucidate the effects of matrix stiffness on glioblastoma cell behavior using PEG-based hydrogels. *Molecular Pharmaceutics*, 2014. **11**(7): pp. 2115–25.

83. O'Connor, S.M., et al., Survival and neurite outgrowth of rat cortical neurons in three-dimensional agarose and collagen gel matrices. *Neuroscience Letters*, 2001. **304**(3): pp. 189–93.

84. Hopkins, A.M., et al., Silk hydrogels as soft substrates for neural tissue engineering. *Advanced Functional Materials*, 2013. **23**(41): pp. 5140–9.

85. Tang-Schomer, M.D., et al., Bioengineered functional brain-like cortical tissue. *Proceedings of the National Academy of Sciences of the United States of America*, 2014. **111**(38): pp. 13811–6.

86. Johnson, B.N., et al, 3D printed anatomical nerve regeneration pathways. *Advanced Functional Materials*, 2015. **25**(39): pp. 6205–17.

87. Luo, C.X., et al., Differentiating stem cells on patterned substrates for neural network formation. *Microelectronic Engineering*, 2011. **88**(8): pp. 1707–10.

88. Wang, X.C., et al., A 3D-printed scaffold with MoS2 nanosheets for tumor therapy and tissue regeneration. *Npg Asia Materials*, 2017. **9**: p. 376.

89. Akkineni, A.R., et al., Highly concentrated alginate-gellan gum composites for 3D plotting of complex tissue engineering scaffolds. *Polymers*, 2016. **8**(5): p. 170.

90. Wu, D.W., et al., 3D bioprinting of gellan gum and poly (ethylene glycol) diacrylate based hydrogels to produce human-scale constructs with high-fidelity. *Materials & Design*, 2018. **160**: pp. 486–95.

91. Ning, L.Q., et al., 3D bioprinting of scaffolds with living Schwann cells for potential nerve tissue engineering applications. *Biofabrication*, 2018. **10**(3): p. 035014.

92. Akkineni, A.R., et al., A versatile method for combining different biopolymers in a core/shell fashion by 3D plotting to achieve mechanically robust constructs. *Biofabrication*, 2016. **8**(4): p. 045001.

93. Visser, J., et al., Biofabrication of multi-material anatomically shaped tissue constructs. *Biofabrication*, 2013. **5**(3): p. 035007.

94. Melchels, F.P.W., et al., Additive manufacturing of tissues and organs. *Progress in Polymer Science*, 2012. **37**(8): pp. 1079–104.

95. Derby, B., Printing and prototyping of tissues and scaffolds. *Science*, 2012. **338**(6109): pp. 921–6.

96. Ahlfeld, T., et al., Design and fabrication of complex scaffolds for bone defect healing: Combined 3D plotting of a calcium phosphate cement and a growth factor-loaded hydrogel. *Annals of Biomedical Engineering*, 2017. **45**(1): pp. 224–36.

97. Heinemann, S., et al., Properties of injectable ready-to-use calcium phosphate cement based on water-immiscible liquid. *Acta Biomaterialia*, 2013. **9**(4): pp. 6199–207.

98. Lode, A., et al., Fabrication of porous scaffolds by three-dimensional plotting of a pasty calcium phosphate bone cement under mild conditions. *Journal of Tissue Engineering and Regenerative Medicine*, 2014. **8**(9): pp. 682–93.

99. Li, H.J., C. Tan, and L. Li, Review of 3D printable hydrogels and constructs. *Materials & Design*, 2018. **159**: pp. 20–38.

100. Chia, H.N. and B.M. Wu, Recent advances in 3D printing of biomaterials. *Journal of Biological Engineering*, 2015. **9**: pp. 1–4.

101. Gao, T., et al., Optimization of gelatin-alginate composite bioink printability using rheological parameters: a systematic approach. *Biofabrication*, 2018. **10**(3): p. 034106.

102. Holzl, K., et al., Bioink properties before, during and after 3D bioprinting. *Biofabrication*, 2016. **8**(3): p. 032002.

103. Chawla, S., et al., Silk-Based Bioinks for 3D Bioprinting. *Advanced Healthcare Materials*, 2018. **7**(8): p. 1701204.

104. Donderwinkel, I., J.C.M. van Hest, and N.R. Cameron, Bio-inks for 3D bioprinting: Recent advances and future prospects. *Polymer Chemistry*, 2017. **8**(31): pp. 4451–71.

105. Lozano, R., et al., 3D printing of layered brain-like structures using peptide modified gellan gum substrates. *Biomaterials*, 2015. **67**: pp. 264–73.

106. Hong, S.M., et al., 3D printing of highly stretchable and tough hydrogels into complex, cellularized structures. *Advanced Materials*, 2015. **27**(27): pp. 4035–40.

107. Pati, F., et al., Printing three-dimensional tissue analogues with decellularized extracellular matrix bioink. *Nature Communications*, 2014. **5**: pp. 1–11.

108. Zhang, K., et al., 3D bioprinting of urethra with PCL/PLCL blend and dual autologous cells in fibrin hydrogel: an in vitro evaluation of biomimetic mechanical property and cell growth environment. *International Journal of Urology*, 2017. **24**: p. 16–16.

109. Costa, J.B., et al., Fast setting silk fibroin bioink for bioprinting of patient-specific memory-shape implants. Advanced Healthcare Materials, 2017. **6**(22): p. 1701021.

110. Tao, J., et al. 3D-printed nerve conduits with live platelets for effective peripheral nerve repair. *Advanced Functional Materials*, 2020. **30**(42): p. 2004272.

111. Vijayavenkataraman, S., et al., 3D-printed PCL/rGO conductive scaffolds for peripheral nerve injury repair. *Artificial Organs*, 2019. **43**(5): pp. 515–23.

112. Badea, A., et al., 3D-printed pHEMA materials for topographical and biochemical modulation of dorsal root ganglion cell response. *ACS Applied and Material Interfaces*, 2017. **9**(36): pp. 30318–28.

113. Vijayavenkataraman, S., et al., Electrohydrodynamic jet 3D-printed PCL/PAA conductive scaffolds with tunable biodegradability as nerve guide conduits (NGCs) for peripheral nerve injury repair. *Materials & Design*, 2019. **162**: pp. 171–84.

114. Xu, X., et al. 3D printing of nerve conduits with nanoparticle-encapsulated RGFP966. *Applied Materials Today*, 2019. **16**: pp. 247–56.

115. Vijayavenkataraman, S., et al., 3D-printed PCL/PPy conductive scaffolds as three-dimensional porous nerve guide conduits (NGCs) for peripheral nerve injury repair. *Frontiers Bioengineering and Biotechnology*, 2019. **7**: pp. 266.

116. Uz, M., et al., Development of gelatin and graphene-based nerve regeneration conduits using three-dimensional (3D) printing strategies for electrical transdifferentiation of mesenchymal stem cells. *Industrial & Engineering Chemistry Research*, 2019. **58**(18): pp. 7421–7.

117. Anu, K.R., et al., Neurodegenerative pathways in Alzheimer's disease: A review. Current Neuropharmacology, 2021;19(5):679–692.

118. Kurita, H., M. Inden, and I. Hozumi, Review of relevance between metal homeostasis and neurodegenerative disease. *Nihon Yakurigaku Zasshi*, 2017. **150**(1): pp. 29–35.

119. Mangale, V., et al., Promoting remyelination through cell transplantation therapies in a model of viral-induced neurodegenerative disease. Dev Dyn, 2019. **248**(1): pp. 43–52.

120. Zhang, K.L., et al., 3D bioprinting of urethra with PCL/PLCL blend and dual autologous cells in fibrin hydrogel: An in vitro evaluation of biomimetic mechanical property and cell growth environment. *Acta Biomaterialia*, 2017. **50**: pp. 154–64.

121. Yamamoto, H., et al., A single-cell based hybrid neuronal network configured by integration of cell micropatterning and dynamic patch-clamp. *Applied Physics Letters*, 2018. **113**(13): pp. 133703.

122. Hsieh, F.Y., H.H. Lin, and S.H. Hsu, 3D bioprinting of neural stem cell-laden thermoresponsive biodegradable polyurethane hydrogel and potential in central nervous system repair. *Biomaterials*, 2015. **71**: pp. 48–57.

123. Oliveira, E.P., et al., Advances in bioinks and in vivo imaging of biomaterials for CNS applications. *Acta Biomaterialia*, 2019. **95**: pp. 60–72.

124. Lee, S.J., et al., Fabrication of a highly aligned neural scaffold via a table top stereolithography 3D printing and electrospinning. *Tissue Engineering Part A*, 2017. **23**(11–12): pp. 491–499.

125. Gu, Q., et al., Functional 3D neural mini-tissues from printed gel-based bioink and human neural stem cells. *Advanced Healthcare Materials*, 2016. **5**(12): pp. 1429–38.

126. Frega, M., et al., Network dynamics of 3D engineered neuronal cultures: A new experimental model for in-vitro electrophysiology. *Scientific Reports*, 2014. **4**: pp. 1–4.

127. Chae, D.S., et al. The functional effect of 3D-printing individualized orthosis for patients with peripheral nerve injuries: Three case reports. *Medicine (Baltimore)*, 2020. **99**(16): pp. e19791.

128. Petcu, E.B., et al., 3D printing strategies for peripheral nerve regeneration. *Biofabrication*, 2018. **10**(3): p. 032001.

129. Ye, W.S., et al., 3D printing of gelatin methacrylate-based nerve guidance conduits with multiple channels. *Materials & Design*, 2020. **192**: pp. 108757.

130. Zhu, W., et al., Rapid continuous 3D printing of customizable peripheral nerve guidance conduits. *Materials Today*, 2018. **21**(9): pp. 951–9.

131. Evangelista, M.S., et al., Single-lumen and multi-lumen poly(ethylene glycol) nerve conduits fabricated by stereolithography for peripheral nerve regeneration in vivo. *Journal of Reconstructive Microsurgery*, 2015. **31**(5): pp. 327–35.

132. Tetsuka, H. and S.R. Shin. Materials and technical innovations in 3D printing in biomedical applications. *Journal of Materials Chemistry B*, 2020. **8**(15): pp. 2930–50.

133. Lee, J.M. and W.Y. Yeong. Design and printing strategies in 3D bioprinting of cell-hydrogels: A review. *Advanced Healthcare Materials*, 2016. **5**(22): pp. 2856–65.

134. Poomathi, N., et al., 3D printing in tissue engineering: A state of the art review of technologies and biomaterials. *Rapid Prototyping Journal*, 2020. **26**(7): pp. 1313–34.

135. Saroia, J., et al. A review on biocompatibility nature of hydrogels with 3D printing techniques, tissue engineering application and its future prospective. *Bio-Design and Manufacturing*, 2018. **1**(4): pp. 265–79.

136. Dorweiler, B., et al., The future of vascular medicine - Role of 3D printing. *Zentralbl Chir*, 2020. **145**(05): pp. 448–55.

137. Tao, J., et al., 3D-printed nerve conduit with vascular networks to promote peripheral nerve regeneration. *Medical Hypotheses*, 2019. **133**: pp. 109395.

138. Rabionet, M., et al., 3D-printed tubular scaffolds for vascular tissue engineering. *19th Cirp Conference on Electro Physical and Chemical Machining*, 23–27 April 2017, Bilbao, Spain.

139. Costantini, M., et al., Co-axial wet-spinning in 3D bioprinting: State of the art and future perspective of microfluidic integration. *Biofabrication*, 2019. **11**(1): pp. 012001.

140. Hsieh, F.Y. and S.H. Hsu, 3D bioprinting: A new insight into the therapeutic strategy of neural tissue regeneration. *Organogenesis*, 2015. **11**(4): pp. 153–8.

8 Progress in Biomaterials for Application of Esophageal Stents

Yachen Hou, Jingan Li, Aqeela Yasin, and Mujiahid Iqbal
Zhengzhou University

CONTENTS

8.1 INTRODUCTION: ESOPHAGEAL CANCER

Esophageal cancer is the ninth most common cancer in the world and the fifth most common cancer in developed countries.[1] In the United States, the incidence of esophageal cancer continues to rise and is by far the fastest-growing cancer, with an estimated 14,550 new cases diagnosed in 2006 and 13,770 cancer-related deaths.[2] Overall, 482,300 new esophageal cancer cases were estimated in 2008 and 406,800 deaths were recorded in the same year.[3] Until 2018, there were 572,034 new diagnoses and 508,585 deaths from esophageal cancer worldwide.[4] The overall 5-year survival rate of patients who are amenable to definitive treatment ranges from 5% to 30%. There are two main subtypes of esophageal cancer: squamous cell carcinoma (OSCC) and adenocarcinoma (OAC). OSCC accounts for nearly 90% of esophageal cancers worldwide and is extremely prevalent in China, which is mainly related to smoking and alcohol abuse.[5] OAC mainly occurs in Western males.[6]

Poor prognosis has been reported because esophageal malignancies have no specific symptoms in the early stage. Moreover, 60%–80% of esophageal cancers are diagnosed as intermediate to advanced stage,[7] while less than 50% of patients with esophageal carcinoma are suitable for surgery at the time of diagnosis. Most of these patients present with locally advanced or metastatic disease and/or significant comorbidities.[8] Radical treatment regimens are not suitable for most patients as their expected survival is short which is determined on a monthly basis; thus, the primary aim of treatment is to reduce morbidity and mortality in patients.[9] Traditionally, surgery has been considered the best treatment for esophageal cancer, which removes the tumor, the esophagus, the lymphatic drainage, and the surrounding tissue to restore continuity of the alimentary tract. Studies have found that the survival of esophageal malignancies is zero without intervention, while the resectability, postoperative mortality, and morbidity have been reported to be 54%–69%, 4%–10%, and 26%–41%, respectively, with 5-year survival of 15%–24% after surgery alone.[10] In cases where the cancer is unresectable, dysphagia is the main symptom. Many patients with dysphagia can only receive palliative therapy to ameliorate symptoms of dysphagia to maintain oral intake, which ultimately improves quality of life.[11] Implantation of esophageal stents in patients with advanced esophageal cancer may improve quality of life, but it does not significantly extend survival. These palliative treatments can extend survival. The most common means of palliation includes self-expanding metal stents (SEMSs) to relieve malignant dysphagia. Besides, irradiation stent has been developed to prolong life-span, and this stent can effectively prevent restenosis and avoid the side effects of systemic chemotherapy.[12] The classical esophageal lesion and treatment options are shown in Figure 8.1.

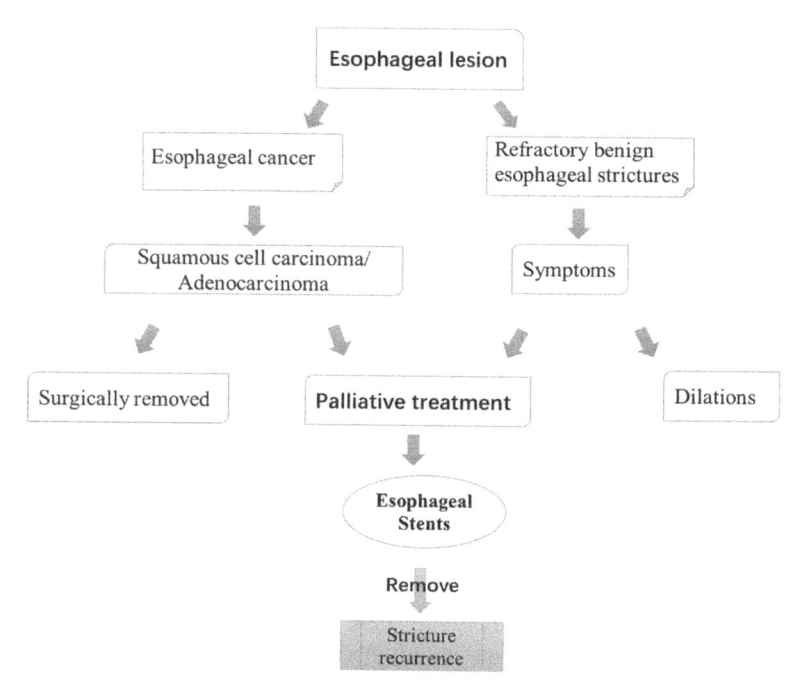

FIGURE 8.1　Classical esophageal lesion and treatment options.

8.1.1 REFRACTORY BENIGN ESOPHAGEAL STRICTURES (RBES)

Stents are used to palliate malignant dysphagia, and are also increasingly used for the treatment of refractory esophageal benign strictures.[13] RBES are defined as those that persist after three or more dilations. It is hypothesized that temporary stent placement would promote tissue remodeling to yield durable palliation of RBES.[14] Contrary to esophageal cancer, RBES of the esophagus is a sequela of esophageal injury, which stimulates fibrous tissue hyperplasia and deposition of collagen production.[15] The symptoms of dysphagia caused by these strictures may seriously impair quality of life. The treatments for RBES are challenging and time-consuming as these problems may relate to the depth fibrotic reaction, the submucosa, and the muscularis propria. Surgery is the primary choice to remove hyperplasia tissue, while the morbidity and mortality after operations remain high, which makes surgery unsuitable for a benign condition. When conventional therapy for benign esophageal strictures is unsuccessful, stent placement has been proposed for patients who are poor candidates for surgery to restore lumen patency and resolve dysphagia symptoms.[16] After initial dilation, stricture recurrence is frequent, especially in patients who have severe, long, and tight strictures at presentation.[17–19]

8.2 SELECTION OF COMMERCIAL ESOPHAGEAL STENTS

The following patients are suitable for stent implantation, according by Kochman et al.,[20] the result of either an inability to successfully remediate the anatomic problem to a diameter of 14 mm over five sessions at 2-week intervals, or as a result of an inability to maintain a satisfactory luminal diameter for 4 weeks once the target diameter of 14 mm has been achieved. Carotid stenting of the esophagus is a minimally invasive intervention, which has been used as expansion and perforation and narrow fistula treatment. SEMSs are the current endoscopic standard for palliation of dysphagia resulting from malignant esophageal stenosis. SEMSs have also been used with variable success in the treatment of benign strictures. Complications of uncovered or partially covered SEMSs include difficulty in stent extraction, development of secondary strictures, necrosis, and ulceration from the stents themselves.

Some results founded that utilizing SEMS to treat REBS may result in a number of adverse events, including stricture formation, stent migration, fatal bleeding, perforation, and other complications requiring additional interventions.[13] In 1983, Frimberger[21] treated esophageal stenosis with a metal stent. Placement of metal stents for esophageal stenosis has gained gradual popularity. The SEMS has been used successfully for palliative treatment of malignant esophageal obstruction.[22] Self-expandable plastic stents (SEPSs) have been used for the management of benign esophageal conditions, such as tracheoesophageal fistulas, benign esophageal strictures, esophageal perforations, and leaks. From the available research results, few studies have demonstrated which kind of stent is more suitable for esophageal cancer or REBS. The stent migration rate in RBES is higher than that of the cancer.[23] The classification of the esophageal stents is shown in Figure 8.2 and Table 8.1. Therefore, discussing the characteristics of each kind of stent may guide individual patients in choosing the most appropriate stents for different diseases.

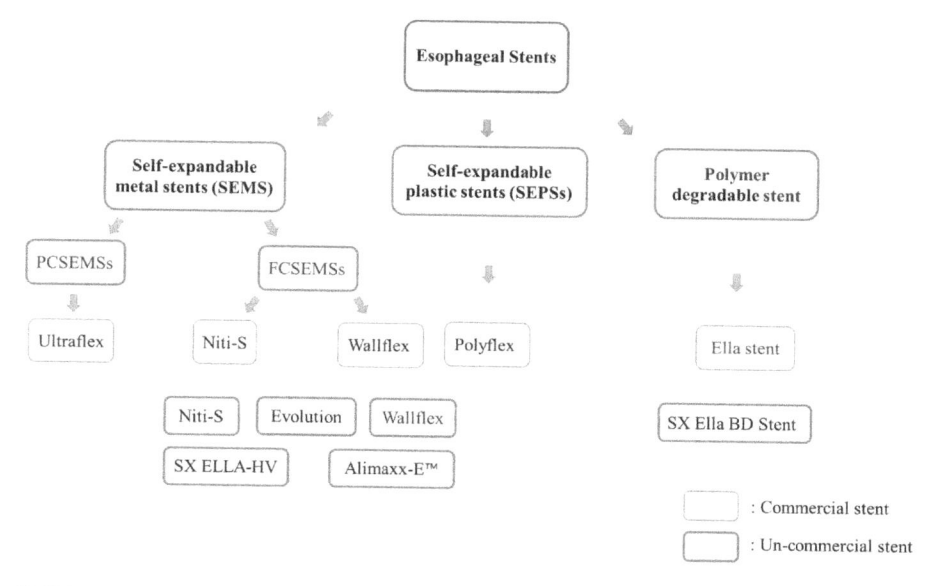

FIGURE 8.2   Classification of the esophageal stents.

8.2.1   SELF-EXPANDABLE METAL STENTS (SEMS)

Currently, three different types of metal stents are available: uncovered SEMSs, partially covered SEMSs (PCSEMSs), and fully covered SEMSs (FCSEMSs). Various types of SEMS, either fully covered or partially covered, have been used for the palliation of RBES and MOS.

For uncovered SEMS, the complications, such as bleeding, fistulae, and recurrence of tissue growth, are the main problems to reduce the expansion effect. Tissue grows through the stent mesh, which inserts the SEMS into the tumor tissue. Although the tissue can fix the stent on the esophagus wall, they also lead in new stenosis or occlusion in stent. To improve the complication, covered polymer on the stent is an efficient method.

Based on the uncovered SEMS, PCSEMSs and FCSEMSs were discovered. The major limitation of PCSEMS has been recurrent dysphagia due to tissue in- and overgrowth in the anchored stent. For the PCSEMS, the uncovered ends (the proximal and distal portions of the stent) quickly embed in the esophageal wall to fix, and the radial force of the stent causes stent embedding in the esophageal wall to avoid migration.[24,25] In combination with its nitinol material, which may reactive tissue in- and overgrowth to firm stent anchoring.[26] Therefore, some researchers have strongly recommended not to use PCSEMS to treat RBES.[27] The main problem about benign esophageal disorders is endoscopic removal of the stent, while the uncovered parts of the PCSEMS can be embedded into the esophageal wall to prevent stent removal and influence the stent removal from the esophageal wall after treatment process.[28] After removing the stent, the esophageal wall may post-procedure stenoses from extensive mucosal damage in some patients[29] and may result a new stricture formation.[30] Besides, some studies have reported that PCSEMS should not be implanted

TABLE 8.1

Overview of SEMS, SEPS, and BEST Used in Clinics

		Product	Manufacturer	Size	Material	Coating	Advantages	Drawbacks	Ref.
SEBS	FC	Wallflex	Boston Scientific	Diameter: 18, 23 mm Proximal flare: 23, 28 mm Length: 10, 12, 15 mm	Nitinol	Permalume silicone	1. Low-profile delivery system for tight strictures	/	[35, 46]
		Niti-S	Taewoong Medical	Diameter: 16–20 mm; Length: 60, 80, 100, 120, 150 mm	Nitinol	Inner polyurethane layer	1. Available with an inner and outer metal framework to reduce migration 2. Antireflux valve available 3. Prevent tumor ingrowth	/	[45]
		Alimaxx-E	Alveolus (Charlotte, NC)	Diameter: 18-22 mm; Length: 70, 100, 120 mm	Nitinol	Polyurethane	1. Smaller flexible delivery system (GW system) 2. Antimigration struts on the outside	High migration rate	[49, 57, 58]
		Endomaxx	Merit Medical (South Jordan, UT)	/	Nitinol	Polyurethane	1. Improvement in dysphagia score	/	[52]
		Choo stent	M.I. Tech (Seoul, Korea)	Diameter: 18 mm; Length: 40, 70, 100, 120 mm	Nitinol	Polyurethane	1. Anti-reflux valve available 2. Retrievable	/	[59, 60]
		SX-ELLA-HV	Ella-CS (Hradec Kralove, Czech Republic)	Diameter: 20 mm Proximal flare: 25 mm Length: 80–150mm	Nitinol	Polyurethane	1. With antimigration collar 2. Improve the flexibility 3. Reduced hyperplastic tissue overgrowth	Corrosive strictures have poorer outcomes	[61]
	PC	Ultraflex	Boston Scientific (Natick, MA)	Diameter: 18, 23 mm Proximal flare: 23,28 mm Length: 10,12,15 mm	Nitinol	Polyurethane	1. Stent foreshortens up to 30%–40% 2. Implant the stent without fluoroscopy guidance 3. Most commonly used	/	[62, 63]

(*Continued*)

TABLE 8.1 (*Continued*)
Overview of SEMS, SEPS, and BEST Used in Clinics

	Product	Manufacturer	Size	Material	Coating	Advantages	Drawbacks	Ref.
SEPS	Polyflex	Boston Scientific (Natick, MA)	Diameter: 16, 18, 21 mm; Length: 90, 120, 150 mm	Polyester mesh	Silicone membrane	1. Lower cost, ease of placement and retrieval 2. Providing alleviation of dysphagia 3. Removable	1. limited local tissue reaction 2. stent migration 3. the recurrence of dysphagia after stent removal	[64]
BDS	SX-Ella-BD	Ella-CS (Hradec Kralove, Czech Republic)	Diameter: 31 mm; Proximal flare: 25 mm; Length: 60 mm	Polydioxanone	Uncovered	1. Overcome the overgrowth of reactive tissue 2. Biodegradable	quick loss of mechanical support	[65]
Irradiation Stent	Stents loaded with 125-iodine seeds	Micro-tech [Nanjing] Co. Ltd; Shanghai GMS Pharmaceutical Co., Ltd.	/	Nitinol alloy	Silicone membrane; polytetra-fluoroethylene membrane iodine seeds.	1. Prolong life-span of the MOS patients 2. Decreases the general side effect of chemotherapy 3. The radiating distance is short	Complication existed	[12]

for more than 6 weeks to prevent removal-related complications.[31] Moreover, it is difficult to remove the entire stent for many small nitinol fragments of the PCSEMS will remain embedded in the esophageal wall.[29] Until now, the popular commercial PCSEMS is named Ultraflex, which is made of nitinol alloy and is covered with a polyurethane coating.[29] A prospective controlled trial was conducted to compare Ultraflex with Polyflex.[32] No difference was seen in the remission of dysphagia between the two stents. However, less complications were observed in the Ultraflex group (33%), especially late stent migration.[32]

FCSEMS can effectively palliate inoperable esophageal cancer or RBES.[33] Although SEMS have no direct antitumor activity, they can probably extend the survival of symptomatic, inoperable patients by improving nutritional intake and preventing starvation, dehydration, and aspiration.[33] Besides, the main advantage of FCSEMS is the lower risk of stent embedding and the ease of stent removal, along with a higher migration rate (36.3%), which are mostly distal migrations, and respiratory distress were the principal major complications of FCSEMS.[31,34] In some patients, the FCSEMS were moved to the stomach which requires a second operation to remove; thus, this kind stent can be removed up to 12 weeks.[35] To prevent stent migration, the endoscopic suturing of FCSEMSs (S-FCSEMSs) to fixed stent on the esophageal wall is a novel technique.[36,37] Some studies have found that the migration rate for FCSEMSs compared with 74% for stents placed without suture fixation that of the anchored stent was 33% in the same patients.[38,39]

The FDA has approved two FCSEMS: Niti-S (TaeWoong) and Wallflex (Boston Scientific).[40] Current European guidelines recommend full coverage rather than partial coverage.[41] Esophageal FCSEMSs did not reveal a lower recurrent obstruction rate compared with PCSEMSs in the palliative management of malignant dysphagia.[42] In several clinical series, however, significant problems were encountered after stent placement, including difficulty in removing the stent and ingrowth of granulation tissue with subsequent obstruction of the uncovered part of the stent as well as pain.[43] A well-known drawback of FCSEMSs is their high migration rate, varying from 31% to 39% in recent reports.

The Niti-S stents (Taewoong Medical, Seoul, Korea) have an inner polyurethane layer and an outer uncovered nitinol wire to prevent migration,[24] which has proven its effectiveness in the palliation of malignant dysphagia. Moreover, the double-layered design is probably important in preventing migration (6%) and can maintain its good advantage of lower incidence of tumor ingrowth (2%),[44] and the complete covering of the Niti-S stent may be a factor in preventing tissue overgrowth at both ends of the stent (7%).[45] The Wallflex FC stent (Boston Scientific, Natick, Mass) was designed to prevent migration by increasing the outer stent resistance by using internal covering and distinct shouldering at each stent ends. The Wallflex stent is made of a multiple wire of nitinol alloy and was fully covered by Permalume silicone internal coating.[46] A removal suture at the proximal end can be used to pull the stent and reposition or remove it in case of need.[46,47] For malignant strictures, the Wallflex exhibited good ability to improve the dysphagia scores and low migration (9%) and bleeding (6%) in a single-center study of 48 patients.[47] In another multicenter center study involving 82 patients with RBES,[46] the results showed that the Wallflex stent is secure and can effectively palliate dysphagia, with low migration rates (12.2%)

and minor complications (9.8%). Therefore, the Wallflex stent is safe and effective to release malignant dysphagia, with migration (12.2%) and tissue overgrowth rates comparable to previously reported data on partially covered stents.[46] The two stents offer similar degrees of palliation of dysphagia with no statistically significant differences in the occurrence of complications.[46,48] A multicenter retrospective study found that compared to the Endomaxx stents and Evolution stents, low migration for the Wallflex stents were reported, while these differences were not statistically significant ($P = 0.19$).[35]

Except the Niti-S and Wallflex, the Alimaxx-E stent and Endomaxx stent are also the main types of FCSEMS. The Alimaxx-E stent (Alveolus Inc., Charlotte, North Carolina, USA) has been recently developed, which is made of nitinol and is fully covered with polyurethane to resist tissue ingrowth.[49] A research studied the efficacy and security of the Alimaxx-E™ stent, and evaluated the tissue ingrowth and the risk of stent migration. A total of 22 patients (22/45) developed recurrent dysphagia, particularly 16 patients involved in stent migration (16/45). A high risk of stent migration was noted and was shown in a larger prospective follow-up study.[49] Another perspective study by Lakhtakia[50] was related by the Alimaxx-E stent in nine patients with RBES, and the mean pre-stent dysphagia score decreased from $3.2 \pm 0.7SD$ to $0.7 \pm 0.8SD$, which was better than the pre-stent scores. The study also revealed that the Alimaxx-E stent was easy to place and could be removed by endoscopically. Therefore, some studies have indicated that the Alimaxx-E could be a safer treatment for benign esophageal disorders as it prevents stent embedding to the esophageal contour.[34]

The Endomaxx has a favorable safety and efficacy profile. This stent is potentially removable and can be used for various benign and malignant esophageal indications.[51] Nineteen Endomaxx stents were placed in 17 RBES patients, and the dysphagia score was improved (from 3.3 to 1.5) after stent therapy in patients.[52] Evolution stent had a higher rate of clinically relevant migration when compared to the Wallflex and Endomaxx stents.[35] Recently, to reduce malignant dysphagia, a new SX-ELLA stent Esophageal HV (Ella-CS, Hradec Kralove, Czech Republic) has been developed, which is a fully covered nitinol wire stent with an antimigration ring to resist migration.[78] Compared with migration rates of other fully covered stents, the use of SX-ELLA stents may not reduce the migration rate significantly, indicating that the circumferential antimigration ring plus the flared ends are not effective to prevent migration.[53,54] The most common symptoms following SX-ELLA placement were stent migration (36.3%) and chest pain (36.3%).[60] In a study involving 45 RBES patients, the recurrent dysphagia due to tissue growth and stent migration was reduced, although 40% of the patients needed a reintervention for recurrent dysphagia or complications.[80]

A retrospective review of PCSEMS and FCSEMS showed that the complete cover membrane of the Choostent may cause less granulation tissue and allows easier removability a few weeks later,[8] and the researchers believed that the RBES can be effectively decreased by implanted FCSEMS in case of non-corrosive esophageal strictures.[60] Therefore, FCSEMSs are better than uncovered stents as recurrent dysphagia due to tumor ingrowth is common with uncovered stent for treating esophageal cancer.[55] The PCSEMSs are superior to uncovered SEMSs in the palliation of dysphagia due to unresectable esophageal tumor.[56] Esophageal FCSEMSs did not reveal a lower recurrent obstruction rate compared with PCSEMSs in the palliative management of malignant dysphagia.[42]

8.2.2 SELF-EXPANDABLE PLASTIC STENTS (SEPSs)

SEMSs have also been considered as dilation therapy for the treatment of anastomotic strictures. Some studies have found that plastic stents and biodegradable stents can preclude these serious complications caused by the metal stent, including the problems of metal stent-induced hyperplasticity and overgrowth.[26] In several clinical series, however, significant problems were encountered after stent placement. These included difficulty in removing the stent and ingrowth of granulation tissue with subsequent obstruction of the uncovered part of the stent as well as pain. To address this situation, SEPSs were developed to preclude these complications, which have been proposed for use in benign esophageal lesions for their advantages over metallic stents, including ease of placement and retrieval, as well as limited local tissue reaction while still providing alleviation of dysphagia. Some studies have found that SEPS overcomes perforation, bleeding, and difficulty in retrieval.[66]

Until now, the only commercially available stent made of plastic is the Polyflex (Boston Scientific Corp, Natick, MA), which is made of a smooth silicone lining covered with a polyester mesh.[67] The Polyflex stent is available in various sizes with diameters of 16, 18, and 21 mm and lengths of 9, 12, and 15 cm.[68] Some studies have found that a variety of benign and malignant strictures patients with esophageal perforation or fistulas can use Polyflex stents.[69] Other studies have proposed that the Polyflex stents may be more appropriate for the management of malignant dysphagia in patients with locally advanced esophageal cancer.[64] A study reported no stent migration or complications in six patients, and all these patients were maintaining adequate nutrition during neoadjuvant therapy with near-normal dysphagia scores.[70] Therefore, placement of Polyflex stent immediately after staging of locally advanced esophageal malignancies is feasible and effective.

However, the data on the efficacy of these stents in RBES patients are mixed, and a relatively high rate of stent migration has been reported. Some studies have demonstrated that Polyflex stents can provide satisfactory palliation of dysphagia in patients with RBES, while stricture recurrence was common after stent removal.[14] A total of 21 consecutive patients with RBES were treated by Polyflex, and it was found that the placement may lead to long-term benefits compared to the data from a study reporting that maybe less than 1 year treatment by SEPSs is sufficient and shows lasting improvement.[71] Alessandro and his team implanted Polyflex into 15 patients with RBES and found that 12 had no symptoms and did not require any other treatment during the follow-up period (19–27 months),[13] implying that Polyflex can completely solve the difficulty of swallowing. Besides, the Polyflex stent can be easily and safely removed or replaced after a reasonable duration without the fear of long-term complications associated with metal stents. In other studies, 58 stents were placed in 38 patients, and the complications included migration of 38 stents in 1–353 days.[72]

As discussed above, covered SEMS offer effective palliation of esophageal strictures. Some data have confirmed that Polyflex is a suitable alternative to SEMS, as it is equally effective in the palliation of dysphagia. Moreover, the absence of a metal mesh and the completely covering silicone membrane of the Polyflex can reduce hyperplasia after removal, even if Polyflex has been implanted for a few months. The relatively higher migration rate of Polyflex compared to Ultraflex is the main disadvantage.[62,71] Moreover, SEPS placement did not result in stricture resolution or stabilization after SEPS removal in a study.[26,73]

The main disadvantage of the SEPS is the migration, with migration rates ranging from 5% to 23%. Although the first results were promising, several studies on SEPSs have now revealed a long-term clinical success rate of well below 50%, a migration rate of about 50%, and severe complications in 6% of patients.[22,74] While, some clinical studies found Polyflex has shown poor outcomes as it is difficult to place in a complex stricture. The wider delivery system sometimes requires pre-stenting dilatation. Another major drawback is their high frequency of migration. Stent removal may lead to serious trauma. Therefore, Polyflex may be responsible for poor long-term outcomes. Some researchers have found that the use of SEPS appears to be the least desirable for RBES because they are associated with frequent stent migration, more reintervention, and little long-term improvement [35]. Regarding cost, some studies have indicated that compared with the Ultraflex metallic stent, the charges for all sizes of Polyflex stents are $2,775, which varies in cost from $1,825 to $2,183.[69]

8.2.3 POLYMER DEGRADABLE STENT

Biodegradable esophageal stents (BESTs) have recently been developed. First cases using stents made from biodegradable materials were reported from 1997.[75] The prolonged dilatory effect before stent absorption and progressive stent degradation could represent a more favorable solution for RBES patients compared with SEMSs and SEPSs in RBES patients. In 2008, a new biodegradable stent, the SX-ELLA-BD Stent (Ella-CS, Hradec Kralove, Czech Republic), was developed and became available commercially for clinical use. Those stents biodegrade after 11–12 weeks, thus making them appealing alternatives for both benign esophageal strictures and malignant ones, or as a bridge for more radical interventions.

Theoretically, compared with the temporary metal or plastic stent, the biodegradable stent is ideal for the treatment of RBES as it becomes embedded in the esophageal wall, reducing migration rates, dissolving spontaneously after placement, and reducing the need for reinterventions to remove the stent. Furthermore, a stent made from a material with good tissue compatibility should overcome/reduce the in- and overgrowth of reactive tissue.[76] Biodegradable esophageal stents show poor corrosion resistance and quick loss of mechanical support *in vivo*. The short life-span of BD stents has frequently been reported to be a major restriction of this stent type. As the expansion force of BD stents decreases over time, its impact on stricture remodeling may be suboptimal compared to other stent types. Some studies have indicated that the effectiveness of biodegradable stents ranges from more than one-third to a quarter of cases, fairly similar to other types of stents used for the same indication.[77] Polymer stent could maintain the initial radial force in the first 6–8 weeks after implantation. Because the expansive force of polymer stent decreases with time, its effect on stenosis remodeling may not be optimal. The main limitations of the polymer stent is the initial disintegration occurring at 11–12 weeks after initial stent placement, and the low pH levels of the environment may accelerate the disintegration rate.[74] Besides, the disintegration process can increase the formation of local proliferative tissue.[74] While this disadvantage endows the polymer stent a property, the polymer stent could be an alternative to repeated endoscopic dilatation therapy.[78]

ELLA-CS-BD stent is the first commercially available biodegradable stent for REBS (without FDA approval) made of polydioxanone (PDO). As no subsequent removal is required for biodegradable stents, sequential biodegradable stent placement in the esophagus may be a feasible solution.[78] According to Fuccio et al.,[79] clinical success rate after biodegradable stent placement is comparable to other stent types. Canena et al.[80] compared outcomes of biodegradable stents ($n = 10$), plastic stents ($n = 10$), and FCSEMS ($n = 10$) and found that there were no significant differences in the incidence of adverse events among the three different stent types. Moreover, SX-ELLA stent is promising for its efficacy and safety in patients with dysphagia caused by benign anastomotic esophageal stenosis.[74] Repici et al.[81] conducted a prospective study of 21 patients with benign esophageal strictures refractory to standard dilation therapy with SX-ELLA stent, and found a low rate of stent migration, and dysphagia scores increased significantly, with 45% of patients being dysphagia-free at the end of the study. Compared with the Polyflex stent, low migration rates with the ELLA stent were observed between the two stents, as well as a significantly lower reintervention rate for the ELLA stent group.[82]

PDO has been widely used as an absorbable suture in various clinical cases due to its degradability and biocompatibility.[82] PDO is a semicrystalline, biodegradable polymer belonging to the polyester family. It degrades by random hydrolysis of its molecular ester bonds. The degradation accelerates at low pH.[81] The degradation product glyoxylic acid is the primary precursor of oxalic acid and is an intermediate in the conversion of glycolic acid to glycine. None of the degradation products or intermediates are harmful.[81] Because we used a biodegradable stent, we cannot exclude the possibility that the chemical dissolution of the stent may have also influenced tissue hyperplasia.[74]

As discussed before, the SEMS was found to provide more long-term relief of symptoms compared to other stents.[61] The main complications of the esophageal stents are demonstrated in Tables 8.2 and 8.3. The ease of delivery and no requirement of extensive dilation are the main advantages of the metal stent. The incidence of complications with metal stents is no less and the research results have not been shown to be better than SEPS. The BDS is a novel stent with lower rate of overgrowth compared with the Polyflex and Niti-S, which may be the larger midsection size.[53] Biodegradable stents are ideal therapy for benign esophageal strictures (BOS), although this stent requires frequent dilatation.[81]

8.3 IMPROVEMENT OF THE ESOPHAGEAL STENT

In a recent overview, hyperplastic tissue ingrowth or overgrowth was the cause of recurrent dysphagia in 17% of patients treated with a partially covered or uncovered SEMS for benign esophageal strictures.[43] It is speculated that this hyperplasia is related to the radial force, the size of the stent, and the duration of stenting. Most of

TABLE 8.2
The Main Complications of the Esophageal Stents

Name	Number (Patient/ Stent)	Median Survival	Dysphagia Score (before/after)	Disease	Early Complications			Late Complications				Ref.
					Bleeding	Pain	Death	Dysphagia	Obstruction	migration	fistula	
Wallflex FC	82/81	/	3–1	RBESs	3	8	12	19	7	10	1	[46]
	48	68 day	/	MOS (33) / BOS (15)	6%	20%	/	15%	3%	9%	6%	[47]
Niti-S	100	74 day	1.3±0.7	RBESs	2	12	/	19	9	6	/	[44]
	55		2.8–1.3	RBESs	1	17	/	38	15	14	/	[23]
Alimaxx-E	45	/	/	MOS	2	3		22	7	16	2	[49]
	9/13	/	3.2±0.7– 0.7±0.8	RBESs	/	1	/	/	/	4	/	[50]
Endomaxx	17/19	/	3.33–1.5	RBESs	/	/	/	/	1	3	2	[52]
SX-ELLA Stent Esophageal HV	45	107 day	3–1	MOS	10	12	5	12	/	6	/	[83]
	11		0	RBESs	/	4	/	/	2	4	/	[61]
	45/46	110 day	3–1	MOS	8	6	/	/	2	6	2	[54]
Ultraflex	2	/	/	RBESs								[84]
Polyflex	30/83	/	/	RBESs	/	23	4	/	/	18	13	[85]
	30/37	/	/	MOS / BOS	/	11	/	/	/	9	3	[69]
	40	/	3.0±0.8– 0.6±0.7	RBESs	3	4	/	/	/	8	1	[86]
SX-ELLA BD	21	/	3–1	RBESs	1	3	/	9	1	2	/	[81]
	2	/	/	MOS / BOS	/	1	/	/	/	1	/	[76]
	10	/	2.5–1	MOS	/	2	/	/	4	/	/	[74]

RBESs: refractory benign esophageal strictures; BOS: benign esophageal strictures; MOS: malignant esophageal stricture; uMOS: unresectable malignant esophageal strictures; The ability to swallow was assessed by the dysphagia score (graded as: 0=ability to eat a normal diet; 1=ability to eat some solid food; 2=ability to eat some semi-solids only; 3=ability to swallow liquids only; and 4=complete dysphagia)

TABLE 8.3

The Comparation of Different Esophageal Stents

Ref.	Name	Number (Patient/ Stent)	Median Survival	Dysphagia Score (before/ after)	Disease	Major Complications						
						Death	Obstruction	Migration	Dysphagia	Severe Pain	Bleeding	Fistula
[35]	Wallflex	218/218	/	/	BOSs (161)	/	/	15% 7%	/	/	/	/
	Endomaxx	96/96	/	/	MOS (208)	/	/	19% 12%	/	/	/	/
	Evolution	55/55	/	/		/	/	25% 29%	/	/	/	/
[8]	Ultraflex	33	/	1.9±0.3	uMOS	/	/	/	/	3	/	/
	Choostent	32	/	2.1±0.4		/	/	/	/	/	/	/
[63]	Ultraflex	23	177±109	1.9±0.77	uMOS	/	3	2	/	1	/	/
	Esophacoil	27				/	1	/	/	9	1	1
[42]	fully covered	49	/	/	RBESs	/	19%	/	/	/	/	/
	partially covered	49	/	/		/	22%	/	/	/	/	/
[32]	Polyflex	47	134	/	MOS	/	20	/	/	/	2	1
	Ultraflex	54	122	/		/	18	/	/	/		1
[87]	Irradiation stent	73	177	/	MOS	66	/	/	21	17	5	6
	Self-expandable covered nitinol stent	75	147	/		64	/	/	20	15	5	5

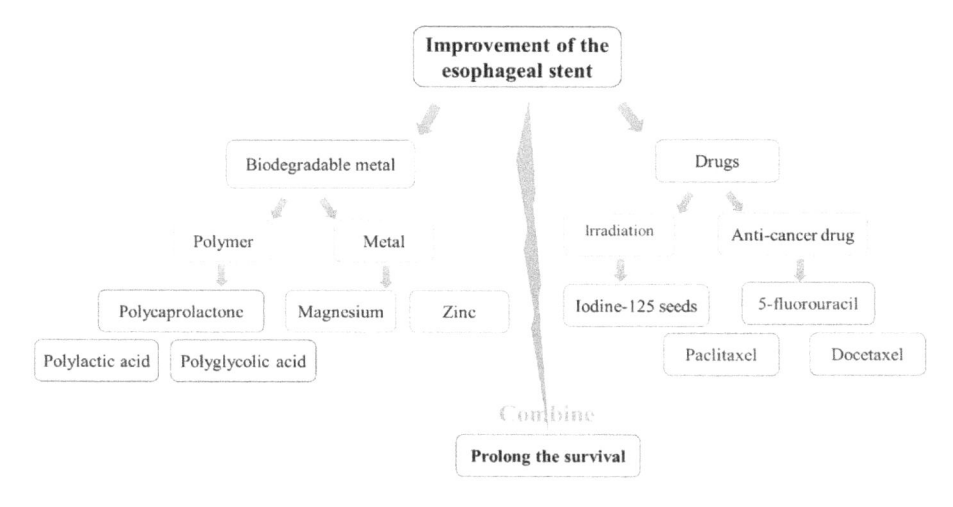

FIGURE 8.3   Candidate of the stent improving line.

the work has focused on covering materials. Stent shape is also considered to be an important factor affecting stent migration.[46] To solve the problems discussed before, there are two main stent designs: utilizing new materials and adding suitable drugs on the stent surface.

Therefore, the biodegradable metal material and drug delivery esophageal stents are promising to improve the stent treatment effect. Innovative biodegradable stents are typically manufactured from materials including polylactic acid, polyglycolic acid, polycaprolactone, especially magnesium and zinc alloy, to improve the radial force and control the degradation period.[81] Besides, another method is adding drugs on stent coating. The main targets of the release stent were not only keeping the esophagus open after placement inside the esophagus which is partly blocked by the tumor but also releasing the antitumor drugs directed to the tumor around the implanted site. Figure 8.3 shows a candidate of the stent improving line. This system can provide sustained and prolonged local chemotherapy with high antitumor efficacy and low systemic toxicity.[88–90]

8.3.1   DEGRADABLE STENT

Based on the material of ELLA stent, many improvements have been made to increase the properties of polystent. PDO and poly(L-lactic acid) (PLLA) sheath-core biphasic monofilament was designed to develop an esophageal stent with improved mechanical properties and controlled biodegradability.[91] The degradation behavior of pure Mg in artificial saliva was studied and found that a dense degradation product film was formed on the surface, which provided Mg the potential to make up the esophageal stent.[92] The hardness testing showed that Mg-Zn-Y-Nd alloy had less mechanical properties compared with the commercial esophageal stent material, 317L stainless steel (317L SS), as well as inhibited adhesion and proliferation of tumor cells, fibroblasts, and epithelial cells. A study suggested potential application of Mg-Zn-Y-Nd alloy as a novel material for BEST.[93] Zn-0.1Li alloy could partly inhibit L929 cell proliferation, which might be beneficial for esophageal cancer treatment.[94]

Elastic, PCL, and PTMC as the coated membrane on Mg alloy stents allowed fabricating a fully BEST, which provided reliable support for at least 4 weeks, without causing severe injury or collagen deposition.[95] Silicone-covered magnesium stents covered with a silicon membrane through the dipping and spinning method, which have poor corrosion resistance and rapid loss of mechanical support, was shown in rabbits.[96,97] Although the results of BDS appear promising, further developments are needed. More information is needed on the safety of the material used.

8.3.2 DRUG-ELUTING STENTS

The main problems after stent implantation are low tissue adhesion[65] and tissue hyperplasia. Many complications can be improved by surface modification through adding 5-fluorouracil (5-FU), paclitaxel (PTX), and docetaxel (DTX) on the surface.[98,99] Drug-eluting stents (DESs) are widely used in blood vessels, but the development of DES for non-vascular organs (such as the esophagus) has been slow, and there are no clinically applicable DESs for esophageal cancer. High dose of 5-FU or paclitaxel are useful in the treatment of esophageal cancer. Stent loaded with the drug could inhibit the cancer process and decrease side effects compared with systemic administration.[88,89,100] The PTX or 5-FU/stent was prepared by covering a nitinol stent with a bi-layered polymer film consisting of a layer of 50% PTX or 5-FU and a layer of drug-free backing. A type of esophageal stent coating, composed of one 5-FU containing ethylene-vinyl acetate (EVA) copolymer layer and one drug-free EVA protective layer, behaved in a unidirectional release fashion.[101] Triplet therapy, with the addition of epirubicin to cisplatin and 5-FU, has been shown to be superior to cisplatin and 5-fluorouracil (CF) alone.[102,103] A novel 5-FU-containing EVA copolymer layer and one drug-free EVA protective layer were coated on the commercial self-expandable nitinol stent, which create a long-term local drug delivery system with great treat efficiency..[90] To increase the cell apoptosis and necrosis and decrease the restenosis in the stent, 5-FU was coated onto the PDA/PEI layers to manufacture the PDA/PEI/5-FU layers, which exhibited suppressed esophageal tumor cells, epithelial cells, and fibroblasts.[104]

Additionally, docetaxel delivery films were prepared using PurSil AL 20 (PUS), which can be used as a covering material for SEMS, exhibiting sustained release (>30 days) and minimal DTX permeation through esophageal tissues in vitro.[105] PDA/PEI layers significantly improve Eca109 cells apoptosis and necrosis, suggesting excellent anticancer function.[106] Development of a soft and flexible multifunctional bilayer membrane carrying paclitaxel, and the use of solution-casting and electrospinning to form this material into an esophageal stent coating, the bilayer membrane increases the concentration of drug aggregation at the tumor site, achieving an effective antitumor effect and reducing the side effects of PTX.[99] A paclitaxel-eluting metallic SEMS was inserted into the lower esophagus of rabbits and showed an antitumor effect on esophageal tissue.[107]

8.3.3 IRRADIATION STENT

Interventional therapy with a metal stent can help patients with advanced-stage esophageal carcinoma to rebuild swallowing function. However, the conventional metal stent provides only palliative treatment in mechanical support and improved eating ability, whereas intraluminal radioactive stent placement can treat the esophageal stricture much more effectively. In addition to providing mechanical expansion, intraluminal irradiation inhibits tumor growth via continuous low-dose irradiation from iodine-125 seeds.[85] A novel esophageal stent loaded with iodine-125 seeds has been developed. The system of metal stent combined with intraluminal irradiation of iodine-125 seeds is composed of three parts: esophageal nitinol stent, covering of silicone membrane or polytetrafluoroethylene membrane, and nitinol sheaths fixed outside the membrane containing iodine seeds.[12] A clinical trial demonstrated that dysphagia grades significantly improved in both groups within the first month after stent placement, but were better in the irradiation stent group than in the control stent group after 2 months.[12,87,108]

8.4 CONCLUSION

Over the past 30 years, esophageal stents have rapidly evolved from rigid, plastic tubes to partially or fully covered SEMS in the 1990s and SEPS in the beginning of the 21st century. The process of developing specific stent characteristics to reduce complications of stent placement, such as migration, reflux esophagitis, and hyperplastic tissue in- or overgrowth, continues. An optimal stent design should be flexible, nontraumatic, and should have an internal diameter large enough to allow normal food passage yet minimize the risks of perforation, pain, and hemorrhage. Furthermore, placement, repositioning, and removal of the stent should be easy, without risks of stent migration, as well as nontumoral and tumoral tissue in- or overgrowth. Although the ideal stent does not exist, most currently used stents fulfill at least some of these criteria.

SEMSs have proven benefit in patients with malignant esophageal disease and have been used for palliation of symptoms related to esophageal obstruction. The benefit of metal stents in benign disease is limited because of difficulties during removal and tissue hyperplasia that leads to stents embedding in benign tissue. SEPSs and biodegradable stents have also been tried in the treatment of refractory benign esophageal stricture. SEPSs have become less popular due to relatively high migration rates. Furthermore, the use of PCSEMS has been discouraged as embedment of the uncovered stent flares may result in recurrence of dysphagia and may complicate stent removal. Consequently, FCSEMS are currently the mainstay in the treatment of benign esophageal strictures. Moreover, BEST coated with suitable drugs are the promising candidate to release the restenosis and avoid the burden of subsequent stent removal and the potential risk of adverse events.

To enhance the properties of the stent, novel materials and suitable drugs are promising candidates. Biodegradable Mg and Zn alloys are alternative material of PDO, and the two mentals could eliminate the collapse of polymer material. From the market perspective, FDA-approved materials and established methods can reduce the certification process. In summary, we suggest that patients with benign strictures should be considered for biodegradable stent insertion if conventional dilatation has had no significant improvement or the result was short-lived.

REFERENCES

1. C. Mariette, G. Piessen, J.P. Triboulet. Therapeutic strategies in oesophageal carcinoma: role of surgery and other modalities. *Lancet Oncology* 8(6) (2007) 545–553.
2. Tarver, Talicia. American cancer society cancer facts & figures 2014. *Journal of Consumer Health on the Internet* 16(3) (2012) 366–367.
3. A. Jemal, F. Bray, M.M. Center, J. Ferlay, D. Forman. Global cancer statistics. *CA Cancer Journal for Clinicians* 6(2) (2011) 169–190.
4. F. Bray, J. Ferlay, I. Soerjomataram, R.L. Siegel, L.A. Torre, A. Jema. Global cancer statistics 2018: GLOBOCAN estimates of incidence and mortality worldwide for 36 cancers in 185 countries. *CA Cancer Journal for Clinicians* 68 (2018) 394–424.
5. M. Arnold, I. Soerjomataram, J. Ferlay, D. Forman. Global incidence of oesophageal cancer by histological subtype in 2012. *Gut* 64(3) (2015) 381–387.
6. H. Jiang, K. Patil, A. Vashi, Y. Wang, E. Strickland, S.B. Pai. Cellular molecular and proteomic profiling deciphers the SIRT1 controlled cell death pathways in esophageal adenocarcinoma cells. *Cancer Treatment & Research Communications* 26 (2020) 100271.
7. G.J. Huang, L.J. Wang, J.S. Liu, G.Y. Cheng, D.W. Zhang, G.Q. Wang, R.G. Zhang, Surgery of esophageal carcinoma. *Surgery of Esophageal Carcinoma* 1 (1985) 74–83.
8. D. Bona, L. Laface, L. Bonavina, E. Abate, R. Carrinola. Covered nitinol stents for the treatment of esophageal strictures and leaks. *World Journal of Gastroenterology* 16(18) (2010) 2260–2264.
9. A. Eroglu, A. Turkyilmaz, M. Subasi, N. Karaoglanoglu. The use of self-expandable metallic stents for palliative treatment of inoperable esophageal cancer. *Diseases of the Esophagus* 23(1) (2010) 64–70.
10. J.F. Bosset, M. Gignoux, J.P. Triboulet, E. Tiret, G. Mantion, D. Elias, P. Lozach, J.C. Ollier, J.J. Pavy, M. Mercier, T. Sahmoud. Chemoradiotherapy followed by surgery compared with surgery alone in squamous-cell cancer of the esophagus. *New England Journal of Medicine* 337 (1997) 161–167.
11. B.T. Deressa, W. Tigeneh, N. Bogale, M. Buwenge, A.G. Morganti, E. Farina. Short-course 2-dimensional radiation therapy in the palliative treatment of esophageal cancer in a developing country: a phase II study (Sharon project). *International Journal of Radiation Oncology*Biology*Physics* 106(1) (2020) 67–72.
12. W. Zhongmin, H. Xunbo, C. Jun, H. Gang, C. Kemin, L. Yu, L. Fenju. Intraluminal radioactive stent compared with covered stent alone for the treatment of malignant esophageal stricture. *Cardiovascular Interventional Radiology* 35(2) (2012) 351–358.
13. A. Repici, M. Conio, C.D. Angelis, E. Battaglia, G. Saracco. Temporary placement of an expandable polyester silicone-covered stent for treatment of refractory benign esophageal strictures. *Gastrointestinal Endoscopy* 60 (2004) 513–519.
14. Y.S. Oh, M.L. Kochman, N.A. Ahmad, G.G. Ginsberg. Clinical outcomes after polyflex stent placement forrefractory benign esophageal stricture (RBES). *Gastrointestinal Endoscopy* 65(5) (2007) AB132.
15. T. Yano, Y. Yoda, S. Nomura, K. Toyosaki, H. Hasegawa, H. Ono, M. Tanaka, H. Morimoto, T. Horimatsu, S. Nonaka. Prospective trial of biodegradable stents for refractory benign-esophageal strictures after curative treatment ofesophageal cancer. *Gastrointestinal Endoscopy* 86(3) (2017) 492–499.

16. P.D. Siersema. How to approach a patient with refractory or recurrent benign esophageal stricture. *Gastroenterology* 156(1) (2019) 7–10.

17. S.L. Broor, G.S. Raju, P.P. Bose, D. Lahoti, G.N. Ramesh, A. Kumar, G.K. Sood. Long term results of endoscopic dilatation for corrosive oesophageal strictures. *Gut* 34(11) (1993) 1498–1501.

18. D.J. Patterson, D.Y. Graham, J.L. Smith, J.T. Schwartz, E. Alpert, F.L. Lanza, G.D. Cain. Natural history of benign esophageal stricture treated by dilatation. *Gastroenterology* 85(2) (1983) 346–350.

19. R.J. Lew, M.L. Kochman. A review of endoscopic methods of esophageal dilation. *Journal of Clinical Gastroenterology* 35(2) (2002) 117–126.

20. M.L. Kochman, S.A. McClave, H.W. Boyce. The refractory and the recurrent esophageal stricture: a definition. *Gastrointestinal Endoscopy* 62(3) (2005) 474–475.

21. E. Frimberger. Endoscopic treatment of benign esophageal stricture. *Endoscopy* 15(1) (1983) 199.

22. G.S. Sandha, N.E. Marcon. Expandable metal stents for benign esophageal obstruction. *Gastrointestinal Endoscopy Clinics of North America* 9(3) (1999) 437–446.

23. J.H. Kim, H.Y. Song, E.K. Choi, K.R. Kim, J.H. Shin, J.O. Lim. Temporary metallic stent placement in the treatment of refractory benign esophageal strictures: results and factors associated with outcome in 55 patients. *European Radiology* 19(2) (2009) 384–390.

24. M. Conio, S. Blanchi, R. Filiberti, A. Repici, M. Barbieri, C. Bilardi, P.D. Siersema. A modified self-expanding Niti-S stent for the management of benign hypopharyngeal strictures. *Gastrointestinal Endoscopy* 65(4) (2007) 714–720.

25. J.E. Sousa, A.G.M.R. Sousa, M.A. Costa, A.C. Abizaid, F. Feres. Use of rapamycin-impregnated stents in coronary arteries. *Transplantation Proceedings* 35(3) (2003) S165–S170.

26. F.P. Vleggaar, P.D. Siersema. Stents for benign esophageal strictures. *Techniques in Gastrointestinal Endoscopy* 12(4) (2010) 231–236.

27. D. Chauhan. Esophageal perforation due to removal of partially covered self-expanding metal stents placed for a benign perforation or leak. *Endoscopy* 43(2) (2010) 156–159.

28. Y.S. Seo, J.J. Park, B.G. Kim, J.H. Kim, J.H. Kim, C.H. Kim, J.Y. Kim, K.S. Byun, Y.T. Bak. Segmental amputation of esophagus with bronchial-wall rupture during removal of a stent for benign esophageal stricture. *Gastrointestinal Endoscopy* 64(1) (2006) 141–143.

29. P.D. Siersema, M.Y.V. Homs, J. Haringsma, H.W. Tilanus, E.J. Kuipers. Use of large-diameter metallic stents to seal traumatic nonmalignant perforations of the esophagus. *Gastrointestinal Endoscopy* 58(3) (2003) 356–361.

30. R.P. Wadhwa, R.A. Kozarek, R.E. France, Use of self-expandable metallic stents in benign GI diseases, *Gastrointestinal Endoscopy* 58 (2003) 207–212.

31. P. Didden, M.C.W. Spaander, M.J. Bruno, E.J. Kuipers. Esophageal stents in malignant and benign disorders. *Current Gastroenterology Reports* 15(4) (2013) 1–9.

32. M. Conio, A. Repici, G. Battaglia, G. De Pretis, L. Ghezzo, M. Bittinger, H. Messmann, J.-F. Demarquay, S. Blanchi, M. Togni, R. Conigliaro, R. Filiberti. A randomized prospective comparison of self-expandable plastic stents and partially covered self-expandable metal stents in the palliation of malignant esophageal dysphagia. *American Journal of Gastroenterology* 102(12) (2007) 2667–2677.

33. R.E. White, R.K. Parker, J.W. Fitzwater, Z. Kasepoi, M. Topazian. Stents as sole therapy for oesophageal cancer: a prospective analysis of outcomes after placement. *The Lancet Oncology* 10(3) (2009) 240–246.

34. J.C. Bakken, L.M. Wong Kee Song, P.C. de Groen, T.H. Baron, Use of a fully covered self-expandable metal stent for the treatment of benign esophageal diseases. *Gastrointestinal Endoscopy* 72(4) (2010) 712–720.

35. S. Thomas, A.A. Siddiqui, L.J. Taylor, S. Parbhu, C. Cao, D. Loren, T. Kowalski, D.G. Adler. Fully-covered esophageal stent migration rates in benign and malignant disease: a multicenter retrospective study. *Endosc Int Open* 7(6) (2019) E751–E756.
36. B.L. Bick, T.F. Imperiale, C.S. Johnson, J.M. Dewitt. Endoscopic suturing of esophageal fully covered self-expanding metal stents reduces rates of stent migration. *Gastrointestinal Endoscopy* 86(6) (2017) 1015–1021.
37. P.D. Siersema. Esophageal Stents: Malignancy, Springer Link, 2012.
38. L.L. Fujii, E.A. Bonin, T.H. Baron, C.J. Gostout, K.S. Wong, Louis M.. Utility of an endoscopic suturing system for prevention of covered luminal stent migration in the upper GI tract. *Gastrointestinal Endoscopy* 78(5) (2013) 787–793.
39. J. Yang, A.A. Siddiqui, T.E. Kowalski, D.E. Loren, A. Khalid, A. Soomro, S.M. Mazhar, J. Rose, L. Isby, M. Kahaleh, A. Kalra, A.M. Sarkisian, N.A. Kumta, J. Nieto, R.Z. Sharaiha. Esophageal stent fixation with endoscopic suturing device improves clinical outcomes and reduces complications in patients with locally advanced esophageal cancer prior to neoadjuvant therapy: a large multicenter experience. *Surgical Endoscopy* 31(3) (2017) 1414–1419.
40. S. Prateek, K. Richard. Role of esophageal stents in benign and malignant diseases. *The American Journal of Gastroenterology* 105(2) (2010) 258–273.
41. M.C.W. Spaander, T.H. Baron, P.D. Siersema. Esophageal stenting for benign and malignant disease: European Society of Gastrointestinal Endoscopy (ESGE) clinical guideline. *Endoscopy* 48(10) (2016) 939–948.
42. H.D.D. Reus, I.V.D. Hal. Fully vs. partially covered selfexpandable metal stent for palliation of malignant esophageal strictures: a randomized trial (the COPAC study). *Endoscopy* 50(10) (2018) 961–971.
43. P.D. Siersema. Stenting for benign esophageal strictures. *Endoscopy* 41(4) (2009) 363–373.
44. S.J. Choi, J.H. Kim, J.W. Choi, S.G. Lim, S.J. Shin, K.M. Lee, K. Lee. S1494: fully covered, retrievable self-expanding metal stents (Niti-S) in palliation of malignant dysphagia long-term results of a prospective study (10 years). *Scandinavian Journal of Gastroenterology* 71(7–8) (2011) AB176–AB177.
45. E.M.L. Verschuur, M.Y.V. Homs, E.W. Steyerberg, J. Haringsma, P.J. Wahab, E.J. Kuipers, P.D. Siersema. A new esophageal stent design (Niti-S stent) for the prevention of migration: a prospective study in 42 patients. *Gastrointestinal Endoscopy* 63(1) (2006) 134–140.
46. A. Repici, M. Jovani, C. Hassan, B. Solito, R.D. Mitri, F. Buffoli, G. Macrì, D. Fregonese, V. Cennamo, M.D. Bellis. Management of inoperable malignant oesophageal strictures with fully covered WallFlex® stent: a multicentre prospective study. *Digestive & Liver Disease* 46(12) (2014) 1093–1098.
47. M.M. Hirdes, P.D. Siersema, F.P. Vleggaar. A new fully covered metal stent for the treatment of benign and malignant dysphagia: a prospective follow-up study. *Gastrointestinal Endoscopy* 75(4) (2012) 712–718.
48. P.D. Siersema, W.C.J. Hop, M. van Blankenstein, A.J.P. van Tilburg, D.-J. Bac, M.Y.V. Homs, E.J. Kuipers. A comparison of 3 types of covered metal stents for the palliation of patients with dysphagia caused by esophagogastric carcinoma: a prospective, randomized study. *Gastrointestinal Endoscopy* 54(2) (2001) 145–153.
49. M.J. Uitdehaag, J.E. van Hooft, E.M.L. Verschuur, A. Repici, E.W. Steyerberg, P. Fockens, E.J. Kuipers, P.D. Siersema. A fully-covered stent (Alimaxx-E) for the palliation of malignant dysphagia: a prospective follow-up study. *Gastrointestinal Endoscopy* 70(6) (2009) 1082–1089.
50. S. Lakhtakia, N.D. Reddy, K.S. Dua. Refractory benign esophageal strictures: continuous, non-permanent dilatation with a self-expandable metal esophageal stent (Alimaxx-E). *Gastrointestinal Endoscopy* 65(5) (2007) PAB284.

51. S.U. Latif, K.S. Dua, J.F. Yang, Y. Oh, A.H. Khan. Efficacy and safety of EndoMAXX, a new non-foreshortening fully covered nitinol esophageal stent. *Gastroenterology* 144(5) (2013) 483.

52. D. Chavalitdhamrong, P.V. Draganov, M.S. Wagh. Sa1553 efficacy and safety of the fully covered esophageal EndoMAXX stent: a prospective study. *Gastrointestinal Endoscopy* 79(5) (2014) AB253.

53. E.M.L. Verschuur, E.W. Steyerberg, E.J. Kuipers, P.D. Siersema. Effect of stent size on complications and recurrent dysphagia in patients with esophageal or gastric cardia cancer. *Gastrointestinal Endoscopy* 65(4) (2007) 592–601.

54. M.J. Uitdehaag, P.D. Siersema, M.C.W. Spaander, F.P. Vleggaar, E.M.L. Verschuur, E.W. Steyerberg, E.J. Kuipers. A new fully covered stent with antimigration properties for the palliation of malignant dysphagia: a prospective cohort study. *Gastrointestinal Endoscopy* 71(3) (2010) 600–605.

55. N. Vakil. A prospective, randomized, controlled trial of covered expandable metal stents in the palliation of malignant esophageal obstruction at the gastroesophageal junction. *American Journal of Gastroenterology* 96(6) (2001) 1791–1796.

56. D. Saranovic, A. Djuric-Stefanovic, A. Ivanovic, D. Masulovic, P. Pesko. Fluoroscopically guided insertion of self-expandable metal esophageal stents for palliative treatment of patients with malignant stenosis of esophagus and cardia: comparison of uncovered and covered stent types. *Diseases of the Esophagus* 18(4) (2010) 230–238.

57. M. Uitdehaag, J.V. Hooft, E.M. Verschuur, A. Repici, E.W. Steyerberg, P. Fockens, E.J. Kuipers, P.D. Siersema, A Fully-covered stent (Alimaxx-E) for the palliation of dysphagia from esophageal and gastric cardia cancer: a prospective study. *Gastrointestinal Endoscopy* 67(5) (2008) PAB250.

58. S. Jaganmohan, G.S. Raju. Tissue ingrowth in a fully covered self-expandable metallic stent (with videos). *Gastrointestinal Endoscopy* 68(3) (2008) 602–604.

59. D. Bona, L. Laface, S. Siboni, M. Schaffer, D. Baldoli, A. Sironi, F. Sorba, L. Bonavina. Self-expanding oesophageal stents: comparison of Ultraflex and Choostent. *Chirurgia Italiana* 61(5–6) (2009) 641–646.

60. D.J. van Westerloo, M.J. Bruno, J.F.W.M. Bartelsman, J.J.G.H.M. Bergman, G.N.J. Tytgat. Efficacy and complications of a modified Gianturco-Z stent (Choo stent) used in the palliation of esophagogastric malignancies. *European Journal of Gastroenterology & Hepatology* 11(12) (1999) A29.

61. V. Kahalekar, D.T. Gupta, P. Bhatt, A. Shukla, S. Bhatia. Fully covered self-expanding metallic stent placement for benign refractory esophageal strictures. *Indian Journal of Gastroenterology* 36(3) (2017) 197–201.

62. M.D. Bellis, P. Marone, G.B. Rossi, G.D. Nardo, A. Crispo, M. Esposito, R. Aprea, A. Tempesta. Comparison of polyflex and ultraflex stent for palliation of inoperable neoplastic esophageal strictures. A single center prospective study. *Gastrointestinal Endoscopy* 65(5) (2007) AB149.

63. M.E. Riccioni, S.K. Shah, A. Tringali, S. Ciletti, M. Mutignani, V. Perri, G. Zuccalà, R. Coppola, G. Costamagna, Endoscopic palliation of unresectable malignant oesophageal strictures with self-expanding metal stents: comparing Ultraflex and Esophacoil stents. *Digestive and Liver Disease* 34 (2002) 356–363.

64. J. García-Cano. Dilation of benign strictures in the esophagus and colon with the polyflex stent: a case series study. *Digestive Diseases & Eences* 53(2) (2008) 341–346.

65. A. Repici, N. Pagano, G. Rando, A. Carlino, E. Vitetta, E. Ferrara, G. Strangio, A. Zullo, C. Hassan. A retrospective analysis of early and late outcome of biodegradable stent placement in the management of refractory anastomotic colorectal strictures. *Surgical Endoscopy* 27(7) (2013) 2487–2491.

66. Y. Kang. A review of self-expanding esophageal stents for the palliation therapy of inoperable esophageal malignancies. *BioMed Research International* 2019 (2019) 9265017.
67. S. Buhner, Q. Li, S. Vignali, R. Langer, G. Barbara, R.D. Giorgio, V. Stanghellini, F. Zeller, K. Michel, M. Schemann. Failure of self-expanding plastic stents in treatment of refractory benign esophageal strictures. *Endoscopy* 38(5) (2006) 533–537.
68. L.H, Moyes, C. K, Mackay, M. J, F.J. Diagnostic, T. Endoscopy. The use of self-expanding plastic stents in the management of oesophageal leaks and spontaneous oesophageal perforations. *Diagnostic & Therapeutic Endoscopy* 2011 (2011) 418103.
69. M. Karbowski, D. Schembre, R. Kozarek, K. Ayub, D. Low. Polyflex self-expanding, removable plastic stents: assessment of treatment efficacy and safety in a variety of benign and malignant conditions of the esophagus. *Surgical Endoscopy* 22(5) (2008) 1326–1333.
70. S. Komanduri, V. Villaflor, B. John. Polyflex stent placement immediately following endoscopic ultrasound staging of advanced esophageal malignancy: a feasible and effective alternative to surgical jejunostomy. *Gastrointestinal Endoscopy* 63(5) (2006) AB131.
71. S. Evrard, O.L. Moine, G. Lazaraki, A. Dormann, J. Devière, Self-expanding plastic stents for benign esophageal lesions. *Gastrointestinal Endoscopy* 60 (2004) 894–900.
72. A. Pennathur, A.C. Chang, K.M. Mcgrath, G. Steiner, M. Alvelo-Rivera, O. Awais, W.E. Gooding, N.A. Christie, S. Gilbert, R.J. Landreneau. Polyflex expandable stents in the treatment of esophageal disease: initial experience. *Annals of Thoracic Surgery* 85(6) (2008) 1968–1973.
73. J.S. Barthel, S.T. Kelley, J.B. Klapman. Management of persistent gastroesophageal anastomotic strictures with removable self-expandable polyester silicon-covered (Polyflex) stents: an alternative to serial dilation. *Gastrointestinal Endoscopy* 67(3) (2008) 546–552.
74. J.E. van Hooft, M.I. van Berge Henegouwen, E.A. Rauws, J.J. Bergman, O.R. Busch, P. Fockens. Endoscopic treatment of benign anastomotic esophagogastric strictures with a biodegradable stent. *Gastrointestinal Endoscopy* 73(5) (2011) 1043–1047.
75. S.W. Fry, D.E. Fleischer. Management of a refractory benign esophageal stricture with a new biodegradable stent. *Gastrointestinal Endoscopy* 45(2) (1997) 179–182.
76. S.M. Stivaros, L.R. Williams, C. Senger, L. Wilbraham, H.U. Laasch. Woven polydioxanone biodegradable stents: a new treatment option for benign and malignant oesophageal strictures. *European Radiology* 20(5) (2010) 1069–1072.
77. P. Gkolfakis, P.D. Siersema, G. Tziatzios, K. Triantafyllou, I.S. Papanikolaou. Biodegradable esophageal stents for the treatment of refractory benign esophageal strictures. *Annals of Gastroenterology* 33(4) (2020) 330–337.
78. P. Hommes, S. Berlin, H.U. Reissig. Single and sequential biodegradable stent placement for refractory benign esophageal strictures: a prospective follow-up study. *Gastrointestinal Endoscopy* 75(7) (2012) 452–452.
79. L. Fuccio, C. Hassan, L. Frazzoni, R. Miglio, A. Repici. Clinical outcomes following stent placement in refractory benign esophageal stricture: a systematic review and meta-analysis. *Endoscopy* 48(2) (2015) 141–148.
80. J.M.T. Canena, M.J.A. Liberato, R.A.N. Rio-Tinto, P.M. Pinto-Marques, C.M.M. Romão, A.V.M.P. Coutinho, B.A.H.C. Neves, M.F.C.N. Santos-Silva. A comparison of the temporary placement of 3 different self-expanding stents for the treatment of refractory benign esophageal strictures: a prospective multicentre study. *BMC Gastroenterology* 12(1) (2012) 70–70.
81. A. Repici, F.P. Vleggaar, C. Hassan, P.G. van Boeckel, F. Romeo, N. Pagano, A. Malesci, P.D. Siersema. Efficacy and safety of biodegradable stents for refractory benign esophageal strictures: the BEST (Biodegradable Esophageal Stent) study. *Gastrointestinal Endoscopy* 72(5) (2010) 927–934.

82. Petra G.A. van Boeckel, Frank P. Vleggaar, Peter D. Siersema, A Comparison of temporary self-expanding plastic and biodegradable stents for refractory benign esophageal strictures. *Clinical Gastroenterology & Hepatology* 9(8) (2011) 653–659.
83. M. Uitdehaag, M. Spaander, F.P. Vleggaar, E.M. Verschuur, E.W. Steyerberg, P.D. Siersema, E.J. Kuipers. A new design fully covered metal stent (SX-ELLA Stent Esophageal HV) for the palliation of malignant dysphagia: a prospective follow-up study. *Gastrointestinal Endoscopy* 69(5) (2009) AB357–AB358.
84. T. Tanaka, M. Takahashi, N. Nitta, A. Furukawa, A. Andoh, Y. Saito, Y. Fujiyama, K. Murata. Newly developed biodegradable stents for benign gastrointestinal tract stenoses: a preliminary clinical trial. *Digestion* 74(3–4) (2006) 199–205.
85. A.N. Holm, J.G. de la Mora Levy, C.J. Gostout, M.D. Topazian, T.H. Baron. Self-expanding plastic stents in treatment of benign esophageal conditions. *Gastrointestinal Endoscopy* 67(1) (2008) 20–25.
86. K.S. Dua, F.P. Vleggaar, R. Santharam, P.D. Siersema. Removable self-expanding plastic esophageal stent as a continuous, non-permanent dilator in treating refractory benign esophageal strictures: a prospective two-center study. *American Journal of Gastroenterology* 103(12) (2008) 2988–2994.
87. H. Zhu, J. Guo, A. Mao, W. Lv, J. Ji, W. Wang, B. Lv, R. Yang, W. Wu, C. Ni. Conventional stents versus stents loaded with (125)iodine seeds for the treatment of unresectable oesophageal cancer: a multicentre, randomised phase 3 trial. *Lancet Oncology* 15(6) (2014) 612–619.
88. L. Lei, X. Liu, S. Guo, M. Tang, L. Cheng, L. Tian. 5-Fluorouracil-loaded multilayered films for drug controlled releasing stent application: drug release, microstructure, and ex vivo permeation behaviors. *Journal of Controlled Release* 146(1) (2010) 45–53.
89. Q.H. Guo, S.R. Guo, Z.M. Wang. Estimation of 5-fluorouracil-loaded ethylene-vinyl acetate stent coating based on percolation thresholds. *International Journal of Pharmaceutics* 333(1–2) (2007) 95–102.
90. E.G. Torfason, S. Gunadóttir. In vivo evaluation of 5-Fluorouracil-containing self-expandable nitinol stent in rabbits: efficiency in long-term local drug delivery. *Journal of Pharmaceutical Sciences* 99(1–2) (2010) 3009–3018.
91. H.C. Min, L. Eugene, C.S. Ki, B.T. M., L.Y. Jae, P. Wooram, H.D. Keun, S.J. Sik, J.Y. Ki. Biodegradable sheath-core biphasic monofilament braided stent for bio-functional treatment of esophageal strictures. *Journal of Industrial and Engineering Chemistry* 67 (2018) 396–406.
92. Z.R. Chang, L.X. Ting, L.L. Jun, L.S. Qi, Z. Fen. In vitro degradation of pure Mg for esophageal stent in artificial saliva. *Journal of Materials Science & Technology* 32(5) (2016) 437–444.
93. S. Wang, X. Zhang, J. Li, C. Liu, S. Guan. Investigation of Mg-Zn-Y-Nd alloy for potential application of biodegradable esophageal stent material. *Bioactive Materials* 5(1) (2020) 1–8.
94. H. Guo, Y. He, Y. Zheng, Y. Cui. In vitro studies of biodegradable Zn-0.1Li alloy for potential esophageal stent application. *Materials Letters* 275 (2020) 128190.
95. T. Yuan, Y. Jia, J. Cao, G. Fei, Y. Zhu, Y. Cheng, W. Cui. Fabrication of a delaying biodegradable magnesium alloy-based esophageal stent via coating elastic polymer. *Materials* 9(5) (2016) 384.
96. K. Yang, J. Cao, T.W. Yuan, Y.Q. Zhu, Y.S. Cheng. Silicone-covered biodegradable magnesium stent for treating benign esophageal stricture in a rabbit model. *World Journal of Gastroenterology* 25(25) (2019) 3207–3217.
97. Y.Q. Zhu, K. Yang, L. Edmonds, L.M. Wei, R. Zheng, R.Y. Cheng, W.G. Cui, Y.S. Cheng. Silicone-covered biodegradable magnesium-stent insertion in the esophagus: a comparison with plastic stents. *Therapeutic Advances in Gastroenterology* 10(1) (2017) 11–19.

98. J. Liu, Z. Wang, K. Wu, J. Li, W. Chen, Y. Shen, S. Guo, Paclitaxel or 5-fluorouracil/ esophageal stent combinations as a novel approach for the treatment of esophageal cancer. *Biomaterials* 53 (2015) 592–599.

99. Q. Xia, N. Zhang, J. Li, H. Wang, C. Wang, Z. Zhang. J.G. Gu, M. Wang, C.C. Han, S. Xu, Y. Liu. Dual-functional esophageal stent coating composed of paclitaxel-loaded electrospun membrane and protective film. *Journal of Biomedical Nanotechnology* 15(13) (2019) 2108–2120.

100. E.G. Torfason, S. Guðnadóttir, Polymerase chain reaction for laboratory diagnosis of orf virus infections. *Journal of Clinical Virology* 99 (2002) 3009–3018.

101. Q. Guo, S. Guo, Z. Wang. A type of esophageal stent coating composed of one 5-fluorouracil-containing EVA layer and one drug-free protective layer: in vitro release, permeation and mechanical properties. *Journal of Controlled Release* 118(3) (2007) 318–324.

102. J. Lagergren, E. Smyth, D. Cunningham, P. Lagergren. Oesophageal cancer. *The Lancet* 390(10110) (2017) 2383–2396.

103. D. Alderson, D. Cunningham, M. Nankivell, J.M. Blazeby, S.M. Griffin, A. Crellin, H.I. Grabsch, R. Langer, S. Pritchard, A. Okines, R. Krysztopik, F. Coxon, J. Thompson, S. Falk, C. Robb, S. Stenning, R.E. Langley. Neoadjuvant cisplatin and fluorouracil versus epirubicin, cisplatin, and capecitabine followed by resection in patients with oesophageal adenocarcinoma (UK MRC OE05): an open-label, randomised phase 3 trial. *The Lancet Oncology* 18(9) (2017) 1249–1260.

104. Y. Bai, K. Zhang, R. Xu, H. Liu, F. Guan, H. Luo, Y. Chen, J. Li. Surface modification of esophageal stent materials by a drug-eluting layer for better anti-restenosis function. *Coatings* 8(6) (2018) 215.

105. M. Shaikh, N.R. Choudhury, R. Knott, S. Garg. Engineering stent based delivery system for esophageal cancer using docetaxel. *Molecular Pharmaceutics* 12(7) (2015) 2305–2317.

106. K. Zhang, Y. Bai, X. Wang, Q. Li, F. Guan, J. Li. Surface modification of esophageal stent materials by a polyethylenimine layer aiming at anti-cancer function. *Journal of Materials Science: Materials in Medicine* 28(8) (2017) 125.

107. Y. Zhang, Y. Gao, J. Chen, L. Ma, L. Liu, X. Wang, Z. Fan. Effect of a paclitaxel-eluting metallic stent on rabbit esophagus. *Experimental & Therapeutic Medicine* 12(5) (2016) 2928–2936.

108. J.H. Guo, G.J. Teng, G.Y. Zhu, S.C. He, G. Deng, J. He. Self-expandable stent loaded with 125I seeds: feasibility and safety in a rabbit model. *European Journal of Radiology* 61(2) (2007) 356–361.

9 High-Performance Materials for Targeted and Controlled Drug Delivery Systems

Jinjie Zhang
Zhengzhou University

CONTENTS

DOI: 10.1201/9781003161981-9

9.1 INTRODUCTION

The ultimate goal of drug delivery is to maximize the therapeutic efficacy of drugs while minimizing side effects [1]. With increasing recognition of the importance of biodistribution and pharmacokinetics for safe and effective treatment, targeted and controlled drug delivery systems (DDSs) are considered as the best candidates for the goal because of their ability to deliver the necessary amount of drug to the targeted site and realize appropriate drug release from dosage form, both precisely and efficiently [2]. Particle-based DDSs with particle size within the nanometer to micrometer range, including microspheres [3,4], microcapsules [5,6], nanoparticles [7–9], liposomes [10,11], and microemulsions [12,13], are well known for addressing the inefficiencies of conventional drug administration and enhancing drug safety and patient adherence. In particular, the short half-life and potential toxicity of macro-molecular drugs [14], such as proteins, peptides, and nucleic acids, provide further impetus for the design of optimal DDSs, which can protect them from degradation and control their release in a constant manner [15].

DDSs with sustained or controlled-release properties can maintain effective blood drug concentrations, reduce the frequency of administration, and enhance the thera-peutic index [16]. In addition, developing targeting strategies utilizing DDS, such as targeting tumor sites, can lower the therapeutic dose, achieve desired efficacy, as well as reduce unwanted toxicities. Some researchers have also classified the targeted DDS as a directional controlled-release system [17]. It should be noted that the choice of carrier materials is the most critical element of efficient fabrication of DDS. The development of biodegradable/biocompatible materials that can be degraded into non-toxic products in vivo has received the most attention. In this chapter, we focus on high-performance drug carriers along with recent research in the construction of targeted and controlled DDSs. First, we introduce the development of biodegrad-able materials fabricated for targeted and controlled DDSs with special emphasis on their advantages and limitations. Several kinds of targeted and controlled DDSs through common routes of administration, including oral, intravenous, and transder-mal routes, are then highlighted. In addition, the techniques utilized in micro and nanoscale production of these DDSs are summarized. At the end, the future pros-pects of this field are discussed.

9.2 BIODEGRADABLE POLYMERS USED FOR CONSTRUCTION OF SUSTAINED/CONTROLLED DRUG DELIVERY SYSTEMS

Since the first introduction of controlled-release formulations in 1960s [18], numer-ous controlled drug delivery formulations have been developed and marketed for convenient dosing schedules and improved patient compliance, leading to more effi-cacious treatment [18]. In parallel, notable researchers such as Folkman, Zaffaroni,

TABLE 9.1

Development of Controlled Drug Delivery Systems Since 1950

First-Generation (1G) (1950s–1970s)	Second-Generation (2G) (1980s–2000s)	Third-Generation (3G) (2010s–2030s)
Basics of controlled-release	*Smart delivery systems*	*Modulated delivery systems*
Oral delivery:	Zero-order release	On-off insulin release:
Twice-a-day, once-a-day	Smart polymers and hydrogels:	Glucose-sensitive release
Transdermal delivery:	Environment-sensitive,	Targeted delivery:
Once-a-day, once-a-week	Self-regulated release	Anticancer drugs, siRNA
Drug delivery mechanisms:	Nanoparticles:	Long-term delivery systems:
Dissolution, diffusion, osmosis,	Tumor-targeted delivery	12 months delivery with minimal
and ion-exchange	Gene delivery	initial burst effect
		In vitro-in vivo correlation:
		Prediction of PK profiles from in
		vitro release study

Michaels, Higuchi, and Langer have made significant contributions [19–21]. Tremendous advances in this field have revolutionized the drug delivery technology for both old and new drugs.

Table 9.1 describes the technologies developed since the early 1960s until 2020 [18], and the technologies necessary for treating various diseases in the next 10 years [22]. Controlled-release formulations are often known as sustained-release formulations, extended-release preparations, retard preparations, and prolonged-action preparations [20]. In this chapter, we use these terms interchangeably. With the development of controlled DDSs, numerous natural and synthetic biomaterials have been studied and investigated for their biocompatibility and utilization as drug delivery carriers. Here, we present a brief overview of biodegradable biomaterials (either synthetic or natural) commonly used for delivering medication at a controlled rate, summarize the formulation of several types of sustained-release DDSs, and discuss the main drug delivered problems and resolutions.

9.2.1 Natural and Synthetic Biomaterials for Controlled-release DDS

The biodegradable polymers generally fall into two categories according to their origin [23], namely, natural and synthetic, as listed in Figure 9.1.

9.2.1.1 Synthetic Polymers

The synthetic polymers commonly used in fabricating micro/nanocarriers include polyesters [24], polyanhydrides [25–27], poly(ortho esters) [28–30], polyphosphazenes [31], and polysaccharides [32, 33]. Their chemical structures are provided in Figure 9.2.

Aliphatic polyesters have received significant attention and gained wide acceptance in pharmaceutical technology due to their remarkable biocompatibility and biodegradability [34–36]. While the action of enzymes in biodegradation of aliphatic

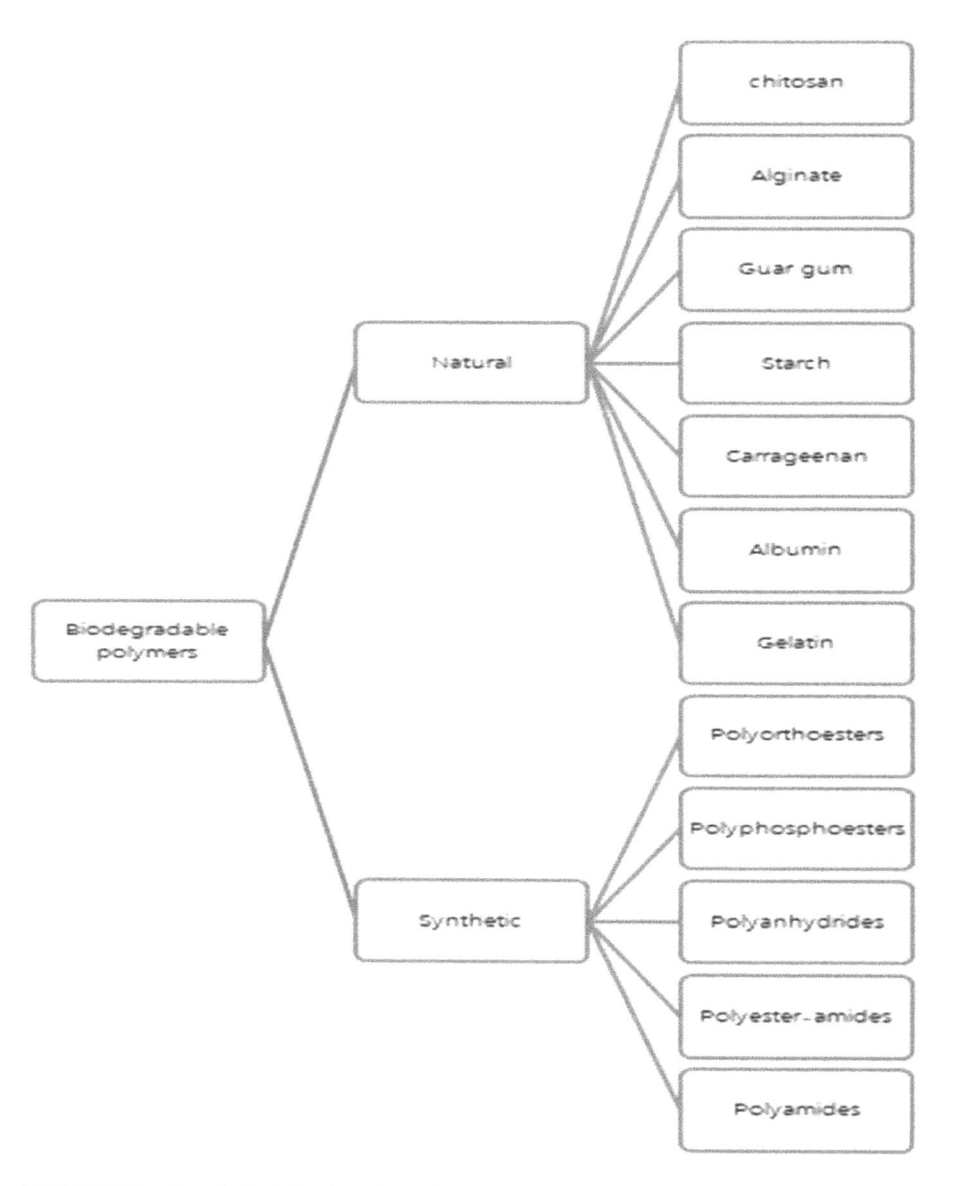

FIGURE 9.1   Broad classification of biodegradable polymer.

polyesters remains unclear, they can degrade by the hydrolysis of the ester bonds in their polymer chain [37]. Chemical structures of several representative polyesters, such as poly(ε-caprolactone) (PCL), poly(lactic-co-glycolic acid) (PLGA), and poly(phosphoesters), are shown in Figure 9.3.

Among them, PLGA copolymers are the most widely explored polymers and reported as the most effective micro/nanocarriers [38–40]. PLGA polymers degrade into water-soluble monomeric acids (i.e., lactic and glycolic acids), which can further

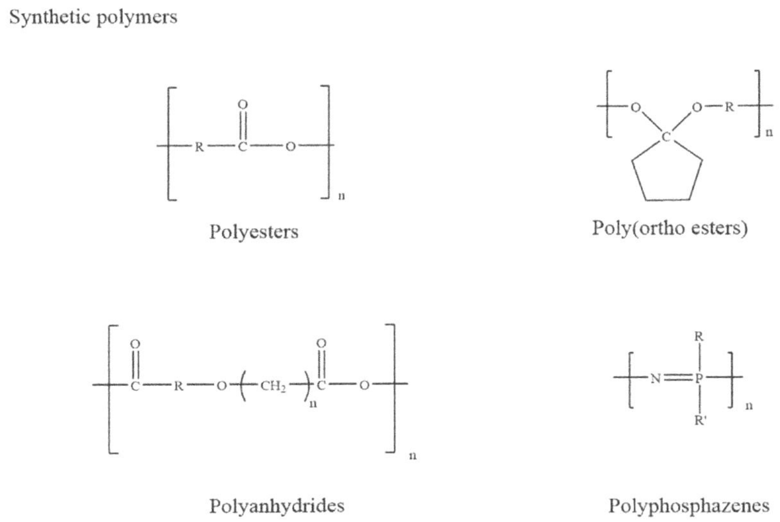

Synthetic polymers

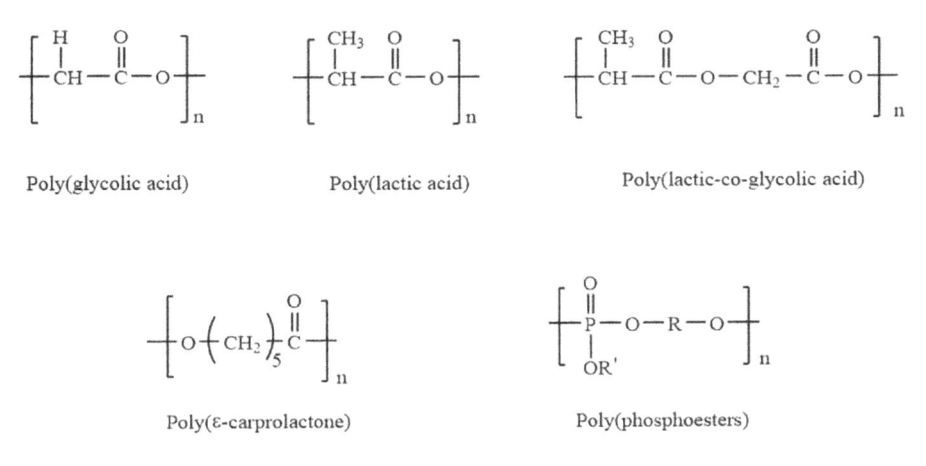

Polyesters

Poly(ortho esters)

Polyanhydrides

Polyphosphazenes

FIGURE 9.2 Chemical structures of several synthetic polymers.

Poly(glycolic acid)

Poly(lactic acid)

Poly(lactic-co-glycolic acid)

Poly(ε-carprolactone)

Poly(phosphoesters)

FIGURE 9.3 Chemical structures of polyesters.

be metabolized to carbon dioxide and water [41–43]. These naturally existing metabolites are readily excreted from or resorbed by the body [44]. Therefore, PLGA is one of the few biocompatible polymers that has been generally regarded as safe for controlled drug delivery [45,46]. More importantly, it is the only FDA-approved intra-articular injected drug carrier [44].

PLGA carriers can provide controlled drug release from periods of a few days up to several months [47,48]. The degradation rate and mechanical properties of PLGA are tunable by altering the lactic acid/glycolic acid ratio and the molecular weight of the polymers, which are also critical for determining the release rate of the encapsulated drugs [47,49]. In general, PLGA copolymers composed of high percentage of glycolic acid copolymers (up to 70%) are amorphous in nature and degrade more rapidly. As the molecular weight of the polymer decreases, the degradation becomes faster due to the higher content of carboxylic groups at the end of their backbone which accelerate acid-catalyzed degradation. Despite these promising drug delivery properties, studies have demonstrated that PLGA copolymers significantly impair the stability and bioactivity of biomacromolecules, mainly due to the hydrophobicity of the polymers and the presence of acidic degradation products [43,50].

Due to the complexity and poor reproducibility of the synthetic process, the biomedical application of polyanhydrides, poly(ortho esters), polyphosphazenes, and polysaccharides are limited. Their properties and other related information can be seen in review articles [51–53] and are not discussed further here.

9.2.1.2 Natural Biomaterials

Despite increasing numbers of synthetic biodegradable polymers developed for controlled DDSs, the use of natural biodegradable polymers has attracted significant attention due to good biocompatibility, ease of modification by simple chemistry, and their widespread abundance in nature [54]. Natural polymers include protein-based polymers (e.g., collagen, gelatin, and albumin) [23] and polysaccharides (e.g., chitosan, hyaluronic acid, cyclodextrin, starch, and dextran) [55]. Figure 9.4 shows the chemical structure of several most commonly used natural polymers. The applications of protein-based polymers have been limited because of their low mechanical properties, high cost, and potential immunogenicity [56,57]. In contrast, polysaccharides show great promise as drug carriers because they are low-cost, amenable to chemical modifications, and exhibit low immunogenicity [58, 59]. For example, chitosan, one of the most abundant naturally occurring polysaccharide, is obtained from the deacetylation of chitin [60]. Chitosan is mainly composed of 2-amino-2-deoxy-β-D-glucopyranose (D-glucosamine) (Figure 9.4). Due to the active functional

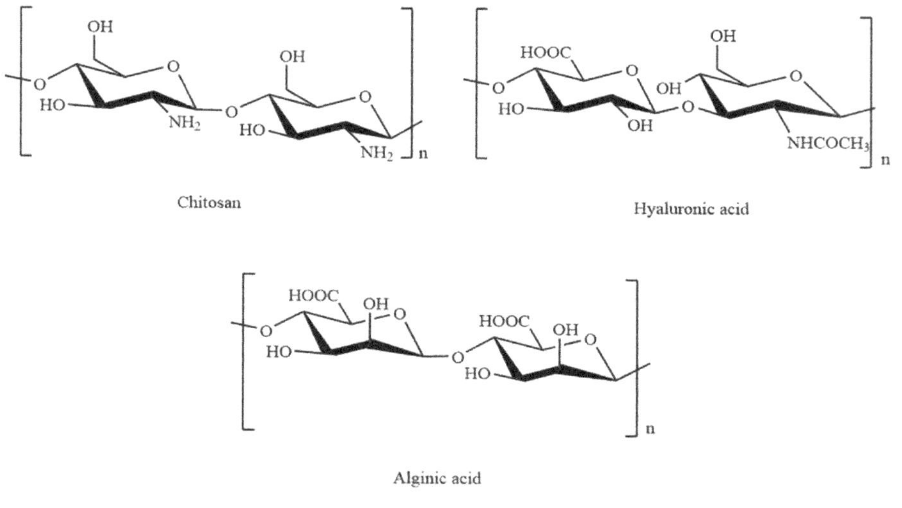

FIGURE 9.4 Chemical structures of several natural polymers.

groups of chitosan, chitosan derivatives can be readily synthesized through chemical reactions [61]. Chitosan and its derivatives play a potential role in biomedical applications due to their good biodegradability, biocompatibility, low immunogenicity, and significant biological activities [62,63]. It is worth noting that that the biodegradability of chitosan can be precisely controlled through chemical conjugation with acetic anhydride [64]. Additionally, they exhibit positive charge on the surfaces in biological fluids due to protonation of primary amino groups in their main backbone. Therefore, chitosan-based biodegradable microparticles can be readily prepared by treating them with various biocompatible polyanionic substances such as sulfate, citrate, and tripolyphosphate [65,66]. These outstanding features of chitosan have driven and broadened the development of delivery systems for biological macromolecules.

9.2.2 FORMULATION OF DIFFERENT TYPES OF CONTROLLED-RELEASE DRUG DELIVERY SYSTEMS

9.2.2.1 Sustained-Release Matrix Tablets

Among various types of controlled-release DDS, the sustained-release matrix tablets are relatively low-cost, easy to carry, and exhibit high patient compliance. Sustained-release matrix tablets is defined as a solid preparation made by mixing drugs with one or more inert matrix materials and other excipients [67]. The matrix tablets have different bioavailability due to different matrix materials or different preparation processes. Various matrix materials can be used to make hydrophilic gel matrix, insoluble matrix, and bioerodible matrix. Here, we will introduce commonly used matrix materials for matrix tablets according to their properties.

9.2.2.1.1 Hydrophilic Gel Matrix Materials

Hydrophilic gel matrix materials refer to substances that swell when exposed to water or digestive juice to form a gel barrier and therefore can control the dissolution of drugs. There are many varieties of materials, which can be roughly divided into four categories, including natural gums (such as sodium alginate, agar, and tragacanth), cellulose derivatives (such as methyl cellulose, hydroxyethyl cellulose, and sodium carboxymethyl cellulose), non-cellulosic polysaccharides (such as chitosan, galactose, and mannitol), and ethylene polymers and acrylic resins (polyvinyl alcohol and polyvinyl) [68].

The ratio of materials to the drug can adjust the drug release rate of the formulations. For example, the changes in the content of methoxy and hydroxypropyl substituents in hydroxypropyl methylcellulose (HPMC) change its viscosity and hydration speed [69]. The greater the hydration rate, the easier it is to form a gel layer on the surface of the preparation to achieve controlled drug release [70]. HPMA has been included in the US Pharmacopoeia from the 19th edition. The main HPMC products currently available for medicinal use in the domestic and foreign markets are shown in Table 9.2.

Another classic example is sodium alginate. Sodium alginate is polysaccharide extracted from kelp or seaweed. As a natural product, the place of production and the production process have a great impact on the physical and chemical properties

TABLE 9.2

Hydroxypropyl Methyl Cellulose (HPMC) of Medicinal Specification

Product	Application	viscosity/10^{-9}(Pa s)
METHOCEL E4 CR PREMIUM	Super-grade (controlled-release) powdered HPMC	4,000
METHOCEL E10M CR PREMIUM	Super-grade (controlled-release) powdered HPMC	10,000
METHOCEL K100-LV PREMIUM	Superior-grade powdered HPMC	100
METHOCEL K100-LV CR PREMIUM	Super-grade (controlled-release) powdered HPMC	100
METHOCEL K4M PREMIUM	Superior-grade powdered HPMC	4,000
METHOCEL K4M CR PREMIUM	Super-grade (controlled-release) powdered	4,000
METHOCEL K15M PREMIUM	Superior-grade powdered HPMC	15,000
METHOCEL K15M CR PREMIUM	Super-grade (controlled-release) powdered	15,000
METHOCEL K100M CR PREMIUM	Superior-grade powdered HPMC	100,000
METHOCEL K100M CR PREMIUM	Super-grade (controlled-release) powdered	100,000

of sodium alginate [71], which greatly affects its application in sustained-release preparations. There is a linear relationship between the molecular weight of sodium alginate and the drug release rate [72]. The larger the molecular weight of sodium alginate, the slower the drug release rate. In addition, for the same sodium alginate matrix, the dissolution rate of water-soluble drugs is greater than that of insoluble drugs. The dissolution rate of cationic drugs is slower than that of anionic drugs. Therefore, when using sodium alginate, it is necessary to consider the molecular weight of the drug and sodium alginate.

9.2.2.1.2 Insoluble Matrix Materials

Insoluble matrix materials refer to high-molecular polymers that are insoluble in water or have very little water solubility. Commonly used insoluble matrix materials include polyethylene, polyvinyl chloride, methacrylic acid-methyl acrylate copolymer, ethyl cellulose, etc. [73]. Because the release rate of poorly soluble drugs from the matrix is very slow, only water-soluble drugs can be loaded in such sustained-release tablets. Factors that affect the release rate of the drug include the properties and amount of the matrix materials and drugs, the size of the drug particle, and the preparation process.

9.2.2.1.3 Bioerodible Matrix Tablets

The erodible matrix tablets consists of insoluble but erodible inert wax, fatty acid, and its esters and other excipients such as beeswax, carnauba wax, stearic acid, hydrogenated vegetable oil, polyethylene glycol, and triglycerides [74]. There are many factors that affect the release of corrosive matrix tablets, such as the nature of the matrix material, the ratio of drug/matrix and the molecular weight of the matrix polymer, drug content, drug solubility, and formulation factors. For example, the release of bovine serum albumin from the fumaric acid polyester hydrogel cross-linked with N-vinylpyrrolidone showed a significant degree of cross-linking dependence [75]. When the degree of cross-linking is low, the hydrogel rapidly swells and hydrolyzes, leading to quick drug release. When the degree of cross-linking is high, the hydrogel swells slowly when it absorbs water. Therefore, the degradation of the hydrogel and the release of the drug reduce.

9.2.2.2 Biomaterials Used for Bioadhesive Drug Delivery System

Research on controlled-release preparations not only requires local targeted drug delivery in the spatial direction but also requires control of drug release in the body in the time direction. For example, an oral preparation originally designed for 24-hour drug release may only reach the colon in half of the designed time due to gastric emptying or rapid small intestinal peristalsis, resulting in a decrease in systemic blood concentration and a large waste of drugs. Therefore, it is necessary to extend the retention of sustained and controlled-release preparations at the absorption site. Utilizing the principle of biological mucosal adhesion in the field of biology, using polymer materials to play a positioning role, and administering through the mucosa, the preparation has the dual characteristics of local targeting and long-term administration.

Bioadhesion refers to the ability of natural or synthetic macromolecule substances to adhere to the surface of mucus or epithelial cells in the lumen [76]. When the bioadhesive substrate is mucus, it is called mucosal adhesion. When the substrate is cell membrane, it is called cell adhesion. The use of bioadhesive polymers in DDSs is called bioadhesive DDSs. Some small-molecule drugs or peptide protein drugs are rapidly metabolized after oral administration and have low bioavailability. The bioavailability of these drugs can be improved when they are administered to the mucosal membrane. Drug delivery to human mucosal systems, including eyes, nasal cavity, lung, vagina, gastrointestinal tract, etc., can use bioadhesion to allow the controlled release of drugs. Currently, these mucosal systems are research hotspots to achieve non-invasive drug delivery. Illustration of oral drug absorption and mucosal absorption can be seen in Figure 9.5.

There are many types of bioadhesive materials. According to their sources, bioadhesive materials can be divided into natural bioadhesive materials, semi-synthetic adhesive materials, and synthetic bioadhesive materials. Natural bioadhesive materials include vegetable glues, animal tissue gelatin, chondroitin sulfate, heparin, and hyaluronic acid, among others. Semi-synthetic adhesive materials include cellulose derivatives and chitosan derivatives. Synthetic bioadhesive materials include acrylics, methacrylic acid, and vinyl polymer materials. In addition to the above types, new adhesive materials can also be obtained through chemical modification or re-synthesis.

9.2.2.3 Biomaterials Used for Membrane-Controlled Sustained-Release Preparation

Membrane-controlled sustained-release preparations refer to preparations in which tablets, capsules, or pellets are coated by one or more coating materials to control the dissolution and diffusion of drugs [77]. Membrane-controlled sustained-release

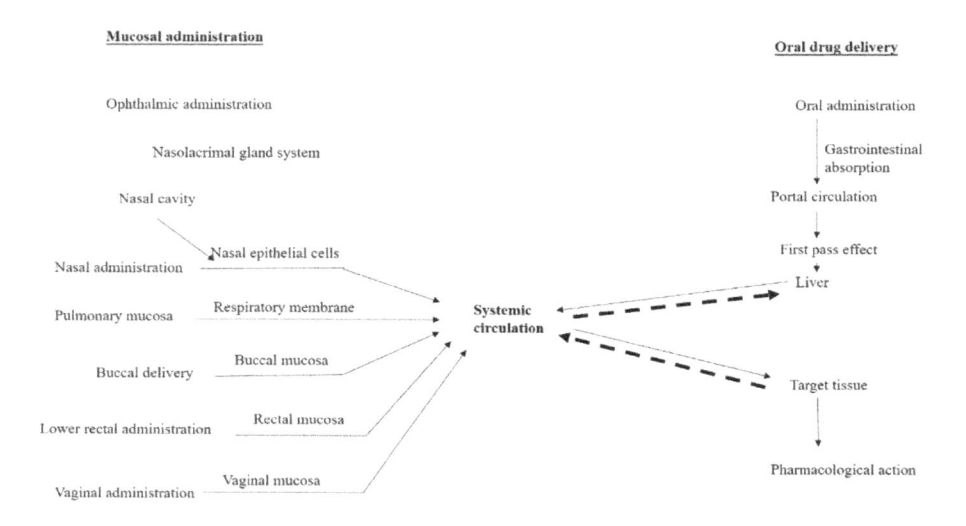

FIGURE 9.5   Illustration of oral and mucosal absorption routes of drugs.

preparations are divided into two types according to different polymer structures, as shown in Figure 9.6. The coating preparation is composed of a drug-containing tablet core and a coating material. The tablet core is generally composed of drugs and some excipients. Commonly used membrane-controlled-release coating materials are high-molecular polymers, most of which are difficult to dissolve in water, but they are non-toxic, not interfered by gastrointestinal fluids or body fluids, and have good film-forming properties and mechanical properties [78]. The application of biomaterials mainly considers the release site of the coating material in the gastrointestinal tract, solubility in solvents and digestive juices, permeability, viscosity, and mechanical properties. Among them, cellulose acetate, ethyl cellulose, and polyacrylic resin are widely used due to their stable properties.

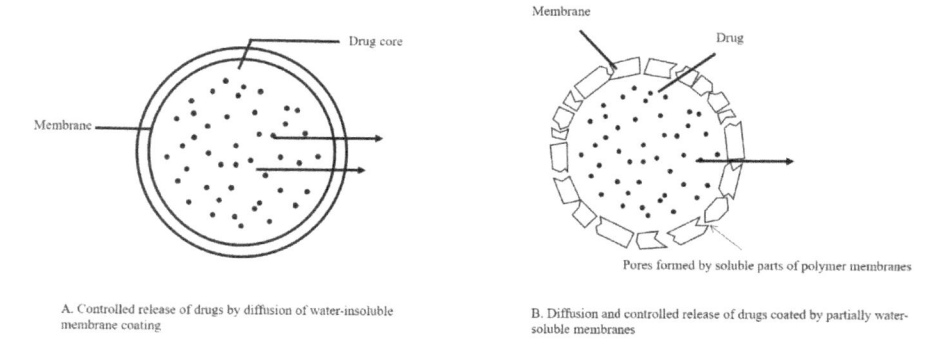

A. Controlled release of drugs by diffusion of water-insoluble membrane coating

B. Diffusion and controlled release of drugs coated by partially water-soluble membranes

FIGURE 9.6   Structural representations of membrane-controlled sustained-release preparations. (a) controlled release of drugs by diffusion of water-insoluble membrane coating, (b) diffusion and controlled release of drugs coated by partially water-soluble membranes.

9.2.3 PROBLEMS AND SOLUTIONS

Reducing the burst release and achieving zero-order drug release have been two major difficulties in obtaining the sustained release of drugs. In addition, maintaining the long circulation of particles in the body and enhancing their adhesion to target disease site are still not well resolved.

9.2.3.1 How to Eliminate Sudden Release of Drug from the Carriers?

Many research studies have centered on developing new biomaterial-based controlled drug delivery, but less attention has paid to controlling initial burst drug release from controlled drug delivery till today. Generally, drugs are released from micro/nanocarriers by drug leaching from the polymer or by degradation of the polymer matrix [79]. Due to the influence of the preparation procedure or intrinsic drug-carrier interaction for drug loading, some drugs can be released directly from the surface of the particles or through the micro/nanopores of the carrier at the initial stage of release, resulting in a sudden increase in blood concentration, which is called sudden release [80,81]. Sudden drug release not only reduces the amount of drug reaching the target site but also increases the blood concentration of drug, leading to potential adverse effects in the body [82,83]. Through washing, extraction, and other methods, reducing the amount of drug attached to the particle surface can reduce the burst release. However, at the same time, these methods can decrease the drug loading efficiency and need high solvent consumption [84].

Currently, the main methods to solve the sudden-release problem include optimizing the preparation process parameters [85], improving the process [86], and improving the drug distribution in the carrier [87]. The drug release characteristics of the particles are controlled by parameters such as particle size, molecular weight of polymer, ratio of carrier material to drug, cross-linking degree, stirring speed, and temperature [88]. The preparation of bilayer microspheres can encapsulate drugs with different solubilities to reduce sudden release rate. For example, double-layer microspheres composed of poly(l-lactic acid) (PLA) shells/PLGA cores can effectively reduce the sudden release of water-soluble drugs [89, 90]. Another example is the preparation of POE (core)/PLGA (shell) double-layer microspheres [91]. The addition of water-soluble protein BSA in the shell can adjust the porosity of the shell, resulting in the controlled release of water-insoluble protein. For water-insoluble drugs, solid dispersion technology is used before drug encapsulation [92], which can improve the bioavailability of drugs and help to adjust the release rate of drugs. In addition, the existing form of carrier materials and the properties of drugs should also be considered. Kim and Park [93] found that the degradation rate of semi-crystalline PLA was significantly lower than that of amorphous PLGA. Due to improved slow-release performance, the rapid degradation of some protein drugs caused by the acidic environment inside the microspheres could be avoided.

Utilization of excipients to improve the distribution of drugs in the carrier has attracted much attention because of its ease of application. Yamaguchi et al. [94] used multiemulsion solvent evaporation method to prepare PLGA microspheres. The addition of hydrophilic polar solvents such as glycerol or ethanol in the organic phase can reduce the distribution of amphoteric drugs (such as protein) on the surface of microspheres and therefore reduce sudden release rate. However, the effectiveness of this method is also related to the properties of drugs. For example, spray drying method is used to prepare PLGA microspheres encapsulating water-soluble drugs [95]. Addition of ethanol in the organic phase causes uneven drug distribution and unstable microsphere structure due to phase separation, resulting in an increase in burst release of drug [95]. However, Wang et al. added 0.2% glucose to the internal aqueous phase in the double emulsion solvent evaporation method, which reduced the burst release rate of PLGA microspheres containing water-soluble drugs [96]. The reason may be that glucose rearranges the polymer microstructure and reduces the permeability of PLGA microspheres.

9.2.3.2 Long Circulating Properties of DDS

Intravenous administration of long-circulating drug carriers can avoid the degradation of gastrointestinal enzymes and the first-pass intestinal and liver metabolism caused by oral administration. For drugs that are unstable in the gastrointestinal tract and need long-term administration, it is more suitable to be administered as parenteral dosage forms. However, the micro/nanocarriers are easily engulfed by macrophages in the reticuloendothelial tissue (RES) after intravenous injection, leading to undesired side effects on off-target organs. The particle size and surface properties are the main factors affecting the clearance rate [97]. In addition, the properties of plasma protein adsorbed on the particle surface also affect the clearance rate [98].

Many studies have been carried out to reduce the clearance rate of particles by RES and achieve long circulation in vivo to target non-RES-related tissues. The particle size ranging between 50 and 200 nm has a good long cycle effect [99, 100]. Gaur et al. used hydrophilic polyvinylpyrrolidone (PVP) as the carrier material to construct gel nanoparticles containing hydrophilic drugs. To improve long-circulating ability in vivo, the nanoparticles were prepared by adjusting particle size (<100 nm) to avoid RES recognition. Particles with surface-modified hydrophilic groups (such as active groups of PEO, PEG, and poloxamers) can reduce the adsorption of plasma proteins, thus avoiding phagocytosis of macrophages. PEG is the most commonly used material. The modification methods include physical adsorption of PEG onto the surface of nano/microparticles, or embedding PEG into lipid nanoparticles [99], or covalent binding of PEG hydroxyl group with the active group of carrier material to achieve different circulating time by regulating the length of PEG chain [101] and the ratio of carrier material to PEG [102]. However, these methods have their own disadvantages. On one hand, physical adsorption is not stable. On the other hand, it is difficult to attach PEG to the surface of the inert particles.

Recently, Kim et al. skillfully modified polystyrene particles with inert surface by PEG [65]. First, polystyrene was used to strongly adsorb the protein drug, and then the nanoparticles with a diameter of 60 nm were obtained by covalent binding between the amino group of protein and mPEG5000 activated by cyanuric chloride. The experimental results of intravenous injection of nanoparticles separated by hydrophobic chromatography showed that the nanoparticles with strong hydrophilic surface had good "avoidance" performance.

9.2.3.3 How to Improve Controlled-Release Performance by Bioadhesion Polymers?

Bioadhesion refers to the adhesion between natural or synthetic polymer materials and biological tissues (mainly epithelial cells or mucous membranes, or both) [103]. The particles prepared by dispersing or confining drugs in adhesive carriers or coating with adhesive materials can reduce the clearance effect of our body on particles, prolong the residence time of drugs in absorption sites, and improve the bioavailability of drugs. Most macromolecules with bioadhesive properties have negatively charged hydrophilic groups (such as hydroxyl, carboxyl, amino, etc.). They interact with the adhesive layer to form non-covalent bonding forces such as hydrogen bond [104]. Chitosan, carbopol, hydroxypropyl cellulose, and sodium alginate are well-known bioadhesive materials [105]. Mumuni et al. [106] prepared insulin-loaded nanoparticles via self-gelation of natural polymers, aqueous soluble snail mucin, and chitosan. The strong adhesive effect of such insulin-loaded nanoparticles on intestinal tract resulted in good insulin absorption and excellent hypoglycemic effect in diabetic rats after oral administration. This kind of adhesive material is mainly activated by wetting, but the adhesion is non-selective, and the adhesion performance is mostly affected by environmental factors, such as pH and enzymes [107]. In addition, suitable modification of carrier materials, such as sulfhydrylation [108], or preparation of PEGylated drugs, can enhance the adhesion ability by forming disulfide bonds or controlling the hydrolysis rate of the prodrugs [109]. Particles modified with plant lectin [110], bacterial adhesion [111], ligands, or antibodies can also achieve targeted adhesion, which has attracted wide attention as the second generation of bioadhesive DDS [76]. The traditional methods to evaluate the bioadhesive properties of DDS include Wilhelm plate method, shear stress method, rheology method, residence time method, and isotope tracer method [112]. New evaluation methods have been developed, such as Biacore method [113]. However, the main problem is that there is no unified standard for these evaluation methods, which brings challenges to the development of bioadhesive systems.

9.3 APPLICATION OF BIOMATERIALS IN TARGETED DRUG DELIVERY SYSTEM

Targeted DDS can locate the drug in the target area, increase the blood drug concentration, and reduce the side effects of drugs [114]. One of the most significant advantage of targeted DDS is reducing off-target side effects of anticancer drugs during chemotherapy [115, 116]. Widder proposed that there are three levels of drug targeting [117]: tissue-specific distribution (level 1), diseased organ-specific distribution (level 2), and delivery of drugs to diseased cells (level 3). At present, targeted gene therapy systems targeting nuclear repair defects or abnormal genes are being studied, which can be referred to as level 4. Generally, passive targeting and active targeting are the two main ways that can direct particles toward the disease site [118]. The targeting function of particles can also be divided into biophysics, physical mechanics, and biochemistry bioimmune targeting according to the targeting mechanism.

9.3.1 BIOMATERIALS UTILIZED FOR DIFFERENT TARGETING MECHANISM

9.3.1.1 Biophysical Drug Targeting

Biophysical targeted particles can be intercepted and absorbed by different tissue parts of the body due to different particle sizes after injection (intravenous, arterial, or intraperitoneal injection) [119]. Generally, micro/nanocarriers cannot recognize target cells. Most of them selectively gather in liver, lung, lymph, and other parts depending on the physical and physiological functions of the body [120]. In addition, the surface charge, hydrophilicity, and adsorption of macromolecules on the surface of the particles also affect their targeting [121]. This kind of target is a passive target, which requires particle size control [122]. Besides, the particle distribution is greatly affected by the microenvironment of the disease site [123]. At present, more attention is being paid to the modification of the targeted DDS to achieve long circulation by escaping from the RES tissue (see Section 9.2.2.2 of this chapter), or to make them have the active targeting function of magnetism, intelligent response, and affinity with the receptors at the disease site.

9.3.1.2 Physical and Mechanical Targeting

At the end of 1970s, magnetic particles (including magnetic nanoparticles) which rely on external forces to achieve drug targeting distribution in vivo were developed [124]. First, chemotherapy drugs are encapsulated in biocompatible magnetic particles. Using the external magnetic field, the particles are concentrated in the lesion site for drug release, which can effectively reduce the toxicity of drugs to normal cells and reduce the dosage of drugs [125]. The targeting efficiency of magnetic particles is affected by many physical and mechanical parameters and hydrodynamic parameters, such as magnetic field intensity and gradient, blood flow velocity during intravenous and pulse injection, magnetic fluid concentration, circulation time, etc. [126–128]. Meanwhile, some physiological parameters, such as the distance from the drug delivery site to the target area, tumor size, and drug-carrier binding degree, should also be considered [129]. Some studies have shown that in areas with slow blood flow velocity, especially when the target is very close to the magnetic source, the targeting function of magnetic particles is the best [130]. Generally, larger particles (1 μm level) can resist blood fluid dynamics, especially in the static and arterial with larger diameter [131], but the particle size to a certain extent can lead to vascular embolism or cause immune response or even inflammation of the body [79]. Therefore, the particle size also needs to be strictly controlled. Considering the magnetic effect of the particles, combined with other surface properties such as particle size, charge, or hydrophilicity, the clearance rate of macrophages can be reduced [132,133].

9.3.1.3 Biochemical Targeting

According to the special biochemical environment of some parts of the body or lesion area (such as pH, temperature, and the difference of the concentration of released biological substances) [134], the drugs loaded in environment-responsive particles can be released in the special environment after administration to avoid the stimulation and side effects of drugs on other parts [135]. More studies have focused on targeting pH-responsive particles in the gastrointestinal tract [136] or tumor [137]. Usually, the pH of gastric juice in human digestive tract is 0.9–1.5, 6–6.8 in the small intestine, and 6.5–7.5 in the colon [136]. Most tumor sites are acidic. pH-responsive targeted DDS can be designed directly using pH-sensitive materials, such as pH-sensitive hydrogels, which have weak acid or alkaline groups on the skeleton, ionized by the influence of external environment pH and ionic strength, and then expanding and releasing drugs [138].

Latest literature has reported several targeted DDS based on poly(methyl methacrylate) (PMMA) [139,140], polyacrylic acid (PAA) [141,142], and natural polysaccharide chitosan [143,144]. Another preparation method is to cross-link or graft pH-sensitive polymer onto the surface of micro/nanocarriers. For example, polyacrylamide guar gum (pAAm-g-GG) has better thermal stability than guar gum [145]. Soppimath used this graft polymer to prepare hydrogel microspheres, producing carboxyl groups through hydrolysis and ionization, so that it has pH sensitivity [146]. Polyvinyl alcohol (PVA)/polyacrylic acid (PAA) prepared by cross-linking emulsification method has a similar pH sensitivity to the network hydrogel microspheres [147], which can achieve the release of drugs in the intestinal tract (pH 7.4). In addition, nanoscale polymer micelles prepared by block copolymers can also be sensitive to acidic pH to achieve targeted drug release [148]. However, the pH difference between tissues in the body is not significant, and it is seriously disturbed by the external environment. For example, the pH environment of small intestine and colon is very similar, which brings some difficulties to the pH-responsive particle DDS.

9.3.1.4   Bioimmune Targeting

Because some antigens or receptors are specifically expressed or overexpressed on the surface of tumor cells, surface modification of the corresponding antibodies or ligands, preparation of immune or affinity-specific particles, can be recognized by tumor tissues or cells, achieving targeted delivery of therapeutic drugs. This kind of targeting overcomes the disadvantage of poor sensitivity of biochemical targeting. Particles prepared from dendrimers (such as polyamide amine dendrimer (PMAMA)) have the advantages of high branching, multivalent state, self-assembled nanospherical structure [149], and therefore are widely used in bioimmune targeting. Thomas et al. linked monoclonal antibodies 60bca and J591 that specifically bind to CD14 and prostate cancer antigen (PSMA) to PMAMA, respectively [150]. In vitro experiments showed that they could target antigen-secreting cells. However, there are still many problems in antibody-modified carriers, such as the decrease in the specificity and the enhancement in the antigenicity after antibody cross-linking. More importantly, there are individual differences in tumors, and monoclonal antibodies can only target specific tumors. In addition, the particle size can be increased after modification, making it difficult to penetrate the tumor. Another difficulty is that there is a great difference in the results of experiments in vivo and in vitro. In contrast, the receptors secreted by tumors are widely distributed. For example, folate receptor is overexpressed in many kinds of tumor cells, and the binding between folate receptor and ligand has the characteristics of specificity, selectivity, and strong affinity. Yi cross-linked folate on the fifth-generation PMAMA (g5-PMAMA) and cross-linked fluorescein (FI) as a detection agent to prepare a multifunctional dendritic nanocarrier, which can effectively target methotrexate (MTX) to KB cells overexpressing folate receptor [151].

9.3.2 DIFFERENT TYPES OF CARRIERS

Targeted DDS mainly includes liposomes, microspheres, nanoparticles, nanocapsules, monoclonal antibody conjugates, and other carriers. Here, recent development of several targeted drug carriers is reviewed.

9.3.2.1 Liposomes

Liposomes can achieve targeted drug delivery through passive targeting and active targeting [152]. Passive targeting can be achieved using conventional liposomes that have not been modified on the surface as a carrier to encapsulate drugs, which can accumulate in different tissues according to different particle sizes. To improve the targeting efficiency and stability of conventional liposomes, more and more liposomes are modified through attachment of antibodies, receptors, sugar residues, etc., on their surface to perform active targeting on specific organs. For example, Shavi et al. [153] developed conventional and PEGylated liposomes loaded with anastrozole for breast cancer therapy. Using thin film hydration method, PEGylated liposomes were successfully prepared by the addition of polyethylene glycol-distearyl phosphatidylethanolamine (PEG-DSPE) in the formulation of conventional liposomes, and the resulting liposomes were characterized by various techniques. The tumor inhibition effect of the stealth liposome and conventional liposome was investigated on BT-549 and MCF-7 cell lines using in vitro cytotoxicity studies. The results showed that the antitumor activity and targeting of anastrozole-loaded stealth liposomes were significantly higher than those of common liposomes.

Apart from PEGylated liposomes, thermosensitive liposomes have also received significant attention for decades [154]. Phospholipids with higher Tc such as dipalmitic acid toluene phosphatidylcholine (Tc was $42°C$) were the most commonly used carrier. By raising the temperature above the phase transition temperature of liposomes on the tumor surface or in the focus, the drug is released rapidly in the target area and the drug concentration is increased. A recent study reported a long-circulating thermosensitive liposome (LCTL) for targeted delivery of oxaliplatin [155]. The in vivo results indicated LCTL could target tumors and exhibit long systemic circulation for more than 24 hours, thereby improving antitumor efficacy on 4T1-bearing mice.

In addition to the above two types of liposomes, there are magnetic liposomes, precursor liposomes, and immune liposomes, among others. Although magnetic liposomes have some advantages, they do not have enough energy in the magnetic field to make the drug stay in the target area and easily cause embolism [156]. At present, the research is limited to animal experiments, and clinical application is challenging [157]. The application of immune liposome also has some shortcomings, such as sensitivity to pH change, thermal instability, and variability in the process of purification [158, 159], causing formidable hurdles for the wide application of immune liposomes.

9.3.2.2   Nanoparticles

Nanoparticles refer to a kind of solid colloidal particles with a particle size of 1 mm–1,000 nm, which can be divided into two types: skeleton solid nanospheres and membrane drug library nanocapsules [160]. They have the advantages of improving the water solubility of insoluble drugs, prolonging the half-life of drugs, slow and controlled release, and can overcome the shortcomings of easy leakage of drugs by carriers such as emulsions and liposomes. For example, hydroxycamptothecin (HPT) is a anticancer monomer with a lactone structure that inhibits the activity of DNA topoisomerase I [161]. HPT exists in the form of lactone under acidic conditions and is hydrolyzed to carboxylate under alkaline conditions. Because lactone is poorly soluble in water, its carboxylate form is often used in clinic at present. However, its carboxylate form has lower structural activity and higher toxicity than lactone. To overcome the above shortcomings, Wang et al. designed novel folate-coated human serum albumin nanoparticle-loaded HPT [162]. In addition to the improved stability and sustained-release properties, the functional nanoparticles showed stronger anti-tumor efficacy than HPT both in vitro and in vivo.

9.3.2.3   Microspheres

Microsphere system refers to the particle dispersion system formed by drug molecules dispersed or adsorbed in polymer carriers [163]. The microsphere has the characteristics of slow-release, long-term effect, targeting, embolism, and so on. The system includes magnetic albumin microspheres, gelatin microspheres, ethyl cellulose microspheres, and starch microspheres. More research and review of microspheres can be seen in the literature [164–166].

9.4   FUTURE PERSPECTIVES

The development of biodegradable and biocompatible materials makes micro/nanocarriers have great potential in targeted and controlled-release DDS. In addition, micro/nanocarriers can deliver bioactive macromolecules and have unique functions in maintaining drug activity and stability. However, there are still some problems to be solved.

The main problem in all carriers is stability, including physical, chemical, and biological stability. By optimizing the particle size, pH value, and ionic strength of the carrier, adding antioxidants, chelating agents, etc., or adding cryoprotectant, the carrier can be made into frozen or freeze-dried products. The carrier can be stabilized for several years. In addition, all kinds of carriers will be cleared by various physiological barriers in the process of drug administration. Due to the effects of albumin, opsins, and antibodies in the blood, some carriers are prone to rupture and rapid leakage of encapsulated drugs, which are quickly recognized and absorbed by the RES, which can be easily deposited in the RES, thus affecting stability and limiting its targeting. Targeted DDS also causes embolism, toxicity, and other problems. However, there is no good quality standard to evaluate it at present.

In addition, there are other problems that cannot be ignored, such as complex production process, poor inter-batch repeatability, poor stability, residual organic solvents during the production process, and high cost of industrial production. Improving the existing technology, reducing the influence of parameter changes, analyzing the particle release behavior using the transfer theory, or developing new technology and new drug carriers can be used as solutions. The development of parenteral drug delivery particles, such as the drug delivery particles of mucosal system, is one of the development directions of DDSs in the future. However, the long-term toxicity to mucosa is also worth considering. The sensitivity and specificity of biochemical targeting DDS are still low, and the development of bacteria-triggered and enzyme-triggered colon DDS will receive more and more attention. The preparation of composite particles should also be explored. Many in vitro and animal experiments of these carriers have shown the desired results, but clinical application in the human body is still challenging due to the large differences in race and individuals, as well as the problems that have been listed above.

REFERENCES

1. P. Davoodi, L. Lee, Q. Xu, V. Sunil, Y. Sun, S. Soh, C. Wang. Drug delivery systems for programmed and on-demand release. *Advanced Drug Delivery Reviews* 132 (2018) 104–138.
2. Y.H. Bae, K. Park. Advanced drug delivery 2020 and beyond: Perspectives on the future. *Advanced Drug Delivery Reviews* 158 (2020) 4–16.
3. T. He, W. Wang, B. Chen, J. Wang, Q. Liang, B. Chen. 5-Fluorouracil monodispersed chitosan microspheres: Microfluidic chip fabrication with crosslinking, characterization, drug release and anticancer activity. *Carbohydrate Polymers* 236 (2020) 116094.
4. J. Andhariya, R. Jog, J. Shen, S. Choi, Y. Wang, Y. Zou, D. Burgess. In vitro-in vivo correlation of parenteral PLGA microspheres: Effect of variable burst release. *Journal of Controlled Release: Official Journal of the Controlled Release Society* 314 (2019) 25–37.
5. T. Bollhorst, K. Rezwan, M. Maas. Colloidal capsules: Nano- and microcapsules with colloidal particle shells. *Chemical Society Reviews* 46(8) (2017) 2091–2126.
6. S. Cao, R. Tang, G. Sudlow, Z. Wang, K. Liu, J. Luan, S. Tadepalli, A. Seth, S. Achilefu, S. Singamaneni. Shape-dependent biodistribution of biocompatible silk microcapsules. *ACS Applied Materials & Interfaces* 11(5) (2019) 5499–5508.
7. J. Peng, Q. Yang, K. Shi, Y. Xiao, X. Wei, Z. Qian. Intratumoral fate of functional nanoparticles in response to microenvironment factor: Implications on cancer diagnosis and therapy. *Advanced Drug Delivery Reviews* 143 (2019) 37–67.
8. X. Fu, J. Cai, X. Zhang, W. Li, H. Ge, Y. Hu. Top-down fabrication of shape-controlled, monodisperse nanoparticles for biomedical applications. *Advanced Drug Delivery Reviews* 132 (2018) 169–187.
9. S. Deka, S. Yadav, D. Kumar, S. Garg, M. Mahato, A. Sharma. Self-assembled dehydropeptide nano carriers for delivery of ornidazole and curcumin. *Colloids and Surfaces. B. Biointerfaces* 155 (2017) 332–340.
10. W. Chen, E. Goldys, W. Deng. Light-induced liposomes for cancer therapeutics. *Progress in Lipid Research* 79 (2020) 101052.
11. L. Mu, R. Ju, R. Liu, Y. Bu, J. Zhang, X. Li, F. Zeng, W. Lu. Dual-functional drug liposomes in treatment of resistant cancers. *Advanced Drug Delivery Reviews* 115 (2017) 46–56.
12. P. Degot, V. Huber, E. Hofmann, M. Hahn, D. Touraud, W. Kunz. Solubilization and extraction of curcumin from Curcuma Longa using green, sustainable, and food-approved surfactant-free microemulsions. *Food Chemistry* 336 (2021) 127660.

13. J. Zhang, Q. Peng, S. Shi, Q. Zhang, X. Sun, T. Gong, Z. Zhang. Preparation, characterization, and in vivo evaluation of a self-nanoemulsifying drug delivery system (SNEDDS) loaded with morin-phospholipid complex. *International Journal of Nanomedicine* 6 (2011) 3405–3414.

14. Q. Guo, C. Jiang. Delivery strategies for macromolecular drugs in cancer therapy. *Acta Pharmaceutica Sinica. B* 10(6) (2020) 979–986.

15. A. Mahmood, A. Bernkop-Schnürch. SEDDS: A game changing approach for the oral administration of hydrophilic macromolecular drugs. *Advanced Drug Delivery Reviews* 142 (2019) 91–101.

16. X. Shi, Y. Ye, H. Wang, F. Liu, Z. Wang. Designing pH-responsive biodegradable polymer coatings for controlled drug release via vapor-based route. *ACS Applied Materials & Interfaces* 10(44) (2018) 38449–38458.

17. H. Dong, Q. Li, C. Tan, N. Bai, P. Cai. Bi-directional controlled release of ibuprofen and Mg(2+) from magnesium alloys coated by multifunctional composite. *Materials Science & Engineering. C. Materials for Biological Applications* 68 (2016) 512–518.

18. Y. Yun, B.K. Lee, K. Park. Controlled drug delivery systems: The next 30 years. *Frontiers of Chemical Science and Engineering* 8(3) (2014) 276–279.

19. A.S. Hoffman. The origins and evolution of "controlled" drug delivery systems. *Journal Controlled Release* 132(3) (2008) 153–163.

20. J. Heller. Controlled release of biologically active compounds from bioerodible polymers. *Biomaterials.* 1(1) (1980) 51–57.

21. G. Castro, B. Panilaitis, E. Bora, D. Kaplan. Controlled release biopolymers for enhancing the immune response. *Molecular Pharmaceutics* 4(1) (2007) 33–46.

22. I. Kwon, S. Lee, B. Han, K. Park. Analysis on the current status of targeted drug delivery to tumors. *Journal of Controlled Release: Official Journal of the Controlled Release Society* 164(2) (2012) 108–114.

23. A. George, P. Shah, P. Shrivastav. Natural biodegradable polymers based nanoformulations for drug delivery: A review. *International Journal of Pharmaceutics* 561 (2019) 244–264.

24. R.A. Jain. The manufacturing techniques of various drug loaded biodegradable poly(lactide-co-glycolide) (PLGA) devices. *Biomaterials.* 21(23) (2000) 2475–2490.

25. J. Jain, D. Chitkara, N. Kumar. Polyanhydrides as localized drug delivery carrier: An update. *Expert Opinion on Drug Delivery* 5(8) (2008) 889–907.

26. A. Basu, A. Domb. Recent advances in polyanhydride based biomaterials. *Advanced Materials (Deerfield Beach, Fla.)* 30(41) (2018) e1706815.

27. M. Torres, A. Determan, G. Anderson, S. Mallapragada, B. Narasimhan. Amphiphilic polyanhydrides for protein stabilization and release. *Biomaterials* 28(1) (2007) 108–116.

28. C. Wang, Q. Ge, D. Ting, D. Nguyen, H. Shen, J. Chen, H. Eisen, J. Heller, R. Langer, D. Putnam. Molecularly engineered poly(ortho ester) microspheres for enhanced delivery of DNA vaccines. *Nature Materials* 3(3) (2004) 190–196.

29. R. Ji, J. Cheng, T. Yang, C. Song, L. Li, F. Du, Z. Li. Shell-sheddable, pH-sensitive supramolecular nanoparticles based on ortho ester-modified cyclodextrin and adamantyl PEG. *Biomacromolecules* 15(10) (2014) 3531–3539.

30. J. Heller, J. Barr. Poly(ortho esters)--From concept to reality. *Biomacromolecules* 5(5) (2004) 1625–1632.

31. S. Rothemund, I. Teasdale. Preparation of polyphosphazenes: A tutorial review. *Chemical Society Reviews* 45(19) (2016) 5200–5215.

32. Y. Li, G. Qin, C. Cheng, B. Yuan, D. Huang, S. Cheng, S. Cao, G. Chen. Purification, characterization and anti-tumor activities of polysaccharides from Ecklonia kurome obtained by three different extraction methods. *International Journal of Biological Macromolecules* 150 (2020) 1000–1010.

33. C. Pandeirada, É. Maricato, S. Ferreira, V. Correia, B. Pinheiro, D. Evtuguin, A. Palma, A. Correia, M. Vilanova, M. Coimbra, C. Nunes. Structural analysis and potential immunostimulatory activity of Nannochloropsis oculata polysaccharides. *Carbohydrate Polymers* 222 (2019) 114962.

34. A.F. Lima, I.R. Amado, L.R. Pires. Poly(d, l-lactide-co-glycolide) (PLGA) nanoparticles loaded with proteolipid protein (PLP)-exploring a new administration route. *Polymers-Basel* 12(12) (2020) 3063.

35. T. Kissel, Y.X. Li, F. Unger. ABA-triblock copolymers from biodegradable polyester A-blocks and hydrophilic poly(ethylene oxide) B-blocks as a candidate for in situ forming hydrogel delivery systems for proteins. *Advanced Drug Delivery Reviews* 54(1) (2002) 99–134.

36. G.A. Abraham, A. Gallardo, J.S. Roman, A. Fernandez-Mayoralas, M. Zurita, J. Vaquero. Polymeric matrices based on graft copolymers of PCL onto acrylic backbones for releasing antitumoral drugs. *Journal of Biomedical Materials Research A* 64a(4) (2003) 638–647.

37. J.H. Park, M.L. Ye, K. Park. Biodegradable polymers for microencapsulation of drugs. *Molecules* 10(1) (2005) 146–161.

38. Y. Cui, X. Li, K. Zeljic, S. Shan, Z. Qiu, Z. Wang. Effect of PEGylated magnetic PLGA-PEI nanoparticles on primary hippocampal neurons: Reduced nanoneurotoxicity and enhanced transfection efficiency with magnetofection. *ACS Applied Materials & Interfaces* 11(41) (2019) 38190–38204.

39. V. Durán, H. Yasar, J. Becker, D. Thiyagarajan, B. Loretz, U. Kalinke, C. Lehr. Preferential uptake of chitosan-coated PLGA nanoparticles by primary human antigen presenting cells. *Nanomedicine: Nanotechnology, Biology and Medicine* 21 (2019) 102073.

40. F. Qi, J. Wu, H. Li, G. Ma. Recent research and development of PLGA/PLA microspheres/ nanoparticles: A review in scientific and industrial aspects. *Frontiers of Chemical Science and Engineering* 13(1) (2019) 14–27.

41. M.C. Hamoudi-Ben Yelles, V. Tran Tan, F. Danede, J.F. Willart, J. Siepmann. PLGA implants: How Poloxamer/PEO addition slows down or accelerates polymer degradation and drug release. *Journal Controlled Release* 253 (2017) 19–29.

42. E. Fortunati, L. Latterini, S. Rinaldi, J.M. Kenny, I. Armentano. PLGA/Ag nanocomposites: In vitro degradation study and silver ion release. *Journal of Materials Science: Materials in Medicine* 22(12) (2011) 2735–2744.

43. B.S. Zolnik, D.J. Burgess. Effect of acidic pH on PLGA microsphere degradation and release. *Journal Controlled Release* 122(3) (2007) 338–344.

44. M. Rai, C. Pham. Intra-articular drug delivery systems for joint diseases. *Current Opinion in Pharmacology* 40 (2018) 67–73.

45. T. Ahmed. Review: Approaches to develop PLGA based in situ gelling system with low initial burst. *Pakistan Journal of Pharmaceutical Sciences* 28(2) (2015) 657–665.

46. G. Burdock, I. Carabin. Generally recognized as safe (GRAS): History and description. *Toxicology Letters* 150(1) (2004) 3–18.

47. Y. Xu, C.-S. Kim, D.M. Saylor, D. Koo. Polymer degradation and drug delivery in PLGA-based drug–polymer applications: A review of experiments and theories. *Journal of Biomedical Materials Research Part B: Applied Biomaterials* 105(6) (2017) 1692–1716.

48. M. Mir, N. Ahmed, A.u. Rehman. Recent applications of PLGA based nanostructures in drug delivery. *Colloids and Surfaces B: Biointerfaces* 159 (2017) 217–231.

49. A.N. Ford Versypt, D.W. Pack, R.D. Braatz. Mathematical modeling of drug delivery from autocatalytically degradable PLGA microspheres--a review. *Journal Controlled Release* 165(1) (2013) 29–37.

50. R. Jalil, J.R. Nixon. Biodegradable poly(lactic acid) and poly(lactide-co-glycolide) microcapsules: Problems associated with preparative techniques and release properties. *Journal of Microencapsulation* 7(3) (1990) 297–325.
51. C. Chen, P. Huang, W. Law, C. Chu, N. Chen, L. Lo. Biodegradable polymers for gene-delivery applications. *International Journal of Nanomedicine* 15 (2020) 2131–2150.
52. A. Lima, H. Ferreira, R. Reis, N. Neves. Biodegradable polymers: An update on drug delivery in bone and cartilage diseases. *Expert Opinion on Drug Delivery* 16(8) (2019) 795–813.
53. S. Doppalapudi, A. Jain, A. Domb, W. Khan. Biodegradable polymers for targeted delivery of anti-cancer drugs. *Expert Opinion on Drug Delivery* 13(6) (2016) 891–909.
54. C. Vasile, D. Pamfil, E. Stoleru, M. Baican. New developments in medical applications of hybrid hydrogels containing natural polymers. *Molecules (Basel, Switzerland)* 25(7) (2020) 1539.
55. V. Gopinath, S. Saravanan, A. Al-Maleki, M. Ramesh, J. Vadivelu. A review of natural polysaccharides for drug delivery applications: Special focus on cellulose, starch and glycogen. *Biomedicine & Pharmacotherapy = Biomedecine & Pharmacotherapie* 107 (2018) 96–108.
56. N. Domeradzka, M. Werten, F. de Wolf, R. de Vries. Cross-linking and bundling of self-assembled protein-based polymer fibrils via heterodimeric coiled coils. *Biomacromolecules* 17(12) (2016) 3893–3901.
57. B. Chalermthai, W. Chan, J. Bastidas-Oyanedel, H. Taher, B. Olsen, J. Schmidt. Preparation and characterization of whey protein-based polymers produced from residual dairy streams. *Polymers-Basel* 11(4) (2019) 722.
58. J. Liu, X. Wang, H. Yong, J. Kan, C. Jin. Recent advances in flavonoid-grafted polysaccharides: Synthesis, structural characterization, bioactivities and potential applications. *International Journal of Biological Macromolecules* 116 (2018) 1011–1025.
59. X. Cui, S. Wang, H. Cao, H. Guo, Y. Li, F. Xu, M. Zheng, X. Xi, C. Han. A review: The bioactivities and pharmacological applications of Polygonatum sibiricum polysaccharides. *Molecules (Basel, Switzerland)* 23(5) (2018) 1170.
60. P. Bakshi, D. Selvakumar, K. Kadirvelu, N. Kumar. Chitosan as an environment friendly biomaterial - a review on recent modifications and applications. *International Journal of Biological Macromolecules* 150 (2020) 1072–1083.
61. W. Wang, Q. Meng, Q. Li, J. Liu, M. Zhou, Z. Jin, K. Zhao. Chitosan derivatives and their application in biomedicine. *International Journal of Molecular Sciences* 21(2) (2020) 487.
62. J. Park, Y. Cho, H. Chung, I. Kwon, S. Jeong. Synthesis and characterization of sugar-bearing chitosan derivatives: Aqueous solubility and biodegradability. *Biomacromolecules* 4(4) (2003) 1087–1091.
63. B. Sultankulov, D. Berillo, K. Sultankulova, T. Tokay, A. Saparov. Progress in the development of chitosan-based biomaterials for tissue engineering and regenerative medicine. *Biomolecules* 9(9) (2019) 470.
64. H. Sashiwa, H. Saimoto, Y. Shigemasa, R. Ogawa, S. Tokura. Lysozyme susceptibility of partially deacetylated chitin. *International Journal of Biological Macromolecules* 12(5) (1990) 295–296.
65. S. Kim, J. Park, Y. Cho, H. Chung, S. Jeong, E. Lee, I. Kwon. Porous chitosan scaffold containing microspheres loaded with transforming growth factor-beta1: Implications for cartilage tissue engineering. *Journal of Controlled Release: Official Journal of the Controlled Release Society* 91(3) (2003) 365–374.
66. T. Ahmed, B. Aljaeid. Preparation, characterization, and potential application of chitosan, chitosan derivatives, and chitosan metal nanoparticles in pharmaceutical drug delivery. *Drug Design, Development and Therapy* 10 (2016) 483–507.

67. M. Teixeira, L. Sa-Barreto, S. Taveira, T. Gratieri, G. Gelfuso, R. Marreto, I. Silva, M. Cunha-Filho. The influence of matrix technology on the subdivision of sustained release matrix tablets. *AAPS PharmSciTech* 21(1) (2019) 8.

68. M. Rabisková, L. Vostalová, G. Medvecká, D. Horácková. [Hydrophilic gel matrix tablets for oral administration of drugs]. *Ceska a Slovenska farmacie: casopis Ceske farmaceuticke spolecnosti a Slovenske farmaceuticke spolecnosti* 52(5) (2003) 211–217.

69. M. Ghimire, L. Hodges, J. Band, B. O'Mahony, F. McInnes, A. Mullen, H. Stevens. In-vitro and in-vivo erosion profiles of hydroxypropylmethylcellulose (HPMC) matrix tablets. *Journal of Controlled Release: Official Journal of the Controlled Release Society* 147(1) (2010) 70–75.

70. R. Hamed, T. Al Baraghthi, S. Sunoqrot. Correlation between the viscoelastic properties of the gel layer of swollen HPMC matrix tablets and their in vitro drug release. *Pharmaceutical Development and Technology* 23(9) (2018) 838–848.

71. S. Fu, I. Buckner, L. Block. Inter-grade and inter-batch variability of sodium alginate used in alginate-based matrix tablets. *AAPS PharmSciTech* 15(5) (2014) 1228–1237.

72. C. Liew, L. Chan, A. Ching, P. Heng. Evaluation of sodium alginate as drug release modifier in matrix tablets. *International Journal of Pharmaceutics* 309 (2006) 25–37.

73. H. Ehmann, S. Winter, T. Griesser, R. Keimel, S. Schrank, A. Zimmer, O. Werzer. Dissolution testing of hardly soluble materials by surface sensitive techniques: Clotrimazole from an insoluble matrix. *Pharmaceutical Research* 31(10) (2014) 2708–2715.

74. J. He, C. Zhong, J. Mi. Modeling of drug release from bioerodible polymer matrices. *Drug Delivery* 12(5) (2005) 251–259.

75. T. Ouchi, T. Saito, T. Kontani, Y. Ohya. Encapsulation and/or release behavior of bovine serum albumin within and from polylactide-grafted dextran microspheres. *Macromolecular Bioscience* 4(4) (2004) 458–463.

76. K. Kumar, N. Dhawan, H. Sharma, S. Vaidya, B. Vaidya. Bioadhesive polymers: Novel tool for drug delivery. *Artificial Cells, Nanomedicine and Biotechnology* 42(4) (2014) 274–283.

77. S. Klein, N. Seeger, R. Mehta, S. Missaghi, R. Grybos, A. Rajabi-Siahboomi. Robustness of barrier membrane coated metoprolol tartrate matrix tablets: Drug release evaluation under physiologically relevant in vitro conditions. *International Journal of Pharmaceutics* 543 (2018) 368–375.

78. M. Choi, D. Choi, J. Hong. Multilayered controlled drug release silk fibroin nanofilm by manipulating secondary structure. *Biomacromolecules* 19(7) (2018) 3096–3103.

79. S. Freiberg, X. Zhu. Polymer microspheres for controlled drug release. *International Journal of Pharmaceutics* 282(1–2) (2004) 1–18.

80. H. Soleymani Abyaneh, M. Vakili, F. Zhang, P. Choi, A. Lavasanifar. Rational design of block copolymer micelles to control burst drug release at a nanoscale dimension. *Acta Biomaterialia* 24 (2015) 127–139.

81. S. Allison. Analysis of initial burst in PLGA microparticles. *Expert Opinion on Drug Delivery* 5(6) (2008) 615–628.

82. A. Thote, J. Chappell, R. Gupta, R. Kumar. Reduction in the initial-burst release by surface crosslinking of PLGA microparticles containing hydrophilic or hydrophobic drugs. *Drug Development and Industrial Pharmacy* 31(1) (2005) 43–57.

83. Z. Xiang, P. Sarazin, B. Favis. Controlling burst and final drug release times from porous polylactide devices derived from co-continuous polymer blends. *Biomacromolecules* 10(8) (2009) 2053–2066.

84. H. Gasmi, F. Siepmann, M. Hamoudi, F. Danede, J. Verin, J. Willart, J. Siepmann. Towards a better understanding of the different release phases from PLGA microparticles: Dexamethasone-loaded systems. *International Journal of Pharmaceutics* 514(1) (2016) 189–199.

85. Y. Zheng, F. Sheng, Z. Wang, G. Yang, C. Li, H. Wang, Z. Song. CoShear speed-regulated properties of long-acting docetaxel control release poly (lactic--glycolic acid) microspheres. *Frontiers in Pharmacology* 11 (2020) 1286.

86. J. Li, L. Yang, C. Zhu, T. Peng, D. Huang, X. Ma, X. Pan, C. Wu. Release mechanisms of bovine serum albumin loaded-PLGA microspheres prepared by ultra-fine particle processing system. *Drug Delivery and Translational Research* 10(5) (2020) 1267–1277.

87. G. Jung, Y. Na, M. Park, C. Park, P. Myung. Preparation of sustained release microparticles with improved initial release property. *Archives of Pharmacal Research* 32(3) (2009) 359–365.

88. H. Abdeltawab, D. Svirskis, M. Sharma. Formulation strategies to modulate drug release from poloxamer based in situ gelling systems. *Expert Opinion on Drug Delivery* 17(4) (2020) 495–509.

89. T.H. Lee, J. Wang, C.-H. Wang. Double-walled microspheres for the sustained release of a highly water soluble drug: Characterization and irradiation studies. *Journal of Controlled Release* 83(3) (2002) 437–452.

90. N.A. Rahman, E. Mathiowitz. Localization of bovine serum albumin in double-walled microspheres. *Journal of Controlled Release* 94(1) (2004) 163–175.

91. M. Shi, Y.-Y. Yang, C.-S. Chaw, S.-H. Goh, S.M. Moochhala, S. Ng, J. Heller. Double walled POE/PLGA microspheres: Encapsulation of water-soluble and water-insoluble proteins and their release properties. *Journal of Controlled Release* 89(2) (2003) 167–177.

92. F. Cui, M. Yang, Y. Jiang, D. Cun, W. Lin, Y. Fan, Y. Kawashima. Design of sustained-release nitrendipine microspheres having solid dispersion structure by quasi-emulsion solvent diffusion method. *Journal of Controlled Release* 91(3) (2003) 375–384.

93. H. Kim, T. Park. Comparative study on sustained release of human growth hormone from semi-crystalline poly(L-lactic acid) and amorphous poly(D, L-lactic-co-glycolic acid) microspheres: Morphological effect on protein release. *Journal of Controlled Release: Official Journal of the Controlled Release Society* 98(1) (2004) 115–125.

94. Y. Yamaguchi, M. Takenaga, A. Kitagawa, Y. Ogawa, Y. Mizushima, R. Igarashi. Insulin-loaded biodegradable PLGA microcapsules: Initial burst release controlled by hydrophilic additives. *Journal of Controlled Release* 81(3) (2002) 235–249.

95. F.-J. Wang, C.-H. Wang. Sustained release of etanidazole from spray dried microspheres prepared by non-halogenated solvents. *Journal of Controlled Release* 81(3) (2002) 263–280.

96. J. Wang, B.M. Wang, S.P. Schwendeman. Mechanistic evaluation of the glucose-induced reduction in initial burst release of octreotide acetate from poly(d, l-lactide-co-glycolide) microspheres. *Biomaterials* 25(10) (2004) 1919–1927.

97. J. Javidi, A. Haeri, F. Nowroozi, S. Dadashzadeh. Pharmacokinetics, tissue distribution and excretion of AgS quantum dots in mice and rats: The effects of injection dose, particle size and surface charge. *Pharmaceutical Research* 36(3) (2019) 46.

98. K.-i. Ogawara, K. Furumoto, Y. Takakura, M. Hashida, K. Higaki, T. Kimura. Surface hydrophobicity of particles is not necessarily the most important determinant in their in vivo disposition after intravenous administration in rats. *Journal of Controlled Release* 77(3) (2001) 191–198.

99. D. Hoarau, P. Delmas, E. Roux, J.-C. Leroux. Novel long-circulating lipid nanocapsules. *Pharmaceutical Research* 21(10) (2004) 1783–1789.

100. I. Brigger, C. Dubernet, P. Couvreur. Nanoparticles in cancer therapy and diagnosis. *Advanced Drug Delivery Reviews* 54(5) (2002) 631–651.

101. U. Gaur, S. Sahoo, T. De, P. Ghosh, A. Maitra, P. Ghosh. Biodistribution of fluoresceinated dextran using novel nanoparticles evading reticuloendothelial system. *International Journal of Pharmaceutics* 202 (2000) 1–10.

102. K. Avgoustakis, A. Beletsi, Z. Panagi, P. Klepetsanis, E. Livaniou, G. Evangelatos, D. Ithakissios. Effect of copolymer composition on the physicochemical characteristics, in vitro stability, and biodistribution of PLGA-mPEG nanoparticles. *International Journal of Pharmaceutics* 259 (2003) 115–127.

103. J.W. Lee, J.H. Park, J.R. Robinson. Bioadhesive-based dosage forms: The next generation. *Journal of Pharmaceutical Sciences* 89(7) (2000) 850–866.

104. J.D. Smart. The basics and underlying mechanisms of mucoadhesion. *Advanced Drug Delivery Reviews* 57(11) (2005) 1556–1568.

105. M. Stie, J. Gätke, F. Wan, I. Chronakis, J. Jacobsen, H. Nielsen. Swelling of mucoadhesive electrospun chitosan/polyethylene oxide nanofibers facilitates adhesion to the sublingual mucosa. *Carbohydrate Polymers* 242 (2020) 116428.

106. M. Mumuni, F. Kenechukwu, K. Ofokansi, A. Attama, D. Díaz. Insulin-loaded mucoadhesive nanoparticles based on mucin-chitosan complexes for oral delivery and diabetes treatment. *Carbohydrate Polymers* 229 (2020) 115506.

107. J. Xu, M. Tam, S. Samaei, S. Lerouge, J. Barralet, M. Stevenson, M. Cerruti. Mucoadhesive chitosan hydrogels as rectal drug delivery vessels to treat ulcerative colitis. *Acta Biomaterialia* 48 (2017) 247–257.

108. W. Suchaoin, I. Pereira de Sousa, K. Netsomboon, J. Rohrer, P. Hoffmann Abad, F. Laffleur, B. Matuszczak, A. Bernkop-Schnürch. Mucoadhesive polymers: Synthesis and in vitro characterization of thiolated poly(vinyl alcohol). *International Journal of Pharmaceutics* 503 (2016) 141–149.

109. B. Lele, A. Hoffman. Mucoadhesive drug carriers based on complexes of poly(acrylic acid) and PEGylated drugs having hydrolysable PEG-anhydride-drug linkages. *Journal of Controlled Release: Official Journal of the Controlled Release Society* 69(2) (2000) 237–248.

110. M. Jepson, M. Clark, B. Hirst. M cell targeting by lectins: A strategy for mucosal vaccination and drug delivery. *Advanced Drug Delivery Reviews* 56(4) (2004) 511–525.

111. J.K. Vasir, K. Tambwekar, S. Garg. Bioadhesive microspheres as a controlled drug delivery system. *International Journal of Pharmaceutics* 255(1) (2003) 13–32.

112. A. Hoffmann, R. Daniels. A novel test system for the evaluation of oral mucoadhesion of fast disintegrating tablets. *International Journal of Pharmaceutics* 551 (2018) 141–147.

113. H. Takeuchi, J. Thongborisute, Y. Matsui, H. Sugihara, H. Yamamoto, Y. Kawashima. Novel mucoadhesion tests for polymers and polymer-coated particles to design optimal mucoadhesive drug delivery systems. *Advanced Drug Delivery Reviews* 57(11) (2005) 1583–1594.

114. J. Majumder, O. Taratula, T. Minko. Nanocarrier-based systems for targeted and site specific therapeutic delivery. *Advanced Drug Delivery Reviews* 144 (2019) 57–77.

115. T. Souho, L. Lamboni, L. Xiao, G. Yang. Cancer hallmarks and malignancy features: Gateway for improved targeted drug delivery. *Biotechnology Advances* 36(7) (2018) 1928–1945.

116. Q. Liu, M. Das, Y. Liu, L. Huang. Targeted drug delivery to melanoma. *Advanced Drug Delivery Reviews* 127 (2018) 208–221.

117. K. Widder, P. Marino, R. Morris, D. Howard, G. Poore, A. Senyei. Selective targeting of magnetic albumin microspheres to the Yoshida sarcoma: Ultrastructural evaluation of microsphere disposition. *European Journal of Cancer & Clinical Oncology* 19(1) (1983) 141–147.

118. R. Das, V. Gandhi, B. Singh, A. Kunwar. Passive and active drug targeting: Role of nanocarriers in rational design of anticancer formulations. *Current Pharmaceutical Design* 25(28) (2019) 3034–3056.

119. W. Yu, R. Liu, Y. Zhou, H. Gao. Size-tunable strategies for a tumor targeted drug delivery system. *ACS Central Science* 6(2) (2020) 100–116.

120. B. Sharma, C. Peetla, I. Adjei, V. Labhasetwar. Selective biophysical interactions of surface modified nanoparticles with cancer cell lipids improve tumor targeting and gene therapy. *Cancer Letters* 334(2) (2013) 228–236.

121. H. Ren, Y. He, J. Liang, Z. Cheng, M. Zhang, Y. Zhu, C. Hong, J. Qin, X. Xu, J. Wang. Role of liposome size, surface charge, and PEGylation on rheumatoid arthritis targeting therapy. *ACS Applied Materials & Interfaces* 11(22) (2019) 20304–20315.

122. J. Heo, S. Kang, Y. Kim, S. You, K. Jin, S. Kim, H. Jung, K. Jung, C. Lee, M. Kim, S. Sung, B. Kim, I. Choi, H. Youn, J. Chung, S. Kim, Y. Kim. Toward redesigning the PEG surface of nanocarriers for tumor targeting: Impact of inner functionalities on size, charge, multivalent binding, and biodistribution. *Chemical Science* 8(7) (2017) 5186–5195.

123. Y. Huang, K. Jiang, X. Zhang, E. Chung. The effect of size, charge, and peptide ligand length on kidney targeting by small, organic nanoparticles. *Bioengineering & Translational Medicine* 5(3) (2020) e10173.

124. D. Devineni, A. Klein-Szanto, J. Gallo. Tissue distribution of methotrexate following administration as a solution and as a magnetic microsphere conjugate in rats bearing brain tumors. *Journal of Neuro-Oncology* 24(2) (1995) 143–152.

125. J. Connell, P. Patrick, Y. Yu, M. Lythgoe, T. Kalber. Advanced cell therapies: Targeting, tracking and actuation of cells with magnetic particles. *Regenerative Medicine* 10(6) (2015) 757–772.

126. M. Saadat, M. Manshadi, M. Mohammadi, M. Zare, M. Zarei, R. Kamali, A. Sanati-Nezhad. Magnetic particle targeting for diagnosis and therapy of lung cancers. *Journal of Controlled Release: Official Journal of the Controlled Release Society* 328 (2020) 776–791.

127. S. Odenbach. Fluid mechanics aspects of magnetic drug targeting. *Biomedizinische Technik. Biomedical Engineering* 60(5) (2015) 477–483.

128. E. Cherry, P. Maxim, J. Eaton. Particle size, magnetic field, and blood velocity effects on particle retention in magnetic drug targeting. *Medical Physics* 37(1) (2010) 175–182.

129. K. Choi, K. Nam, L. Malkinski, E. Choi, J. Jung, B. Park. Size-dependent photodynamic anticancer activity of biocompatible multifunctional magnetic submicron particles in prostate cancer cells. *Molecules (Basel, Switzerland)* 21(9) (2016) 1187.

130. P.A. Voltairas, D.I. Fotiadis, L.K. Michalis. Hydrodynamics of magnetic drug targeting. *Journal of Biomechanics* 35(6) (2002) 813–821.

131. V. Cardoso, A. Francesko, C. Ribeiro, M. Bañobre-López, P. Martins, S. Lanceros-Mendez. Advances in magnetic nanoparticles for biomedical applications. *Advanced Healthcare Materials* 7(5) (2018) 1700845.

132. B. Partain, M. Unni, C. Rinaldi, K. Allen. The clearance and biodistribution of magnetic composite nanoparticles in healthy and osteoarthritic rat knees. *Journal of Controlled Release: Official Journal of the Controlled Release Society* 321 (2020) 259–271.

133. M. Longmire, P. Choyke, H. Kobayashi. Clearance properties of nano-sized particles and molecules as imaging agents: Considerations and caveats. *Nanomedicine (London, England)* 3(5) (2008) 703–717.

134. A. Chung, J. Lee, N. Ferrara. Targeting the tumour vasculature: Insights from physiological angiogenesis. *Nature Reviews. Cancer* 10(7) (2010) 505–514.

135. T. Lammers, F. Kiessling, W. Hennink, G. Storm. Drug targeting to tumors: Principles, pitfalls and (pre-) clinical progress. *Journal of Controlled Release: Official Journal of the Controlled Release Society* 161(2) (2012) 175–187.

136. S. Hua. Advances in oral drug delivery for regional targeting in the gastrointestinal tract - influence of physiological, pathophysiological and pharmaceutical factors. *Frontiers in Pharmacology* 11 (2020) 524.

137. M. Kanamala, W. Wilson, M. Yang, B. Palmer, Z. Wu. Mechanisms and biomaterials in pH-responsive tumour targeted drug delivery: A review. *Biomaterials* 85 (2016) 152–167.

138. S. Solomevich, P. Bychkovsky, T. Yurkshtovich, N. Golub, P. Mirchuk, M. Revtovich, A. Shmak. Biodegradable pH-sensitive prospidine-loaded dextran phosphate based hydrogels for local tumor therapy. *Carbohydrate Polymers* 226 (2019) 115308.

139. C. Ferguson, A. Al-Khalaf, R. Isaac, O. Cayre. pH-responsive polymer microcapsules for targeted delivery of biomaterials to the midgut of Drosophila suzukii. *PLoS One* 13(8) (2018) e0201294.

140. S. Cai, B. Luo, X. Zhan, X. Zhou, F. Lan, Q. Yi, Y. Wu. pH-responsive superstructures prepared via the assembly of FeO amphipathic Janus nanoparticles. *Regenerative Biomaterials* 5(5) (2018) 251–259.

141. J. Weng, Z. Huang, X. Pu, X. Chen, G. Yin, Y. Tian, Y. Song. Preparation of polyethylene glycol-polyacrylic acid block copolymer micelles with pH/hypoxic dual-responsive for tumor chemoradiotherapy. *Colloids and Surfaces. B Biointerfaces* 191 (2020) 110943.

142. S. Saroj, S. Rajput. Tailor-made pH-sensitive polyacrylic acid functionalized mesoporous silica nanoparticles for efficient and controlled delivery of anti-cancer drug Etoposide. *Drug Development and Industrial Pharmacy* 44(7) (2018) 1198–1211.

143. J. Qu, X. Zhao, P. Ma, B. Guo. pH-responsive self-healing injectable hydrogel based on N-carboxyethyl chitosan for hepatocellular carcinoma therapy. *Acta Biomaterialia* 58 (2017) 168–180.

144. Y. Wang, A. Khan, Y. Liu, J. Feng, L. Dai, G. Wang, N. Alam, L. Tong, Y. Ni. Chitosan oligosaccharide-based dual pH responsive nano-micelles for targeted delivery of hydrophobic drugs. *Carbohydrate Polymers* 223 (2019) 115061.

145. K. Soppirnath, T. Aminabhavi. Water transport and drug release study from crosslinked polyacrylamide grafted guar gum hydrogel microspheres for the controlled release application. *European Journal of Pharmaceutics and Biopharmaceutics: Official Journal of Arbeitsgemeinschaft fur Pharmazeutische Verfahrenstechnik e.V* 53(1) (2002) 87–98.

146. K. Soppimath, A. Kulkarni, T. Aminabhavi. Chemically modified polyacrylamide-g-guar gum-based crosslinked anionic microgels as pH-sensitive drug delivery systems: Preparation and characterization. *Journal of Controlled Release: Official Journal of the Controlled Release Society* 75(3) (2001) 331–345.

147. M. Kurkuri, T. Aminabhavi. Poly(vinyl alcohol) and poly(acrylic acid) sequential interpenetrating network pH-sensitive microspheres for the delivery of diclofenac sodium to the intestine. *Journal of Controlled Release: Official Journal of the Controlled Release Society* 96(1) (2004) 9–20.

148. C.-H. Wang, C.-H. Wang, G.-H. Hsiue. Polymeric micelles with a pH-responsive structure as intracellular drug carriers. *Journal of Controlled Release* 108(1) (2005) 140–149.

149. E.R. Gillies, J.M.J. Fréchet. Dendrimers and dendritic polymers in drug delivery. *Drug Discovery Today* 10(1) (2005) 35–43.

150. T.P. Thomas, A.K. Patri, A. Myc, M.T. Myaing, J.Y. Ye, T.B. Norris, J.R. Baker. In vitro targeting of synthesized antibody-conjugated dendrimer nanoparticles. *Biomacromolecules* 5(6) (2004) 2269–2274.

151. Y.-S. Yi. Folate receptor-targeted diagnostics and therapeutics for inflammatory diseases. *Immune Network* 16(6) (2016) 337–343.

152. M. Riaz, M. Riaz, X. Zhang, C. Lin, K. Wong, X. Chen, G. Zhang, A. Lu, Z. Yang. Surface functionalization and targeting strategies of liposomes in solid tumor therapy: A review. *International Journal of Molecular Sciences* 19(1) (2018) 195.

153. G. Shavi, M. Sreenivasa Reddy, R. Raghavendra, U. Nayak, A. Kumar, P. Deshpande, N. Udupa, G. Behl, V. Dave, K. Kushwaha. PEGylated liposomes of anastrozole for long-term treatment of breast cancer: In vitro and in vivo evaluation. *Journal of Liposome Research* 26(1) (2016) 28–46.

154. Y. Dou, K. Hynynen, C. Allen. To heat or not to heat: Challenges with clinical translation of thermosensitive liposomes. *Journal of Controlled Release: Official Journal of the Controlled Release Society* 249 (2017) 63–73.
155. A. Haeri, L. Pedrosa, T. Ten Hagen, S. Dadashzadeh, G. Koning. A Novel Combined Approach of short-chain sphingolipids and thermosensitive liposomes for improved drug delivery to tumor cells. *Journal of Biomedical Nanotechnology* 12(4) (2016) 630–644.
156. A. T S, K. Shalumon, J. Chen. Applications of magnetic liposomes in cancer therapies. *Current Pharmaceutical Design* 25(13) (2019) 1490–1504.
157. Y. Deng, J. Ling, M. Li. Physical stimuli-responsive liposomes and polymersomes as drug delivery vehicles based on phase transitions in the membrane. *Nanoscale* 10(15) (2018) 6781–6800.
158. J. Kuai, Q. Wang, A. Zhang, J. Zhang, Z. Chen, K. Wu, X. Hu. Epidermal growth factor receptor-targeted immune magnetic liposomes capture circulating colorectal tumor cells efficiently. *World Journal of Gastroenterology* 24(3) (2018) 351–359.
159. S. Ambati, A. Ferarro, S. Kang, J. Lin, X. Lin, M. Momany, Z. Lewis, R. Meagher. Dectin-1-targeted antifungal liposomes exhibit enhanced efficacy. *mSphere* 4(1) (2019) 1–15.
160. N. Erdoğar, S. Akkın, E. Bilensoy. Nanocapsules for drug delivery: An updated review of the last decade. *Recent Patents on Drug Delivery & Formulation* 12(4) (2018) 252–266.
161. X. Pu, L. Zhao, J. Li, R. Song, Y. Wang, K. Yu, X. Hou, P. Qiao, L. Zong, S. Chang. A polymeric micelle with an endosomal pH-sensitivity for intracellular delivery and enhanced antitumor efficacy of hydroxycamptothecin. *Acta Biomaterialia* 88 (2019) 357–369.
162. W. Wang, H. Liang, B. Sun, J. Xu, Z. Zeng, X. Zhao, Q. Li. Pharmacokinetics and tissue distribution of folate-decorated human serum albumin loaded with nano-hydroxycamptothecin for tumor targeting. *Journal of Pharmaceutical Sciences* 105(6) (2016) 1874–1880.
163. J. Andhariya, D. Burgess. Recent advances in testing of microsphere drug delivery systems. *Expert Opinion on Drug Delivery* 13(4) (2016) 593–608.
164. C. Lin, S. Lin, S. Yang, D. Wang, H. Cheng, M. Yeh. Biodegradable polymeric microsphere-based vaccines and their applications in infectious diseases. *Human Vaccines & Immunotherapeutics* 11(3) (2015) 650–656.
165. Q. He, J. Zhang, Y. Liao, E. Alakpa, V. Bunpetch, J. Zhang, H. Ouyang. Current advances in microsphere based cell culture and tissue engineering. *Biotechnology Advances* 39 (2020) 107459.
166. C. Wong, H. Al-Salami, C. Dass. Microparticles, microcapsules and microspheres: A review of recent developments and prospects for oral delivery of insulin. *International Journal of Pharmaceutics* 537 (2018) 223–244.

10 Wearable/Attachable Sensors and Biosensors

Jingwen Li, Haiyang Liu, and Yifeng Lei
Wuhan University

CONTENTS

10.1 INTRODUCTION

Wearable or attachable sensors and biosensors represent a novel non-invasive approach for human health evaluation as well as diagnosis of diseases [1–4]. Wearable sensors and biosensors can be conformably contacted to different sites of the human body in the form of wearable patches, bands, and pads, and enable real-time health monitoring of biological signals tightly associated with health conditions, including information from physical activities (such as body motion, heart rate, breath rate, wrist pulse, pulse pressure, body temperature, etc.) [1,2], or from biochemical signals (such as glucose levels, pH value, ion concentrations, etc.) [3,4].

In this chapter, we review the recent state of the art of the wearable biosensors, and their applications in health monitoring. We present a summary of different materials and related working principles used for wearable biosensors, and analyze their applications in monitoring health signals. We also include the most recent representative progress of wearable sensors for measurement of physical signals and chemical signals. Finally, the challenges and future perspectives of wearable biosensors for monitoring of various kinds of human activities and biochemical signals are discussed.

10.2 MATERIALS FOR BIOSENSOR DEVICES

Wearable biosensors for health signal monitoring involve complex integrated systems, which generally consist stretchable substrates with good flexibility, conducting electrodes with excellent conductivity, and sensing materials with high sensitivity and specificity [5]. Researchers need to pay special attention to the different roles of each component, and their interactions with each other, as well as understand how these interactions affect the performance of the sensor systems. To achieve mechanical flexibility, two approaches have been mostly used, either with elastic materials or with stretchable/wearable materials. The intrinsically wearable materials have been widely investigated in wearable biosensor applications, such as elastic films, conducting polymers, organic semiconductors, liquid metal, and ionic liquid. Another important approach for high flexibility is to design materials with special structures, for example, in serpentine, helix, and other micro/nanostructures.

10.2.1 WEARABLE SUBSTRATES

Flexible substrate materials play an important role in the construction of sensor devices [5]. Generally, metal foils, rubbers, and polymers are employed as wearable substrates because of their mechanical flexibility, good chemical resistance, and thermal stability. Among polymer substrates, polyimide (PI) is widely used as it exhibits high tensile strength, great flexibility, very low creep, and can be used above the temperatures of 452°C. Moreover, it also resists acids, alkalis, and commonly used organic solvents, which make PI a compatible substrate material during sensor manufacturing.

Moreover, some particular applications need substrates with good transparency and low birefringence. Polyethylene naphthalate (PEN) and polyethylene terephthalate (PET) are transparent materials with transmittance greater than 85% in the visible wavelength region, and can be used for this purpose.

Fiber and textiles are also widely employed as substrates for wearable sensor devices because they are the most natural materials close to human skin. By integration with multifunctional wearable electronics, novel textiles have both the functionalities of wearable electronics and the characteristics of clothing-like textiles.

It should be noted that polydimethylsiloxane (PDMS) has been abundantly used as a substrate material in wearable sensor systems because of its advantage of intrinsic high stretchability and good biocompatibility. To improve the adhesion between the

PDMS substrate and the attached skin surface, various surface treatment technologies have been employed to improve the surface property of PDMS, including chemical functionalization, ultraviolet exposure, and oxygen plasma, and others. Furthermore, the microstructured PDMS film is a popular wearable substrate to integrate with sensitive nanomaterials for wearable sensing systems.

10.2.2 CONDUCTING ELECTRODES

Conducting electrodes are essential elements which can be encapsulated in or on the surface of the above-described elastic substrates of wearable sensor devices [5]. Conventional materials, including gold (Au), platinum (Pt), and films of indium tin oxide, have been proven to construct highly sensitive wearable sensors as the materials of conducting electrodes. However, these materials are usually rigid and brittle, leading to their cracking during deformation, which limits their applications in wearable sensor devices. Nanostructured materials, such as nanotube and nanowire networks, are considered promising substitutes to replace these rigid conducting materials because of their stretchable, electrically stable, mechanically durable, and transparent properties. Metal nanowires (for example, Au, Ag, Cu, etc.) have been widely used as conducting electrode materials to construct wearable sensor devices.

Carbon-based nanomaterials, such as carbon nanotube (CNT) and graphene, have also demonstrated unprecedented performance as wearable conducting elements due to their excellent physical and chemical properties. In fact, in the past decade, significant efforts have been made to fabricate composites of CNTs with polymers for stretchable conductors.

10.2.3 SENSING MATERIALS

Sensing materials are crucial for wearable sensor devices [5]. For sensing materials, semiconducting polymers and nanowires are promising in biosensing applications. Polymers, including polyaniline (PANI), poly(3,4-ethylenedioxythiophene)-poly(styrenesulfonate) (PEDOT:PSS), polypyrrole (PPy), and poly(3-hexylthiophene) (P3HT) have been widely used as sensing materials for construction of wearable electronics. These polymers are attractive due to their highly adjustable physical and chemical properties by varying their molecular structures and compositions. Semiconducting polymers also possess mechanical properties comparable to that of insulated polymer substrates, making them easy to integrate with polymer substrates. In addition, the elasticity modulus of semiconducting polymers is close to the skin, giving them the ability for integration in wearable or attachable sensing applications on the skin.

10.3 PHYSICAL BIOSENSORS

Wearable physical sensors can be employed for monitoring various physical parameters, including pressure or strain generated by the body (such as motion, heart rate, breath rate, blood pressure, wrist pulse, etc.) and body temperature. Monitoring such physical signals provides a prominent approach for health assessment, as well as diagnosis and prevention of various diseases.

Wearable physical sensors can monitor the signals produced by various human activities, and attract great attention due to their unique properties, such as ultra thin, light weight, low modulus, and high flexibility to human skin. Wearable physical sensors can firmly attach on the skin surface, providing monitoring of human activity and personal health information.

In the last decade, considerable research efforts have been made to develop wearable physical sensors (Figure 10.1). Here, the most representative wearable physical sensors are reviewed. We illustrate the recent representative work of wearable physical sensors for the detection of pressure, strain, and temperature, as well as the novel structures and technological innovations involved in the development. Recent progress regarding physical sensors for various physical signals are reviewed in detail.

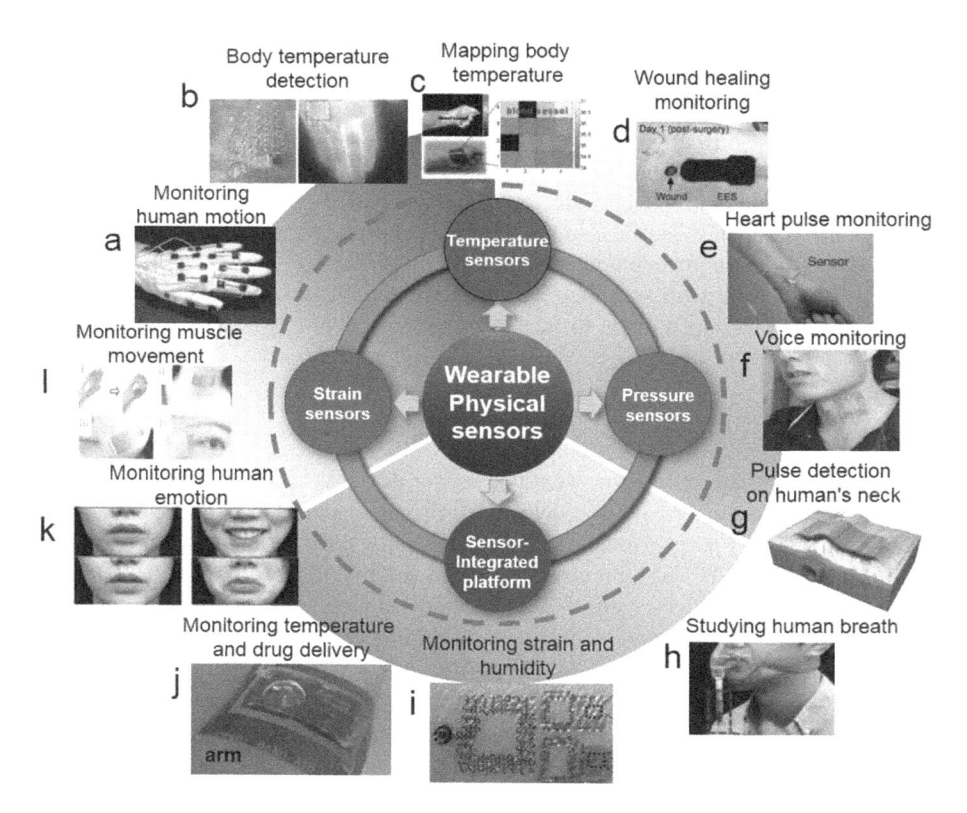

FIGURE 10.1 Wearable physical biosensors for monitoring of human activities and healthcare. (a) Strain sensors for monitoring human motions. (b) Temperature sensors for body temperature detection. (c) Mapping body temperature. (d) Wound healing monitoring. (e) Pressure sensors for heart pulse monitoring. (f) Voice monitoring. (g) Pulse detection on human's neck. (h) Human breath monitoring. (i) Monitoring strain and humidity. (j) Integrated sensor platform for both of temperature monitoring and drug delivery. (k) Monitoring human emotion. (l) Monitoring muscle movements. ((a)–(l) Adapted with permission from ref. [1]. Copyright 2016, John Wiley and Sons.)

10.3.1 WORKING PRINCIPLES OF PHYSICAL BIOSENSORS

In physical biosensing, pressure and strain sensors are generally employed to detect the pressure and strain applied on the sensing devices. Different transduction principles are used for these sensors, including piezoelectricity, piezoresistivity, capacitance, and triboelectricity [1,2,5]. These sensors can convert signals of mechanical motion (pressure or strain) into electrical signals. Among them, piezoelectric or piezoresistive pressure/strain sensors are most commonly used.

10.3.1.1 Piezoelectricity-Based Sensors

The working principle of piezoelectric type of pressure/strain sensors is based on piezoelectric materials and their piezoelectricity effect [6]. The external pressure/strain on the materials can be converted into electrical charges by piezoelectricity [6]. Piezoelectric materials instantaneously generate electricity when the materials experienced pressure or strain; therefore, piezoelectric-type sensors have been widely developed using piezoelectric materials with high piezoelectric constants. Most commonly used piezoelectric materials are lead zirconium titanate (PZT) [7], which are widely used for the construction of pressure sensors due to their high piezoelectric constants. However, PZT is generally rigid and brittle.

Polymer-based piezoelectric materials, such as polyvinylidene fluoride (PVDF), more wearable PZT materials in the forms of nanowires and thin ribbons, ZnO nanowires [8], and the composites of polymers and inorganic piezoelectric materials, have also been widely used as piezoelectric materials due to their mechanical flexibility and cost-effectiveness. These materials take advantages of the mechanical flexibility of polymers and the high performance of piezoelectric inorganics, and are therefore more advantageous than rigid piezoelectric materials.

10.3.1.2 Piezoresistivity-Based Sensor

Piezoresistivity is another commonly used property for pressure/strain sensors [5]. In a piezoresistive sensor, the resistance of the sensor significantly changes when the sensor is stretched or compressed, and the resistance change is directly proportional to the strain caused by external pressure. This phenomena is also known as piezoresistive effect [5], which refers to the change in the electrical resistivity of a material when mechanical strain is applied. The electrical resistance changes are mainly due to two reasons, either geometry change or conductivity change of the materials. Generally, this resistance change is much more significant for semiconductors than for metals.

Therefore, to effectively realize the piezoresistive effect of the materials, there are two critical parameters to regulate: (1) soft and wearable substrate; and (2) special micro- or nanoscaled structures of the sensing materials.

Generally, polymers show a mechanical hysteresis, which affects the sensing performance of wearable pressure/strain sensors with long response time and long recovery times. Conductive materials with special structures and their integration into polymer matrix can enable their deformation upon stretching or compression of polymer matrix, leading to an increase in the conductivity of the entire structure.

10.3.1.3 Capacitance-Based Sensor

Wearable capacitive type-based sensors are also used for pressure and strain sensing [5]. Typically, a capacitor is featured by two parallel electrodes which are sandwiched by a dielectric layer (as shown in Figure 10.2a). The capacitance (*C*) of the capacitor is calculated according to the following equation:

$$C = \varepsilon A / d$$

where ε is the effective dielectric constant of the dielectric layer, and A and d are the effective area and the distance between the two electrodes, respectively. When pressure or strain is applied on the capacitor (Figure 10.2b), the distance, area, or the dielectric constant changes, leading to the changes in capacitance readout.

Generally, Au films are used as the top and bottom electrodes to construct the capacitive sensing devices. Recently, Ag nanowire and CNT networks have been embedded into PDMS substrates for construction of elastic conducting films. The embedded CNT network can achieve a stretching strain of up to 700%, leading to a significantly increased resistance.

John Rogers of Northwestern University [9], Zhenan Bao from Stanford University [10], and others have pioneered the research of wearable physical biosensors for monitoring various physical activities, with different transduction principles and materials integrated in the sensing systems. In the following section, we summarize the recent studies of wearable or attachable physical sensing systems, their working principles, and examples in monitoring of physical signals of human activities.

10.3.2 MOTION

The various motions of the human body, including the motion of limbs, walking, flexing of muscles, and finger movement, become energy sources which can be employed to power the above-described physical sensing systems. The mechanical energy generated during these motions can vary over several orders of magnitude and can be harvested using wearable piezoelectric sensors, piezoresistive sensors, and recently developed triboelectric generators [8]. These physical biosensors are employed to harvest energy from the motion of joints including knees, elbows, wrists, and fingers and transfer the mechanical energy into different forms of signal readouts.

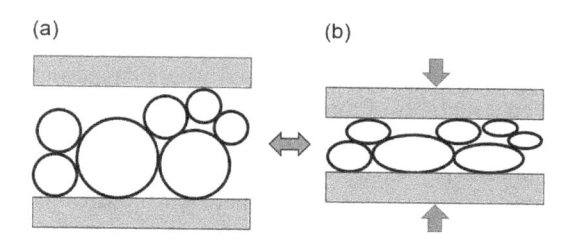

FIGURE 10.2 Schematic illustration of capacitor and its working principles. (a) Structure of capacitor. (b) A capacitor under pressure.

Zhenan Bao from Stanford University has developed wearable physical sensing systems, such as pressure and strain sensor, tactile-sensing control, and so on [10]. Recently, the research group developed a soft and stretchable skin-like electronics which can firmly contact the human skin, and applied them for health monitoring, biological investigations, and medical treatments [10]. A transistor array with a record density of 347 transistors/cm² were fabricated with intrinsically stretchable polymers. The transistors showed high stretchability (up to 100%) and enabled various applications, such as tactile sensor, strain sensors, inverter, NAND gate, and signal amplifier [10].

Based on piezoelectric nanogenerators [8], Zhonglin Wang from Georgia Institute of Technology developed a series of piezoelectric and triboelectric sensors for monitoring human motion as well as physiological signals [11]. Recently, the group fabricated a large-area wearable pressure sensor array on common fabric substrates. The textile sensors achieved a high sensitivity of 14.4 kPa^{-1}, a low detection limit of 2 Pa, with fast response of 24 ms, low power consumption of less than 6 µW, and good mechanical stability. These textile sensors can recognize motions such as hand gestures, finger movement, real-time pulse waves, and acoustic vibrations [11]. Furthermore, the same group demonstrated a wearable mechano-sensation sensor based on shape memory polymers for monitoring body motion [12]. Based on shape memory polymer and conductive liquid, the obtained sensor can harvest biomechanical energy from biomechanical motions. Moreover, the sensor can transform its shape according to different requirements, and its form of a shape-adaptive wrist splint has been developed for detection of the motion of a human twist [12].

Recently, Xingyu Jiang and coworkers developed a series of pintable metal-polymer conductors (MPCs) and applied them for stretchable biosensor devices [13]. MPCs and elastomeric block copolymer were employed to fabricate the multilayered integration of the electronic sensors [13], which is highly stretchable with a maximum strain of 800%, conformal, and sticky to the skin [13]. The wearable tattoo enables the crease amplification effect, and amplifies the output signals of integrated strain sensors, which can be applied for monitoring different movements, as well as for the remote control of robots [13].

10.3.3 HEART RATE

Monitoring heart rate is important in personal healthcare management. Development of non-invasive, user-friendly, and low-cost heart rate monitoring systems is highly required.

In 2011, John Rogers from Northwestern University first reported skin-like epidermal electronic system for physiological measurement [9], including heart rate monitoring. Ultrathin, low modulus, lightweight, and stretchable membranes were fabricated on a sacrificial and water-soluble film of polyvinyl alcohol (PVA). The device can firmly contact the surface of the skin after dissolving the PVA. The systems incorporate with strain, electrophysiological, and temperature sensors, and can be used to measure electrical activity produced by the brain (electroencephalograms (EEGs)), the heart (electrocardiograms (ECGs)), and the skeletal muscles (electromyograms (EMGs)) [9].

In 2017, Zhonglin Wang and coworkers developed a body sensor network with triboelectric effect for monitoring human heart rate [14]. The sensor device consists of a heart rate sensor, a downy-structure-based triboelectric nanogenerator (D-TENG), and wireless data transmission module. By harvesting human biomechanical energy from mechanical movements, a maximum power of 2.28 mW, with a total conversion efficiency of 57.9%, is delivered from the wearable triboelectric nanogenerator, which can drive the entire sensor system [14]. The obtained heart rate signals by the sensor are then processed, transmitted via the Bluetooth module, and displayed via personal cell phone to achieve real-time analysis of human heart rate information. This sensor device provides a better solution for personal monitoring of human heart rates.

10.3.4 RESPIRATORY RATE

Detection of respiratory rate is critical for assessment of human lung states in healthy subjects as well as in patients with pulmonary diseases, such as pneumonia, COVID-19 diseases, or acute respiratory distress syndrome.

Dong Wang and coworkers have reported a stretchable electric material integrated into a waistband for human breathing rate detection [15]. The PPy/PU elastomers can stretch when breathing out, and can release when breathing in, which changes the resistance of circuit, bringing various electrical signals and effectively detecting breathing rate [15]. Recently, Michelle Khine and coworkers reported a wearable sensor capable of monitoring respiration rates based on piezoresistive stain sensors [16]. The disposable respiration sensor has a format of Band-Aid©, and can detect both respiration rate and respiratory volume, simply from measuring the local strain of the abdomen and ribcage during normal breathing. Moreover, these observations are in good correlation with the clinical measurements from spirometer [16].

Xu Yong and coworkers developed a series of ultra-sensitive sensors for continuous monitoring of respiratory rate and heart rates (Figure 10.3a) [17]. The sensors are based on piezoelectric PZT materials with an asymmetric gapped cantilever structure (Figure 10.3b). The asymmetric gapped cantilever structure enhanced the sensitivity of the sensor compared with conventional structures (Figure 10.3c). The piezoelectric PZT layer can transfer the strain coming from biomechanical energy (such as acoustic vibration) to electric charge due to the piezoelectric effect of PZT. The obtained sound sensors exhibit an ultra-high sensitivity of 86 V/g in frequency less than 1,000 Hz, which makes them suitable for monitoring weak physiological signals [18], especially for weak respiratory sound monitoring [18]. When applied on a healthy subject, the sound sensor can detect the weak signals of lung sounds with high sensitivity (Figure 10.3d), and normal heart sounds (S1 and S2) can be clearly detected from the monitored heart sound waveform (Figure 10.3e). Moreover, the sensor device is applied on patients with pneumonia. Increased respiratory rate (Figure 10.3f) and heart rate (Figure 10.3g) are observed in pneumonia patients, which indicate lung injury and heart injury of pneumonia patients. Compared with conventional medical instruments, such as CT imaging and lung ultrasound for lung evaluation and ECG and cardiac magnetic resonance imaging for heart evaluation,

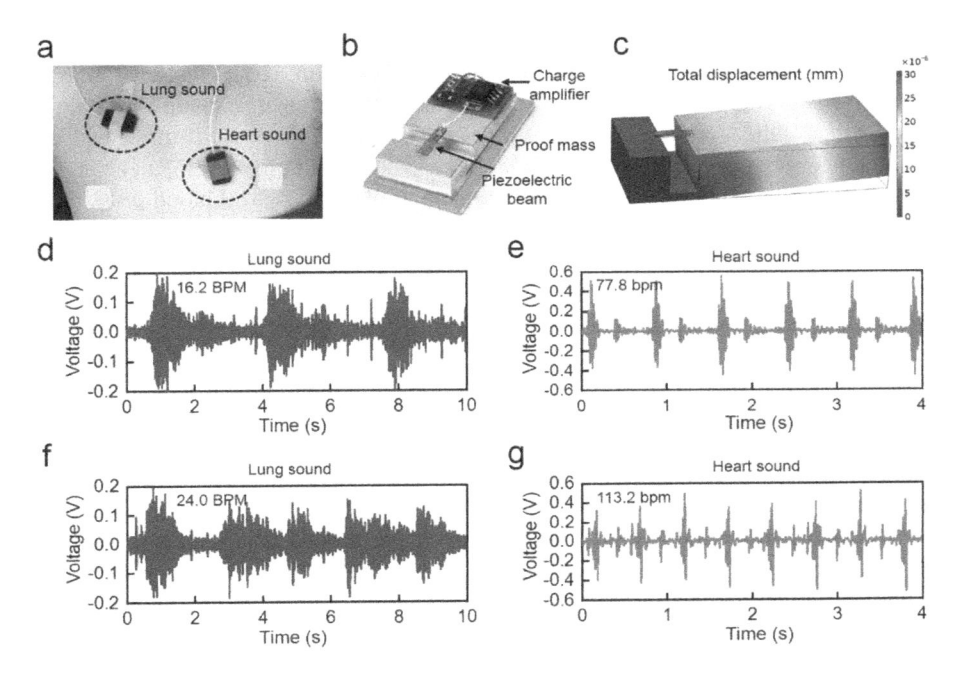

FIGURE 10.3 Attachable physical biosensors for lung and heart sound monitoring. (a) Placement of physical sensors on the human body. (b) Inside view of the sensor with printed circuit board. (c) Simulation of the strain distributed on piezoelectric PZT cantilever of the sensor. (d and e) Lung and heart sound waveforms monitored on healthy subject. (f and g) Lung and heart sound monitoring on patient with pneumonia.

these sensor devices provide ultra-sensitive detection of lung and heart sounds, providing a cost-effective alternative approach for the diagnosis of pneumonia, and has potential in clinical and home-use health monitoring.

10.3.5 BLOOD PRESSURE

Real-time monitoring of blood pressure from various vessels has clinical values for the assessment of personal health status as well as for the detection of cardiovascular diseases. Conventional pulse sensors, such as photoplethysmography and tonometry, can only enable the measurement to the superficial peripheral vasculatures, and show significant disadvantages of power consumption issues which hinder the sustainable operation of sensor devices.

Recently, Keon Jae Lee and coworkers developed an ultrathin piezoelectric sensor for real-time wearable monitoring of arterial pulses [19]. The pressure sensor consists of a thin film of inorganic piezoelectric PZT, which is deposited on a sapphire wafer, and further transferred onto an ultrathin substrate of PET. The sensor has a high sensitivity of $0.018\,kPa^{-1}$, a fast response time of 60 ms, and has good mechanical stability. Moreover, the wearable sensor can conformably contact on human wrist, and demonstrate the possibility of real-time monitoring of arterial pulse signals in near-surface arteries, including radial/carotid pulses [19].

More recently, Sheng Xu and coworkers designed a stretchable ultrasonic sensor device for wearable measurement of central blood pressure [20]. This sensor device hybridizes high performance and rigid 1–3 kinds of piezoelectric composites, which are further embedded in a soft epoxy matrix. The wearable device is ultrathin (with a thickness of only 240 μm), highly stretchable (with strain up to 60%), and can conformably contact the skin, thus enabling the monitoring of central blood pressure by capturing the diameters of the pulsating vessels, including deeply embedded arteries and veins [20].

Zhonglin Wang and coworkers reported a wearable weaving constructed pressure sensor for non-invasive monitoring of human blood pressure as well as pulse wave velocity [21]. Relying on the rational weaving structure design and plasma etching techniques, polymer nanowires are created on the flexible surface. The designed device shows superior capacity in capturing and converting the weak change of blood pressure into electrical signals than commercial devices. The wearable sensor has an ultra-high sensitivity of 45.7 mV/Pa, an ultrafast response time of less than 5 ms, and good mechanical stability after 40,000 motion cycles. The sensor system precisely monitors the pulse wave and blood pressure from the ankles, wrist, fingertip, and ear of the people with different ages and different health states, and these results are consistent with commercialized electronic sphygmomanometer. This wearable sensor is a great potential alternative to the currently used complex cardiovascular monitoring systems [21].

10.3.6 TEMPERATURE

Body temperature is an important vital sign of the human body, and body temperature measurement is critical for home-use and clinical assessment of human health condition, such as detection of fever and infection. Commercial temperature sensors use thermometer based on the thermoresistive effect of pure metal (such as Hg); however, these rigid materials are not very compatible with human skin. Wearable temperature sensing systems may overcome the above problems due to their mechanical flexibility and biocompatibility.

Various materials are promising for the construction of skin-compatible wearable thermoresistive sensors [5], including metal and Si nanoribbons, nanocrystals (NCs) and nanoparticles (NPs), CNT, graphene, etc. The resistivity of thermoresistive materials varies according to the temperature because of the variation in charge carrier density or mobility. With increasing temperature, charge hopping dominant materials or semiconductors show decreased resistivity due to the enhanced thermally assisted charge carrier hopping or the improved charge carrier density, respectively. These types of temperature sensors contain Ag nanocrystal/PDMS, CNT/polymer composite, PEDOT:PSS/CNT films, polyaniline nanofibers, reduced graphene oxide (rGO), etc. Engineered material structures, such as serpentine, buckling, net-shaped metals, nanowire (NW), nanomesh, and nanowalls, have been widely demonstrated to improve the flexibility and resistivity with the change in temperature.

Recently, Kilwon Cho and coworkers demonstrated an rGO-based thermoresistive sensor for temperature monitoring [22]. The sensor achieved a very high sensitivity of 0.83% $°C^{-1}$, with optimization of the reduction degree of rGO which affects the charge carrier hopping [22]. More recently, Soong Ju Oh and coworkers fabricated wearable temperature sensor on PDMS substrate by integration of Ag NC film [23]. The charge transport properties of Ag NC film can be controlled by ligand treatment and nanocracks induced by thermal expansion of PDMS. By doing this, the temperature sensor demonstrates a high sensitivity of 50% $°C^{-1}$ [23].

In addition to thermoresistive effect, thermoelectric effect is also employed in temperature sensors, in which electricity (voltage or currents) is generated upon variations in temperature [5]. For example, Daoben Zhu and coworkers fabricated a wearable temperature sensor based on porous polyurethane (PU) and PEDOT:PSS materials, where the last one is a thermoelectric material. The obtained sensor demonstrated a high temperature detection resolution of less than 0.1 K, and a fast response time of less than 2 s [24]. Moreover, a 12×12 sensor array can be attached to a hand, and can detect the distribution of temperature on human hand [24].

10.4 CHEMICAL BIOSENSORS

Compared to the above-described physical biosensors for monitoring physical activities and signals of the body, chemical biosensors can detect the biochemical information from the body; therefore, these sensors can help in accurate monitoring of human health condition and in the diagnosis of various diseases. More specifically, wearable chemical biosensors are attracting great attention due to their potential in providing real-time and continuous biochemical information via non-invasive, dynamic detection of biomarkers on human body interfaces, and represent a potential alternative to characterize the biochemical factors in the body.

Generally, wearable chemical sensors are employed to monitor analytes from different human body fluids, including sweat, interstitial fluid (ISF), blood, saliva, tears, and so on. Various biomarkers or metabolites, such as glucose, pH, various ions, uric acid, tyrosine, and lactate, can be detected via electrochemical and optical biosensor technologies (Figure 10.4).

John Rogers from Northwestern University [25,26], Joseph Wang from University of California, San Diego (UCSD) [27–29], Ali Javey of University of California, Berkeley [30,31], Wei Gao from California Institute of Technology [32–34], and others have pioneered in the researches of such wearable biosensor devices for sensitive detection of various analytes in different biofluids to make real-time evaluation of the physiological health condition of the human body.

This section illustrates the working principles of different chemical biosensors, and summarizes the most recent advances in wearable chemical biosensors for their application in analysis of glucose, pH, and ion sensing.

10.4.1 WORKING PRINCIPLES OF CHEMICAL SENSORS

Chemical sensor devices mainly include electrochemical devices, chemiresistor-based sensors, and transistor-based sensors. When exposed to the targeted chemical analytes, these sensor devices generally show variations in potential, current, or resistance.

Electrochemical sensors generally consist of working electrode (WE), reference electrode (RE), and counter electrode (CE). When electrochemical sensors are

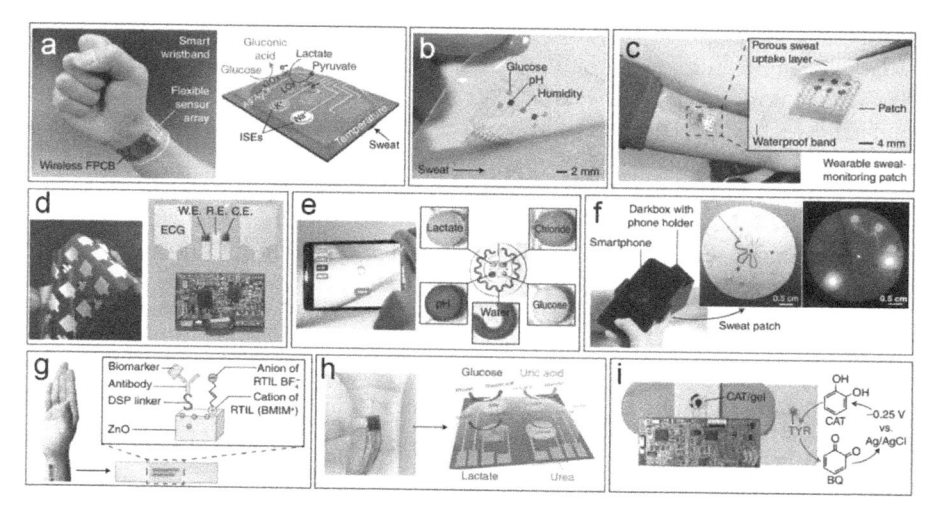

FIGURE 10.4   Wearable chemical biosensors for non-invasive monitoring of different analytes in human body [3]. (a) A wearable sensor array for sweat analysis on human wrist for multiplex monitoring of lactate, glucose, K+, Na+, and temperature [32]. (b) A graphene-based wearable electrochemical sensor device for diabetes monitoring on human arm. Simultaneous tests of pH, humidity, and temperature are carried out for correction of obtained glucose signals [35]. (c) Wearable sweat-based glucose monitoring device, together with drug delivery attached on human arm [36]. (d) A wearable patch array of chemical-electrophysiological hybrid sensors for real-time monitoring of sweat lactate levels and heart rate of human body [27]. (e) A wearable biosensor for sweat sampling and colorimetric monitoring of multiple analytes in sweat, including lactate, chloride, glucose, and pH [25]. (f) Wearable fluorometric microfluidic sensor for monitoring of chloride, sodium, and zinc in sweat [42]. (g) An ionic liquid-based and antibody-based wearable biosensor on human arm for the diagnostic detection of various analytes in human sweat [43]. (h) Wearable multifunctional biosensors for simultaneous monitoring of analytes in sweat (including glucose, uric acid, urea, and lactate) based on piezoelectric-enzymatic reaction [44]. (i) Wearable bandage sensor for non-invasive screening of tyrosinase biomarkers [45]. ((a)–(i) Reproduced with permission from ref. [3]. Copyright 2019, Nature Publishing Group.)

exposed to target analytes, a variation of potential or current is induced between different electrodes. Chemiresistors contain a sensing element between two electrodes. The resistance of the sensing element varies upon the exposure to target analytes. Transistor-type chemical sensors consist of three electrodes, a semiconducting layer, and a dielectric layer. Transistors can serve as chemiresistors which are modified with additional gate electrode and dielectric layer, which allow high sensitivity and signal amplification of the sensor.

The application of chemical biosensors generally needs sampling of biofluids for analysis. The methods used for sampling biofluids include iontophoresis, reverse iontophoresis, and so on. Iontophoresis typically depends on the topical current applied on the skin for local sweat stimulation, and delivers the stimulated factors with the help of an electrical current (Figure 10.5a). During iontophoresis, current is applied between hydrogels or hydrogels encapsulated with sweat-stimulating drugs. The

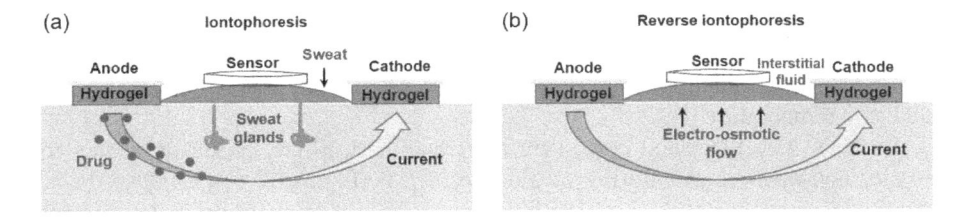

FIGURE 10.5 Schematic illustration and working principles of iontophoresis (a) and reverse iontophoresis (b).

drugs are driven under the skin surface and trigger adjacent glands to secrete sweat, where wearable sensors can then access (Figure 10.5a). In contrast, reverse iontophoresis utilizes the current to drive the ISF electro-osmotically from the epidermis to the surface of the skin (Figure 10.5b). In reverse iontophoresis, hydrogels isolate the current-applying electrodes from the surface of the skin to prevent irritation to the skin, and analytes are transported to the surface of the skin along with ISF flow, which can further be detected by wearable sensors (Figure 10.5b). Generally, iontophoresis is used for sweat sampling, whereas reverse iontophoresis is used for ISF acquisition and chemical sensing.

10.4.2 GLUCOSE

Glucose is an essential nutrient for human body. Blood glucose levels in the human body is a key indicator of health, particularly for diseases such as obesity, diabetes, and cancers. Traditionally, people use finger-prick blood testing with a glucose meter. However, this method is painful to patients and have the risk of infection during the process of blood acquisition. Recently, wearable sensing devices have been abundantly developed for analysis of human glucose levels [32,35,36].

Joseph Wang and coworkers pioneered the development of a series of electrochemical glucose sensors for wearable diabetes management [28,29]. Various wearable glucose monitoring devices have been developed based on advanced flexible nanomaterials, alternative body fluids, innovative sensing principles, and platforms. For minimally invasive continuous glucose monitoring which can achieve real-time readouts for interstitial glucose levels, the group focused on the integration of biocompatible material coatings to protect the electrochemical glucose sensors from *in vivo* biofouling [3]. For non-invasive, real-time glucose monitoring, the group developed various paper-based glucose sensing platforms and realized multiple detection of diabetes-related biomarkers from various body fluids [28,29].

In 2016, Dae-Hyeong Kim and coworkers developed a graphene-based electrochemical sensor device integrated with microneedle patches for simultaneous glucose monitoring and drug delivery in diabetes (Figure 10.4b) [35]. The Au-doped graphene was combined with a gold mesh, which could enhance the electrochemical readout of the devices during the detection of important biomarkers upon human sweat. The hybrid graphene interconnections transmit the signal efficiently through the stretchable microneedle array and supplementary electrochemical glucose sensors [35]. More recently, the same group developed a sweat-based sensing system for the electrochemical analysis of sweat glucose levels and continuous monitoring of vital signals, including blood oxygen saturation level, physical activity, heart rate, and skin temperature [36].

In 2017, Xue Feng and coworkers fabricated a skin-like biosensor system for in situ non-invasive monitoring of glucose in ISF (Figure 10.6) [37]. The device consisted of an ultrathin skin-like biosensor with electrochemical twin channels (ETCs) (Figure 10.6a), which act through hyaluric acid penetration into the ISF. The ETCs drive the intravascular blood glucose out of the blood vessels, and further transport the glucose to the surface of human skin (Figure 10.6a). The glucose sensor has a sensing element with ultrathin nanostructures (~3 mm) (Figure 10.6b), along with a high sensitivity of 130.4 mA/mM. Profiting from extreme conformability, the wearable glucose sensor can fully absorb and measure the glucose from ISF (Figure 10.6c and d). The results of non-invasive measurements of intravascular

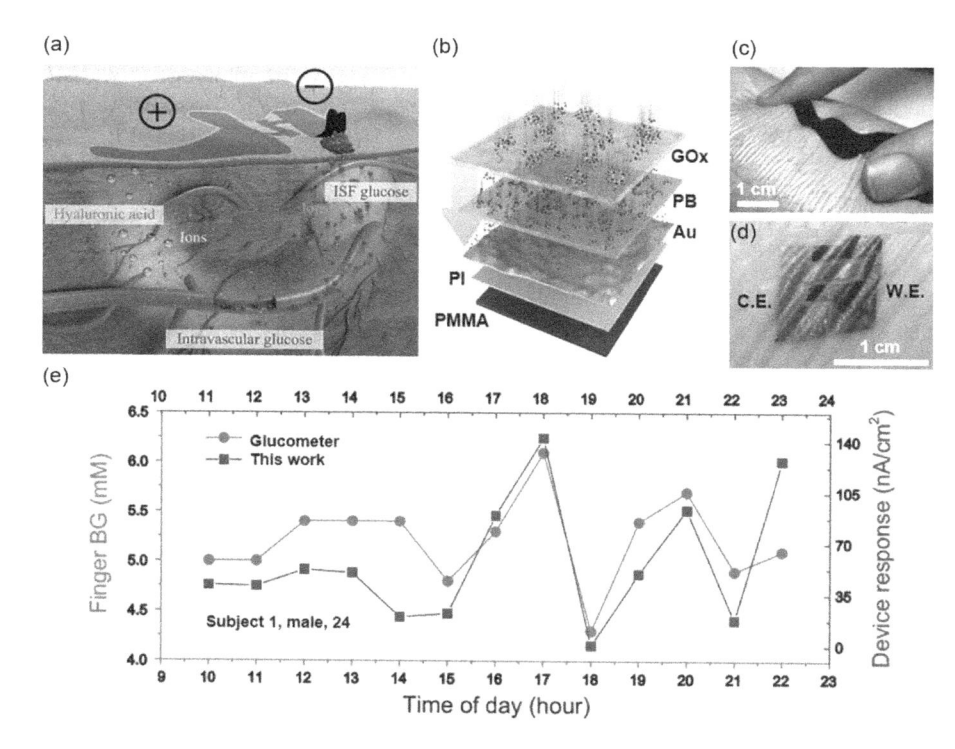

FIGURE 10.6 Wearable biosensors for non-invasive and continuous monitoring of glucose in ISF [37]. (a) Working principle of the glucose sensor. ETCs increase the transportation of intravascular glucose into the ISF, increasing the electro-osmotic flux of reverse iontophoresis. (b) Multilayers of ultrathin skin-like electrochemical sensor. (c) Wearable paper battery on the skin for glucose measurement. (d) Dual electrochemical electrodes of the sensor on the skin. (e) Glucose monitoring by developed wearable glucose sensor (curve with square) compared with a glucometer (curve with circle). ((a)–(e) Reproduced from open-access article of ref. [37], under the terms of the Creative Commons-Attribution-Non Commercial license.)

blood glucose have a high correlation (>0.9) with clinical measurements of blood glucose levels by finger-prick. During a one-day period of testing on humans, the results of the ETC-based glucose monitoring were concurrent with finger-pricked blood glucose measurements (Figure 10.6e). The system provides a new prospect for non-invasive continuous monitoring of glucose.

In 2018, Park and coworkers reported a soft and smart contact lens for glucose monitoring and display [38]. In the contact lens device, a glucose sensor displays pixels to visualize sensing signals in real-time, and wireless power transfer circuits are completely integrated using stretchable and transparent nanostructures. This device can monitor the health condition of the wearer wirelessly through the LED pixel. The rectified power can turn on the glucose sensor and LED pixel. Because this smart contact lens is transparent, it provides a clear observation by matching the refractive indices of the locally patterned areas. The obtained contact lens provides wireless operation and real-time monitoring of glucose concentration in tears [38]. When exposed to tear fluid with a concentrated glucose solution above the threshold, the resistance of the parallel circuit of the LED and the sensor reduces. The difference in the bias applied to the LED pixel then turns it on. After the detection of glucose levels in tear fluid above the threshold, the LED pixel turns off [38].

10.4.3 Ion

Ions, such as Ca^{2+}, Na^+, and K^+, are essential elements for human mineral homeostasis and metabolism. Aberrant variations of ion levels in human body may induce harmful effects on the structure and functions of many systems and organs in the body, leading to diseases such as acid-base balance disorder, hyperparathyroidism, and renal failure. Wearable ion sensors have become important approaches for application in personal health assessment [30,32].

In 2016, Wei Gao and Ali Javey developed a fully integrated wearable sensor array for real-time monitoring of multiple analytes in sweat, including electrolytes (K^+ and Na^+), sweat metabolites (glucose and lactate), and skin temperature (Figure 10.4a) [32]. The sensors were fabricated on the mechanically wearable substrate of PET, and could form a stable contact between the sensor and human skin. The target analytes and skin temperature were measured to facilitate the understanding of human physiological states. The measurement of ion levels (including K^+ and Na^+) is carried out using ion-selective electrodes (ISEs), which is coupled with an RE to maintain a stable potential in solutions with different ionic concentrations. Using PEDOT:PSS as an ion-to-electron transducer in the ISEs, the potentiometric sensors with voltage output are obtained for continuous and long-term monitoring of these ions (Figure 10.4a) [32]. Meanwhile, amperometric sensors with current output for glucose and lactate are based on glucose oxidase and lactate oxidase, respectively, with the enzymes being immobilized within a permeable film of linear polysaccharide chitosan [32]. In addition, a resistance-based temperature sensor is obtained by integration of Cr/Au metal microwires in the device [32].

Moreover, Ali Javey and coworkers developed a wearable electrochemical sensor device for simultaneous measurement of ionized calcium (Ca^{2+}) and pH in various kinds of body fluids (Figure 10.7a) [30]. The wearable system consists of wearable

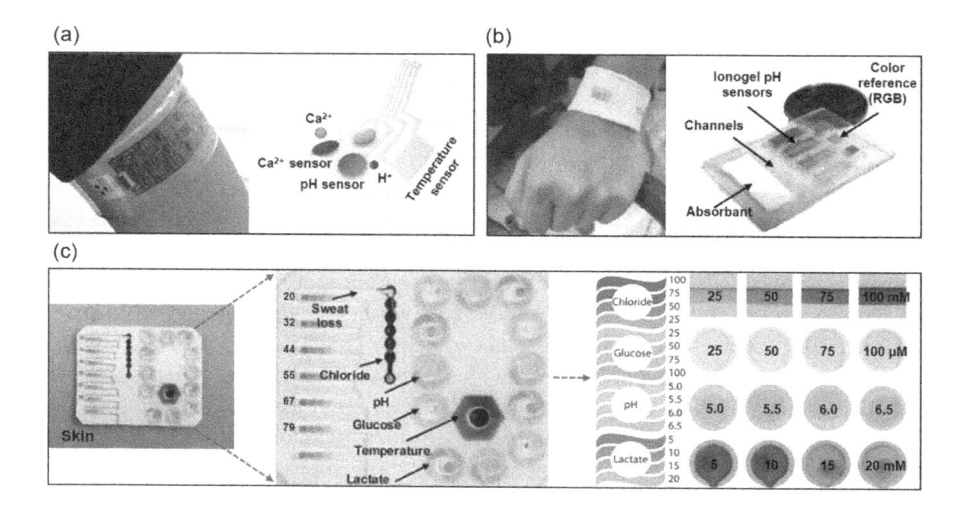

FIGURE 10.7 Wearable biosensor devices for pH sensing. (a) A wearable sensing device on human arm for monitoring of Ca^{2+}, pH, and temperature. (Adapted with permission from ref. [30]. Copyright 2016, American Chemical Society.) (b) A microfluidic-based sensor device for sweat routing and colorimetric measurement of pH. (Reproduced with permission from ref. [39]. Copyright 2012, Elsevier.) (c) Soft, flexible microfluidic device for colorimetric analysis of sweat on the skin, including chloride, pH, glucose, and lactate. (Modified with permission [40]. Copyright 2019, American Chemical Society.)

sensors of a Ca^{2+} ion sensor, a pH sensor, and a skin temperature sensor. They are fabricated on a wearable PET substrate. Monitoring of Ca^{2+} levels and pH values are based on ISEs, coupled with RE of Ag/AgCl. The differences in electrical potentials between two electrodes are measured, which is essentially linear to the strengths of respective target ions. Moreover, accurate analysis of Ca^{2+} concentrations and pH value are realized in various kinds of body fluids, including sweat, tears, and urine [30].

10.4.4 pH

pH is an important indicator to assess body's health condition as it can affect many important physiological processes, such as inflammatory response, wound healing, tumor microenvironment, and blood vessel formation. Monitoring of pH values of the human body can provide early warning of infection risk, provide indicators for different healing stages, and help in effective wound management.

In the last decades, various investigations have been conducted for wearable sensing of pH in the body (Figure 10.7). Benito-Lopez and coworkers developed a real-time wearable monitoring system of sweat pH based on a chemical barcode microfluidic platform (Figure 10.7b) [39]. A disposable and wearable chemical barcode device was developed based on a microfluidic platform, which incorporated ionic liquid polymer gels (ionogels). The obtained sensor device can be incorporated directly into clothing, wristbands, or on human head, allowing conformal contact with the skin, and therefore enables real-time monitoring of pH in the sweat, even during exercise. Moreover, due to the microfluidic structure of the sensing device, fresh sweat can be continuously passed through the sensing area of the device, therefore providing the possibility of continuous and real-time analysis [39].

Recently, John Rogers and coworkers developed a soft, wearable microfluidic system for colorimetric sweat analysis on the skin surface, including pH, chloride, glucose, and lactate (Figure 10.7c) [40]. This work integrated the multiple sweat sensing capabilities in a skin-interfaced, flexible microfluidic platform. The sensing platform enabled separate reactions of multiple assays in a single device, and achieved real-time measurements of electrolytes and metabolites in sweat with physiologically relevant ranges (Figure 10.7c). Moreover, color calibration flags enable precise readout by digital image analysis (Figure 10.7c), which made the sensor applicable in various conditions.

Recently, Zhang Lei and coworkers developed an intelligent zwitterionic hydrogels, which are attachable on the diabetic wound, and simultaneously detect two different parameters of the wound, including pH value and blood glucose concentrations [41]. Phenol red, which served as a pH indicator dye, and two enzymes associated with glucose sensing were encapsulated into the matrix of hydrogels [41]. Visible images of the obtained hydrogels were collected using a smartphone, and further converted into RGB signals for the quantification of wound parameters. When pH is detected, the indicator dye encapsulated in the hydrogel showed sensitive color changes in the pH range of the wound environment [41], providing pH value in intelligent wound dressing.

10.5 CONCLUSION AND PERSPECTIVES

In this chapter, we review the recent advances in wearable physical and chemical biosensors and their applications in wearable/attachable health monitoring. We introduce various materials (inorganic materials, polymers, and nanomaterials, etc.) and their working principles in wearable sensing devices, including piezoresistive, piezoelectrical, and capacitive-based physical biosensors; electrochemical, chemiresistor, and transistor-based chemical biosensors; iontophoresis for biofluid sampling; and reverse iontophoresis for ISF acquisition and chemical biosensing. In detail, we summarize the most recent representative progress of wearable physical sensors for health monitoring of motion, heart rate, breath rate, blood pressure, and body temperature. We also summarize the recent advances of wearable chemical biosensors for monitoring of various analytes, including glucose levels, ion concentrations, and pH in different kinds of body fluids. Their underlying sensing principle, adopted materials, and fabrication process, as well as their applications are described. All these novel sensor devices can be utilized in wearable healthcare monitoring systems and promote their applications in medicine.

Despite abundant materials, structures and engineered technologies have been devoted to improve the performance of wearable/attachable biosensors, there are still a series of challenges that need to be figured out for the practical applications of these wearable sensing devices.

For physical biosensors, several challenges should be addressed to achieve good flexibility and high performance of the sensing devices. First, fabrication of sensors with high uniformity is important for sensor efficiency. For a sensor array, the sensor-to-sensor variability should be considered and eliminated; for composite sensors, the inconsistent dispersion and aggregation of conductive materials in the matrix of elastomer may also induce sensor-to-sensor variability. To solve these problems, uniform dispersion techniques are needed for controlled dispersion to ensure uniformity in sensor materials. Second, scalable fabrication of wearable device in microscales and nanoscales should be considered to improve the efficiency of the sensor devices. To date, stretchable conductors, semiconductors, and dielectrics were investigated separately; nevertheless, their integration in a single device need to be considered. To date, wearable sensors were mainly p-type semiconductors, and the development of wearable and stable n-type semiconductors may direct new applications in wearable biosensor systems. In addition, actually it is hard to distinguish the physiological signals from noisy background signals, therefore, high-performance sensors with high signal-to-noise readout are needed to achieve their high sensitivity to target physical activities when placed on the human body. To achieve successful practical applications of the wearable biosensing devices, cost-effective manufacturing and packaging methods, together with large-scale and mass customizations, should be addressed during the fabrication process of wearable sensor devices.

For chemical biosensors, many measurements of analytes are strongly dependent on the sampling of various body fluids. One of the biggest inherent challenges of wearable chemical sensors is to correct the confounding factors induced by diluted or filtered analytes from the body. A better understanding of the correlations between the concentrations of analytes in the blood and in the non-invasive body fluids is needed to enhance the reliability of the wearable chemical sensors. An expanded set of on-body affinity assays and more sensing strategies are also needed to make more biomarkers accessible to the wearable monitoring. In practical applications, the chemical sensors should exhibit high sensitivity, high selectivity, low limit of detection, and excellent repeatability. More validation studies of wearable biosensor performance will be needed before they are accepted for clinical use. Precise and reliable real-time continuous sensing of biological signals using wearable biosensors have great potential for monitoring health condition in our daily lives.

ACKNOWLEDGEMENT

The authors thank the financial supports from National Natural Science Foundation of China (NSFC, grant no. 81871484), Natural Science Foundation of Guangdong Province (grant no. 2021A1515012183), and research start-up fund of Wuhan University (20035).

REFERENCES

1. Trung TQ, Lee N-E. Flexible and stretchable physical sensor integrated platforms for wearable human-activity monitoring and personal healthcare. *Adv Mater.* 2016;28:4338–72.
2. Amjadi M, Kyung KU, Park I, Sitti M. Stretchable, skin-mountable, and wearable strain sensors and their potential applications: a review. *Adv Funct Mater.* 2016;26:1678–98.
3. Kim J, Campbell AS, de Ávila BE-F, Wang J. Wearable biosensors for healthcare monitoring. *Nat Biotechnol.* 2019;37:389–406.

4. Yang YR, Gao W. Wearable and flexible electronics for continuous molecular monitoring. *Chem Soc Rev.* 2019;48:1465–91.

5. Yang TT, Xie D, Li ZH, Zhu HW. Recent advances in wearable tactile sensors: materials, sensing mechanisms, and device performance. *Mater Sci Eng R-Reports.* 2017;115:1–37.

6. Chorsi MT, Curry EJ, Chorsi HT, Das R, Baroody J, Purohit PK, Ilies H, Nguyen TD. Piezoelectric biomaterials for sensors and actuators. *Adv Mater.* 2019;31:15.

7. Saito Y, Takao H, Tani T, Nonoyama T, Takatori K, Homma T, Nagaya T, Nakamura M. Lead-free piezoceramics. *Nature.* 2004;432:84–7.

8. Wang ZL, Song J. Piezoelectric nanogenerators based on zinc oxide nanowire arrays. *Science.* 2006;312:242–6.

9. Kim DH, Lu N, Ma R, Kim YS, Kim RH, Wang S, Wu J, Won SM, Tao H, Islam A, Yu KJ, Kim TI, Chowdhury R, Ying M, Xu L, Li M, Chung HJ, Keum H, McCormick M, Liu P, Zhang YW, Omenetto FG, Huang Y, Coleman T, Rogers JA. Epidermal electronics. *Science.* 2011;333:838–43.

10. Wang S, Xu J, Wang W, Wang GN, Rastak R, Molina-Lopez F, Chung JW, Niu S, Feig VR, Lopez J, Lei T, Kwon SK, Kim Y, Foudeh AM, Ehrlich A, Gasperini A, Yun Y, Murmann B, Tok JB, Bao Z. Skin electronics from scalable fabrication of an intrinsically stretchable transistor array. *Nature.* 2018;555:83–8.

11. Liu M, Pu X, Jiang C, Liu T, Huang X, Chen L, Du C, Sun J, Hu W, Wang ZL. Large-area all-textile pressure sensors for monitoring human motion and physiological signals. *Adv Mater.* 2017;29:1703700.

12. Liu RY, Kuang X, Deng JN, Wang YC, Wang AC, Ding WB, Lai YC, Chen J, Wang PH, Lin ZQ, Qi HJ, Sun BQ, Wang ZL. Shape memory polymers for body motion energy harvesting and self-powered mechanosensing. *Adv Mater.* 2018;30:8.

13. Tang L, Shang J, Jiang X. Multilayered electronic transfer tattoo that can enable the crease amplification effect. *Sci Adv.* 2021;7:eabe3778.

14. Lin ZM, Chen J, Li XS, Zhou ZH, Meng KY, Wei W, Yang J, Wang ZL. Triboelectric nanogenerator enabled body sensor network for self-powered human heart-rate monitoring. *ACS Nano.* 2017;11:8830–7.

15. Li MFF, Li HY, Zhong WB, Zhao QH, Wang D. Stretchable conductive polypyrrole/polyurethane (PPy/PU) strain sensor with netlike microcracks for human breath detection. *ACS Appl Mater Interfaces.* 2014;6:1313–9.

16. Chu M, Nguyen T, Pandey V, Zhou Y, Pham HN, Bar-Yoseph R, Radom-Aizik S, Jain R, Cooper DM, Khine M. Respiration rate and volume measurements using wearable strain sensors. *NPJ Digit Med.* 2019;2:8.

17. Hu YT, Xu Y. An ultra-sensitive wearable accelerometer for continuous heart and lung sound monitoring. *34th Annual International Conference of the IEEE Engineering in Medicine and Biology Society.* 2012: 694–7. San Diego, CA.

18. Resnekov L. Understanding heart sounds and murmurs, with an introduction to lung sounds. *JAMA.* 1985;254:124–5.

19. Park DY, Joe DJ, Kim DH, Park H, Han JH, Jeong CK, Park H, Park JG, Joung B, Lee KJ. Self-powered real-time arterial pulse monitoring using ultrathin epidermal piezoelectric sensors. *Adv Mater.* 2017;29:1702308.

20. Wang C, Li X, Hu H, Zhang L, Huang Z, Lin M, Zhang Z, Yin Z, Huang B, Gong H, Bhaskaran S, Gu Y, Makihata M, Guo Y, Lei Y, Chen Y, Wang C, Li Y, Zhang T, Chen Z, Pisano AP, Zhang L, Zhou Q, Xu S. Monitoring of the central blood pressure waveform via a conformal ultrasonic device. *Nat Biomed Eng.* 2018;2:687–95.

21. Meng K, Chen J, Li X, Wu Y, Fan W, Zhou Z, He Q, Wang X, Fan X, Zhang Y, Yang J, Wang ZL. Flexible weaving constructed self-powered pressure sensor enabling continuous diagnosis of cardiovascular disease and measurement of cuffless blood pressure. *Adv Funct Mater.* 2019;29:1806388.

22. Bae GY, Han JT, Lee G, Lee S, Kim SW, Park S, Kwon J, Jung S, Cho K. Pressure/temperature sensing bimodal electronic skin with stimulus discriminability and linear sensitivity. *Adv Mater.* 2018;30:1803388.

23. Bang J, Lee WS, Park B, Joh H, Woo HK, Jeon S, Ahn J, Jeong C, Kim T-i, Oh SJ. Highly sensitive temperature sensor: ligand-treated Ag nanocrystal thin films on PDMS with thermal expansion strategy. *Adv Funct Mater.* 2019;29:1903047.

24. Zhang F, Zang Y, Huang D, Di C-a, Zhu D. Flexible and self-powered temperature–pressure dual-parameter sensors using microstructure-frame-supported organic thermoelectric materials. *Nat Commun.* 2015;6:8356.

25. Koh A, Kang D, Xue Y, Lee S, Pielak RM, Kim J, Hwang T, Min S, Banks A, Bastien P, Manco MC, Wang L, Ammann KR, Jang K-I, Won P, Han S, Ghaffari R, Paik U, Slepian MJ, Balooch G, Huang Y, Rogers JA. A soft, wearable microfluidic device for the capture, storage, and colorimetric sensing of sweat. *Sci Transl Med.* 2016;8:366ra165.

26. Bandodkar AJ, Gutruf P, Choi J, Lee K, Sekine Y, Reeder JT, Jeang WJ, Aranyosi AJ, Lee SP, Model JB, Ghaffari R, Su C-J, Leshock JP, Ray T, Verrillo A, Thomas K, Krishnamurthi V, Han S, Kim J, Krishnan S, Hang T, Rogers JA. Battery-free, skin-interfaced microfluidic/electronic systems for simultaneous electrochemical, colorimetric, and volumetric analysis of sweat. *Sci Adv.* 2019;5:eaav3294.

27. Imani S, Bandodkar AJ, Mohan AMV, Kumar R, Yu S, Wang J, Mercier PP. A wearable chemical–electrophysiological hybrid biosensing system for real-time health and fitness monitoring. *Nat Commun.* 2016;7: 11650.

28. Kim J, Sempionatto JR, Imani S, Hartel MC, Barfidokht A, Tang G, Campbell AS, Mercier PP, Wang J. Simultaneous monitoring of sweat and interstitial fluid using a single wearable biosensor platform. *Adv Sci.* 2018;5:1800880.

29. Teymourian H, Barfidokht A, Wang J. Electrochemical glucose sensors in diabetes management: an updated review (2010–2020). *Chem Soc Rev.* 2020;49:7671–709.

30. Nyein HY, Gao W, Shahpar Z, Emaminejad S, Challa S, Chen K, Fahad HM, Tai LC, Ota H, Davis RW, Javey A. A Wearable electrochemical platform for noninvasive simultaneous monitoring of Ca^{2+} and pH. *ACS Nano.* 2016;10:7216–24.

31. Bariya M, Nyein HYY, Javey A. Wearable sweat sensors. *Nat Electron.* 2018;1:160–71.

32. Gao W, Emaminejad S, Nyein HYY, Challa S, Chen K, Peck A, Fahad HM, Ota H, Shiraki H, Kiriya D, Lien DH, Brooks GA, Davis RW, Javey A. Fully integrated wearable sensor arrays for multiplexed in situ perspiration analysis. *Nature.* 2016;529:509–14.

33. Yang Y, Song Y, Bo X, Min J, Pak OS, Zhu L, Wang M, Tu J, Kogan A, Zhang H, Hsiai TK, Li Z, Gao W. A laser-engraved wearable sensor for sensitive detection of uric acid and tyrosine in sweat. *Nat Biotechnol.* 2020;38:217–24.

34. Yu Y, Nassar J, Xu C, Min J, Yang Y, Dai A, Doshi R, Huang A, Song Y, Gehlhar R, Ames AD, Gao W. Biofuel-powered soft electronic skin with multiplexed and wireless sensing for human-machine interfaces. *Sci Robot.* 2020;5:eaaz7946.

35. Lee H, Choi TK, Lee YB, Cho HR, Ghaffari R, Wang L, Choi HJ, Chung TD, Lu N, Hyeon T, Choi SH, Kim DH. A graphene-based electrochemical device with thermoresponsive microneedles for diabetes monitoring and therapy. *Nat Nanotechnol.* 2016;11:566–72.

36. Lee H, Song C, Hong YS, Kim MS, Cho HR, Kang T, Shin K, Choi SH, Hyeon T, Kim DH. Wearable/disposable sweat-based glucose monitoring device with multistage transdermal drug delivery module. *Sci Adv.* 2017;3:e1601314.

37. Chen Y, Lu S, Zhang S, Li Y, Qu Z, Chen Y, Lu B, Wang X, Feng X. Skin-like biosensor system via electrochemical channels for noninvasive blood glucose monitoring. *Sci Adv.* 2017;3:e1701629.

38. Park J, Kim J, Kim S-Y, Cheong WH, Jang J, Park Y-G, Na K, Kim Y-T, Heo JH, Lee CY, Lee JH, Bien F, Park J-U. Soft, smart contact lenses with integrations of wireless circuits, glucose sensors, and displays. *Sci Adv.* 2018;4:eaap9841.

39. Curto VF, Fay C, Coyle S, Byrne R, O'Toole C, Barry C, Hughes S, Moyna N, Diamond D, Benito-Lopez F. Real-time sweat pH monitoring based on a wearable chemical barcode micro-fluidic platform incorporating ionic liquids. *Sens Actuators B: Chem.* 2012;171–172:1327–34.

40. Choi J, Bandodkar AJ, Reeder JT, Ray TR, Turnquist A, Kim SB, Nyberg N, Hourlier-Fargette A, Model JB, Aranyosi AJ, Xu S, Ghaffari R, Rogers JA. Soft, skin-integrated multifunctional microfluidic systems for accurate colorimetric analysis of sweat bio-markers and temperature. *ACS Sens.* 2019;4:379–88.

41. Zhu Y, Zhang J, Song J, Yang J, Du Z, Zhao W, Guo H, Wen C, Li Q, Sui X, Zhang L. A Multifunctional pro-healing zwitterionic hydrogel for simultaneous optical monitoring of pH and glucose in diabetic wound treatment. *Adv Funct Mater.* 2019;30:1905493.

42. Sekine Y, Kim SB, Zhang Y, Bandodkar AJ, Xu S, Choi J, Irie M, Ray TR, Kohli P, Kozai N, Sugita T, Wu Y, Lee K, Lee K-T, Ghaffari R, Rogers JA. A fluorometric skin-interfaced microfluidic device and smartphone imaging module for in situ quantitative analysis of sweat chemistry. *Lab on a Chip.* 2018;18:2178–86.

43. Munje RD, Muthukumar S, Jagannath B, Prasad S. A new paradigm in sweat based wearable diagnostics biosensors using room temperature ionic liquids (RTILs). *Sci Rep.* 2017;7:1950.

44. Morris D, Coyle S, Wu Y, Lau KT, Wallace G, Diamond D. Bio-sensing textile based patch with integrated optical detection system for sweat monitoring. *Sens Actuators B: Chem.* 2009;139:231–6.

45. Ciui B, Martin A, Mishra RK, Brunetti B, Nakagawa T, Dawkins TJ, Lyu M, Cristea C, Sandulescu R, Wang J. Wearable wireless tyrosinase bandage and microneedle sensors: toward melanoma screening. *Adv Healthc Mater.* 2018;7:1701264.

11 Micro/Nanobiomaterials

Shuo Wang
University of Tsukuba

CONTENTS

11.1 INTRODUCTION

As people pay more attention to health, biomaterials, an emerging technology, has become more and more important. It can not only overcome some limitations of traditional materials but also bring better therapeutic effect [1]. As the most basic structure and functional unit of an organism, the effect of material on cell function is very important for biomaterials [2]. The function of cells is affected by physical, chemical, and biological factors [3–6]; hence, it is very important to study how these factors affect the function of cells. As Figure 11.1 shows, with the rapid development of micro and nanotechnology, people can more accurately prepare related materials, change the physical factors such as the morphology and size of materials

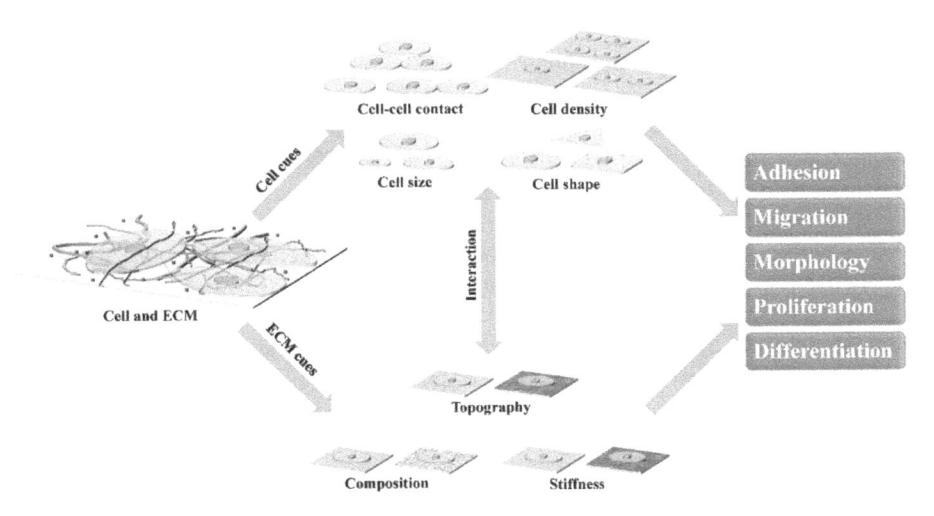

FIGURE 11.1 Effect of cell microenvironment on cell behavior.

DOI: 10.1201/9781003161981-11

through the preparation of micropatterns [7], nanoparticles [8], nanotubes [9], and other materials with different micro and nanoscales [10] to study the cell functions such as adhesion [11], proliferation [12], migration [13], and diffusion [14] on a scale closer to the cell size [15].

In this chapter, we briefly introduce the emerging field of micro/nanobiomaterials through the research of micropattern, nanomedicine, micro/nanobiological devices, and their applications in related fields.

11.2 MICROPATTERN IN BIOMATERIAL

The microenvironment around the cell plays an important role in its function, and micropatterns can accurately regulate the cell microenvironment and influence the related functions of the cell [16]. As a kind of vascular scaffold material, the surface of material plays an important role in regulating the behavior of endothelial cells (ECs) [17]. Li et al. prepared hyaluronic acid microstrips on the surface of titanium alloy to obtain endothelial cells under simulated blood flow shear stress [18]. The effects of endothelial cell morphology on the release of functional factors such as nitric oxide (NO), von Willebrand factor (vWF), prostacyclin (PGI2), thrombomodulin (TM), tissue factor pathway inhibitor (TFPI), E-selectin, and fibronectin (FN) were studied. It was found that the morphology of endothelial cells was elongated, which regulated the release of functional factors, indicating that the function of EC could be regulated by changing its shape. Extracellular matrix (ECM) of endothelial cells has a very significant effect on improving the biocompatibility of cardiovascular scaffold materials [19]; therefore, Li et al. prepared hyaluronic acid microstrip on the surface of titanium alloy, and obtained endothelial cell ECM on this surface by acellular method, thus preparing hyaluronic acid micropattern and ECM biomimetic coating [20]. The co-culture of endothelial cells, smooth muscle cells, and macrophages showed that the coating promoted endothelium, anti-proliferation, and anti-inflammation. On this basis, to obtain more ECM of endothelial cells, Li et al. prepared a biomimetic ECM surface on 316L SS with hyaluronic acid micropattern by multiple layer-by-layer decellularization [21]. A series of *in vitro* blood experiments, *in vitro* cell experiments, and *in vivo* animal experiments showed that the bionic ECM surface could inhibit the adhesion and activation of platelets, promote the proliferation of endothelial cells and the release of NO, inhibit the adhesion and activation of macrophages, and possess good anticoagulant, endothelium promoting, and anti-inflammatory effects, as well as good histocompatibility.

The human bone itself contains various micronanostructures, so the micropattern can better regulate the function of related bone cells [22,23]. Zhao et al. prepared various micropatterns on bioceramics using a micropattern nylon sieve [24]. The adhesion, proliferation, and osteogenic differentiation of bone marrow mesenchymal stem cells (BMSCs) were studied. It was observed that the wettability and surface of micropatterns were better and could promote the related functions of BMSCs. Later, Zhao et al. prepared micro nanohybrid structure patterns on hydroxyapatite (HA) bioceramics [24]. The effects of different structures on the integrin expression, bone morphogenetic protein-2 (BMP2) signaling pathway, and intercellular communication of BMSCs through adhesion, proliferation, alkaline phosphatase activity, integrin, and related gene expression experiments were tested. It was found that the micro/nanohybrid pattern could promote the adhesion, proliferation, and osteogenic gene expression of BMSCs by activating integrin, BMP2 signaling pathway, and intercellular communication, which had a synergistic effect on regulating the behavior of BMSCs. Periosteum plays an important role in bone regeneration [25]. To simulate the natural periosteum, Yang et al. prepared mineralized hydroxyapatite nanoparticles (HANPs) micropatterns by printing method [26]. Apatite and growth factors were co-precipitated on the micropatterns by selective mineralization to prepare biomimetic periosteum. The biomimetic membrane was co-cultured with rat BMSCs. It was found that biomimetic membrane could promote angiogenesis and osteogenesis. The experiment of repairing rat skull defect showed that biomimetic membrane with mineralized micropattern could regulate vascularized bone formation. This biomimetic membrane had a good application prospect in the field of bone repair.

Micropatterns can also be used to study the related functions of cells at the single-cell level. Peng et al. prepared an arginine-glycine-aspartate (RGD) micropattern on polyethylene glycol (PEG) hydrogel [27]. The effects of aspect ratio on osteogenic and adipogenic differentiation of single mesenchymal stem cells were studied. It was found that when the aspect ratio was 1, the adipogenic differentiation was good, and the osteoblast differentiation was better when the aspect ratio was 2. Yan et al. prepared a series of microislands with different areas and studied the critical area of cell adhesion [28]. Through semi-quantitative calculation of the number and area of cell adhesion, they defined the critical area A_{C1} for single cell from apoptosis to survival, A_{C2} for single-cell adhesion to multiple cells, and A_Δ for more than one cell adhesion. This provided a theoretical basis for the reasonable design of micropattern size. Based on this study, Yao et al. prepared RGD circular microislands to study the adhesion and proliferation of different cells on the micropattern [29]. They set up a series of microislands with different areas to control the adhesion area. By calculating the proliferation rate of cells on different microislands, the authors found a significant relationship between the proliferation of cells and the diffusion area of cells. Two critical regions of cell proliferation were proposed for the first time: A_P, a critical region from almost no proliferation to limited proliferation, and A_{FP}, a critical region from limited proliferation to free proliferation. In addition to the single-cell-level study, Liu et al. also studied the effect of nuclear geometry on adipogenic and osteogenic differentiation of BMSCs from the cellular substructure level by preparing microcolumn [30]. They found that larger nuclear deformation could promote osteogenic differentiation but inhibit adipogenic differentiation, which also provided new evidence for the effect of cell substructure on cell differentiation.

11.3 NANOMEDICINE IN BIOMATERIAL

Cancer is the main cause of human death globally [31]. People have been committed to the development of cancer treatment drugs [32]. In recent years, with the development of nanotechnology, more and more nanomedicines come into people's sight [33]. Two-dimensional nanomaterials have always been a research hotspot in the field of nanotechnology because of their special physical and chemical properties [34–36]. The development of nanomedicines using graphene, transition metal dihaloalkanes (TMDs), and other two-dimensional nanomaterials is also a hot field in nanomedicine [37,38]. Antimony two-dimensional nanomaterials have more excellent properties than graphene and TMDs, and antimony drugs are also widely used in the clinic, which shows that antimony nanomedicine has a better application prospect [39,40]. Tao et al. developed a new two-dimensional antimony nanosheet photonic drug delivery platform, and studied its biocompatibility, degradation, *in vitro*, and *in vivo* properties, as well as the intracellular mechanism of two-dimensional nanomaterials [41]. The experimental results showed that the platform had excellent photothermal performance, high drug loading, and excellent multi-mode imaging characteristics, as well as could inhibit tumor growth without obvious side effects. A high concentration of NO could induce apoptosis of tumor cells in target cells, which has an anticancer effect [42,43]. Jia et al. combined the enzyme-sensitive NO-release prodrug NPQ in tumor with an organic silica nanocarrier of a redox reaction to prepare a double tumor redox/enzyme reaction NO-release nanomedicine [44]. The redox, drug release *in vitro*, cytotoxicity to cancer cells and normal cells *in vitro* and tumor therapeutic effect *in vivo* were tested in detail. It was found that nanomedicine could reach tumor tissue effectively and release a large amount of NO to kill tumor cells, with fewer side effects on normal tissue and good targeted therapeutic effect.

During drug delivery for tumor-targeted therapy, the structure, size, and loading capacity of nanocarriers affect the drug delivery efficiency, and porous nanomaterials are the best choice as carriers because of their high specific surface area, porosity, and low density [45–47]. Metal organic framework (MOF) is a new type of porous nanomaterial, which is composed of metal ions or metal clusters and organics [48,49]. By combining with other nanostructures, MOF could give new nanoformulations collective functionality and synergy, which could not be obtained from single component nanostructures, so it has been widely studied in the biomedical field [50–52]. Chu et al. developed coordination driven self-assembled metal organic nanostructures with multifunctional nanotechnology, and prepared zinc (II) coordination nanostructures capable of loading indocyanine green (ICG) and therapeutic genes to realize fluorescence and PA image-guided light/gene combination therapy [53]. The results showed that the synergistic effect of phototherapy and gene therapy realized by this simple, stable, and multifunctional platform is better than that of single therapy. Chen et al. combined MOF with hollow organic silica nanoparticles (HMONs) to a prepare tumor-thermosensitive universal nanoplatform, which not only could achieve large drug loading but also had a good photothermal effect, dual-mode imaging ability, and excellent biocompatibility [54]. Microwave thermal therapy (MTT) is a kind of clinical treatment method with simple operation, high efficiency, fewer side effects, and application prospects [55,56]. However, the limited ablation area of tumor results in a high recurrence rate after traditional MTT treatment and improves the curative effect of MTT combined with other methods. To combine MTT with microwave dynamic therapy (MDT), Fu et al. prepared Mn-doped MOF nanocubes (Mn ZrMOF NCS) by hydrothermal method and tested its hyperthermia effect *in vitro*, and microwave dynamic experiment, biodegradability, cytotoxicity and tumor treatment effect *in vivo* [57]. The results showed that Mn ZrMOF NCS with high porosity, high specific surface area, and high thermal conversion efficiency had excellent biocompatibility and biodegradability, which was expected to become a new nanomedicine for the synergistic treatment of tumor by MTT and MDT. Abazari et al. used FOLA as a molecular localizer to prepare pH-responsive MOFs for the delivery of 5-fluorouracil (5-FU) as an anticancer drug to cancer cells [58]. The drug release, reactive oxygen species release, apoptosis rate of cancer cells, wound healing ability, and anticancer ability of the nanomedicine were tested. It was found that the nanomedicine could inhibit the growth of cancer cells without significantly affecting normal cell behavior. Biomarker microRNAs (miRNAs) can detect the development stage of cancer, which has attracted widespread attention [59]. However, there are few studies on the use of miRNAs as triggers of anticancer drug release. Chen et al. loaded doxorubicin onto uio-68 metal organic framework nanoparticles (NMOFs) and used structural engineering to lock the double-stranded nucleic acid structure [60]. The two chains were connected with NMOFs and anchored chain, respectively. The second strand is not only complementary to the anchoring sequence but also complementary to the specific miRNA biomarkers of MCF-7 breast cancer cells or OVCAR-3 ovarian cancer cells. Cell experiments showed that miRNA could unlock NMOF and inhibit MCF-7 or OVCAR-3 cancer cells. Janus nanoparticles (JNPs) are new multi-component hybrid nanoparticles with different compositions and chemical and physical properties, which have been widely used in biomedicine due to their unique properties [61,62]. One-dimensional gold nanorods/MOFs JNP (AuNR/ ZIF-8) modified with lactic acid (LA) were synthesized by Zhang et al. [63]. The photothermal properties, drug loading, pH/NIR stimulated drug release, cytotoxicity, and blood compatibility of the JNP were tested. The results showed that the JNP had good photothermal properties, high drug loading, effective pH, NIR-stimulated drug release, good cell safety and blood compatibility, excellent photothermal and chemotherapeutic effects, and clear *in vivo* imaging characteristics. These results indicated that LA- AuNR/ZIF-8 could introduce DOX into tumor sites to induce chemotherapy, which showed good photothermal therapeutic effect under near-infrared laser irradiation, and had good biocompatibility and application prospects. Zhang et al. developed a UFO-like cyclodextrin palladium nanosheets/zeolite imidazole framework-8 Janus nanoparticles (CD-PdNS/ZIF-8 JNP) [64]. Hydrophobic 10 hydroxycamptothecin (HCPT) was loaded on CD-PdNS, and DOX was loaded on PAA-ZIF-8. Through the accurate synthesis of this nanostructure, the combination of 2D metal, MOFs, and organic CD were realized to achieve a synergistic therapeutic effect. Because PdNSs had a wide near-infrared absorption band, the photothermal effect of the JNPs in near-infrared-II biofilm was studied. *In vitro* and *in vivo* experimental results showed that JNPs loaded with two drugs could effectively treat cancer through the synergistic effect of chemotherapy and photothermal therapy. In addition, this method could also be extended to the synthesis of other Janus nanostructured materials, which had broad application prospects.

The complex microenvironment around tumor can affect the behavior of tumor cells, so it is very important to simulate the tumor microenvironment *in vivo* for the research of anticancer drugs. The current two-dimensional (2D) culture system and animal model cannot well simulate the tumor environment *in vivo*, so a more reliable and effective screening method is needed to evaluate the drug response. Microfluidic technology can accurately control the relevant conditions so that cells can coexist in the three-dimensional complex microenvironment, which is a new and effective research method. To simulate the microenvironment of a colon tumor, Carvalho et al. developed a three-dimensional microfluidic chip model that can reconstruct the physiological function of microvessels to evaluate the delivery efficiency of anticancer nanomedicines [65]. The invasion of endothelial cells, the formation of nanoparticle gradient, drug screening performance, gene expression, and immunocytochemistry of the microfluidic chip were tested. The results showed that the three-dimensional microfluidic chip could better screen drugs to achieve better results. The tumor microenvironment will affect the diffusion of nanomedicines, which may lead to nanomedicines that cannot completely penetrate the tumor, thus reducing the therapeutic effect. Therefore, it is very important to study the penetration of nanomedicines into the tumor. The traditional strategy of drug diffusion is to promote its movement in tumor ECM to enhance the effect of drug diffusion, but there are still some problems in the movement of nanomedicines in ECM. As a kind of cell behavior, transcytosis can break through the limitation of ECM and provide a driving force for the penetration of nanomedicines. Liu et al. used modified upconversion nanoparticles (UCNs) with the ability of photodynamic therapy (PDT) as model nanomedicines [66]. Through UCN emission, quantitative internalization and excretion of UCNs, intracellular transport, tumor tissue observation, blocking cell transport, and other tests, we found that the interaction of nanoparticles between cells and transcytosis occurred in the interaction of cells and nanoparticles, which indicated that the permeability of tumor depends on the transport of nanomedicines. Transcytosis could improve the therapeutic effect of a tumor by enhancing the permeability of nanomedicines.

11.4 MICRO/NANOBIODEVICES IN BIOMATERIAL

Cancer cell detection technology is very important in the early diagnosis of cancer [67]. Aptamer is a kind of synthetic nucleic acid with molecular recognition ability, which can specifically modify various functional ligands [68]. Due to its good stability and specificity, aptamer is widely used in the biomedical field [69]. Ou et al. designed a DNA tetrahedral-connected aptamer electrochemical cell sensor based on MOFs PCN-224 [70]. First, a tetrahedral DNA nanostructure was fixed on the surface of the gold electrode to connect the aptamer. Then, PCN-224 was modified by g-tetramer/heme DNase, horseradish peroxidase, and the aptamer. The results of electrochemical test, cell capture, cell release, and cell activity analysis showed that the sensor can detect breast cancer MCF-7 cells with high selectivity, and could be extended to other cancer cells with specific aptamers, which provided a new and effective method for cancer cell detection and had a good application prospect in cancer diagnosis. Folate receptor (FR) is highly expressed in various malignant tumors, so FR is often used as a tool for targeted therapy and imaging [71,72]. Graphene quantum dots (GQDs) can be used for real-time monitoring of cell–cell interactions and biological functions due to their unique fluorescence properties [73]. Soleymani et al. prepared folate (FA)-modified nitrogen-doped graphene quantum dots (N-GQDs) cell sensor targeting MKN45 cells to achieve rapid and accurate detection of FR expression in cancer cells [74]. Through cell fluorescence imaging, cytotoxicity, apoptosis, tumor cell-selective detection, and adriamycin treatment effect, it was found that the cell sensor had good cell compatibility and detection ability, which provided a new idea for the development of tumor diagnosis biological device.

Cell microenvironment can guide cell tissue and improve the role of synthetic tissue in biosensor and regenerative medicine [75]. ECM in natural tissue has an ideal structure and function and can guide cell tissue to achieve regeneration and maintain tissue function [76]. Inspired by the microstructure of ECM, Fujie et al. developed an independent ultra-thin polymer film (nanofilm) with flexibility, cell adhesion, and surface morphology tailorability [77]. The nanofilm was used as a flexible substrate, and the fibronectin combined with carbon nanotubes was fixed on the nanofilm by microcontact printing (μCP) to prepare the micro nanohybrid pattern of cell adhesion. Co-culture with C2C12 skeletal myoblasts showed that the nanomembrane could enhance cell elongation and differentiation. This kind of functional nanofilm with easy preparation, good flexibility, cell adhesion, and surface morphology tailorability was an effective platform to study the interaction between cells and substrate and had a strong guiding significance for the development of related biodevice.

In addition to the medical field, biodevice is also widely used in other fields. After wastewater treatment, the persistence and biological effect of water will produce alkylphenols and bisphenol endocrine disruptors [78]. Phenol is famous for its persistence in the environment and toxicity to organisms [79]. The detection and quantification of phenol in water are crucial for the protection of human health. To develop an economic, reliable, and durable biological device for the detection and monitoring of phenols and phenolic endocrine disruptors in water samples, Penu et al. modified tyrosinase and reduced graphene oxide gold nanoparticles on an indium tin oxide electrode (ITO) to prepare a reagent free amperometric device [80]. It was found that the synergistic effect of RGO and nanocrystalline GNP layer on ITO surface significantly improved the electrode conductivity and promoted the electron transfer reaction. The nanostructured layer provided a good microenvironment for the maintenance of tyrosinase catalytic specificity. The biological device had the characteristics of high sensitivity, simple operation, low cost, fast speed, high precision, and sensitivity. It was a reliable tool to evaluate the content of phenolic endocrine disruptors and had application value in monitoring the concentration of phenolic endocrine disruptors.

11.5 CONCLUSION

Micro/nanotechnology has brought new vitality and vigor to biomaterials. Micro/nanobiomaterials prepared by combining biomaterials with micro/nanotechnology have achieved many functions that traditional biomaterials cannot, which plays an important role in promoting the development of biomaterials. More and more researchers have begun to pay attention to micro/nanobiomaterials, and it is believed that micro/nanobiomaterials will make more valuable contributions to human health and social development in the near future.

REFERENCES

1. S. Mitragotri, J. Lahann. Physical approaches to biomaterial design. *Nature Materials* 8(1) (2009) 15–23.
2. A.J. García. Get a grip: Integrins in cell–biomaterial interactions. *Biomaterials* 26(36) (2005) 7525–7529.
3. P. Bornstein, E.H. Sage. Matricellular proteins: Extracellular modulators of cell function. *Current Opinion in Cell Biology* 14(5) (2002) 608–616.
4. C.J. Bettinger, R. Langer, J.T. Borenstein. Engineering substrate topography at the micro- and nanoscale to control cell function. *Angewandte Chemie International Edition* 48(30) (2009) 5406–5415.
5. W. Dröge. Free radicals in the physiological control of cell function. *Physiological Reviews* 82(1) (2002) 47–95.
6. A.M. Kloxin, A.M. Kasko, C.N. Salinas, K.S. Anseth. Photodegradable hydrogels for dynamic tuning of physical and chemical properties. *Science* 324(5923) (2009) 59.
7. M. Moffa, A.G. Sciancalepore, L.G. Passione, D. Pisignano. Combined nano- and micro-scale topographic cues for engineered vascular constructs by electrospinning and imprinted micro-patterns. *Small* 10(12) (2014) 2439–2450.
8. A. Taglietti, C.R. Arciola, A. D'Agostino, G. Dacarro, L. Montanaro, D. Campoccia, L. Cucca, M. Vercellino, A. Poggi, P. Pallavicini, L. Visai. Antibiofilm activity of a monolayer of silver nanoparticles anchored to an amino-silanized glass surface. *Biomaterials* 35(6) (2014) 1779–1788.
9. Q. Huang, Y. Yang, D. Zheng, R. Song, Y. Zhang, P. Jiang, E.A. Vogler, C. Lin, Effect of construction of TiO_2 nanotubes on platelet behaviors: Structure-property relationships. *Acta Biomaterialia* 51 (2017) 505–512.
10. M.C. Phipps, W.C. Clem, J.M. Grunda, G.A. Clines, S.L. Bellis. Increasing the pore sizes of bone-mimetic electrospun scaffolds comprised of polycaprolactone, collagen I and hydroxyapatite to enhance cell infiltration. *Biomaterials* 33(2) (2012) 524–534.
11. A. Tourovskaia, T. Barber, B.T. Wickes, D. Hirdes, B. Grin, D.G. Castner, K.E. Healy, A. Folch. Micropatterns of chemisorbed cell adhesion-repellent films using oxygen plasma etching and elastomeric masks. *Langmuir* 19(11) (2003) 4754–4764.
12. P. Zapata, J. Su, A.J. García, J.C. Meredith. Quantitative high-throughput screening of osteoblast attachment, spreading, and proliferation on demixed polymer blend micropatterns. *Biomacromolecules* 8(6) (2007) 1907–1917.
13. G. Kumar, C.C. Ho, C.C. Co. Retracted: Guiding cell migration using one-way micropattern arrays. *Advanced Materials* 19(8) (2007) 1084–1090.
14. J.T. Groves, S.G. Boxer. Micropattern formation in supported lipid membranes. *Accounts of Chemical Research* 35(3) (2002) 149–157.
15. D. Falconnet, G. Csucs, H. Michelle Grandin, M. Textor. Surface engineering approaches to micropattern surfaces for cell-based assays. *Biomaterials* 27(16) (2006) 3044–3063.
16. G. Huang, F. Li, X. Zhao, Y. Ma, Y. Li, M. Lin, G. Jin, T.J. Lu, G.M. Genin, F. Xu. Functional and biomimetic materials for engineering of the three-dimensional cell microenvironment. *Chemical Reviews* 117(20) (2017) 12764–12850.
17. P. Wang, P. Xiong, J. Liu, S. Gao, T.F. Xi, Y. Cheng. A silk-based coating containing GREDVY peptide and heparin on Mg-Zn-Y-Nd alloy: Improved corrosion resistance, hemocompatibility and endothelialization. *Journal of Materials Chemistry B* 6(6) (2018) 966–978.
18. J. Li, K. Zhang, P. Yang, W. Qin, G. Li, A. Zhao, N. Huang. Human vascular endothelial cell morphology and functional cytokine secretion influenced by different size of HA micro-pattern on titanium substrate. *Colloids and Surfaces B Biointerfaces* 110 (2013) 199–207.

19. E. Kniazeva, A.J. Putnam. Endothelial cell traction and ECM density influence both capillary morphogenesis and maintenance in 3-D. *American Journal of Physiology-Cell Physiology* 297(1) (2009) C179–C187.

20. J. Li, K. Zhang, J. Wu, L. Zhang, P. Yang, Q. Tu, N. Huang, Tailoring of the titanium surface by preparing cardiovascular endothelial extracellular matrix layer on the hyaluronic acid micro-pattern for improving biocompatibility. *Colloids and Surfaces B Biointerfaces* 128 (2015) 201–210.

21. D. Zou, X. Luo, C.-z. Han, J.-a. Li, P. Yang, Q. Li, N. Huang. Preparation of a biomimetic ECM surface on cardiovascular biomaterials via a novel layer-by-layer decellularization for better biocompatibility. *Materials Science and Engineering: C* 96 (2019) 509–521.

22. L. Zhao, S. Mei, P.K. Chu, Y. Zhang, Z. Wu. The influence of hierarchical hybrid micro/nano-textured titanium surface with titania nanotubes on osteoblast functions. *Biomaterials* 31(19) (2010) 5072–5082.

23. A. Gao, R. Hang, X. Huang, L. Zhao, X. Zhang, L. Wang, B. Tang, S. Ma, P.K. Chu. The effects of titania nanotubes with embedded silver oxide nanoparticles on bacteria and osteoblasts. *Biomaterials* 35(13) (2014) 4223–4235.

24. C. Zhao, X. Wang, L. Gao, L. Jing, Q. Zhou, J. Chang, The role of the micro-pattern and nano-topography of hydroxyapatite bioceramics on stimulating osteogenic differentiation of mesenchymal stem cells. *Acta Biomaterialia* 73 (2018) 509–521.

25. M.R. Allen, J.M. Hock, D.B. Burr. Periosteum: Biology, regulation, and response to osteoporosis therapies. *Bone* 35(5) (2004) 1003–1012.

26. G. Yang, H. Liu, Y. Cui, J. Li, X. Zhou, N. Wang, F. Wu, Y. Li, Y. Liu, X. Jiang, S. Zhang. Bioinspired membrane provides periosteum-mimetic microenvironment for accelerating vascularized bone regeneration. *Biomaterials* 268 (2020) 120561.

27. R. Peng, X. Yao, J. Ding. Effect of cell anisotropy on differentiation of stem cells on micropatterned surfaces through the controlled single cell adhesion. *Biomaterials* 32(32) (2011) 8048–8057.

28. C. Yan, J. Sun, J. Ding. Critical areas of cell adhesion on micropatterned surfaces. *Biomaterials* 32(16) (2011) 3931–3938.

29. X. Yao, R. Liu, X. Liang, J. Ding. Critical areas of proliferation of single cells on micropatterned surfaces and corresponding cell type dependence. *ACS Applied Materials & Interfaces* 11(17) (2019) 15366–15380.

30. X. Liu, R. Liu, B. Cao, K. Ye, S. Li, Y. Gu, Z. Pan, J. Ding. Subcellular cell geometry on micropillars regulates stem cell differentiation. *Biomaterials* 111 (2016) 27–39.

31. K.D. Miller, L. Nogueira, A.B. Mariotto, J.H. Rowland, K.R. Yabroff, C.M. Alfano, A. Jemal, J.L. Kramer, R.L. Siegel. Cancer treatment and survivorship statistics, 2019. *CA: A Cancer Journal for Clinicians* 69(5) (2019) 363–385.

32. C. Holohan, S. Van Schaeybroeck, D.B. Longley, P.G. Johnston. Cancer drug resistance: An evolving paradigm. *Nature Reviews Cancer* 13(10) (2013) 714–726.

33. B.Y.S. Kim, J.T. Rutka, W.C.W. Chan. Nanomedicine. *New England Journal of Medicine* 363(25) (2010) 2434–2443.

34. Y. Chen, Y. Wu, B. Sun, S. Liu, H. Liu. Two-dimensional nanomaterials for cancer nanotheranostics. *Small* 13(10) (2017) 1603446.

35. C. Tan, X. Cao, X.-J. Wu, Q. He, J. Yang, X. Zhang, J. Chen, W. Zhao, S. Han, G.-H. Nam, M. Sindoro, H. Zhang. Recent advances in ultrathin two-dimensional nanomaterials. *Chemical Reviews* 117(9) (2017) 6225–6331.

36. S. Su, Q. Sun, X. Gu, Y. Xu, J. Shen, D. Zhu, J. Chao, C. Fan, L. Wang, Two-dimensional nanomaterials for biosensing applications. *TrAC Trends in Analytical Chemistry* 119 (2019) 115610.

37. D. Chimene, D.L. Alge, A.K. Gaharwar. Two-dimensional nanomaterials for biomedical applications: Emerging trends and future prospects. *Advanced Materials.* 27(45) (2015) 7261–7284.

38. Z. Mohammadpour, K. Majidzadeh-A. Applications of two-dimensional nanomaterials in breast cancer theranostics. *ACS Biomaterials Science & Engineering* 6(4) (2020) 1852–1873.

39. Z. Miao, L. Fan, X. Xie, Y. Ma, J. Xue, T. He, Z. Zha. Liquid exfoliation of atomically thin antimony selenide as an efficient two-dimensional antibacterial nanoagent. *ACS Applied Materials & Interfaces* 11(30) (2019) 26664–26673.

40. Y. Yang, H. Hou, G. Zou, W. Shi, H. Shuai, J. Li, X. Ji. Electrochemical exfoliation of graphene-like two-dimensional nanomaterials. *Nanoscale* 11(1) (2019) 16–33.

41. W. Tao, X. Ji, X. Zhu, L. Li, J. Wang, Y. Zhang, P.E. Saw, W. Li, N. Kong, M.A. Islam, T. Gan, X. Zeng, H. Zhang, M. Mahmoudi, G.J. Tearney, O.C. Farokhzad. Two-dimensional antimonene-based photonic nanomedicine for cancer theranostics. *Advanced Materials* 30(38) (2018) e1802061.

42. S. Singh, A.K. Gupta. Nitric oxide: Role in tumour biology and iNOS/NO-based anti-cancer therapies. *Cancer Chemotherapy and Pharmacology* 67(6) (2011) 1211–1224.

43. S. Kudo, Y. Nagasaki. A novel nitric oxide-based anticancer therapeutics by macrophage-targeted poly(l-arginine)-based nanoparticles. *Journal of Controlled Release* 217 (2015) 256–262.

44. X. Jia, Y. Zhang, Y. Zou, Y. Wang, D. Niu, Q. He, Z. Huang, W. Zhu, H. Tian, J. Shi, Y. Li. Dual intratumoral redox/enzyme-responsive NO-releasing nanomedicine for the specific, high-efficacy, and low-toxic cancer therapy. *Advanced Materials* 30(30) (2018) e1704490.

45. M. Arruebo. Drug delivery from structured porous inorganic materials. *WIREs Nanomedicine and Nanobiotechnology* 4(1) (2012) 16–30.

46. E.J. Anglin, L. Cheng, W.R. Freeman, M.J. Sailor. Porous silicon in drug delivery devices and materials. *Advanced Drug Delivery Reviews* 60(11) (2008) 1266–1277.

47. J. Li, S. Wu, C. Wu, L. Qiu, G. Zhu, C. Cui, Y. Liu, W. Hou, Y. Wang, L. Zhang. I.t. Teng, H.-H. Yang, W. Tan. Versatile surface engineering of porous nanomaterials with bioinspired polyphenol coatings for targeted and controlled drug delivery. *Nanoscale* 8(16) (2016) 8600–8606.

48. J. Lee, O.K. Farha, J. Roberts, K.A. Scheidt, S.T. Nguyen, J.T. Hupp. Metal–organic framework materials as catalysts. *Chemical Society Reviews* 38(5) (2009) 1450–1459.

49. Q.-L. Zhu, Q. Xu. Metal–organic framework composites. *Chemical Society Reviews* 43(16) (2014) 5468–5512.

50. S. Wuttke, A. Zimpel, T. Bein, S. Braig, K. Stoiber, A. Vollmar, D. Müller, K. Haastert-Talini, J. Schaeske, M. Stiesch, G. Zahn, A. Mohmeyer, P. Behrens, O. Eickelberg, D.A. Bölükbas, S. Meiners. Validating metal-organic framework nanoparticles for their nanosafety in diverse biomedical applications. *Advanced Healthcare Materials* 6(2) (2017) 1600818.

51. S. Keskin, S. Kızılel. Biomedical applications of metal organic frameworks. *Industrial & Engineering Chemistry Research* 50(4) (2011) 1799–1812.

52. S. Zhang, X. Pei, H. Gao, S. Chen, J. Wang. Metal-organic framework-based nanomaterials for biomedical applications. *Chinese Chemical Letters* 31(5) (2020) 1060–1070.

53. C. Chu, E. Ren, Y. Zhang, J. Yu, H. Lin, X. Pang, Y. Zhang, H. Liu, Z. Qin, Y. Cheng, X. Wang, W. Li, X. Kong, X. Chen, G. Liu. Zinc(II)-Dipicolylamine coordination nanotheranostics: Toward synergistic nanomedicine by combined photo/gene therapy. *Angewandte Chemie International Edition* 58(1) (2019) 269–272.

54. L. Chen, J. Zhang, X. Zhou, S. Yang, Q. Zhang, W. Wang, Z. You, C. Peng, C. He. Merging metal organic framework with hollow organosilica nanoparticles as a versatile nanoplatform for cancer theranostics. *Acta Biomaterialia* 86 (2019) 406–415.

55. Q. Wu, N. Xia, D. Long, L. Tan, W. Rao, J. Yu, C. Fu, X. Ren, H. Li, L. Gou, P. Liang, J. Ren, L. Li, X. Meng. Dual-functional supernanoparticles with microwave dynamic therapy and microwave thermal therapy. *Nano Letters* 19(8) (2019) 5277–5286.

56. H. Zhou, C. Fu, X. Chen, L. Tan, J. Yu, Q. Wu, L. Su, Z. Huang, F. Cao, X. Ren, J. Ren, P. Liang, X. Meng. Mitochondria-targeted zirconium metal–organic frameworks for enhancing the efficacy of microwave thermal therapy against tumors. *Biomaterials Science* 6(6) (2018) 1535–1545.

57. C. Fu, H. Zhou, L. Tan, Z. Huang, Q. Wu, X. Ren, J. Ren, X. Meng. Microwave-activated Mn-doped zirconium metal-organic framework nanocubes for highly effective combination of microwave dynamic and thermal therapies against cancer. *ACS Nano* 12(3) (2018) 2201–2210.

58. R. Abazari, F. Ataei, A. Morsali, A.M.Z. Slawin, L. Carpenter-Warren, C. A luminescent amine-functionalized metal-organic framework conjugated with folic acid as a targeted biocompatible pH-responsive nanocarrier for apoptosis induction in breast cancer cells. *ACS Applied Materials and Interfaces* 11(49) (2019) 45442–45454.

59. R. Garzon, G.A. Calin, C.M. Croce. MicroRNAs in cancer. *Annual Review of Medicine* 60(1) (2009) 167–179.

60. W.H. Chen, G.F. Luo, Y.S. Sohn, R. Nechushtai, I. Willner. miRNA-specific unlocking of drug-loaded metal-organic framework nanoparticles: Targeted cytotoxicity toward cancer cells. *Small* 15(17) (2019) e1900935.

61. C. Lu, M.W. Urban. Tri-phasic size- and Janus balance-tunable colloidal nanoparticles (JNPs). *ACS Macro Letters* 3(4) (2014) 346–352.

62. T. Parpaite, B. Otazaghine, A.S. Caro, A. Taguet, R. Sonnier, J.M. Lopez-Cuesta, Janus hybrid silica/polymer nanoparticles as effective compatibilizing agents for polystyrene/polyamide-6 melted blends. *Polymer* 90 (2016) 34–44.

63. H. Zhang, Q. Zhang, C. Liu, B. Han. Preparation of a one-dimensional nanorod/metal organic framework Janus nanoplatform via side-specific growth for synergistic cancer therapy. *Biomaterials Science* 7(4) (2019) 1696–1704.

64. L. Zhang, S. Li, X. Chen, T. Wang, L. Li, Z. Su, C. Wang. Tailored surfaces on 2D material: UFO-like cyclodextrin-Pd nanosheet/metal organic framework Janus nanoparticles for synergistic cancer therapy. *Advanced Functional Materials* 28(51) (2018) 1803815.

65. M.R. Carvalho, D. Barata, L.M. Teixeira, S. Giselbrecht, R.L. Reis, J.M. Oliveira, R. Truckenmüller, P. Habibovic. Colorectal tumor-on-a-chip system: A 3D tool for precision onco-nanomedicine. *Science Advances* 5(5) (2019) eaaw1317.

66. Y. Liu, Y. Huo, L. Yao, Y. Xu, F. Meng, H. Li, K. Sun, G. Zhou, D.S. Kohane, K. Tao. Transcytosis of nanomedicine for tumor penetration. *Nano Letters* 19(11) (2019) 8010–8020.

67. C.D. Medley, S. Bamrungsap, W. Tan, J.E. Smith. Aptamer-conjugated nanoparticles for cancer cell detection. *Analytical Chemistry* 83(3) (2011) 727–734.

68. I. Willner, M. Zayats. Electronic aptamer-based sensors. *Angewandte Chemie International Edition* 46(34) (2007) 6408–6418.

69. S. Song, L. Wang, J. Li, C. Fan, J. Zhao. Aptamer-based biosensors. *TrAC Trends in Analytical Chemistry* 27(2) (2008) 108–117.

70. D. Ou, D. Sun, Z. Liang, B. Chen, X. Lin, Z. Chen. A novel cytosensor for capture, detection and release of breast cancer cells based on metal organic framework PCN-224 and DNA tetrahedron linked dual-aptamer. *Sensors and Actuators B: Chemical* 285 (2019) 398–404.

71. J. Sudimack, R.J. Lee. Targeted drug delivery via the folate receptor. *Advanced Drug Delivery Reviews* 41(2) (2000) 147–162.

72. A.R. Hilgenbrink, P.S. Low. Folate receptor-mediated drug targeting: From therapeutics to diagnostics. *Journal of Pharmaceutical Sciences* 94(10) (2005) 2135–2146.

73. X.T. Zheng, A. Ananthanarayanan, K.Q. Luo, P. Chen. Glowing graphene quantum dots and carbon dots: Properties, syntheses, and biological applications. *Small* 11(14) (2015) 1620–1636.

74. J. Soleymani, M. Hasanzadeh, M.H. Somi, S.A. Ozkan, A. Jouyban. Targeting and sensing of some cancer cells using folate bioreceptor functionalized nitrogen-doped graphene quantum dots. *International Journal of Biological Macromolecules* 118(Pt A) (2018) 1021–1034.

75. C.M. Metallo, J.C. Mohr, C.J. Detzel, J.J. de Pablo, B.J. Van Wie, S.P. Palecek. Engineering the stem cell microenvironment. *Biotechnology Progress* 23(1) (2007) 18–23.

76. C. Frantz, K.M. Stewart, V.M. Weaver. The extracellular matrix at a glance. *Journal of Cell Science* 123(24) (2010) 4195.

77. T. Fujie, S. Ahadian, H. Liu, H. Chang, S. Ostrovidov, H. Wu, H. Bae, K. Nakajima, H. Kaji, A. Khademhosseini. Engineered nanomembranes for directing cellular organization toward flexible biodevices. *Nano Letters* 13(7) (2013) 3185–3192.

78. D. Voutsa, P. Hartmann, C. Schaffner, W. Giger. Benzotriazoles, alkylphenols and bisphenol a in municipal wastewaters and in the Glatt River, Switzerland. *Environmental Science and Pollution Research* 13(5) (2006) 333–341.

79. W. Kujawski, A. Warszawski, W. Ratajczak, T. Porębski, W. Capała, I. Ostrowska. Removal of phenol from wastewater by different separation techniques. *Desalination* 163(1) (2004) 287–296.

80. R. Penu, A.C. Obreja, D. Patroi, M. Diaconu, G.L. Radu, Graphene and gold nanoparticles based reagentless biodevice for phenolic endocrine disruptors monitoring. *Microchemical Journal* 121 (2015) 130–135.

12 Bioinspired Design for Medical Applications

Feng Wu
Xuzhou University of Technology

CONTENTS

12.1 INTRODUCTION

Learning from nature provides us with various inspirations for medical applications. The morphology and characteristics of biological materials and structures have been developed in nature for millions of years, with unique characteristics and almost perfect functions to adapt to harsh environments, such as the self-cleaning characteristics of lotus leaves,[1,2] corresponding multiscale structures of water strider,[3–5] and the superhydrophobic butterfly wings.[6,7] These natural functions and strategies have recently emerged as a new source of inspiration to create multifunctional surfaces with high potential that can be applied to biological materials.

Similarly, biological systems can be imitated at different stages of technological innovation (functional and morphological design, principles, strategies, etc.), as well as in different sizes, which makes this concept highly versatile. For instance, although metal biomaterials have been utilized in clinics because of their excellent mechanical properties and durability compared with ceramic and polymer biomaterials, they still lack satisfactory biological functions in certain application areas, such as blood compatibility of blood contact equipment, osteoconductivity in orthopedic applications, ultra-high wear resistance, and corrosion resistance.[8,9] Therefore, bioinspired design exhibits special significance and requirements for improving biomaterials with biological activity and multiple functions to enhance the cell and tissue response.

In this chapter, we focus on the functionalization strategy of bioinspired surface and their application in biomaterials. Section 12.2 presents the physical and chemical properties of biomaterials. Section 12.3 introduces the biomaterial's functionalization bioinspired design for medical devices. Section 12.4 discusses future challenges in the development of bioinspired design for medical applications.

12.2 PHYSICAL AND CHEMICAL PROPERTIES OF BIOMATERIALS

When biomaterials are implanted into living tissues, an interface is formed between the implanted material and the surrounding tissues. It is important to ensure that implants with specific surface characteristics are recognized by the highly precocious ability of the biological system at the implant–tissue interface.[8,10] Implant surfaces with different morphologies, chemical properties, and wettability strongly affect the interaction of materials and cells, thereby affecting the tissue integration at the interface.

12.2.1 BIOMATERIAL TOPOGRAPHY

Biomaterial surface roughness[11] and its morphology[12] and other morphological characteristics can strongly affect protein adsorption,[11,13] cell adhesion,[14] cell migration, and cell differentiation.[15] Generally, biomaterial surface roughness can directly impact cell behavior by enhancing the formation of local contact, or indirectly by selectively adsorbing serum proteins required for cell attachment. The topography of biomaterials with different scales and characteristics directly impacts the ability of cells to produce organized cytoskeletal arrangements.[16] It has been reported that the adhesion and proliferation of vessel cells and bone cells increase on nanoscale surfaces;[12] nonetheless, some reports have not confirmed this significant correlation. Bagherifard et al.[17] proposed considering additional roughness parameters, such as the formation of surface irregularities and their spatial distribution to fully describe the precise morphological characteristics of biomaterials. In addition, different types of cells may respond differently to the same biomaterial topography. For instance, on a 316L surface, osteoblasts can maintain their proliferation and adhesion functions, while the adhesion ability of gram-positive bacteria is significantly reduced.

12.2.2 BIOMATERIAL CHEMISTRY

Chemistry of biomaterials can be modified to induce cell adhesion and diffusion.[18] Many studies have shown that biomaterial functional groups can affect protein adsorption and subsequent cellular responses.[19] Generally, hydrophilic functionality provides low interfacial free energy, leading to reduced protein adsorption, cell adhesion, and blood compatibility.[20,21]

12.2.3 BIOMATERIAL WETTABILITY

Various in vitro studies have reported that adsorption characteristics of protein adsorption and cell attachment can be affected by the wettability of biomaterials.[22] Wetting is a critical implantation process by the physiological fluid.[23]

In aqueous solutions, proteins tend to bind onto hydrophobic biomaterial surfaces and cells usually adhere selectively to hydrophilic areas, although cell behavior also depends on cell type and biomaterials.[24] Generally, few cells can adhere to super-hydrophobic surfaces, on which cells usually adopt a circular shape.[25] The wettability of biomaterials can be tuned preferentially from hydrophobic to hydrophilic by controlling the surface chemistry and morphology.[26] Hence, it is difficult to discuss the influence of wettability without considering these two factors. For instance, when taking the attachment ability of L929 cells on surfaces with different wettability as an example, it can be observed that the hydrophilic biomaterial has more cells attached than the hydrophobic biomaterial. The decrease in contact angle is due to the introduction of more hydrophilic -COOH groups on the biomaterial and the reduction of more hydrophobic -CH3 groups.[27]

12.3 BIOMATERIAL FUNCTIONALIZATION

To meet different clinical needs, various synthetic functionalization methods (mechanical, chemical, and physical) on biomaterials have been proposed.[28] In addition to these methods, nature has developed fascinating strategies over millions of years to display almost perfect multifunctional surfaces. These natural functions and strategies have recently become a new source of inspiration to create multifunctional biomaterials. Bioinspired design may come from two sources: first, the graft structure is inspired by the natural vascular structure; second, the position of the constituent material itself is inspired by the extracellular matrix. Therefore, in the following sections, we will discuss the various functionalizations of biomaterials using bioinspired design.

12.3.1 BIOINSPIRED DESIGN FOR OSTEOINTEGRATION

For bone implants, osteoprogenitor cells migrate to the implantation site and differentiate into osteoblasts, thereby forming bone. Biocompatibility requires that the material should integrate with the bone. Stainless steel and titanium alloys are commonly used clinical fracture fixation materials, on the surface of which new bone can be observed, especially titanium alloys. The natural TiO_2 layer minimizes the release of metal ions and adverse body reactions, thereby improving the biocompatibility of titanium alloys.[29] However, this natural passive oxide layer cannot provide the required osseointegration,[30] so various biomaterial functionalization methods have been proposed to improve osteoconductivity or biological activity.

12.3.1.1 Micro/Nanostructure Surface Design

Biomaterial surface properties, such as morphology, roughness, and wettability, have been thought to affect the response of osteoblasts for titanium implants.[31] Zinger et al. found that the micron and sub-micron-scale topological structures on titanium implants can promote osteoblast differentiation and the production of osteogenic local factors.[32] There is a synergistic effect between the high biomaterial surface energy and morphology of the titanium substrate.[33] Recently, by taking inspiration from the natural layered micro/nanostructure in rat alveolar bone, a combined layered structure composed of micropits staggered self-assembled TiO_2 nanotubes was developed on the Ti surface.[34] Tightly arranged self-assembled TiO_2 nanotubes with a diameter of 30–50 nm on the surface of the bioinspired material are close to the collagen fibers of 60–80 nm in the rat mandible. Compared with the smooth and purely micro-treated counterparts, the larger surface energy and hydrophilicity of the bioinspired micro/nanomaterial surface can provide excellent adhesion and growth of osteoblasts, thereby exhibiting better biological activity and biocompatibility. This bioinspired design on the implants has been successfully applied in a 12-month clinical trial,[35] providing a new strategy for orthopedic applications of biomaterials.

12.3.2 BIOINSPIRED DESIGN FOR BLOOD COMPATIBILITY

Blood compatibility is critical to the success of many clinical procedures, including synthetic vascular grafts, electronic pacemakers, coronary stents, mechanical heart valves, and left ventricular-assist devices.[36] Thrombosis forms when fibrin and platelets adhere to the surface of the synthetic vascular grafts during blood flow. The blood–substance interaction is complex and involves many factors, including surface chemical composition, charge, flexibility, wettability, and blood flow conditions. In general, biologically inert surfaces can enhance blood contact materials by reducing the intrinsic pathway of blood coagulation.[37]

12.3.2.1 Biomolecular Coating Design

Surface biomolecular coating is the most common method to improve the blood compatibility of the stents. Various bioactive agents and molecules, such as heparin, prostaglandins, and hyaluronic acid, have been studied as inhibitors of the coagulation process.[38] In addition, drugs and endothelial cell seeds are also utilized for biomaterial surface coating.[39] The functionalization of the bioinspired material surface with endothelial cells as seeds may be similar to the function of the endothelial surface itself. However, poor adhesion and slow formation of the endothelial layer limit its clinical application, especially in emergencies.[40] Another bioinspired design is to utilize polydopamine, a mussel adhesive and easy-to-deposit protein-activated coating material, which can also be applied to the stents. The surface of the 316L stent modified with polydopamine has been shown to reduce the adhesion and proliferation of human umbilical artery smooth muscle cells while promoting the proliferation of endothelial cells.[41] Polydopamine can also be used as a loading platform to support the strong anchoring of bioactive agents and drugs to further improve blood compatibility.[42,43]

12.3.2.2 Superhydrophobic Surface Design

Inspired by the lotus leaf, superhydrophobic surfaces have been widely studied for various engineering and biomedical applications.[44] It has been proven that superhydrophobic surfaces can strongly affect protein adsorption, thereby significantly reducing the adsorption of bovine serum albumin, and completely inhibiting platelet adhesion and activation.[45,46] For instance, superhydrophobic TiO_2 nanotubes are prepared by electrochemical anodization and then functionalized with perfluorooctyltriethoxysilane (POTS) on Ti implants with low adhesion to improve blood compatibility and anticoagulant properties.[47] The evaluation of blood compatibility in vitro shows that the superhydrophobic TiO_2 nanostructured surface shows good blood compatibility and effectively resists the adhesion and activation of platelets. However, superhydrophobic surfaces rely on trapped air to repel liquids. Under conditions involving high temperature, pressure, humidity, and exposure to low surface tension liquids, superhydrophobic surfaces are prone to failure.[48] Therefore, the utilization of superhydrophobic coatings to prepare ideal antithrombotic surfaces is still a challenge.

12.3.2.3 Liquid Interface Design

The liquid interface in nature plays an important role in the biological organism. For example, the defect-free coating formed by the tear film can prevent bacteria from harming the eyes while maintaining transparency. Due to the fluidity of the liquid, it can repel various liquids and redistribute them in a large range, thereby achieving self-repair and high adaptability. Fewer number of platelets adhere to the sliding interface, and the shape remains circular. Using the model, a liquid interface is constructed in the blood transfusion catheter in pigs as a living body. Even if no anticoagulant is added, blood circulation can be maintained for 8 hours without coagulation and thrombus.[49]

12.3.3 BIOINSPIRED DESIGN TO ENHANCE ANTIBACTERIAL PROPERTIES

Biomaterial-related infections are one of the most common complications of medical implants and devices such as orthopedic implants, cardiovascular stents, and vascular catheters. To prevent infection, at least two bioinspired designs can be used: antibacterial coatings that kill bacteria by contact or release of antimicrobial agents, and anti-adhesive surfaces that reduce or eliminate bacterial adhesion.[50]

12.3.3.1 Antibacterial Coatings Design

Various synthetic methods based on the immobilization or release of bactericidal substances have been widely used in the production of antibacterial coatings.[51] It has been reported that nails coated with antibiotic D-polylactic acid/gentamicin in the bone marrow are associated with clinically positive results within 6 months.[52] However, due to its high toxicity, limited effect, or efficiency on various drug-resistant pathogens, its application in the biomedical field is not entirely satisfactory. In addition to these synthetic methods, some bioinspired designs have also been proposed to prevent bacterial colonization and biofilm formation. Glinel et al.[53] reviewed some bactericidal coatings inspired by these natural defense strategies and mechanisms to deal with the ever-emerging pathogen pressure. These coatings are designed based on bactericidal and biologically active compounds, including antimicrobial peptides and lysozymes secreted or produced by many organisms.[54]

In particular, the surface of orthopedic and dental implants should inhibit bacterial colonization through interaction with proteins, bacteria, and tissue cells, while promoting the function of osteoblasts. Some biomolecules, such as BMP-2[55] and vascular endothelial growth factor (VEGF),[56] can be fixed on the surface of the implant to regulate different cell–cell adhesion. For example, compared with the original titanium alloy, after functionalization with VEGF and carboxymethyl chitosan, the titanium surface showed a lower degree of bacterial colonization but enhanced the proliferation of osteoblasts and calcium mineralization.

12.3.4 CORROSION RESISTANCE

Corrosion is the degradation of metals that interact with the environment through electrochemical processes. Due to the high concentration of chloride ions and pH changes caused by implants, metal biomaterials are corroded by the human environment. Corrosion can produce harmful metal ions, cause toxicity and allergies, and deteriorate the mechanical properties of the implant.[57] Therefore, corrosion resistance has become one of the main selection criteria for biomaterials. Inert biomaterials generally have high corrosion resistance due to the presence of a protective passivation layer.

To improve the corrosion resistance of biomaterials in the body, various methods have been developed, including surface coatings, alloying elements, and surface mechanical treatments. The application of coatings is the most suitable way for implants because the coating can not only provide effective physical protection but also biological functions.

12.4 CONCLUSION

Learning from nature is a continuous process. Bioinspired design provides a new source of inspiration for creating multifunctional surfaces with great potential for biomedical applications. It can improve artificial biocompatible properties to directly or coordinate the functions of biological cells and simulate biological surfaces for solving the obstacles encountered in current medical equipment. Undoubtedly, extensive teamwork is needed in the fields of biomaterials, physical chemistry, biotechnology, medical devices, and medicine to promote the development of basic science and treatment of materials. We hope that this chapter can arouse the interest of scholars in these fields and contribute to the development of bioinspired design for human welfare.

REFERENCES

1. Feng Lin, Li Shuhong, Li Yingshun, Li Huanjun, Zhang Lingjuan, Zhai Jin, Song Yanlin, Liu Biqian, Jiang Lei, Zhu Daoben. Super-hydrophobic surfaces: From natural to artificial. *Advanced Materials*, 2002, 14(24):1857–1860.
2. Long Mengying, Ma Yu, Yang Chao, Zhang Runnan, Jiang Zhongyi. Superwetting membranes: From controllable constructions to efficient separations. *Journal of Materials Chemistry A*, 2021.

3. Bird James C, Dhiman Rajeev, Kwon Hyuk-Min, Varanasi Kripa K. Reducing the contact time of a bouncing drop. *Nature*, 2013, 503(7476):385–388.
4. Xu Wanghuai, Zheng Huanxi, Liu Yuan, Zhou Xiaofeng, Zhang Chao, Song Yuxin, Deng Xu, Leung Michael, Yang Zhengbao, Xu Ronald X. A droplet-based electricity generator with high instantaneous power density. *Nature*, 2020, 578(7795):392–396.
5. Wu Hao, Mendel Niels, van den Ende Dirk, Zhou Guofu, Mugele Frieder. Energy harvesting from drops impacting onto charged surfaces. *Physical Review Letters*, 2020, 125(7):078301.
6. Zheng Yongmei, Gao Xuefeng, Jiang Lei. Directional adhesion of superhydrophobic butterfly wings. *Soft Matter*, 2007, 3(2):178–182.
7. Dai Haoyu, Dong Zhichao, Jiang Lei. Directional liquid dynamics of interfaces with superwettability. *Science Advances*, 2020, 6(37):eabb5528.
8. Nel Andre E, Mädler Lutz, Velegol Darrell, Xia Tian, Hoek Eric MV, Somasundaran Ponisseril, Klaessig Fred, Castranova Vince, Thompson Mike. Understanding biophysicochemical interactions at the nano–bio interface. *Nature Materials*, 2009, 8(7):543–557.
9. Planell Josep A, Navarro Melba, Altankov George, Aparicio Conrado, Engel Elisabeth, Gil Javier, Ginebra Maria Pau, Lacroix Damien. Materials surface effects on biological interactions. *Advances in Regenerative Medicine: Role of Nanotechnology, and Engineering Principles*. Springer. 2010: pp. 233–252.
10. Xie Meihua, Zhang Wei, Fan Chengying, Wu Chu, Feng Qishuai, Wu Jiaojiao, Li Yingze, Gao Rui, Li Zhenguang, Wang Qigang. Bioinspired soft microrobots with precise magneto-collective control for microvascular thrombolysis. *Advanced Materials*, 2020, 32(26):2000366.
11. Deligianni Despina D, Katsala N, Ladas S, Sotiropoulou D, Amedee J, Missirlis YF. Effect of surface roughness of the titanium alloy Ti–6Al–4V on human bone marrow cell response and on protein adsorption. *Biomaterials*, 2001, 22(11):1241–1251.
12. Khang Dongwoo, Lu Jing, Yao Chang, Haberstroh Karen M, Webster Thomas J. The role of nanometer and sub-micron surface features on vascular and bone cell adhesion on titanium. *Biomaterials*, 2008, 29(8):970–983.
13. Chrzanowska Agnieszka, Derylo-Marczewska Anna, Borowski Piotr. Comprehensive characterization of biocomposite surface based on the mesoporous silica and lysozyme molecules: Chemistry, morphology, topography, texture and micro-nanostructure. *Applied Surface Science*, 2020, 525:146512.
14. Li Jingan, Li Guicai, Zhang Kun, Liao Yuzhen, Yang Ping, Maitz Manfred F, Huang Nan. Co-culture of vascular endothelial cells and smooth muscle cells by hyaluronic acid micro-pattern on titanium surface. *Applied Surface Science*, 2013, 273:24–31.
15. Li Jingan, Qin Wei, Zhang Kun, Wu Feng, Yang Ping, He Zikun, Zhao Ansha, Huang Nan. Controlling mesenchymal stem cells differentiate into contractile smooth muscle cells on a TiO_2 micro/nano interface: Towards benign pericytes environment for endothelialization. *Colloids and Surfaces B: Biointerfaces*, 2016, 145:410–419.
16. Shen Xinkun, Ma Pingping, Hu Yan, Xu Gaoqiang, Zhou Jun, Cai Kaiyong. Mesenchymal stem cell growth behavior on micro/nano hierarchical surfaces of titanium substrates. *Colloids and Surfaces B: Biointerfaces*, 2015, 127:221–232.
17. Bagherifard Sara, Hickey Daniel J, de Luca Alba C, Malheiro Vera N, Markaki Athina E, Guagliano Mario, Webster Thomas J. The influence of nanostructured features on bacterial adhesion and bone cell functions on severely shot peened 316L stainless steel. *Biomaterials*, 2015, 73:185–197.
18. Roach Paul, Eglin David, Rohde Kirsty, Perry Carole C. Modern biomaterials: A review—bulk properties and implications of surface modifications. *Journal of Materials Science: Materials in Medicine*, 2007, 18(7):1263–1277.

19. Tang Liping, Thevenot Paul, Hu Wenjing. Surface chemistry influences implant biocompatibility. *Current Topics in Medicinal Chemistry*, 2008, 8(4):270–280.

20. Geetha Manivasagam, Singh Ashok K, Asokamani Rajamanickam, Gogia Ashok K. Ti based biomaterials, the ultimate choice for orthopaedic implants–a review. *Progress in Materials Science*, 2009, 54(3):397–425.

21. Mitrousis Nikolaos, Fokina Ana, Shoichet Molly S. Biomaterials for cell transplantation. *Nature Reviews Materials*, 2018, 3(11):441–456.

22. Han Aifang, Ding Hao, Tsoi James Kit Hon, Imazato Satoshi, Matinlinna Jukka P, Chen Zhuofan. Prolonged UV-C irradiation is a double-edged sword on the zirconia surface. *ACS Omega*, 2020, 5(10):5126–5133.

23. Paital Sameer R, Dahotre Narendra B. Calcium phosphate coatings for bio-implant applications: Materials, performance factors, and methodologies. *Materials Science and Engineering: R: Reports*, 2009, 66(1–3):1–70.

24. Arima Yusuke, Iwata Hiroo. Effect of wettability and surface functional groups on protein adsorption and cell adhesion using well-defined mixed self-assembled monolayers. *Biomaterials*, 2007, 28(20):3074–3082.

25. Song Wenlong, Mano João F. Interactions between cells or proteins and surfaces exhibiting extreme wettabilities. *Soft Matter*, 2013, 9(11):2985–2999.

26. Lai Yuekun, Pan Fei, Xu Cong, Fuchs Harald, Chi Lifeng. In situ surface-modification-induced superhydrophobic patterns with reversible wettability and adhesion. *Advanced Materials*, 2013, 25(12):1682–1686.

27. Wei Jianhua, Yoshinari Masao, Takemoto Shinji, Hattori Masayuki, Kawada Eiji, Liu Baolin, Oda Yutaka. Adhesion of mouse fibroblasts on hexamethyldisiloxane surfaces with wide range of wettability. *Journal of Biomedical Materials Research Part B: Applied Biomaterials: An Official Journal of The Society for Biomaterials, The Japanese Society for Biomaterials, and The Australian Society for Biomaterials and the Korean Society for Biomaterials*, 2007, 81(1):66–75.

28. Hornberger Helga, Virtanen Sannakaisa, Boccaccini Aldo R. Biomedical coatings on magnesium alloys–a review. *Acta Biomaterialia*, 2012, 8(7):2442–2455.

29. Lorenzetti Martina, Dakischew Olga, Trinkaus Katja, Susanne Lips Katrin, Schnettler Reinhard, Kobe Spomenka, Novak Saša. Enhanced osteogenesis on titanium implants by UVB photofunctionalization of hydrothermally grown TiO_2 coatings. *Journal of Biomaterials Applications*, 2015, 30(1):71–84.

30. Liu Xuanyong, Chu Paul K, Ding Chuanxian. Surface modification of titanium, titanium alloys, and related materials for biomedical applications. *Materials Science and Engineering: R: Reports*, 2004, 47(3–4):49–121.

31. Juan Ignacio Rosales-Leal, Miguel A Rodríguez-Valverde, Giuseppe Mazzaglia, Pedro Jesús Ramón-Torregrosa, Lourdes Díaz-Rodríguez, Olga García-Martínez, Manuel Vallecillo-Capilla, Concepción Ruiz, Miguel Ángel Cabrerizo-Vílchez. Effect of roughness, wettability and morphology of engineered titanium surfaces on osteoblast-like cell adhesion. *Colloids and Surfaces A: Physicochemical and Engineering Aspects*, 2010, 365(1–3):222–229

32. Olivier Zinger, Ge Zhao, Zvi Schwartz, Jame Simpson, Marco Wieland, Dieter Landolt, Barbara D Boyan. Differential regulation of osteoblasts by substrate microstructural features. *Biomaterials*, 2005, 26(14):1837–1847.

33. Gliver Zhao, Andrew L Raines, Marco Wieland, Zvi Schwartz, Barbara D Boyan. Requirement for both micron-and submicron scale structure for synergistic responses of osteoblasts to substrate surface energy and topography. *Biomaterials*, 2007, 28(18): 2821–2829.

34. Wang Feng, Shi Liang, He Wen-Xi, Han Dong, Yan Yan, Niu Zhong-Ying, Shi Sheng-Gen. Bioinspired micro/nano fabrication on dental implant–bone interface. *Applied Surface Science*, 2013, 265:480–488

35. Huang Mao-Suan, Chen Li-Kai, Ou Keng-Liang, Cheng Han-Yi, Wang Che-Shun. Rapid osseointegration of titanium implant with innovative nanoporous surface modification: Animal model and clinical trial. *Implant Dentistry*, 2015, 24(4):441–447.
36. Chen Li, Han Dong, Jiang Lei. On improving blood compatibility: From bioinspired to synthetic design and fabrication of biointerfacial topography at micro/nano scales. *Colloids and Surfaces B: Biointerfaces*, 2011, 85(1):2–7.
37. Zhang Zheng, Zhang Min, Chen Shengfu, Horbett Thomas A, Ratner Buddy D, Jiang Shaoyi. Blood compatibility of surfaces with superlow protein adsorption. *Biomaterials*, 2008, 29(32):4285–4291
38. Ma Jun, Zhao Nan, Zhu Donghui. Sirolimus-eluting dextran and polyglutamic acid hybrid coatings on AZ31 for stent applications. *Journal of Biomaterials Applications*, 2015, 30(5):579–588.
39. Wei Yu, Ji Ying, Xiao Lin-Lin, Lin Quan-kui, Xu Jian-ping, Ren Ke-feng, Ji Jian. Surface engineering of cardiovascular stent with endothelial cell selectivity for in vivo re-endothelialisation. *Biomaterials*, 2013, 34(11):2588–2599.
40. Heyligers JMM, Arts CHP, Verhagen HJM, De Groot Ph G, Moll FL. Improving small-diameter vascular grafts: From the application of an endothelial cell lining to the construction of atissue-engineered blood vessel. *Annals of Vascular Surgery*, 2005, 19(3):448–456.
41. Yang Zhilu, Tu Qiufen, Zhu Ying, Luo Rifang, Li Xin, Xie Yichu, Maitz Manfred F, Wang Jin, Huang Nan. Mussel-inspired coating of polydopamine directs endothelial and smooth muscle cell fate for re-endothelialization of vascular devices. *Advanced Healthcare Materials*, 2012, 1(5):548–559.
42. Li Jingan, Wu Feng, Zhang Kun, He Zikun, Zou Dan, Luo Xiao, Fan Yonghong, Yang Ping, Zhao Ansha, Huang Nan. Controlling molecular weight of hyaluronic acid conjugated on amine-rich surface: Toward better multifunctional biomaterials for cardiovascular implants. *ACS Applied Materials & Interfaces*, 2017, 9(36):30343–30358.
43. Wu Feng, Li Jingan, Zhang Kun, He Zikun, Yang Ping, Zou Dan, Huang Nan. Multifunctional coating based on hyaluronic acid and dopamine conjugate for potential application on surface modification of cardiovascular implanted devices. *ACS Applied Materials & Interfaces*, 2016, 8(1):109–121.
44. Zhang Xi, Shi Feng, Niu Jia, Jiang Yugui, Wang Zhiqiang. Superhydrophobic surfaces: From structural control to functional application. *Journal of Materials Chemistry*, 2008, 18(6):621–633
45. Patankar Neelesh A. Mimicking the lotus effect: Influence of double roughness structures and slender pillars. *Langmuir*, 2004, 20(19):8209–8213.
46. Sun Taolei, Tan Hong, Han Dong, Fu Qiang, Jiang Lei. No platelet can adhere—largely improved blood compatibility on nanostructured superhydrophobic surfaces. *Small*, 2005, 1(10):959–963.
47. Yang Yun, Lai Yuekun, Zhang Qiqing, Wu Ke, Zhang Lihai, Lin Changjian, Tang Peifu. A novel electrochemical strategy for improving blood compatibility of titanium-based biomaterials. *Colloids and Surfaces B: Biointerfaces*, 2010, 79(1):309–313.
48. Lafuma Aurélie, Quéré David. Superhydrophobic states. *Nature Materials*, 2003, 2(7):457–460.
49. Leslie Daniel C, Waterhouse Anna, Berthet Julia B, Valentin Thomas M, Watters Alexander L, Jain Abhishek, Kim Philseok, Hatton Benjamin D, Nedder Arthur, Donovan Kathryn. A bioinspired omniphobic surface coating on medical devices prevents thrombosis and biofouling. *Nature Biotechnology*, 2014, 32(11):1134–1140.
50. Zhao Lingzhou, Chu Paul K, Zhang Yumei, Wu Zhifen. Antibacterial coatings on titanium implants. *Journal of Biomedical Materials Research Part B: Applied Biomaterials*, 2009, 91(1):470–480.
51. Lichter Jenny A, Rubner Michael F. Polyelectrolyte multilayers with intrinsic antimicrobial functionality: The importance of mobile polycations. *Langmuir*, 2009, 25(13):7686–7694.

52. Fuchs Thomas, Stange Richard, Schmidmaier Gerhard, Raschke Michael J. The use of gentamicin-coated nails in the tibia: Preliminary results of a prospective study. *Archives of Orthopaedic and Trauma Surgery*, 2011, 131(10):1419–1425.

53. Glinel Karine, Thebault Pascal, Humblot Vincent, Pradier Claire-Marie, Thierry Jouenne. Antibacterial surfaces developed from bio-inspired approaches. *Acta Biomaterialia*, 2012, 8(5):1670–1684.

54. Holmberg Kyle V, Abdolhosseini Mahsa, Li Yuping, Chen Xi, Gorr Sven-Ulrik, Aparicio Conrado. Bio-inspired stable antimicrobial peptide coatings for dental applications. *Acta Biomaterialia*, 2013, 9(9):8224–8231.

55. Shi Zhilong, Neoh Koon Gee, Kang En-Tang, Poh Chyekhoon, Wang Wilson. Titanium with surface-grafted dextran and immobilized bone morphogenetic protein-2 for inhibition of bacterial adhesion and enhancement of osteoblast functions. *Tissue Engineering Part A*, 2009, 15(2):417–426.

56. Hu Xuefeng, Neoh Koon-Gee, Shi Zhilong, Kang En-Tang, Poh Chyekhoon, Wang Wilson. An in vitro assessment of titanium functionalized with polysaccharides conjugated with vascular endothelial growth factor for enhanced osseointegration and inhibition of bacterial adhesion. *Biomaterials*, 2010, 31(34):8854–8863.

57. Jonathan Walczak, Banoo Fariba Shahgaldi , Frederick W Heatley. In vivo corrosion of 316L stainless-steel hip implants: Morphology and elemental compositions of corrosion products. *Biomaterials*, 1998, 19(1–3):229–237.

13 Modeling and Simulation of Biomaterials

Zhe Fang
Zhongyuan University of Technology

Yu Zhao and Hongyan Wang
Zhengzhou University

CONTENTS

13.1 INTRODUCTION

The interaction between material surface and biomolecule covers a lot of content. At present, experiments and simulations are the two major branches of investigating the effect of biomaterial surfaces on the adsorption of biomolecules. Repeated experiments lead to a huge amount of experimental research work; therefore, the gradual development of large-scale parallel supercomputer has ensured the high accuracy of molecular simulation, making the results consistent with experiments and the characteristics to further predict the properties of the research object.

It is crucial to pay attention to the interaction between biomaterials and molecules at the molecular level to prepare functional biological coatings on biomaterials [1]. Although a large number of experimental studies on the adsorption of protein on solid materials have been reported [2–4], the mechanism of recognition and interaction between biomaterial surfaces and biomolecules is still unclear. Theoretical modeling and simulation techniques have been used to explore the binding mechanism between biomaterial surfaces and protein, the binding specificity and determinants of different material surfaces, as well as adsorption thermodynamics and kinetics. Computer simulation, as another scientific research method in addition to experiment and theoretical research, can study the physical and chemical properties of materials in different time and space scales, from electron transfer to intermolecular interaction, from nanoscale defects to several meter-scale bulk materials, with corresponding solutions. There are two types of molecular simulation: one is a quantum chemical simulation based on the principle of quantum mechanics, and the other is a molecular simulation based on the principle of statistical mechanics. Density functional theory (DFT), molecular dynamics (MD), and the Monte Carlo (MC) method can simulate some specific properties of biomaterials.

DFT is usually adopted to calculate the structural changes of biomolecules before and after adsorption, the electronic structural properties of the adsorption surface, and the bond length after stable adsorption. DFT and the recent DFT-D methods (including the dispersive force in Hamiltonian) have been proven to be very successful in describing bond breaking/bonding and analyzing electronic properties, and have been widely used in materials, chemistry, and other fields. DFT calculations can give detailed information regarding all aspects of chemical bonding, such as bonding sites, charge density distribution between surface and adsorbate, involved atomic orbits, and theoretical vibrational spectra.

Some properties of molecules are calculated by the MD method based on classical Newton mechanics and molecular force fields, which originated around 1970. The molecular force field contains various parameters that can be obtained by quantum mechanical calculations or experimental methods. The computational skills of MD simulation have been improved to study the dynamic behavior and thermodynamic properties of complex systems over the years. As MD calculations need to introduce some mathematical integration algorithms, it can only research the motion of the system in a short time and cannot simulate long-term motion problems. Nowadays, scientists are trying to boost their computers to improve calculation methods and computing power to investigate the scope of the movement over a longer duration.

The MC method (also known as the statistical test method) is a basic method to describe various random phenomena during movement, and it is especially suitable for problems that are difficult or impossible to solve by analytical methods.

13.2 DENSITY FUNCTIONAL THEORY

Materials are composed of atoms, and their properties depend on the motion state of atoms and electrons. From an energy point of view, the motion of atoms and electrons of materials in equilibrium should be in the energy steady-state or metastable state of the entire system. Analyzing the properties of materials from the atomic scale, classical Newton mechanics can easily solve millions of atoms; however, it is difficult to solve the electronic state, electronic structure, and bonding information. Therefore, new research methods are needed to obtain the above information.

Quantum mechanics is the basic theory to study the motion law of microparticles (molecules, atoms, nuclei, and basic particles) in the material field. Computational materials science, computational physics, and quantum chemistry established based on quantum mechanics and fast-developing computer technology have promoted the leap-forward development of materials science, physics, and chemistry, as well as provided a theoretical basis and new research methods for the development and design of new materials.

From a theoretical point of view, DFT is a quantum mechanical method to study the electronic structure of a multielectron system. The calculation of real material design in the future is to solve the Schrödinger equation of the system, that is, the first-principles calculation in computational materials science, also known as ab-initio calculation, and its theoretical basis is DFT. This method does not contain any empirical parameters. Based on quantum mechanics, the electronic structure and energy of the studied material system can be obtained by solving the Schrödinger equation, and the basic information of various physical and chemical properties of the system can be calculated using the single-electron approximation. The results present good accuracy. It directly starts from the Schrödinger equation of the many-body problem, uses DFT to solve the wave function and the corresponding eigen energy of the electron, and obtains the total energy of the system and the related physical properties derived from it. Using this method, the electronic motion state and the related microinformation of various systems (atoms, ions, molecules, cluster chemical reaction system, etc.) are obtained, which can reasonably explain and predict the bonding type of atoms, molecular structure, chemical reaction process, material properties, and some information related to the experimental results.

13.2.1 SCHRÖDINGER EQUATION OF MANY-BODY SYSTEM

Materials are composed of a large number of atoms or molecules, which can be further divided into the nucleus and extranuclear electrons. Schrödinger equation describes a multielectron system, which can be expressed as:

$$H\psi(\vec{r},\vec{R}) = E\psi(\vec{r},\vec{R}) \tag{13.1}$$

where ψ represents the eigenfunction, $\vec{r}$ and $\vec{R}$ represent the coordinate set of electron and nucleus, E represents the energy eigenvalue, and H is the Hamiltonian for the multisystem. If the effect of other external field is not considered, H can be expressed by the energy of the electron (H_e), the energy of the nucleus (H_N), and the potential energy between electrons and nucleus interaction (H_{e-N}), as shown in formula (13.2):

$$H = H_e + H_N + H_{e-N} \tag{13.2}$$

where

$$H_e(\vec{r}) = T_e(\vec{r}) + V_e(\vec{e}) = -\sum_i \frac{\hbar^2}{2m_e} \nabla_{r_i}^2 + \frac{1}{2} \sum_{i \neq j} \frac{e^2}{|\vec{r_i} - \vec{r_j}|} \tag{13.3}$$

$$H_N(\vec{R}) = T_N(\vec{R}) + V_N(\vec{R}) = -\sum_j \frac{\hbar^2}{2M_j} \nabla_{R_j}^2 + \frac{1}{2} \sum_{i \neq j} V_N(\vec{R_i} - \vec{R_j}) \tag{13.4}$$

$$H_{e-N}(\vec{r}, \vec{R}) = -\sum_{i,j} V_{e-N}(\vec{r_i} - \vec{R_j}) \tag{13.5}$$

where $T_e(\vec{r})$, $T_N(\vec{R})$, $V_e(\vec{r})$, and $V_N(\vec{R})$ represent electron kinetic energy, nuclear kinetic energy, Coulomb interactions energy by electron-electron, and Coulomb interaction energy by nucleus-nucleus, respectively.

13.2.2 BORN–OPPENHEIMER APPROXIMATION

In the many-body system studied, the mass of the nucleus is much larger than that of the electron, which is about 3~4 orders of magnitude of the electron mass. Under the condition of the same force, the speed of the electron is much faster than that of the nucleus, so the movement of the nucleus and electron can be considered separately. When considering the motion state of electrons, the nucleus is considered to be in a transient state; when considering the motion state of the nucleus, the nucleus is in the static distribution of electrons. This method is known as the Born–Oppenheimer approximation, which is commonly referred to as adiabatic approximation. According to this method, the motion of the nucleus and the electrons can be studied, and the Schrödinger equation of the electron in the many-body system can be written as:

$$\left[-\sum_i \frac{\hbar^2}{2m} \nabla_{r_i}^2 + \sum_i V(\vec{r_i}) + \frac{1}{2} \sum_{i \neq j} \frac{e^2}{|\vec{r_i} - \vec{r_j}|} \right] \phi = \left[\sum_i H_i + \sum_{i,j} H_{i,j} \right] \phi = E_\phi \tag{13.6}$$

13.2.3 Hartree–Fock Approximation

Hartree proposed the one-electron approximation method [5–8] in 1928, that is, the wave function of the multielectron system is expressed by the linear superposition of the antisymmetric product of wave functions of each electron state. The effective potential field is only related to the average density of electrons, but not to the instantaneous position of electrons. Fock improved the one-electron and mean-field method proposed by Hartree in 1930, and the Hartree–Fock equation can be further simplified as follows:

$$\left[-\frac{1}{2} \nabla^2 + V(\vec{r}) + V_{\text{eff}}(\vec{r}) \right] \phi_i(\vec{r}) = E_i \phi_i(\vec{r}) \tag{13.7}$$

The Schrödinger equation of the complex and difficult multielectron system is approximately simplified to a relatively simple single-electron effective potential equation using the Hartree–Fock approximation.

13.2.4 Hohenberg–Kohn Theorem and Kohn-Sham Equation

The Hartree–Fock approximation is a convenient method to deal with a system with fewer atoms. However, the calculation method completely ignores the electron correlation effect, and the amount of calculation increases exponentially with the increase in the number of electrons, which requires computer memory CPU speed. Therefore, it becomes extremely difficult to deal with the system with more atoms, which leads to the emergence of DFT.

Hohenberg and Kohn put forward two basic theorems [9] by deeply researching the Thomas–Fermi model of uniform electron gas in 1964, which laid the foundation of DFT. Hohenberg–Kohn theorem points out that the ground state of the system can be obtained by taking the electron density as the basic variable and using the variational method; however, how to determine the electron density function, kinetic energy functional, and exchange-correlation functional has not been solved. To determine the electron density function and kinetic energy functional, Kohn and sham proposed the Kohn–Sham equation [10].

Compared with the Hartree–Fock approximation method, the Kohn–Sham equation puts all the many-body effects into the specific exchange-correlation functional, which is a big step forward. So far, finding a reasonable exchange-correlation functional expression has become the main problem faced by DFT to improve the accuracy of the problem to be solved as much as possible.

13.2.5 Correlation Exchange Functional

There is no specific model and expression of exchange-correlation functional in the Kohn–Sham equation. If we want to use DFT to solve practical problems, we need to further determine the approximate expression of exchange-correlation functional. The common method is to decompose it into the exchange energy part and correlation energy part. At present, local density approximation (LDA) [11,12] and generalized gradient approximation (GGA) [13] are widely used.

LDA assumes that the distribution of electrons in space is a uniform electron gas, that is, the distribution of electron density changes uniformly in any infinitesimal local area. Based on this, the inhomogeneous system can be approximated by a uniform electron gas exchange-correlation functional with the same density. LDA is widely used because of its simple expression, which can give better results. However, LDA is suitable when electron density changes slowly in space as it is based on the assumption of uniform electron gas. The results are not ideal for other systems where the electron density varies unevenly in space. Generally, the lattice parameters calculated by LDA are smaller than the experimental values, while the dissociation energy and binding energy are higher. Based on LDA processing exchange-correlation functional, to get more accurate results, GGA considers the gradient information of electron density and is a step forward compared with LDA.

To deal with the Van der Waals (VDW) interaction in a multiparticle system, there are many methods, among which DFT-D [14] is a common method, which adds the semi-empirical scattering potential energy to the energy of the Kohn–Sham equation, and Grimme [15] describes the VDW interaction by a simple pairing force field. In 2004, the VDW force density functional proposed by Dion et al. [16] included a dispersive interaction in the exchange-correlation functional, which is a further step forward.

13.3 MOLECULAR DYNAMICS

Based on the classical Newton's equation of motion, MD is a set of computer simulation methods to obtain the physical properties of the studied system by solving the motion of atoms and molecules in the system. In the calculation, the motion state of the electron is ignored and the trajectory of the nucleus is described by the empirical potential function. At the beginning of the MD calculation, the initial velocity of each atom should be given randomly according to the Boltzmann distribution. In molecular simulation, due to the effect of the force field, the structural state of the system changes. A number of samples are taken from the ensemble composed of these different states to integrate the molecular configuration, and then the thermodynamic, kinetic, or other macroscopic properties of materials such as pressure, temperature, energy, and viscosity of the system are obtained by taking the integration results as input parameters. The three-dimensional microstructure of the molecule can also be obtained.

Simulations can reflect the function of the movement of molecules over time, so it is easier to solve specific problems of the nature of the model system than to solve the actual system by experiment. For biological systems, the details of biomolecule function, mechanism and dynamics information obtained through simulation are more meaningful than experimental results. The simulation results can also be compared with the experimental data to verify the accuracy of the simulation results, provide directions and standards for simulation improvement, and reduce the inherent system errors in the simulation [17,18].

The application of simulation methods in the field of macromolecules and mesoscopic systems can be divided into three types. The first application is as a means of sampling, involving the use of MD (often including simulated annealing process) based on experimental data to determine or optimize the structure. The second application is to obtain a description of the state of the system in an equilibrium state through MD, including structural characteristics, motion characteristics, and thermodynamic parameters. In this case, the dynamics need to cover enough sampling space, and each sample must be weighted by the corresponding Boltzmann factor. The third application is to study the actual dynamic processes. In addition to meeting the basic requirements of the second application, the simulation must be able to accurately reflect the changes and development of the system over time. For the first two applications, MC and MD can be satisfied, and in the third application, because the basic requirements of molecular motion change with time need to be met, only molecular kinetics can provide the necessary information. These three applications have promoted the development of simulation methods with accuracy and precision. Although the potential energies used in the simulation are approximate, due to the maneuverability of maneuverability, to study other properties of the system by removing or changing the contribution of the formulation, this is another important application of simulation [17–20].

13.3.1 THE PROCESS OF MD SIMULATIONS

Since the development of MD simulation in the 1970s, researchers are trying to overcome the limitation of using quantum mechanics to describe the motion of macromolecules and reduce the complexity of calculation by simulating the motion of atoms by simple approximations based on Newtonian mechanics. The flow of the kinetic process can be roughly described as:

First, build a computer model of the research object based on data such as nuclear magnetic resonance, crystal structure, and homology modeling. The forces resulting from the interaction between bonded and non-bonded atoms are then estimated. The chemical bonds and bond angles between bonded atoms are modeled by virtual springs, the dihedral angle is modeled by a sine function, and the sine function is an approximation of the energy difference between overlapping and staggered conformations. Non-bonding interactions are represented by VDW force and electrostatic force. VDW interaction is represented by the Lennard–Jones potential energy, while electrostatic interaction is described by the Coulomb's law. Once the force acting on each atom in the system is calculated, the position of the atom can be determined according to Newton's law of motion. The simulation time is also updated, usually, 1fs or 2fs is updated every step, and then the previous process is repeated. This loop repetition usually requires millions of steps, so MD runs on computer clusters and supercomputers. The current popular MD software, NAMD [21,22], GROMACS [23,24], AMBER [25,26], and CHARMM [27,28], have all realized supercomputing and parallel computation on the machine, thus facilitating the study of dynamics.

13.3.2 FORCE FIELD OF MD SIMULATIONS

The force field used for biological macromolecules such as proteins is also called the first type of potential energy function equation:

$$V(r) = \sum_{\text{bonds}} K_b (b - b_0)^2 + \sum_{\text{angles}} K_\theta (\theta - \theta_0)^2 + \sum_{\text{torsions}} K_\phi [1 + \cos(n\phi + \delta)]$$

$$+ \sum_{\text{nonbond pairs}} \left[\frac{q_i q_j}{r_{ij}} + \frac{A_{ij}}{r_{ij}^{12}} - \frac{C_{ij}}{r_{ij}^{6}} \right] \tag{13.8}$$

The first three items are bond length (1–2 interaction), angle item (1–3 interaction), and torsion item (1–4 interaction). The torsion item can include the Improper item. The Improper term is an angle like the torsion term but composed of four non-covalently connected atoms, which can enhance the planarity around the center of sp^2. The last item is a non-key action item, excluding 1–2 and 1–3 action items; usually, independent parameters are used to describe 1–4 actions. Different from the torsion term, the 1–4 effects here are separated by more than three covalent bonds (Figure 13.1).

In the non-bonded interaction, the electrostatic interaction is described by the Coulomb force expression:

$$E_C = \frac{q_i q_j}{4\pi\varepsilon_o r_{ij}} \tag{13.9}$$

VDW interaction is described by the Lennard-Jones expression:

$$E_{LJ} = 4\varepsilon_{ij} \left[\left(\frac{\sigma_{ij}}{r_{ij}} \right)^{12} - \left(\frac{\sigma_{ij}}{r_{ij}} \right)^{6} \right] \tag{13.10}$$

The mixing rule is usually used to calculate the interaction between atoms. There are two commonly used mixing rules, Lorentz–Bertelot mixing rules and geometric average mixing rules, as described below.

Lorentz-Bertelot mixing rules:

$$\sigma_{ij} = \frac{1}{2}(\sigma_{ii} + \sigma_{jj}), \varepsilon_{ij} = (\varepsilon_{ii}\varepsilon_{jj})^{1/2} \tag{13.11}$$

Geometric mean mixing rules:

$$\sigma_{ij} = (\sigma_{ii}\sigma_{jj})^{1/2}, \varepsilon_{ij} = (\varepsilon_{ii}\varepsilon_{jj})^{1/2} \tag{13.12}$$

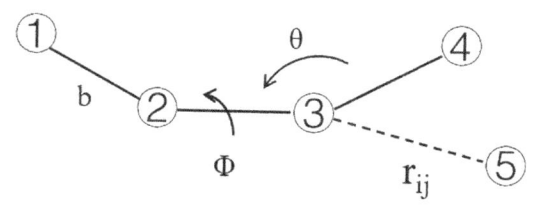

FIGURE 13.1   Principle of potential function.

To reproduce the actual motion of real molecules, each energy item describing the interaction between molecules (bond length, bond angle, dihedral angle, non-bonding interaction, etc.) needs to be parameterized through quantum mechanics calculation and experimental data. Sending some parameterization includes determining the length and elastic coefficient of virtual bombs describing chemical bonds and angles, establishing the best charges of different atoms to accurately calculate the electrostatic interaction energy, and defining the VDW radius for calculating non-bonding interactions. These parameters are called force fields because they objectively describe the contribution of different atoms between atoms to their interaction, and determine the motion of atoms and molecules. In MD simulation, common all-atom force fields include AMBER [29,30], CHARMM [31,32], and OPLS-AA [33]. The difference between the force fields is mainly manifested in the different ways of parameterization.

1. **AMBER force field**

   The AMBER force field was developed by the Kolman research group [29], and the initial design purpose of the force field is to study protein and nucleic acid systems. With subsequent development, it has also been extended to the simulation calculation of biological macromolecules, small organic molecules, and polymers [29,30]. The parameters of the force field all come from experimental values. Both the stretching vibration of the bond length and the bending of the bond angle are calculated using the harmonic oscillator model, while the dihedral torsion term is calculated in the form of the Fourier series. Its potential energy function expression is:

$$E_{\text{Pair}} = \sum_{\text{bonds}} K_r \left(r - r_{\text{eq}}\right)^2 + \sum_{\text{angles}} K_\theta \left(\theta - \theta_{\text{eq}}\right)^2$$

$$+ \sum_{\text{dihedrals}} \frac{V_n}{2}[1 + \cos(n\phi - \gamma)] + \sum_{i<j} \left[\frac{A_{ij}}{R_{ij}^{12}} - \frac{B_{ij}}{R_{ij}^6} + \frac{q_i q_j}{\varepsilon R_{ij}}\right] \quad (13.13)$$

2. **CHARMM force field**

   The CHARM force field was developed by Martin Karpus, the winner of the Nobel Prize in Chemistry in 2013, and is used in the dynamics of biological macromolecules such as proteins, nucleic acids, scales, and lipids, as well as organic molecules and polymers [31]. In addition to the source of experimental data, the parameters of the force field also introduce many calculation results [31,32]. The form of the force field is divided into two parts:

   Describing the part of the intramolecular interaction (bonding interaction):

$$\sum_{\text{bonds}} K_b \left(b - b_0\right)^2 + \sum_{\text{angles}} K_\theta \left(\theta - \theta_0\right)^2 + \sum_{\text{torsions}} K_\phi[1 + \cos(n\phi - \delta)]$$

$$+ \sum_{\text{impropers}} K_\varphi \left(\varphi - \varphi_0\right)^2 + \sum_{\text{Ure-Bradley}} K_{\text{UB}} \left(r_{1,3} - r_{1,3,o}\right)^2 \quad (13.14)$$

The Urey-Bradley term is added to calculate the 1–3 effects, which also includes the correction of the torsion of the skeleton residues.

$$\sum_{\text{residues}} U_{\text{CMAP}}(\phi,\psi) \qquad (13.15)$$

Describing the part of the interaction between molecules (non-bonding interaction):

$$\sum_{\text{nonbonded}} \frac{q_i q_j}{4\pi D r_{ij}} + \varepsilon_{ij}\left[\left(\frac{R_{\min,ij}}{r_{ij}}\right)^{12} - 2\left(\frac{R_{\min,ij}}{r_{ij}}\right)^{6}\right] \qquad (13.16)$$

3. OPLS-AA force field

Based on the AMBER force field, Jorgensen et al. developed the OPLS-AA force field [33]. The expansion and contraction energy of the bond and the opening and closing energy of the bond angle are consistent with the AMBER force field, while the transfer energy within the molecule is described by the Fourier series, where V_1, V_2, and V_3 are Fourier transform coefficients, and f_1, f_2, and f_3 are phase angles.

$$E(\phi) = E_{bond}(\phi) + E_{angle}(\phi) + E_{nonbonded}(\phi) + E_{torsion}(\phi)$$

$$E_{bond} = \sum_{bonds} K_r (r - r_{eq})^2$$

$$E_{angle} = \sum_{angles} K_\theta (\theta - \theta_{eq})^2 \qquad (13.17)$$

$$E_{torsion} = \sum_i \left\{ \frac{V_1^i}{2}\left[1 + \cos\left(\phi_i + f_1^i\right)\right] + \frac{V_2^i}{2}\left[1 - \cos\left(2\phi_i + f_2^i\right)\right] \right.$$

$$\left. + \frac{V_3^i}{2}\left[1 + \cos\left(3\phi_i + f_3^i\right)\right]\right\} \qquad (13.18)$$

The non-bonded interaction includes the electrostatic term in the Coulomb form and the VDW term in the form.

$$E_{ab} = \sum_i^{ona} \sum_j^{onb} \left[\frac{q_i q_j e^2}{r_{ij}} + 4\varepsilon_{ij}\left(\frac{\sigma_{ij}^{12}}{r_{ij}^{12}} - \frac{\sigma_{ij}^6}{r_{ij}^6}\right)\right] f_{ij} \qquad (13.19)$$

In addition to the force fields commonly used for biological macromolecules, there are other force fields, such as MM3, MMFF, UFF, and CFF. These force fields use the second type of potential energy function, which is suitable for different systems, including materials science and transition metals.

13.3.3 MOLECULAR DYNAMICS ALGORITHM

In a system composed of N atoms, the total potential energy of the system can be regarded as the total function $U(r_1 \ldots\ldots r_n)$ of the position of each atom in the system. By solving the classical Newtonian mechanics principle, the force on each atom in the system can be expressed as:

$$\vec{F}_i = -\nabla_i U = -\left(\vec{i}\frac{\partial}{\partial x_i} + \vec{j}\frac{\partial}{\partial y_i} + \vec{k}\frac{\partial}{\partial z_i} \right) U \tag{13.20}$$

Its acceleration is:

$$\vec{a}_i = \frac{\vec{F}_i}{m_i} \tag{13.21}$$

After time t, its speed and position can be expressed as:

$$\vec{v}_i = \vec{v}_i^0 + \vec{a}_i t$$

$$\vec{r}_i = \vec{r}_i^0 + \vec{v}_i^0 t + \frac{1}{2}\vec{a}_i t^2 \tag{13.22}$$

13.3.3.1 Solving the Equation of Motion

In MD simulation, the description of the trajectory of the molecule requires the use of finite difference technology to solve the Newtonian equation of motion to obtain its velocity and position. The basis of solving the equation of motion is to assume that the position and velocity and acceleration of the particles in the system can be expanded using the Taylor series as:

$$\vec{r}(t+\delta t) = \vec{r}(t) + \delta t \vec{v}(t) + \frac{1}{2}\delta t^2 \vec{a}(t) + \frac{1}{6}\delta t^3 \vec{b}(t) + \frac{1}{24}\delta t^4 \vec{c}(t) + \cdots$$

$$\vec{v}(t+\delta t) = \vec{v}(t) + \delta t \vec{a}(t) + \frac{1}{2}\delta t^2 \vec{b}(t) + \frac{1}{6}\delta t^3 \vec{c}(t) + \cdots$$

$$\vec{a}(t+\delta t) = \vec{a}(t) + \delta t \vec{b}(t) + \frac{1}{2}\delta t^2 \vec{c}(t) + \cdots \tag{13.23}$$

In MD simulation, the most used methods are the Verlet algorithm [34] and the Velocity-Verlet algorithm [35] derived from the basic Verlet algorithm and the leap-frog method [36].

1. Verlet algorithm

The core idea is to predict the particle's position at time $t + \delta t$ through the position of the particle at time t and $t - \delta t$. Use the position at time t to denote the positions at time $t + \delta t$ and time $t - \delta t$, respectively, and their respective Taylor expansions are:

$$\vec{r}(t + \delta t) = \vec{r}(t) + \delta t \vec{v}(t) + \frac{1}{2}\delta t^2 \vec{a}(t) + \cdots$$

$$\vec{r}(t - \delta t) = \vec{r}(t) - \delta t \vec{v}(t) + \frac{1}{2}\delta t^2 \vec{a}(t) - \cdots \qquad (13.24)$$

By adding the two formulas and ignoring higher-order terms, the position at time $t + \delta t$ is:

$$\vec{r}(t + \delta t) = 2\vec{r}(t) - \vec{r}(t - \delta t) + \delta t^2 \vec{a}(t) \qquad (13.25)$$

Obviously, the Verlet algorithm [34] only calculates the force once per integration, which is simple and convenient to use, but the disadvantage is that it does not give the speed. Therefore, in a constant temperature system, we can calculate the velocity of the particle by the position of the particle at time $t + \delta t$ and $t - \delta t$:

$$\vec{v}(t) = \frac{\left[\vec{r}(t + \delta t) - \vec{r}(t - \delta t)\right]}{2\delta t} \qquad (13.26)$$

2. Velocity-Verlet algorithm
Based on the Verlet algorithm, the Velocity-Verlet algorithm [35] not only provides the position of the atom but also increases the calculation of velocity and acceleration while ensuring its calculation accuracy.

$$\vec{r}(t + \delta t) = \vec{r}(t) + \delta t \vec{v}(t) + \frac{1}{2}\delta t^2 \vec{a}(t)$$

$$\vec{v}(t + \delta t) = \vec{v}(t) + \frac{1}{2}\delta t[\vec{a}(t) + \vec{a}(t + \delta t)] \qquad (13.27)$$

3. Leap-frog algorithm
In the leap-frog algorithm [36], a velocity of $0.5\delta t$ before and after a certain time is introduced to solve the position:

$$\vec{r}(t + \delta t) = \vec{r}(t) + \delta t \vec{v}\left(t + \frac{1}{2}\delta t\right)$$

$$\vec{v}\left(t + \frac{1}{2}\delta t\right) = \vec{v}\left(t - \frac{1}{2}\delta t\right) + \delta t \vec{a}(t) \qquad (13.28)$$

The solution of the velocity at time t can be expressed using the following formula:

$$\vec{v}(t) = \frac{1}{2}\left[\vec{v}\left(t - \frac{1}{2}\delta t\right) + \vec{v}\left(t + \frac{1}{2}\delta t\right)\right] \tag{13.29}$$

The advantage of the leap-frog method is that it improves the calculation accuracy and provides speed and acceleration information. However, the disadvantage is that the solution of velocity and position is not synchronized, which results in the inability to determine the contribution of velocity to the energy of the system at a certain position.

13.3.3.2 Periodic Boundary Conditions of MD Simulations

Under the existing computer resources, the number of particles that can be processed by MD simulation is limited, and the system studied can be regarded as a reduced version of the macroscopic system. Therefore, the simulated box will produce boundary effects that do not match the actual experiment. Here, we use periodic boundary conditions, and the simulation box is surrounded by its translational mirror image. When any particle in the computing system leaves the box, the corresponding particle must move into the box from the opposite direction in its mirror image, thus maintaining a constant number of particles and a constant density in the system. Therefore, the boundary problem caused by the simulated box is solved by the periodic boundary. When calculating the interaction force between molecules, the nearest mirror image method can be used. In the calculation of non-bonded long-range force field, the method of truncated radius can solve the problem of repeated calculations. If the distance between the molecules is greater than the set cut-off radius, the interaction can be calculated as zero, and the maximum cut-off radius should be less than half the width of the box. Because the potential energy function on the truncation radius is not zero, it will cause discontinuities on the energy curve if it is completely ignored. The switch function is usually multiplied by the original potential energy function to adjust the function curve from the starting point of the switch to the cut-off radius gradually adjusted to zero. The application of periodic boundary conditions facilitates the design of the simulation system, but it also brings some problems, such as the inapplicability to non-periodic research systems and the inability to realize simulation boxes of different shapes.

13.3.3.3 Ensemble of MD Simulations

An ensemble is an aggregation of many possible states of the system under the same macro conditions. According to the needs of the design, MD needs to be implemented in different ensembles. The commonly used ensembles can be divided into equal pressure and equal pressure ensemble, slightly canonical ensemble, canonical ensemble, grand canonical ensemble, and isothermal and equal pressure ensemble according to their different constraints.

1. **Microcanonical ensemble**
   The microcanonical ensemble is a statistical ensemble of isolated conservative systems. Mainly, the number of atoms (N), volume (V) and energy (E)

remain constant, so it can also be called the NVE ensemble. Due to the constant energy, the system moves along a specific energy trajectory in the phase space, and the initial configuration and conditions at the beginning of the simulation are difficult to meet the requirements of the established energy. Therefore, the usual approach is to adjust the appropriate initial structure with a long balance time for energy adjustment to achieve the established energy condition.

2. Canonical ensemble

Different from the microcanonical system, the temperature (T) in the canonical ensemble remains unchanged, and the total momentum is zero, so it can also be called the NVT ensemble. Under constant temperature conditions, the system can exchange energy with the external environment, and it is difficult to keep the temperature constant. The usually adopted solution is to connect to an external thermal bath to maintain the system in thermal equilibrium. Commonly used thermal bath methods are Gaussian thermal bath [37], Nose-Hoover thermal bath [38], and Berendsen thermal bath [39].

3. Isothermal and pressure ensemble

The isothermal and pressure ensemble is an ensemble often used in experiments. Unlike regular ensemble, the pressure (P) of the system remains unchanged, so it is also called the NPT ensemble. Temperature adjustment can be controlled by the Berendsen thermal bath and other methods, while pressure adjustment is usually achieved by controlling the volume of the box. Commonly used methods are the Anderson method [40], the Berendsen method, and the Parrinello–Rahman method [41].

13.3.4 ENHANCED SAMPLING METHODS

MD simulations have become very important research methods, covering millions of systems at the atomic level [42,43]. However, insufficient sampling often limits its application. This limitation is due to the rough energy landscapes of the system, and many local minima are separated by high-energy barriers, causing quasi-ergodic problems, that is, simulations at low temperatures tend to fall into local minimum energy states [44]. These minimum energy points confine the molecule for a long time, which slows down the sampling process, making the sampling unable to span the entire configuration space, leading to the unsatisfactory characterization of protein dynamics. In biological systems, large conformational changes are very important for protein activity.

13.3.4.1 Parallel Tempering

Parallel tempering, also known as replica exchange, is an algorithm that can effectively improve the representativeness of spatial sampling. This algorithm was first proposed by Swendsen and Wang in 1986 [45], mainly for MC simulation, the so-called parallel tempering MC. Later, Sugita and Okamoto extended it to MD simulations, the so-called replica-exchange molecular dynamics (REMD) [46]. The general idea of parallel tempering is simultaneously simulating M copies of the original system, and each copy is at a different temperature; during the simulation process, each copy exchanges conformations with neighboring copies through Metropolis–Hastings criteria [47]. Because high-temperature conditions can sample a wide range of phase space, low-temperature conditions can accurately sample a local area of the phase space. REMD algorithm is generally used to study polymer conformation, peptide/protein folding mechanism, and crystal structure to reduce the relaxation time to the equilibrium state.

13.3.4.2 Simulated Annealing

The simulated annealing algorithm [48] can be considered as an extension of the Markov Chain MC method used to investigate the system state distribution and solve global optimization problems. First, heating the research system to a higher temperature, in which the molecules or atoms inside the system can move freely so that they can find a more suitable position under the action of external and internal forces. When the temperature drops slowly, the kinetic energy of molecules or atoms correspondingly decreases, their movement becomes more and more restricted, and the conformational changes become much smaller. Finally, the system can reach the lowest global energy conformation. Because the conformational energy is very high at the beginning, multiple independent simulations should be able to sample all possible stable conformations of the research system [49].

At present, the commonly used annealing methods are classical simulated annealing (CSA) [48], fast simulated annealing (FSA) [48], and generalized simulated annealing (GSA) [50]. Among them, when the system is large, the efficiency of the GSA method is better than CSA and FSA.

The GSA method can explore the conformational space more uniformly so that a huge jump of the conformational state can be achieved at lower temperatures. The annealing process mainly involves three equations: one is to describe the temperature attenuation, the other is the random variable that guides the system to change after each iteration, and the last one is to describe the probability of acceptance [50]. It is mainly used for global optimization of long-range effects: such as atomic parameterization, gravitational system, and conformation optimization of small molecules and peptides [48]. Simulated annealing is most suitable for characterizing systems with greater flexibility, and conventional simulated annealing can only simulate some small proteins, but the GSA method can be used to simulate large biological macromolecular complexes. The GSA method is expected to study the huge conformational transitions of proteins with very large molecular weights in certain biological processes [48].

13.3.4.3 Umbrella Sampling

Umbrella sampling was first proposed by Torrie and Valleau in 1977 to solve the sampling problem of conventional MD simulation in high free-energy regions [51]. When the two initial and final states to be studied are separated by a high-energy barrier, conventional simulation methods require a long simulation time to sample both states. To solve the sampling problem in the high free-energy region, we can set a reaction coordinate (ξ) between the initial state and the final state, dividing the entire reaction path into multiple regions (windows) [52]. For each window i, add bias potential $\omega_i(\xi)$ that only depends on the reaction coordinate to the research system. When the added bias potential energy is a harmonic potential with intensity K related to the reaction coordinate, for a given position ξ_i, there are:

$$\omega_i(\xi) = \frac{1}{2}K\left(\xi - \xi_i\right)^2 \tag{13.30}$$

Limiting the position of the research system to the vicinity of the center position ξ_i, to enhance the system's sampling in this window. Under the limitation of the corresponding harmonic potential, with MD simulation, a series of biased probability distribution $Pi(\xi)$ of the system on the reaction path can be obtained. Here, the probability distribution of adjacent windows must overlap enough to get an accurate free energy curve. Finally, the weighted histogram analysis method [53] is used to combine the probability distributions of this series to remove the influence of the additional harmonic potential, to obtain the accurate probability distribution of the research system along the reaction coordinate, and then to solve the related free-energy curve.

Because umbrella sampling has a strict theoretical basis, very accurate free-energy data can be obtained. However, this method requires many balanced trajectories and computing resources for data collection, and has a lot of requirements and restrictions on computing resources and the size of the system. For umbrella sampling, the aqueous system of biological macromolecules is very large. In addition, umbrella sampling also requires sufficient energy overlap between adjacent windows. For many systems, it is necessary to make multiple attempts in areas with higher free energy to obtain better sampling. Therefore, in the field of biological macromolecules, umbrella sampling is more used to test the accuracy of the newly proposed free energy calculation method. There is also a variant of umbrella sampling, called adaptive umbrella sampling [54], which can adjust the bias potential energy in time to uniformly distribute the energy between the beginning and the end state.

13.3.4.4 Metadynamics

Metadynamics is based on selected collective variables that can effectively reconstruct the free energy surface of the system under study and accelerate sampling [55,56]. It was first proposed by Laio and Parrinello in 2002 and applied to MD simulation [57]. Metadynamics is informally described as "filling the free energy well with computational sand". The algorithm assumes that the system can be described by some reaction coordinates. In the simulation, the calculation system adds a certain Gaussian repulsive potential to the system at regular intervals, as shown in formula (13.31), so that the free energy surface is gradually filled in. It can prevent the system from revisiting the sampled area on the reaction path, and encourages the research system to continuously move to the high free energy area so that the system can escape from the lowest points of local energy. As the simulation progresses, more and more Gaussians are added to the trajectory until the system detects a sufficient energy landscape. When the modified free energy becomes a constant concerning the reaction coordinate, the reaction coordinate begins to fluctuate greatly. Meanwhile, the energy profile can be restored, which is the opposite of the Gaussian potential sum, as shown in formula (13.32).

The Gaussian potential added in the simulation is as follows:

$$V(S,t) = \sum_{k\tau < t} W(k\tau) \exp\left(-\sum_{i=1}^{d} \frac{\left[S_i\left(q(t)\right) - S_i\left(q(k\tau)\right)\right]^2}{2\sigma_i^2}\right) \qquad (13.31)$$

where, $q(t)$ is the microscopic coordinate of the system corresponding to time t, $S_i(q)$ is the i-th reaction coordinate based on the microscopic coordinate q, σ_i is the width of the Gaussian potential of the i-th reaction coordinate, and d is the number of reaction coordinates. τ is the time interval for adding the Gaussian potential, k is a positive integer, and $W(t)$ is the height of the Gaussian potential at time t.

When the simulation time tends to infinity, all potential wells will be "filled", and the modified free energy becomes a constant function of the reaction coordinate:

$$V(S, t \rightarrow \infty) = -F(S) + C \qquad (13.32)$$

By adjusting the time interval of adding Gaussian potential, as well as the height and width of Gaussian potential, the ratio of accuracy to calculation cost can be optimized.

To solve the various problems and limitations of the metadynamics method (such as convergence, sampling, multiple reaction coordinates, etc.), some new variants have been proposed, such as well-tempered metadynamics with gradually decreasing Gaussian potential [58], multiwalker metadynamics based on multiple copies and the same reaction coordinate [59], based on multiple copies Bias-exchange metadynamics with different reaction coordinates [60], parallel tempering metadynamics based on different temperature copies and the same reaction coordinates [61]. Metadynamics methods are mainly used to study protein folding [60,61], chemical reactions [62], molecular docking [63], and phase transitions [64]. Recently, this method has also been applied to simulate the adsorption of peptides on surfaces [65] and to calculate the free energy of protein-ligand and protein-protein binding [66]. At present, the software specially used for metadynamics simulation is PLUMED [67,68]. Now, this method has been integrated into many commonly used molecular simulation software, such as AMBER [25,26], GROMACS [23,34], LAMMPS [69], and NAMD [21,22].

13.4 MONTE CARLO METHOD

Many problems of the material system are probabilistic and statistical, which require a new method to solve. MC method is based on simple theoretical criteria (such as simple material and material and material environment interaction) and uses a repeated random sampling method to deal with the problem of a complex system, and it adopts random sampling to simulate the probability and statistics of the object. MC simulation method is also called the stochastic simulation method or the statistical simulation method. In MC simulation, through a specific "experimental" method, the frequency of an event (or some eigenvalues of a variable) can be obtained, which can be regarded as the probability of a random event (or the expected value of a random variable) to achieve the purpose of solving related problems. When the MC method is used to simulate a process, it is necessary to generate random variables with various probability distributions. The simplest and most important random variable is the random number uniformly distributed on [1].

The traditional MC method is very simple, it must undergo a lot of sampling to get a more accurate result, so the amount of calculation required is very large. Given this, Metropolis et al. [42] proposed an important sampling method, which is to choose whether to accept the new state with a certain probability. MC simulation is widely used because of its simple algorithm, easy implementation, and rapid development of computer science. For example, it can be used in financial engineering, macroeconomics, computational physics (such as particle transport problems, quantum thermodynamics, aerodynamics), medicine, biology, and prospecting. Nowadays, the MC method is also used to simulate protein adsorption on a solid surface.

Zhou et al. used MC simulation combined with MD simulation to study the adsorption of cytochrome C on the surface of self-assembled membranes at the carboxyl end of differently charged density surfaces, and they also used MC simulation to study the adsorption of antibody molecules on charged surfaces at the same time [70,71]. Carlsson et al. [72] investigated the adsorption of lysozyme on negatively charged surfaces and studied the effects of protein concentration and net charge and solution ionic strength through MC simulation. Anand et al. [73] employed the MC simulation method to research the adsorption and conformational changes of different concentrations of proteins (lysozyme and ribonuclease A, etc.) on the surface of self-assembled membranes with different properties. Some molecular software can perform MC simulation, such as TINKER [74], Materials Studio [75], Macro Model [76], and BOSS [77].

REFERENCES

1. Heinz H., Ramezani-Dakhel H. Simulations of inorganic–bioorganic interfaces to discover new materials: insights, comparisons to experiment, challenges, and opportunities. *Chem. Soc. Rev.*, 2016, 45(2): 412–448.
2. Ozboyaci M., Kokh D. B., Corni S., et al. Modeling and simulation of protein-surface interactions: achievements and challenges. *Q. Rev Biophys.*, 2016, 49: 1–45.
3. Wang W., Anderson C. F., Wang Z. Y., et al. Peptide-templated noble metal catalysts: syntheses and applications. *Chem. Sci.*, 2017, 8(5): 3310–3324.
4. Ariöz C., Wittung-Stafshede P. Folding of copper proteins: role of the metal? *Q. Rev Biophys.*, 2018, 51: 1–39.
5. Hartree D. R. The wave mechanics of an atom with a non-coulomb central field. Part II. Some results and discussion. *Math. Proc. Cambridge.*, 1928, 24: 111–132.
6. Hartree D. R. The wave mechanics of an atom with a non-coulomb central field. Part I. Theory and methods. *Math. Proc. Cambridge.*, 1928, 24: 89–110.
7. Hartree D. The wave mechanics of an atom with a non-coulomb central field. Part III. Term values and intensities in series in optical spectra. *Math. Proc. Cambridge.*, 1928, 24: 426–437.

8. Hartree D. The wave mechanics of an atom with a non-coulomb central field. Part IV. Further results relating to terms of the optical spectrum. *Math. Proc. Cambridge.*, 1929, 25: 310–314.

9. Hohenberg P., Kohn W. Inhomogeneous electron gas. *Phys. Rev.*, 1964, 136(3B): B864.

10. Kohn W., Sham L. J. Self-consistent equations including exchange and correlation effects. *Phys. Rev.*, 1965, 140(4A): A1133–A1138.

11. Ceperley D. M., Alder B. J. Ground state of the electron gas by a stochastic method. *Phys. Rev. Lett.*, 1980, 45(7): 566–569.

12. Perdew J. P., Zunger A. Self-interaction correction to density-functional approximations for many-electron systems. *Phys. Rev. B*, 1981, 23(10): 5048–5079.

13. Perdew J. P., Burke K., Ernzerhof M. Generalized gradient approximation made simple. *Phys. Rev. Lett.*, 1996, 77(18): 3865–3868.

14. Wu X., Vargas M. C., Nayak S., et al. Towards extending the applicability of density functional theory to weakly bound systems. *J. Chem. Phys.*, 2001, 115(19): 8748–8757.

15. Grimme S. Semiempirical GGA-type density functional constructed with a long-range dispersion correction. *J. Comput. Chem.*, 2006, 27(15): 1787–1799.

16. Dion M., Rydberg H., Schröder E., et al. Van der Waals density functional for general geometries. *Phys. Rev. Lett.*, 2004, 92(24): 1–4.

17. Karplus M., Kuriyan J. Molecular dynamics and protein function. *P. Natl. Acad. Sci. USA*, 2005, 102(19): 6679–6685.

18. Karplus M., McCammon J. A. Molecular dynamics simulations of biomolecules. *Nat. Struct. Mol. Biol.*, 2002, 9(9): 646–652.

19. Durrant J. D., McCammon J. A. Molecular dynamics simulations and drug discovery. *BMC Biol.*, 2011, 9(1): 1–9.

20. Hansson T., Oostenbrink C., van Gunsteren W. F. Molecular dynamics simulations. *Curr. Opin. Struc. Biol.*, 2002, 12(2): 190–196.

21. Phillips J. C., Braun R., Wang W., et al. Scalable molecular dynamics with NAMD. *J. Comput. Chem.*, 2005, 26(16): 1781–1802.

22. Nelson M. T., Humphrey W., Gursoy A., et al. NAMD: a parallel, object-oriented molecular dynamics program. *Int. J. High Perform. C.*, 1996, 10(4): 251–268.

23. Berendsen H. J. C., van der Spoel D., van Drunen R. GROMACS: a message-passing parallel molecular dynamics implementation. *Comput. Phys. Commun.*, 1995, 91(1–3): 43–56.

24. Pronk S., Páll S., Schulz R., et al. GROMACS 4.5: a high-throughput and highly parallel open source molecular simulation toolkit. *Bioinformatics*, 2013, 29(7): 845–854.

25. Case D. A., Cheatham III T. E., Darden T., et al. The Amber biomolecular simulation programs. *J. Comput. Chem.*, 2005, 26(16): 1668–1688.

26. Salomon-Ferrer R., Case D. A., Walker R. C. An overview of the Amber biomolecular simulation package. *Wiley Interdisciplinary Reviews: Wires. Comput. Mol. Sci.*, 2013, 3(2): 198–210.

27. Brooks B. R., Bruccoleri R. E., Olafson B. D., et al. CHARMM: a program for macromolecular energy, minimization, and dynamics calculations. *J. Comput. Chem.*, 1983, 4(2): 187–217.

28. Brooks B. R., Brooks III C. L., Mackerell Jr. A. D., et al. CHARMM: the biomolecular simulation program. *J. Comput. Chem.*, 2009, 30(10): 1545–1614.

29. Wang J., Wolf R. M., Caldwell J. W., et al. Development and testing of a general amber force field. *J. Comput. Chem.*, 2004, 25(9): 1157–1174.

30. Maier J. A., Martinez C., Kasavajhala K., et al. ff14SB: improving the accuracy of protein side chain and backbone parameters from ff99SB. *J. Chem. Theory. Comput.*, 2015, 11(8): 3696–3713.

31. Bjelkmar P., Larsson P., Cuendet M. A., et al. Implementation of the CHARMM force field in GROMACS: analysis of protein stability effects from correction maps, virtual interaction sites, and water models. *J. Chem. Theory. Comput.*, 2010, 6(2): 459–466.

32. Vanommeslaeghe K., Hatcher E., Acharya C., et al. CHARMM general force field: a force field for drug-like molecules compatible with the CHARMM all-atom additive biological force fields. *J. Comput. Chem.*, 2010, 31(4): 671–690.

33. Jorgensen W. L., Maxwell D. S., Tirado-Rives J. Development and testing of the OPLS all-atom force field on conformational energetics and properties of organic liquids. *J. Am. Chem. Soc.*, 1996, 118(45): 11225–11236.

34. Verlet L. Computer "experiments" on classical fluids. I. Thermodynamical properties of Lennard-Jones molecules. *Health Phys.*, 1967, 159(1): 98.

35. Swope W. C., Andersen H. C., Berens P. H., et al. A computer simulation method for the calculation of equilibrium constants for the formation of physical clusters of molecules: application to small water clusters. *J Chem. Phys.*, 1982, 76(1): 637–649.

36. Hockney R. W. The potential calculation and some applications. *Methods Comput. Phys.*, 1970, 9: 136.

37. Hoover W. G. *Computational Statistical Mechanics*. Elsevier, Amsterdam, 1991.

38. Nosé S. A unified formulation of the constant temperature molecular dynamics methods. *J Chem. Phys.*, 1984, 81(1): 511–519.

39. Berendsen H. J. C., Postma J. P. M., van Gunsteren W. F., et al. Molecular dynamics with coupling to an external bath. *J Chem. Phys.*, 1984, 81(8): 3684–3690.

40. Andersen H. C. Molecular dynamics simulations at constant pressure and/or temperature. *J Chem. Phys.*, 1980, 72(4): 2384–2393.

41. Parrinello M., Rahman A. Polymorphic transitions in single crystals: a new molecular dynamics method. *J. Appl. Phys.*, 1981, 52(12): 7182–7190.

42. Metropolis N., Rosenbluth A. W., Rosenbluth M. N., et al. Equation of state calculations by fast computing machines. *J. Chem. Phys.*, 1953, 21(6): 1087–1092.

43. Alder B. J., Wainwright T. E. Phase transition for a hard sphere system. *J. Chem. Phys.*, 1957, 27(5): 1208–1209.

44. Xie Y., Zhou J., Jiang S. Y. Parallel tempering monte carlo simulations of lysozyme orientation on charged surfaces. *J. Chem. Phys.*, 2010, 132(6): 065101.

45. Swendsen R. H., Wang J.-S. Replica monte carlo simulation of spin-glasses. *Phys. Rev. Lett.*, 1986, 57(21): 2607–2609.

46. Sugita Y., Okamoto Y. Replica-exchange molecular dynamics method for protein folding. *Chem. Phys. Lett.*, 1999, 314(1–2): 141–151.

47. Earl D. J., Deem M. W. Parallel tempering: theory, applications, and new perspectives. *Phys. Chem. Chem. Phys.*, 2005, 7(23): 3910–3916.

48. Kirkpatrick S., Gelatt C. D., Vecchi M. P. Optimization by simulated annealing. *Science*, 1983, 220(4598): 671–680.

49. Bernardi R. C., Melo M. C. R., Schulten K. Enhanced sampling techniques in molecular dynamics simulations of biological systems. *Biochim. Biophys. Acta*, 2015, 1850(5): 872–877.

50. Szu H., Hartley R. Fast simulated annealing. *Phys. Lett. A*, 1987, 122(3): 157–162.

51. Tsallis C., Stariolo D. A. Generalized simulated annealing. *Physica A*, 1996, 233(1–2): 395–406.

52. Torrie G. M., Valleau J. P. Nonphysical sampling distributions in Monte Carlo free-energy estimation: umbrella sampling. *J. Comput. Phys.*, 1977, 23(2): 187–199.

53. Kästner J. Umbrella sampling. *Wiley Interdiscip. Rev.: Comput. Mol. Sci.*, 2011, 1(6): 932–942.

54. Kumar S., Bouzida D., Swendsen R. H., et al. The weighted histogram analysis method for free-energy calculations on biomolecules. I. The method. *J. Comput. Chem.*, 1992, 13(8): 1011–1021.

55. Bartels C., Karplus M. Probability distributions for complex systems: Adaptive umbrella sampling of the potential energy. *J. Phys. Chem. B*, 1998, 102(5): 865–880.

56. Sutto L., Marsili S., Gervasio F. L. New advances in metadynamics. *Wiley Interdiscip. Rev.: Comput. Mol. Sci.*, 2012, 2(5): 771–779.

57. Barducci A., Bonomi M., Parrinello M. Metadynamics. *Wiley Interdiscip. Rev.: Comput. Mol. Sci.*, 2011, 1(5): 826–843.

58. Laio A., Parrinello M. Escaping free-energy minima. *Proc. Natl. Acad. Sci. USA*, 2002, 99(20): 12562–12566.

59. Barducci A., Bussi G., Parrinello M. Well-tempered metadynamics: a smoothly converging and tunable free-energy method. *Phys. Rev. Lett.*, 2008, 100(2): 020603.

60. Raiteri P., Laio A., Gervasio F. L., et al. Efficient reconstruction of complex free energy landscapes by multiple walkers metadynamics. *J. Phys. Chem. B*, 2006, 110(8): 3533–3539.

61. Piana S., Laio A. A bias-exchange approach to protein folding. *J. Phys. Chem. B*, 2007, 111(17): 4553–4559.

62. Bussi G., Gervasio F. L., Laio A., et al. Free-energy landscape for beta hairpin folding from combined parallel tempering and metadynamics. *J. Am. Chem. Soc.*, 2006, 128(41): 13435–13441.

63. Ensing B., De Vivo M., Liu Z. W., et al. Metadynamics as a tool for exploring free energy landscapes of chemical reactions. *Acc. Chem. Res.*, 2006, 39(2): 73–81.

64. Gervasio F. L., Laio A., Parrinello M. Flexible docking in solution using metadynamics. *J. Am. Chem. Soc.*, 2005, 127(8): 2600–2607.

65. Martonak R., Laio A., Bernasconi M., et al. Simulation of structural phase transitions by metadynamics. *Z. Kristallogr.*, 2005, 220(5–6): 489–498.

66. Deighan M., Pfaendtner J. Exhaustively sampling peptide adsorption with metadynamics. *Langmuir*, 2013, 29(25): 7999–8009.

67. Limongelli V., Bonomi M., Parrinello M. Funnel metadynamics as accurate binding free-energy method. *Proc. Natl. Acad. Sci. USA*, 2013, 110(16): 6358–6363.

68. Bonomi M., Branduardi D., Bussi G., et al. PLUMED: a portable plugin for free-energy calculations with molecular dynamics. *Comput. Phys. Commun.*, 2009, 180(10): 1961–1972.

69. Tribello G. A., Bonomi M., Branduardi D., et al. PLUMED 2: new feathers for an old bird. *Comput. Phys. Commun.*, 2014, 185(2): 604–613.

70. Zhou J., Tsao H. K., Sheng Y. J., et al. Monte Carlo simulations of antibody adsorption and orientation on charged surfaces. *J. Chem. Phys.*, 2004, 121(2): 1050–1057.

71. Zhou J., Zheng J., Jiang S. Y. Molecular simulation studies of the orientation and conformation of cytochrome c adsorbed on self-assembled monolayers. *J. Phys. Chem. B*, 2004, 108(45): 17418–17424.

72. Carlsson F., Hyltner E., Arnebrant T., et al. Lysozyme adsorption to charged surfaces. A Monte Carlo Study. *J. Phys. Chem. B*, 2004, 108(28): 9871–9881.

73. Anand G., Sharma S., Dutta A. K., et al. Conformational transitions of adsorbed proteins on surfaces of varying polarity. *Langmuir*, 2010, 26(13): 10803–10811.

74. Ponder J. W., Richards F. M. An efficient newton-like method for molecular mechanics energy minimization of large molecules. *J. Comput. Chem.*, 1987, 8(7): 1016–1024.

75. Akkermans R. L. C., Spenley N. A., Robertson S. H. Monte Carlo methods in materials studio. *Mol. Simul.*, 2013, 39(14–15): 1153–1164.

76. Mohamadi F., Richards N. G. J., Guida W. C., et al. Macro model-an integrated software system for modeling organic and bioorganic molecules using molecular mechanics. *J. Comput. Chem.*, 1990, 11(4): 440–467.

77. Jorgensen W. L., Tirado-Rives J. Molecular modeling of organic and biomolecular systems using BOSS and MCPRO. *J. Comput. Chem.*, 2005, 26(16): 1689–1700.

Index